Physiotherapy for Respiratory and Cardiac Prol

To John R. Plant

For Churchill Livingstone

Publisher: Mary Law
Project Editor: Dinah Thom
    Copy Editor: Julie Gorman
Production Controller: Mark Sanderson
Sales Promotion Executive: Hilary Brown

Physiotherapy for Respiratory and Cardiac Problems

Edited by

Barbara A. Webber FCSP

Group Superintendent Physiotherapist,
Royal Brompton National Heart and Lung
Hospitals, London

Jennifer A. Pryor MSc FNZSP MCSP

Deputy Group Superintendent Physiotherapist,
Royal Brompton National Heart and Lung
Hospitals, London

Foreword by

Professor Dame Margaret Turner-Warwick

Consulting Physician, Royal Brompton Hospital;
Immediate Past President, Royal College of
Physicians; Emeritus Professor of Medicine,
London University, London

CHURCHILL LIVINGSTONE
EDINBURGH LONDON MADRID MELBOURNE NEW YORK AND TOKYO 1993

CHURCHILL LIVINGSTONE
Medial Division of Longman Group UK Limited

Distributed in the United States of America by Churchill
Livingstone Inc., 650 Avenue of the Americas, New York,
N.Y. 10011, and by associated companies, branches and
representative throughout the world.

First published 1993
  Reprinted 1994

ISBN 0-443-04471-6

British Library of Cataloguing in Publication Data
A catalogue record for this book is available from the British
Library.

Library of Congress Cataloging in Publication Data
Physiotherapy for respiratory and cardiac problems/edited by Barbara
  A. Weber, Jennifer A. Pryor; foreword by Dame Margaret Turner-Warwick.
    p. cm.
  Includes bibliographical references and index.
  ISBN 0-443-04471-6
  1. Cardiopulmonary system — Disease — Physical therapy.
  I. Webber, B. A. (Barbara Anne) II. Pryor, Jennifer A.
  [DNLM: 1. Physical Therapy — methods. 2. Critical Care — methods.
  3. Respiratory Tract Disease   rehabilitation. 4. Heart Diseases—rehabilitation.
    WF 145 P578 1993]
  RC702.P48 1993
  616.1'2062—dc20
  DNLM/DLC
  for Library of Congress   93 – 16683

Produced by Longman Singapore Publishers (Pte) Ltd
Printed in Singapore

Contents

Contributors   vii
Foreword   ix
Preface   xi
Acknowledgements   xiii

SECTION 1
Investigations, patients' problems and techniques

1. Assessment   3
   Sally Parker, Peter G. Middleton

2. Thoracic imaging   23
   Conor D. Collins, David M. Hansell

3. Cardiopulmonary function testing   47
   Michael D. L. Morgan, Sally J. Singh

4. Monitoring and interpreting medical investigations   67
   John S. Turner

5. Mechanical support   83
   John S. Turner

6. Cardiopulmonary resuscitation   93
   John S. Turner

7. Physiotherapy skills: positioning and mobilization of the patient   99
   Elizabeth Dean

8. Physiotherapy skills: techniques and adjuncts   113
   Barbara A. Webber, Jennifer A. Pryor

9. Communication, counselling and health education   173
   Julius Sim

10. Research in cardiopulmonary physiotherapy   187
    Cecily J. Partridge

11. Physiotherapy problems and their management   199
    Jackie Anderson, Susan C. Jenkins

SECTION 2
Patient groups with specific needs

12. Surgical patients and patients requiring intensive care   237
    Marion Kieran, Patricia McCoy, Barbara A. Webber, Jennifer A. Pryor

13. Paediatrics   281
    Annette Parker

14. Cardiac rehabilitation   319
    Helen McBurney

15. Cardiopulmonary transplantation   343
    Catherine E. Bray

16. Spinal injuries   357
    Trudy Ward

17. Care of the dying patient   367
    B. Wendy Burford, Stephen J. Barton

18. Hyperventilation   377
    Diana M. Innocenti

19. Asthma in adults, and the *Aspergillus*   389
    Barbara A. Webber, Jennifer A. Pryor

20. Bronchiectasis, primary ciliary dyskinesia and cystic fibrosis   399
    Barbara A. Webber, Jennifer A. Pryor

21. Immunosuppression or deficiency   419
    Denise Hills

Normal values and abbreviations   429

Index   437

v

Contributors

Jackie Anderson MCSP SRP
Superintendent Physiotherapist, Guy's Hospital, London, UK

Stephen J. Barton RGN RMN
Charge Nurse, Royal Brompton National Heart and Lung Hospitals, London, UK

Catherine E. Bray BAppSc(Phty)
Senior Physiotherapist, Cardiopulmonary Transplant Unit, St Vincent's Hospital, Sydney, Australia

B. Wendy Burford RGN BTTA
Clinical Nurse Specialist, Palliative Care, Royal Brompton National Heart and Lung Hospitals, London, UK

Conor D. Collins BSc MB MRCPI FRCR FFRRCS(Irel)
Senior Registrar in Radiology, Royal Brompton National Heart and Lung Hospitals, London, UK

Elizabeth Dean PhD PT
Associate Professor, School of Rehabilitation Medicine, University of British Columbia, Vancouver, British Columbia, Canada

David M. Hansell MB MRCP FRCR
Consultant Radiologist and Honorary Senior Lecturer, Royal Brompton National Heart and Lung Hospitals, London, UK

Denise Hills MCSP
Superintendent Physiotherapist, Westminster Hospital, London, UK

Diana M. Innocenti MCSP SRP
Superintendent Physiotherapist, Guy's Hospital, London, UK

Susan C. Jenkins PhD MCSP
Senior Lecturer, School of Physiotherapy, Curtin University of Technology, Perth, Western Australia

Marion Kieran GradDP MCSP CertAdvPhys MICSP
Clinical Tutor in Physiotherapy, Dublin School of Physiotherapy, Faculty of Health Sciences, University of Dublin, Dublin, Ireland

Helen McBurney BAppSc (Phty) GradDipPhysio (Cardiothoracic) MAPA
Senior Lecturer in Physiotherapy, Lincoln School of Health Sciences, La Trobe University, Melbourne; Physiotherapist (sessional), Alfred Hospital, Prahran, Victoria, Australia

Patricia McCoy MEd BA MCSP DipTp CertEd(FE)
Senior Lecturer/Senior Course Tutor, Department of Occupational Therapy and Physiotherapy, Faculty of Social and Health Sciences, University of Ulster, Newtonabbey, Co. Antrim, Northern Ireland

Peter G. Middleton MBBS BSc(Med) FRACP
Cystic Fibrosis Research Fellow, Ion Transport Laboratory, National Heart and Lung Institute, London, UK

Michael D. L. Morgan MA MD FRCP (UK)
Consultant Physician and Honorary Senior Lecturer, Department of Respiratory Medicine, Glenfield Hospital, Leicester, UK

Annette Parker MCSP
Superintendent Physiotherapist, King's College Hospital, London, UK

Sally Parker BAppSc(Phty) MSc(Med)
Senior Physiotherapist, Royal Brompton National Heart and Lung Hospitals, London, UK

Cecily J. Partridge PhD FCSP
Reader in Physiotherapy, King's College London,
London, UK

Jennifer A. Pryor MSc FNZSP MCSP
Deputy Group Superintendent Physiotherapist,
Royal Brompton National Heart and Lung
Hospitals, London, UK

Julius Sim BA MSc MCSP
Principal Lecturer in Health Sciences, School of
Health and Social Sciences, Coventry University,
Coventry, UK

Sally J. Singh BA MCSP
Research Physiotherapist, Department of
Respiratory Medicine, Glenfield General
Hospital, Leicester, UK

John S. Turner MBChB MMed(Cape Town) FCP(SA)
Senior Specialist Surgical ICU, Groote Schuur
Hospital, Cape Town, South Africa

Trudy Ward SRP MCSP GradDipPhys
Superintendent Physiotherapist, Duke of
Cornwall Spinal Treatment Centre, Salisbury
District Hospital, Salisbury, UK

Barbara A. Webber FCSP
Group Superintendent Physiotherapist, Royal
Brompton National Heart and Lung Hospitals,
London, UK

Foreword

This book not only demonstrates the art and science of physiotherapy in heart and lung disease, but it also does much more. It emphasizes the essential contribution made by specialist physiotherapists within the whole team of those caring for adults, adolescents and children with cardiac and pulmonary problems. Indeed in many instances physiotherapy assumes a pivotal and life saving role for many very sick patients.

The great tradition of cardiothoracic physiotherapy has been pioneered over decades at the Brompton and London Chest Hospitals and it is therefore fitting that Barbara Webber and Jennifer Pryor were invited to edit this book. It describes the crucial importance of these particular professional skills and the ways in which they integrate with diagnostic and other therapeutic aspects of patient care. It also describes the importance for physiotherapists to understand the pathology and mechanisms of disease as well as the patient's feelings, attitudes and fears.

May I add a personal tribute to the superb physiotherapy teams who have done so much for so many of my own patients over the years and who continue to support tirelessly my medical and surgical colleagues.

M.T–W.

Preface

This book is intended for physiotherapy students, new graduates and postgraduate physiotherapists with an interest in patients with respiratory and cardiac problems.

Assessment of the patient should reveal the patient's problems. If some or all of these problems can be influenced by physical means, physiotherapy is indicated. Physiotherapy is also indicated when potential problems have been identified and preventative measures should be taken. The role of the physiotherapist as an educator in both the prevention and treatment of problems is another important aspect.

Diagnoses will continue to provide useful medical categories, but treatment can become prescriptive and inappropriate or ineffective if given in response to a diagnosis alone. The pathology behind the problem provides the key as to whether it is a physiotherapy problem or a medical problem.

It is by accurate assessment of the patient that short- and long-term patient goals can be identified and agreed, and an effective treatment plan outlined. Continuous reassessment of the patient and the treatment outcomes will identify the need for continuation or modification of treatment.

This book begins with assessment of the patient and the interpretation of medical investigations. This is followed by a section on mechanical support and cardiopulmonary resuscitation.

An important part of our role is communication, counselling and health education. The skills available to the cardiorespiratory physiotherapist are many and varied. Practical skills have been outlined and referenced where possible. All skills are not yet supported by rigorous clinical studies, but it is important that we continue to use them if outcome measures support their place in clinical practice. In the future measurement tools could validate their use. Research should be an integral part of the practice of physiotherapy.

Patients' problems and their management are outlined in the context of differing pathologies. One pathological process may present as several patient problems. Pneumothorax, for example, appears under the problems of both pain and breathlessness. The characteristic problems of some patient groups and diagnostic categories are then discussed detailing the pathology, medical management, physiotherapy and evaluation of treatment.

This book should be read in conjunction with specialized texts on anatomy, physiology and pathology. Further reading is indicated within each chapter. Throughout the text, for simplicity, the patient is referred to as he/him and the physiotherapist as she/her, but it is not intended to imply that all patients are male or that all physiotherapists are female.

It is hoped that the problem orientated approach to physiotherapy practice will facilitate the learning process for the physiotherapist and improve the quality of the care we provide.

London 1993

B.A.W.
J.A.P.

Acknowledgements

We are most grateful to the authors who by their contributions have made this text possible. We would like to thank our secretary Berenice Ebanks, Milena Potucek and Paul Hyett of the Photographic Department, The Royal Marsden Hospital and our staff and friends who have contributed in many ways with their expertise, support and encouragement.

B.A.W.
J.A.P.

Investigations, patients' problems and techniques

1. Assessment

Sally Parker   Peter G. Middleton

INTRODUCTION

The aim of assessment is to define accurately the patient's problems. It is based on both a subjective and an objective assessment of the patient. Without an accurate assessment it is impossible to develop an appropriate plan of treatment. Equally, a sound theoretical knowledge is required to develop an appropriate treatment plan for those problems which may be improved by physiotherapy. Once treatment has commenced it is important to assess regularly its effectiveness in relation to both the problems and goals.

The system of patient management used in this book is based on the problem orientated medical system (POMS) first described by Weed in 1968. This system has three components:

- Problem orientated medical records (POMR)
- Audit
- Educational programme.

The POMR is now widely used as the method of recording the assessment, management and progress of a patient. It is divided into five sections, as shown in Figure 1.1 and summarized below.

1. *Database.* Here personal details, medical history, relevant social history, results of investigations and tests, together with the physiotherapist's assessment of the patient are recorded.

2. *Problem list.* This is a concise list of the patient's problems, compiled after the assessment is complete. Problems are not always written in order of priority. The list includes problems both related and unrelated to physiotherapy. The resolution of problems and the appearance of new ones are noted appropriately.

3. *Initial plan and goals.* A treatment plan is formulated to address the physiotherapy related problems, keeping in mind the patient's other problems. Long- and short-term goals are then formulated. Long-term goals are what the patient and the physiotherapist want to achieve finally and should relate to the problems. Short-term goals are the stages by which the long-term goals should be achieved.

4. *Progress notes.* These are written to document the patient's progress, especially highlighting any changes. The notes are written in the 'subjective, objective, analysis, plan' (SOAP) format for each problem, and provide an up-to-date summary of the patient's progress.

5. *Discharge summary.* This is written when the patient is discharged from treatment or transferred to another institution. It includes presenting problems, treatment given, outcome of treatment, together with any home programme or follow-up instructions.

DATABASE

The database contains a concise summary of the relevant information about the patient taken from the medical notes, together with the subjective and objective assessment made by the physiotherapist. The format may differ from hospital to hospital, but will contain the same information.

The first part contains the patient's personal details including name, date of birth, address, hospital number, and referring doctor. It may also contain the diagnosis and reason for referral. The second part summarizes the history from the medical notes and the physiotherapy assessment.

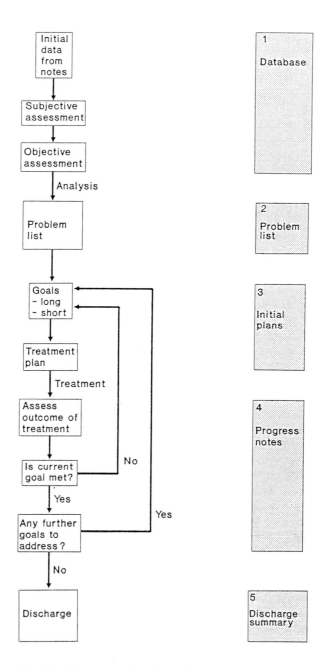

Fig. 1.1   The process of problem oriented medical records.

This is often divided into several sections:

History of presenting condition (HPC) summarizes the patient's current problems, including relevant information from the medical notes.

Previous medical history (PMH) summarizes the entire list of medical and surgical problems that the patient has had in the past. It may be written in disease specific groupings or as a chronological account.

Drug history (DH) is a list of the patient's current medications (including dosage) taken from the medication charts. Drug allergies should also be noted.

Family history (FH) includes a list of any major diseases suffered by members of the immediate family.

Social history (SH) provides a picture of the patient's social situation. It is important to question specifically the patient about the level of support available at home, together with an idea of the patient's expected contribution to household duties. The layout of the patient's home should also be ascertained with particular emphasis on stairs. Occupation and hobbies, both past and present, give further information about the patient's lifestyle. Finally, history of smoking and alcohol use should be noted.

Patient examination includes all information collected in the physiotherapist's subjective and objective assessment of the patient.

Test results contain any significant findings as they become available. These may include arterial blood gases, spirometry, blood tests, sputum analysis, chest radiographs, computerized tomography (CT) and any other relevant tests (e.g. hepatitis B positive).

Subjective assessment

Subjective assessment is based on an interview with the patient. It should generally start with open ended questions — What is the main problem? What troubles you most?—allowing the patient to discuss the problems that are most important to him at that time. Indeed, by asking such questions, previously unmentioned problems may surface. As the interview progresses, questioning may become more focused on those important features that need clarification. There are five main symptoms of respiratory disease:

- Breathlessness (dyspnoea)
- Cough
- Sputum and haemoptysis
- Wheeze
- Chest pain.

With each of these symptoms, enquiries should be made concerning:

- *Duration* — both the absolute time since first recognition of the symptom (months, years) and the duration of the present symptoms (days, weeks).
- *Severity* — in absolute terms and relative to the recent and distant past.
- *Pattern* — seasonal or daily variations.
- *Associated factors* — including precipitants, relieving factors, and associated symptoms, if any.

Breathlessness

Breathlessness is the subjective awareness of an increased work of breathing. It is the predominant symptom of both cardiac and respiratory disease. It also occurs in anaemia where the oxygen-carrying capacity of the blood is reduced, in neuromuscular disorders where the respiratory muscles are affected, and in metabolic disorders where there is a change in the acid–base equilibrium (see Ch.3) or metabolic rate (e.g. hyperthyroid disorders). Breathlessness is also found in the hyperventilation syndrome where it is due to psychological factors (e.g. anxiety).

The pathophysiological mechanisms causing breathlessness are still the subject of intensive investigation. Many factors are involved, including respiratory muscle length–tension relationships, respiratory muscle fatigue, stimulation of pulmonary stretch receptors, and alterations in central respiratory drive.

The duration and severity of breathlessness is most easily assessed through enquiries about the level of functioning in the recent and distant past. For example, a patient may say that 3 years ago he could walk up five flights of stairs without stopping, but now cannot even manage one flight. Some patients may deny feeling breathless as they have (unconsciously) decreased their activity levels so that they do not get breathless. They may only acknowledge breathlessness when it interferes with important activities, e.g. bathing. The physiotherapist should always relate breathlessness to the level of function that the patient can achieve.

Comparison of the severity of breathlessness between patients is difficult because of differences in perception and expectations. To overcome

Table 1.1   The New York Heart Association classification of breathlessness

Class I	No symptoms with ordinary activity, e.g. running up hills, fast bicycling, cross country skiing
Class II	Symptoms with ordinary activity, e.g. walking up stairs, making beds, carrying large amounts of shopping
Class III	Symptoms with mild exertion, e.g. bathing, showering, dressing
Class IV	Symptoms at rest

these difficulties, numerous gradings have been proposed. The New York Heart Association grading (1964) shown in Table 1.1, was developed for patients with cardiac disease, but is also applicable to respiratory patients. No scale is universal and it is important that all staff within one institution use the same scale.

Breathlessness is usually worse during exercise and better with rest. The one exception is hyperventilation syndrome where breathlessness may improve with exercise. Two patterns of breathlessness have been given specific names:

- *Orthopnea* is breathlessness when lying flat.
- *Paroxysmal nocturnal dyspnoea (PND)* is breathlessness that wakes the patient at night. In the cardiac patient, lying flat increases venous return from the legs so that blood pools in the lungs, causing breathlessness. A similar pattern may be described in patients with severe asthma, but here the breathlessness is caused by nocturnal bronchoconstriction.

Further insight into a patient's breathlessness may be gained by enquiring about precipitating and relieving factors. Breathlessness associated with exposure to allergens and relieved by bronchodilators is typically found in asthma.

Cough

Coughing is a protective reflex which rids the airways of secretions or foreign bodies. Any stimulation of receptors located in the pharynx, larynx, trachea, or bronchi may induce cough. Cough is a difficult symptom to clarify as most people cough normally every day, yet a repetitive persistent cough is both troublesome and distressing. Smokers may discount their early morning cough as being 'normal' when in fact it signifies chronic bronchitis.

Important features concerning cough are its effectiveness, and whether it is productive or dry. The severity of cough may range from an occasional disturbance to a continual trouble. It may cause fractured ribs (cough fractures), hernias, and stress incontinence (especially in women). A loud, barking cough, which is often termed 'bovine', may signify laryngeal or tracheal disease. Recurrent coughing after eating or drinking is an important symptom of aspiration. A chronic productive cough every day is a fundamental feature of chronic bronchitis and bronchiectasis. Interstitial lung disease is characterized by a persistent, dry cough. Nocturnal cough is an important symptom of asthma in children and young adults, but in older patients it is more commonly due to cardiac failure. Drugs, especially beta blockers and some other antihypertensive agents, can cause a chronic cough.

Postoperatively, the strength and effectiveness of cough is important for the physiotherapist to assess.

Sputum

In a normal adult, approximately 100 ml of tracheobronchial secretions is produced daily and cleared subconsciously. Sputum is the excess tracheobronchial secretions that are cleared from the airways by coughing. It may contain mucus, cellular debris, microorganisms, blood and foreign particles. Questioning should determine the colour, consistency and quantity of sputum produced each day, which may clarify the diagnosis and the severity of disease (Table 1.2). In general, sputum is described as 'mucoid' (opalescent to white), 'mucopurulent' (thicker and slightly coloured), or 'purulent' (thick, viscous and discoloured). Sputum 'plugs' are hard rubbery casts in the shape of the bronchial tree which may be produced in asthma, allergic bronchopulmonary aspergillosis (ABPA) and occasionally in bronchiectasis.

Haemoptysis is the presence of blood in the sputum. It may range from slight streaking of the sputum to frank blood. Frank haemoptysis can be

Table 1.2 Sputum analysis

	Description	Causes
Saliva	Clear watery fluid	
Mucoid	Opalescent or white	Chronic bronchitis without infection, asthma
Mucopurulent	Slightly discoloured, but not frank pus	Bronchiectasis, cystic fibrosis, pneumonia
Purulent	Thick and viscous: Yellow Dark green/brown Rusty Red currant jelly	 Haemophilus Pseudomonas Pneumococcus, Mycoplasma Klebsiella
Pink or white and frothy		Pulmonary oedema
Haemoptysis	Ranging from blood specks to frank blood, old blood (dark brown)	Infection (tuberculosis, bronchiectasis), infarction, carcinoma, trauma, also coagulation disorders, cardiac disease, vasculitis
Black	Black specks in mucoid secretions	Smoke inhalation (fires, tobacco, heroin), coal dust

life threatening, requiring bronchial artery embolization or surgery. Isolated haemoptysis may be the first sign of bronchogenic carcinoma, even when the chest radiograph is normal. Patients with chronic infective lung disease often suffer from recurrent haemoptyses.

Wheeze

Wheeze is a whistling or musical sound produced by turbulent airflow through narrowed airways. These sounds are generally noted by patients when audible at the mouth. Stridor, the sound of an upper airway obstruction, is often mistakenly called 'wheeze' by patients. Heart failure may also cause wheezing in those patients with significant mucosal oedema. For a full discussion of wheeze see page 18.

Chest pain

Chest pain in respiratory patients usually originates from musculoskeletal, pleural or tracheal inflammation, as the lung parenchyma and small airways contain no pain fibres.

Pleuritic chest pain is caused by inflammation of the parietal pleura, and is usually described as a severe, sharp, stabbing pain which is worse on inspiration. It is not reproduced by palpation.

Tracheitis generally causes a constant burning pain in the centre of the chest, aggravated by breathing.

Musculoskeletal (chest wall) pain may originate from the muscles, bones, joints or nerves of the thoracic cage. It is usually well localized and exacerbated by chest and/or arm movement. Palpation will usually reproduce the pain.

Angina pectoris is a major symptom of cardiac disease. Myocardial ischaemia characteristically causes a dull central retrosternal gripping or band-like sensation which may radiate to either arm, neck or jaw.

Pericarditis may cause pain similar to angina or pleurisy.

A differential diagnosis of chest pain is given in Table 1.3.

Other symptoms

Of the other symptoms a patient may report, a number have particular importance.

Fever (pyrexia) is one of the common features of infection, but low-grade fevers can also occur with malignancy and connective tissue disorders. Equally, infection may occur without fever, especially in immunosuppressed (e.g. chemotherapy) patients or those on corticosteroids. High fevers occurring at night, with associated sweating (night sweats), may be the first indicator of pulmonary tuberculosis.

Table 1.3 Syndromes of chest pain

Condition	Description	Causes
Pulmonary		
Pleurisy	Sharp, stabbing, rapid onset, limits inspiration, well localized, often 'catches' at a certain lung volume, *not* tender on palpation	Pleural infection and inflammation of the pleura, trauma (haemothorax), malignancy
Pulmonary embolus	Usually has pleuritic pain, with or without severe central pain	Pulmonary infarction
Pneumothorax	Severe central chest discomfort, with or without pleuritic component, severity depends on extent of mediastinal shift	Trauma, spontaneous, lung diseases (e.g. cystic fibrosis, AIDS)
Tumours	May mimic any form of chest pain, depending on site and structures involved	Primary or secondary carcinoma, mesothelioma
Musculoskeletal		
Rib fracture	Localized point tenderness, often sudden onset, increases with inspiration	Trauma, tumour, cough fractures (e.g. in chronic lung diseases, osteoporosis)
Muscular	Superficial, increases on inspiration and some body movements, with or without palpable muscle spasm	Trauma, unaccustomed exercise (excessive coughing during exacerbations of lung disease), accessory muscles may be affected
Costochondritis (Tietze's syndrome)	Localized to one or more costochondral joints, with or without generalized, non-specific chest pain	Viral infection
Neuralgia	Pain or paraesthesia in a dermatomal distribution	Thoracic spine dysfunction, tumour, trauma, herpes zoster (shingles)
Cardiac		
Ischaemic heart disease (angina or infarct)	Dull, central, retrosternal discomfort like a weight or band with or without radiation to the jaw and/or either arm, may be associated with palpitations, nausea, or vomiting	Myocardial ischaemia, onset at rest is more suggestive of infarction
Pericarditis	Often retrosternal, exacerbated by respiration, may mimic cardiac ischaemia or pleurisy, often relieved by sitting	Infection, inflammation, trauma, tumour
Mediastinum		
Dissecting aortic aneurysm	Sudden onset, severe, poorly localized central chest pain	Trauma, atherosclerosis, Marfan's syndrome
Oesophageal	Retrosternal burning discomfort, but can mimic all other pains, worse lying flat or bending forward	Oesophageal reflux, trauma, tumour
Mediastinal shift	Severe, poorly localized central discomfort	Pneumothorax, rapid drainage of a large pleural effusion

Headache is an uncommon feature of respiratory disease. Morning headaches in patients with severe respiratory failure may signify nocturnal carbon dioxide retention. Early morning arterial blood gases or nocturnal transcutaneous carbon dioxide monitoring are required for confirmation.

Peripheral oedema in the respiratory patient suggests right heart failure which may be due to cor pulmonale (right ventricular failure secondary to hypoxic pulmonary vasoconstriction).

Peripheral oedema may also occur in patients taking high dose corticosteroids, as a result of salt and water retention.

Functional limitations

It is important to assess the patient as a whole, enquiring about his daily activities. If the patient is employed, what does his job *actually* entail? For example, a surveyor may sit behind a desk all day, or he may be climbing 25-storey buildings. The home situation should also be documented, in particular the number of stairs to the front door and within the house. With whom do they live? What support does this person provide (shopping, housework, cooking)? Finally, questions concerning activities and recreation often reveal areas where significant improvements in quality of life can be made.

Objective assessment

Objective assessment is based on examination of the patient, together with the use of tests such as spirometry, arterial blood gases and chest radiographs. Although a full examination of the patient should be available from the medical notes, it is worthwhile to make a thorough examination at all times as things may have changed since the patient was last examined, and the physiotherapist may need greater detail of certain aspects than is available from the notes. A good examination will provide an objective baseline for the future measurement of the patient's progress. By developing a standard method of examination, the findings are quickly assimilated, and the physiotherapist remains confident that nothing has been forgotten.

General observation

Examination starts by observing the patient from the end of the bed. Is the patient short of breath, sitting on the edge of the bed, distressed? Is he obviously cyanosed? Is he on supplemental oxygen? If so, how much? What is his speech pattern — long fluent paragraphs without discernible pauses for breath, quick sentences, just a few words, or is he too breathless to speak? When he moves around or undresses, does he become distressed? With a little practice, these observations should become second nature and can be noted whilst introducing yourself to the patient.

In the intensive care patient there are a number of further features to be observed. The level of ventilatory support must be ascertained. This includes both the mode of ventilation (e.g. supplemental oxygen, continuous positive airway pressure, intermittent positive pressure ventilation) and the route of ventilation (mask, endotra-

cheal tube, tracheostomy). The level of cardiovascular support should also be noted, including drugs to control blood pressure and cardiac output, pacemakers and other mechanical devices. The patient's level of consciousness should also be noted. Any patient with a decreased level of consciousness is at risk of aspiration and retention of pulmonary secretions. In those patients who are not pharmacologically sedated, the level of consciousness is often measured using the Glasgow Coma Scale (Table 1.4). This gives the patient a score (from 3 to 15) based on his best motor, verbal and eye responses.

The patient's chart should then be examined for recordings of temperature, pulse, blood pressure and respiratory rate. These measurements are usually performed by the nursing staff immediately on admission of the patient and regularly thereafter.

For details of the assessment of the infant and child see page 284.

Body temperature. Body temperature can be measured in a number of ways. Oral temperatures are the most convenient method in adults but should not be performed for at least 15 min after smoking or consuming hot or cold food or drink. Axillary and rectal temperature may also be measured.

Body temperature is maintained within the range 36.5–37.5°C. It is lowest in the early morning and highest in the afternoon.

Fever (pyrexia) is the elevation of the body

Table 1.4 The Glasgow Coma Scale*

Eye opening	Spontaneous	4
	To speech	3
	To pain	2
	None	1
Best verbal response	Oriented	5
	Confused speech	4
	Inappropriate words	3
	Incomprehensible sounds	2
	None	1
Best motor response	Obeys commands	6
	Localizes to pain	5
	Withdraws (generalized)	4
	Flexion	3
	Extension	2
	No response	1

*Maximum total score is 15; minimum total score is 3.

temperature above 37.5°C, and is associated with an increased metabolic rate. For every 0.6°C (1°F) rise in body temperature, there is an approximately 10% increase in oxygen consumption and carbon dioxide production. This places extra demand on the cardiorespiratory system which causes a compensatory increase in heart rate and respiratory rate.

Heart rate. Heart rate is most accurately measured by auscultation at the cardiac apex. The pulse rate is measured by palpating a peripheral artery (radial, femoral or carotid). In most situations, the heart rate and pulse rate are identical; a difference between the two is called the 'pulse deficit'. This indicates that some heart beats have not caused sufficient blood flow to reach the periphery. This is commonly found in atrial fibrillation and some other arrhythmias.

The normal adult heart rate is 60–100 beats per minute.

Tachycardia is defined as a heart rate greater than 100 beats/min at rest. It is found with anxiety, exercise, fever, anaemia and hypoxia. It is also common in patients with cardiac disorders. Medications such as bronchodilators and some cardiac drugs may also increase heart rate.

Bradycardia is defined as a heart rate less than 60 beats/min. It may be a normal finding in athletes and may also be caused by some cardiac drugs (especially beta blockers).

Blood pressure(BP). With every contraction of the heart (systole) the arterial pressure increases. The peak blood pressure is called the 'systolic' pressure. During the relaxation phase of the heart (diastole), the pressure within the arteries drops. The minimum blood pressure is called the 'diastolic' pressure. Blood pressure is usually measured non-invasively by placing a sphygmomanometer cuff around the upper arm, and listening over the brachial artery with a stethoscope. The cuff width should be approximately one-half to two-thirds that of the upper arm length, otherwise readings may be inaccurate. Cuff inflation to above systolic pressure collapses the artery, blocking flow. With release of the air, the cuff pressure gradually falls to a point just below systolic. At this point, the peak pressure within the artery is greater than the pressure outside the artery, so flow recommences. This

turbulent flow is audible through the stethoscope. As the cuff is further deflated the noise continues. When the cuff pressure drops to just below diastolic, the pressure within the artery is greater than that of the cuff throughout the cardiac cycle, so turbulence abates and the noise ceases.

Blood pressure is recorded as systolic/diastolic pressure. Normal adult blood pressure is between 95/60 and 140/90 mmHg.

Hypertension is defined as a blood pressure of greater than 145/95 mmHg is usually due to changes in vascular tone and/or aortic valve disease.

Hypotension is defined as a blood pressure of less than 90/60 mmHg. It is often a normal finding during sleep. Daytime hypotension may be due to heart failure, blood loss or decreased vascular tone.

Postural hypotension is a drop in blood pressure of more than 5 mmHg between lying and sitting or standing, and may be due to decreased circulating blood volume, or loss of vascular tone.

Pulsus paradoxus is the exaggeration of the drop in blood pressure that occurs with inspiration. Normally, during inspiration the negative intrathoracic pressure reduces venous return and drops cardiac output slightly. Exaggeration of this normal response where blood pressure drops by more than 10 mmHg is seen in situations where the intrathoracic pressure swings are greater, as occurs in severe airway obstruction.

Respiratory rate. Respiratory rate should be measured with the patient seated comfortably. The normal adult respiratory rate is approximately 12–16 breaths/min.

Tachypnoea is defined as a respiratory rate greater than 20 breaths/min, and can be seen in any form of lung disease. It may also occur with metabolic acidosis and anxiety.

Bradypnoea is defined as a respiratory rate of less than 10 breaths/min. It is an uncommon finding, and is usually due to central nervous system depression by narcotics or trauma.

Body weight. Weight is often recorded on the observation chart. Respiratory function can be compromised by both obesity and severe malnourishment. As ideal body weight has a large normal range, the body mass index (BMI) has been proposed as an alternative. This is calculated by dividing the weight in kilograms by the square of the height in metres (kg/m^2); the normal range is 20–25 kg/m^2. Patients with values below 20 are underweight, those with values of 25–30 are overweight, and those with values over 30 kg/m^2 are classified as obese.

Malnourished patients often exhibit depression of their immune system with increased risk of infection. They also have weaker respiratory muscles which are more likely to fatigue. Obesity causes an increase in residual volume (RV) and a decrease in functional residual capacity (FRC) (Rubinstein et al 1990). Thus tidal breathing occurs close to closing volumes. This is particularly important postoperatively, where the obese are more prone to subsegmental lung collapse.

An accurate daily weight gives a good estimate of fluid volume changes, as any change in weight of more than 250 g/day is usually due to fluid accumulation or loss. Daily weights are commonly used in intensive care, renal and cardiac patients to assess fluid balance.

Other measures. In the intensive care patient there is a plethora of monitoring that can be performed. As well as the parameters listed above, measures of central venous pressure (CVP), pulmonary artery pressure (PAP), and intracranial pressure (ICP) will need to be reviewed as part of the physiotherapy assessment. Some intensive care units now record this information on bedside computer terminals. Further details of intensive care monitoring can be found in Chapters 4 and 5.

Apparatus. At this point the lines and tubes going into and coming out of the patient should be noted. Venous lines provide constant direct access to the bloodstream, and vary widely in site, complexity and function. The simplest cannula in a small peripheral vein, usually in the forearm, is called a 'drip'. It is used for the administration of intravenous (IV) fluids and most intravenous drugs. At the other end of the spectrum are the multi-lumen lines placed in the subclavian, internal jugular or femoral veins, ending in the vena cavae close to the heart. These central lines allow simultaneous administration of multiple drugs and can be used for central venous pressure monitoring. Central lines can be potentially dangerous, as disconnection of the line can quickly suck air into the central veins, causing an air embolus which may be fatal.

Some patients, especially those in intensive care, may have an arterial line for continuous recording of blood pressure and for repeated sampling of arterial blood. These lines are usually inserted in the radial or brachial artery. If accidentally disconnected, rapid blood loss will occur.

After cardiac surgery, most patients have cardiac pacing wires which exit through the skin overlying the heart. In most cases these wires are not required and are removed routinely before discharge. In the event of clinically significant cardiac arrhythmias, these wires are connected to a pacing box that electrically stimulates the heart. In medical patients, pacemaker wires are introduced through one of the central veins and rest in the apex of the right ventricle. Care must be taken with all pacing wires as dislodgement may be life threatening.

Intercostal drains are placed between two ribs into the pleural space to remove air, fluid or pus which has accumulated. They are also used routinely after cardiothoracic surgery. In general, the tube is attached to a bottle partially filled with sterile water, called an 'underwater seal drain'. The bottle should be positioned at least 0.5 m below the patient's chest (usually on the floor). Bubbling indicates that air is entering the tube from the pleural space at that time. Frequent observations must be made of the fluid level within the tube which should oscillate or 'swing' with every breath. If the fluid does not 'swing' the tube is not patent and requires medical attention. In certain situations the bottle may be connected to continuous suction which will dampen the fluid 'swing'. Those patients who are producing large volumes of fluid or pus may be connected to a double bottle system, where the first bottle acts as a reservoir to collect the fluid and the second provides the underwater seal. More recently, fully enclosed disposable plastic systems have been devised. Any patient with a chest drain should have a pair of large forceps available at all times to clamp the tube if any connection becomes loosened.

Postoperatively, drains may be placed at any operation site (e.g. abdomen) to prevent the collection of fluid or blood. These are generally connected to sterile bags. Nasogastric tubes are placed for two reasons: soft, fine bore tubes are used to facilitate feeding, whilst firm, wider-bore tubes allow aspiration of gastric contents.

The hands. The hands provide a wealth of information. A fine tremor will often be seen in association with high dose bronchodilators. Warm and sweaty hands with an irregular flapping tremor may be due to acute carbon dioxide retention. Weakness and wasting of the small muscles in the hands may be an early sign of an upper lobe tumour involving the brachial plexus (Pancoast's tumour). Examination of the fingers may show nicotine staining from smoking.

Clubbing is the term used to describe the changes in the fingers and toes as shown in Figure 1.2. The first sign of clubbing is the loss of the angle between the nail bed and the nail itself. Later, the finger pad becomes enlarged. The nail bed may also become 'spongy', but this is a difficult sign to elicit. A summary of the diseases associated with clubbing is given in Table 1.5.

The exact cause of clubbing is unknown. It is

Table 1.5   Causes of clubbing

Lung disease	Infective (bronchiectasis, lung abscess, empyema) Fibrotic Malignant (bronchogenic cancer, mesothelioma)
Cardiac disease	Congenital cyanotic heart disease Bacterial endocarditis
Other	Familial Cirrhosis Gastrointestinal disease (Crohn's disease, ulcerative colitis, coeliac disease)

interesting to note that clubbing in cystic fibrosis patients disappears after heart and lung or lung transplant.

The eyes. The eyes should be examined for pallor (anaemia), plethora (high haemoglobin) or jaundice (yellow colour due to liver or blood disturbances). Drooping of one eyelid with enlargement of that pupil suggests Horner's syndrome where there is a disturbance in the sympathetic nerve supply to that side of the head (sometimes seen in cancer of the lung).

Cyanosis. This is a bluish discolouration of the skin and mucous membranes. Central cyanosis, seen on examination of the tongue and mouth, is caused by hypoxaemia where there is an increase in the amount of haemoglobin not bound to oxygen. The degree of blueness is related to the quantity of unbound haemoglobin. Thus a greater degree of hypoxia is necessary to produce cyanosis in an anaemic patient (low haemoglobin), whilst a patient with polycythaemia (increased haemoglobin) may appear cyanosed with only a small drop in oxygen levels. Peripheral cyanosis, affecting the toes, fingers and earlobes may also be due to poor peripheral circulation, especially in cold weather.

Jugular venous pressure. On the side of the neck the jugular venous pressure (JVP) is seen as a flickering impulse in the jugular vein. It is normally seen at the base of the neck when the patient is lying back at 45°. The JVP is usually measured in relation to the sternal angle as this point is relatively fixed in relation to the right atrium. A normal JVP at the base of the neck corresponds to a vertical height approximately

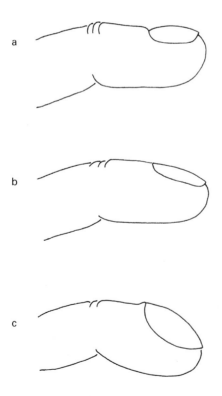

Fig. 1.2   Clubbing. **a** Normal. **b** Early clubbing. **c** Advanced clubbing.

3–4 cm above the sternal angle. The JVP is generally expressed as the vertical height (in centimetres) above normal. The JVP provides a quick assessment of the volume of blood in the great vessels entering the heart. Most commonly it is elevated in right heart failure. This may occur in patients with chronic lung disease complicated by cor pulmonale. In contrast, dehydrated patients may only have a visible JVP when lying flat.

Peripheral oedema. This is an important sign of cardiac failure, but may also be found in patients with a low albumen level, impaired venous or lymphatic function, or those on high dose steroids. When mild it may only affect the ankles, with increasing severity it may progress up the body. In bedbound patients, it is important to check the sacrum.

Observation of the chest

When examining the chest it is important to remember the surface landmarks of the thoracic contents (Fig. 1.3).

Some important points are:

• The oblique fissure, dividing the upper and middle lobes from the lower lobes, runs underneath a line drawn from the spinous process of T2 around the chest to the 6th costochondral junction anteriorly.
• The horizontal fissure on the right, dividing the upper lobe from the middle lobe, runs from the 4th intercostal space at the right sternal edge horizontally to the midaxillary line, where it joins the oblique fissure.
• The diaphragm sits at approximately the 6th rib anteriorly, the 8th rib in the midaxillary line, and the 10th rib posteriorly.
• The trachea bifurcates just below the level of the manubriosternal junction.
• The apical segment of both upper lobes extends 2.5 cm above the clavicles.

Anterior   Posterior

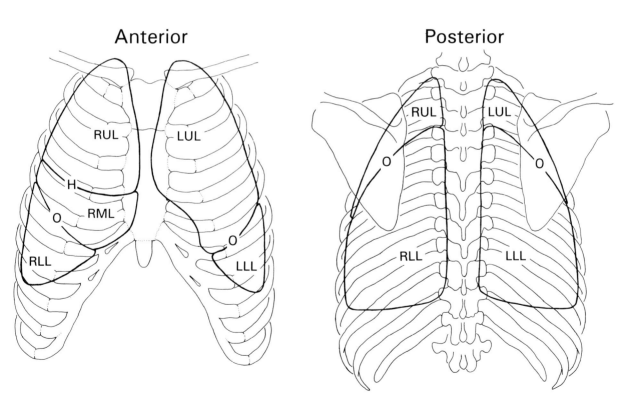

Fig. 1.3   Surface markings of the lungs. H, Horizontal fissure; O, oblique fissures; RUL, right upper lobe; LUL, left upper lobe; RML, right middle lobe; LLL, left lower lobe; RLL, right lower lobe.

Chest shape. The chest should be symmetrical with the ribs, in adults, descending at approximately 45° from the spine. The transverse diameter should be greater than the anteroposterior (AP) diameter. The thoracic spine should have a slight kyphosis. Important common abnormalities include:

Kyphosis, where the normal flexion of the thoracic spine is increased.

Kyphoscoliosis, which comprises both lateral curvature of the spine with vertebral rotation (scoliosis) and an element of kyphosis. This causes a restrictive lung defect which, when severe, may cause respiratory failure.

Pectus excavatum, or 'funnel' chest, is where part of the sternum is depressed inwards. This rarely causes significant changes in lung function but may be corrected surgically for cosmetic reasons.

Pectus carinatum, or 'pigeon' chest, is where the sternum protrudes anteriorly. This may be present in children with severe asthma and rarely causes significant lung function abnormalities.

Hyperinflation, where the ribs lose their normal 45° angle with the thoracic spine and become almost horizontal. The anteroposterior diameter of the chest increases to almost equal the transverse diameter. This is commonly seen in severe emphysema.

Breathing pattern. Observation of the breathing pattern gives further information concerning the type and severity of respiratory disease.

Normal breathing should be regular with a rate of 12–16 breaths/min, as mentioned previously. Inspiration is active and expiration passive. The approximate ratio of inspiratory to expiratory time (I:E ratio) is 1:1.5 to 1:2.

Prolonged expiration may be seen in patients with obstructive lung disease, where expiratory airflow is severely limited by dynamic closure of the smaller airways. In severe obstruction the I:E ratio may increase to 1:3 or 1:4.

Pursed lip breathing is often seen in patients with severe airways disease. By opposing the lips during expiration the airway pressure inside the chest is maintained, preventing the floppy airways from collapsing. Thus overall airflow is increased.

Apnoea is the absence of breathing for more than 15 seconds.

Hypopnoea is diminished breathing with inadequate ventilation. It may be seen during sleep in patients with lung disease.

Kussmaul's respiration is rapid, deep breathing with a high minute ventilation. It is usually seen in patients with metabolic acidosis.

Cheyne–Stokes respiration refers to irregular breathing with cycles consisting of a few relatively deep breaths, progressively shallower breaths (sometimes to the point of apnoea), and then slowly increasing depth of breaths. This is usually associated with severe neurological disturbances or drugs (e.g. narcotics).

Ataxic breathing consists of haphazard, uncoordinated deep and shallow breaths. This may be found in patients with cerebellar disease.

Apneustic breathing is characterized by prolonged inspiration, and is usually the result of brain damage.

Chest movement. During normal inspiration, there are symmetrical increases in the anteroposterior, transverse and vertical diameters of the chest. The increase in vertical diameter is achieved by contraction of the diaphragm, causing the abdominal contents to descend. Sternal and rib movements are responsible for the increases in anteroposterior and transverse diameters of the chest. These movements can be divided into two components (Fig. 1.4). When elevated, the anterior ends of the ribs move forward and upwards with anterior movement of the sternum. This increase in anteroposterior diameter is likened to the movement of an old fashioned 'pump handle'. At the same time, rotation of the ribs causes an increase in the transverse diameter, likened to the movement of a 'bucket handle'.

During normal quiet breathing, the diaphragm is the main inspiratory muscle increasing the vertical diameter. There is also an increase in the lower thoracic transverse diameter due to external intercostal muscle contraction. Expiration is passive, caused by the elastic recoil of the lung and chest wall. When breathing is increased, all the accessory inspiratory muscles (sternomastoid, scalenes, trapezii) contract to increase the anteroposterior and transverse diameters, and the

Pump handle

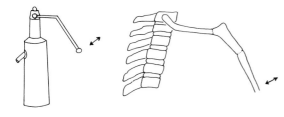

Bucket handle

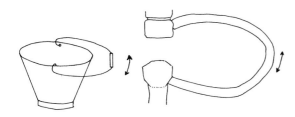

Fig. 1.4 Chest wall movement.

diaphragm activity increases, thus further increasing the vertical dimensions. Expiration may become active with contraction of the abdominal and internal intercostal muscles.

Intercostal indrawing occurs where the skin between the ribs is drawn inwards during inspiration. It may be seen in patients with severe inspiratory airflow resistance. Larger negative pressures during inspiration suck the soft tissues inwards. This is an important sign of respiratory distress in children, but is less often seen in adults.

Palpation

Trachea. Firstly, palpate the trachea to assess its position in relation to the sternal notch. Tracheal deviation indicates underlying mediastinal shift. The trachea may be pulled towards a collapsed or fibrosed upper lobe, or pushed away from a pneumothorax or large pleural effusion.

Chest expansion. This can be assessed by observation, but palpation is more accurate. The patient is instructed to expire slowly to residual volume. At residual volume the examiner's hands

are placed spanning the posterolateral segments of both bases, with the thumbs touching in the midline posteriorly, as shown in Figure 1.5. In obese patients, it helps if the skin of the anterior chest wall is slightly retracted by the finger tips. The patient is then instructed to inspire slowly and the movement of both thumbs is observed. Both sides should move equally, with 3–5 cm being the normal displacement.

A similar technique may be used anteriorly, again to measure basal movements. Measurement of apical movement is more difficult. By placing the hand over the upper chest anteriorly, a qualitative comparison of the two sides can be made. In all cases, diminished movement is abnormal.

Paradoxical breathing is where some or all of the chest wall moves inwards on inspiration and outwards on expiration. It can involve anything from a localized area to the entire chest wall. Localized paradox occurs when the integrity of the chest wall is disrupted. Fractures of multiple ribs with two or more breaks in each rib will result in the central section losing the support usually provided by the rest of the thoracic cage. Thus, during inspiration, this loose segment (often called a 'flail segment') is drawn inwards as the rest of the chest wall moves out. In expiration the reverse occurs.

Paradoxical movement of one hemithorax may be remarkably difficult to observe. It may be caused by unilateral diaphragm paralysis. Paradox of the entire chest wall occurs in bilateral diaphragm weakness or paralysis. It is most apparent when the patient is supine.

Paradoxical movement of the lower chest can occur in patients with severe chronic airflow limitation who are extremely hyperinflated. As the dome of the diaphragm cannot descend any further, diaphragm contraction during inspiration pulls the lower ribs inwards. This is called 'Hoover's sign'.

Surgical emphysema Air in the subcutaneous tissues of the chest, neck or face should also be noted. On palpation there is a characteristic crackling in the skin. This occurs when a pneumomediastinum (air in the mediastinum) has tracked outwards. A chest radiograph must be performed immediately, as a pneumomedi-

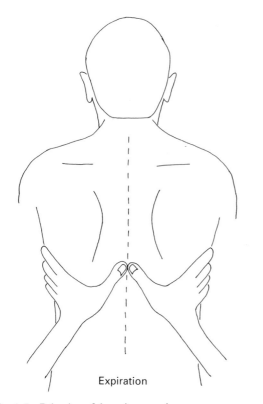

Expiration   Inspiration

Fig. 1.5   Palpation of thoracic expansion.

astinum may be associated with a pneumothorax which may require intervention.

Vocal fremitus. Vocal fremitus is the measure of speech vibrations transmitted through the chest wall to the examiner's hands. It is measured by asking the patient to repeatedly say '99', whilst the examiner's hands are placed flat on both sides of the chest. The hands are moved from apices to bases, anteriorly and posteriorly, comparing the vibration felt. Vocal fremitus is increased when the lung underneath is relatively solid (consolidated), as this transmits sound better. As sound transmission is decreased through any interface between lung and air or fluid, vocal fremitus is decreased in patients with both a pneumothorax or a pleural effusion.

Percussion

Percussion of the chest provides further information that can help in the assessment and localization of lung disease. It is performed by placing the left hand firmly on the chest wall so that the fingers have good contact with the skin. The middle finger of the left hand is struck over the distal interphalangeal joint with the middle finger of the right hand. The right wrist should be relaxed so that the weight of the entire right hand is transmitted through the middle finger. Both sides of the chest from top to bottom should be percussed alternately, paying particular attention to the comparison between sides.

Resonance is generated by the chest wall vibrating over the underlying tissues. Normal resonance is heard over aerated lung, whilst consolidated lung sounds dull, and a pleural effusion sounds 'stony dull'. Increased resonance is heard when the chest wall is free to vibrate over an air-filled space, such as a pneumothorax or bulla. In situations where the chest wall is unable to move freely, as may occur in obese patients, the percussion note may sound dull, even if the underlying lung is normal.

Auscultation

Chest auscultation is the process of listening and interpreting the sounds produced within the thorax. A stethoscope simplifies auscultation and facilitates localization of any abnormalities. It consists of a diaphragm and bell connected by tubing to two ear-pieces. The diaphragm is generally used for listening to breath sounds, whilst the bell is best for the very low frequencies generated by the heart (especially the third and fourth heart sounds). The diaphragm and bell must be intact for a sound to be heard properly, and the tubing relatively short to minimize absorption of the sound. The ear-pieces, made of plastic or rubber, should fit snugly within the ears, pointing slightly forward in order to maximize sound transmission into the auditory canal.

A teaching stethoscope (Fig. 1.6) is a useful tool to allow both the experienced and inexperienced physiotherapist to hear the same sounds simultaneously (Ellis 1985).

Chest auscultation should ideally be performed in a quiet room, with the chest exposed. The patient is instructed to take deep breaths through an open mouth, as turbulence within the nose can interfere with the breath sounds. There is a wide variation in the intensity of breath sounds depending on chest wall thickness. The terms used are described below.

Breath sounds.

Normal breath sounds are generated by turbulent air flow in the trachea and large airways. These sounds, which can be heard directly over the trachea, comprise high, medium and low frequencies. The higher frequencies are attenuated by normal lung tissue so that breath sounds heard over the periphery are softer and lower pitched. Originally it was thought that the higher pitched sounds were generated by the bronchi (bronchial breath sounds) and the lower ones by airflow into the alveoli (vesicular breath sounds). It is now known that normal breath sounds (previously called 'vesicular') simply represent filtering of the 'bronchial' breath sounds generated in the large airways. Although technically incorrect, normal breath sounds are still sometimes referred to as 'vesicular' or 'bronchovesicular'. Normal breath sounds are heard all over the chest wall throughout inspiration and for a short period during expiration.

Bronchial breath sounds are the normal tracheal and large airway sounds, transmitted through airless lung which does not attenuate the higher frequencies. Thus, the sounds heard over an area of consolidated lung are similar to those heard

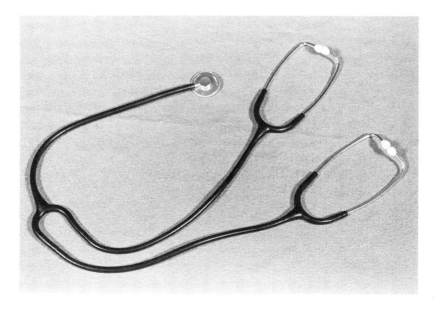

Fig. 1.6 A teaching stethoscope.

over the trachea itself. Bronchial breath sounds are loud and high pitched, with a harsh quality. They are heard equally throughout both inspiration and expiration, with a short pause between the two. Thus in all three respects, bronchial breath sounds differ from normal breath sounds which are faint, lower pitched and absent during the latter half of expiration.

If the bronchus supplying an area of consolidated lung is obstructed (e.g. carcinoma, large sputum plug) bronchial breath sounds may not be heard as the obstruction blocks sound transmission.

Diminished sounds occur when there is a reduction in the initial generation of the sound or when there is an increase in sound attenuation. As the breath sounds are generated by flow-related turbulence, reduced flow causes less sound. Thus patients who will not (e.g. due to pain), or cannot (e.g. due to muscle weakness) breathe deeply, will have globally diminished breath sounds. Similarly, diminished breath sounds are heard in some patients with emphysema where the combination of parenchymal destruction and hyperinflation cause greater attenuation of the normal breath sounds.

Locally diminished breath sounds may represent obstruction of a bronchus by tumour or large sputum plugs. Localized accumulation of air or fluid in the pleural space will block sound transmission so that breath sounds are absent.

Added sounds.

Wheezes, previously called 'rhonchi', are musical tones produced by airflow vibrating a narrowed or compressed airway. A fixed, monophonic wheeze is caused by a single obstructed airway, whilst polyphonic wheezes are due to widespread disease. Any cause of narrowing, for example, bronchospasm, mucosal oedema, sputum or foreign bodies, may cause wheezes. As the airways are normally compressed during expiration, wheezes are first heard at this time. When airway narrowing is more severe, wheezes may also be heard during inspiration. The pitch of the wheeze is directly related to the degree of narrowing, with high pitched wheezes indicating near total obstruction. However, the volume of the wheeze may be misleading as the moderate asthmatic may have loud wheezes whilst the very severe asthmatic may have a 'quiet chest' because he is not generating sufficient airflow to cause wheezes.

Low pitched, localized wheezes are caused by sputum retention and can change or clear after coughing.

Crackles, previously called 'crepitations' or 'râles', are clicking sounds heard during inspiration. They are caused by the opening of previously closed alveoli and small airways during inspiration. Crackles are described as 'early' or 'late', 'fine' or 'coarse', and 'localized' or 'widespread'. Coarse, early inspiratory crackles occur when bronchioles open (often heard in bronchiectasis and bronchitis), whilst fine, late inspiratory crackles occur when alveoli and respiratory bronchioles open (often heard in pulmonary oedema and pulmonary fibrosis). When severe, the late inspiratory crackles of pulmonary oedema and pulmonary fibrosis may become coarser and commence earlier in inspiration.

Localized crackles may occur in dependent alveoli which are gradually closed by compression from the lung above. This early feature of subsegmental lung collapse resolves when the patient breathes deeply or coughs. The crackles of pulmonary oedema are also more marked basally, but only clear transiently after coughing. The differentiation between subsegmental lung collapse and pulmonary oedema may be difficult, and sometimes auscultation will not clarify the situation. Elevation of the jugular venous pressure and peripheral oedema suggest pulmonary oedema, whereas ineffective cough, recent anaesthesia and pyrexia suggest sputum retention which could lead to subsegmental lung collapse (Table 1.6). Postoperative and intensive care patients may have a combination of both pulmonary oedema and sputum retention.

Pleural rub is the creaking or rubbing sound which occurs with each breath when the pleural surfaces are roughened by inflammation, infection or neoplasm. Normally the visceral and parietal pleura slide silently. Pleural rubs range from being localized and soft to being loud and generalized, sometimes even palpable. In certain instances, they may be difficult to differentiate from crackles. An important distinguishing feature is

Table 1.6 Differentiation between pulmonary oedema and sputum retention

Chest sign	Pulmonary oedema	Sputum retention
Auscultation	Fine crackles, especially at bases, with or without wheezes	Scattered or localized crackles, with or without wheezes, may move with coughing
Sputum	Frothy white or pink	Thicker, more viscid, any colour
Other signs	Elevated JVP Peripheral oedema Increased weight, positive fluid balance History of previous cardiac disease	Pyrexia History of intercurrent chest disease, recent anaesthetic, aspiration, respiratory muscle weakness

that pleural rubs are heard equally during inspiration and expiration, with the sounds often recurring in reverse order during expiration.

Vocal resonance. Vocal resonance is the transmission of voice through the airways and lung tissue to the chest wall where it is heard through a stethoscope. It is usually tested by instructing the patient to say '99' repeatedly (like vocal fremitus which is felt with the hands). As mentioned previously, normal lung attenuates the higher frequencies so that the lower frequencies dominate. Thus, speech normally becomes a low pitched mumble. Consolidated lung transmits all sounds better, especially the high frequencies, so the transmitted sound is louder and higher pitched. In this situation speech can actually be understood. Whispered speech lacks the lower frequencies and is normally not transmitted to the chest wall. However, over areas of consolidation the whisper is clearly heard and intelligible — this is called 'whispering pectoriloquy'.

As with auscultation of breath sounds, vocal resonance is decreased when the transmission of sound through the lung or from the lung to chest wall is impeded. This occurs with emphysema, pneumothorax, pleural thickening or pleural effusion.

A summary of the chest examination of selected chest problems is given in Table 1.7.

Heart sounds. The normal heart sounds represent the closure of the four heart valves. The first heart sound is caused by closure of the mitral and tricuspid valves, while the second heart sound is due to closure of the aortic and pulmonary valves. A third heart sound indicates cardiac failure in adults, but may be normal in children. It is attributed to vibration of the ventricular walls caused by rapid filling in early diastole. The fourth heart sound is caused by vibration of the ventricular walls in late diastole as the atria contract. It may be heard in heart failure, hypertension and aortic valve disease.

A murmur is the sound generated by turbulent flow through a valve. The murmur of valvular incompetence is caused by back flow across the valve, whilst stenotic valves generate murmurs by turbulent forward flow.

Sputum

If the patient has already produced some sputum, this should be examined for colour, consistency, and quantity as described on page 6.

Exercise tolerance

For a complete assessment of the respiratory system exercise capacity should also be measured. Depending on the situation, this may vary from a full exercise test for measuring maximum oxygen

Table 1.7 Summary of chest examination in selected chest problems*

Disease	Breath sounds	PN	VF	VR
Consolidation:				
With open airway	Bronchial	Dull	↑	↑
With blocked airway	↓	Dull	↓	↓
Pneumothorax	↓ or Absent	Hyperresonant	↓ or Absent	↓ or Absent
Pleural effusion	↓ or Absent	Stony dull	↓ or Absent	↓ or Absent

*PN, percussion note; VF, vocal fremitus; VR, vocal resonance   ↑, increased; ↓, decreased

uptake, to a simple assessment of breathlessness during normal activities. An exercise test provides the best measure of functional limitation, which may be different from that suggested by a patient's lung function. One of the most common methods used to assess patients with respiratory disease is the 6 min walk test. More recently, the shuttle test has been proposed in place of the 6 min walk. For further details, see Chapter 3.

Test results

The final stage of assessment of a respiratory patient involves the use of tests, in particular spirometry, arterial blood gases, and chest radiography. The following is a brief summary of the application of these tests. A full discussion is given in Chapters 2 and 3.

Spirometry

The forced expiratory volume in 1 second (FEV_1), the forced vital capacity (FVC) and peak expiratory flow (PEF) are important measures of ventilatory function. Normal values, based on population studies, depend on age, height, sex and race. Weight is not an important determinant of lung function, except in the markedly obese or malnourished.

Although often expressed as absolute values, lung function should always be compared with the predicted values and with the previous recordings for that patient. For example a 21-year-old, 6-foot tall male asthmatic changing his spirometry (FEV_1/FVC) from 4.0/5.0 litres to 1.5/3.0 litres should cause concern, whilst a normal 81-year-old, 5-foot female may never manage to blow more than 1.3/1.8 litres!

Arterial blood gases

Arterial blood gases (ABGs) provide an accurate measure of oxygen uptake and carbon dioxide removal by the respiratory system as a whole. The arterial blood is usually sampled from the radial artery at the wrist. Rarely, arterialized capillary samples may be taken from the earlobe. Arterial blood gases are best used as a measure of steady state gas exchange, thus it is imperative that the patient is resting quietly with a constant inspired oxygen level (FiO_2) and mode of ventilation for at least 30 min prior to sampling. When analysing the results, consideration must be given to all these factors.

Normal values for arterial blood gases are:

pH	7.35–7.45	
PaO_2	10.7–13.3 kPa	(80–100 mmHg)
$PaCO_2$	4.7–6.0 kPa	(35–45 mmHg)
HCO_3^-	22–26 mmol	
Base excess	−2 to +2	

Chest radiographs

Chest radiographs are an important aid to physical examination as they provide a clear picture of the extent and severity of disease at that time. In some instances, chest radiographs may show more extensive disease than expected, whilst in others they may underestimate the pathology present. Comparison with previous radiographs provides an excellent measure of improvement or deterioration over time, and an objective assessment of the response to treatment. However, the chest radiograph may sometimes lag 1–2 days behind the clinical findings.

PROBLEM LIST

The second part of the problem oriented medical record (POMR) is the problem list (see Fig. 1.1). The information in the database, together with the subjective and objective assessment are then analysed as a whole, and integrated with the physiotherapist's knowledge of disease processes.

The problem list is then compiled. It consists of a simple, functional and specific list of the patient's problems at that time, not always listed in order of priority. Each problem is numbered and dated at the time of assessment. The problem list should not only include those problems that may improve with physiotherapy (e.g. breathlessness on exertion), but should also include other relevant problems that may have a bearing on the treatment chosen (e.g. anaemia). The problem list should not be a list of signs and symptoms, as this would provide the wrong emphasis for treatment. In the past, disease based treatment tended to result in standardized treatment, ignoring the patient's individual problems. This meant that all chronic airflow limitation patients were given treatment for increased sputum production. All intubated patients also received standard treatment, irrespective of the presence or absence of excess secretions and the patient's ability to clear them. The best system is one that is individualized to each patient.

Problems once resolved should be signed off and dated. Any subsequent problems are added and dated appropriately.

INITIAL PLANS

For each of the problems listed, long- and short-term goals are formulated. A treatment plan is then devised for each of these goals. This process must be performed, where possible, in consultation with the patient. The importance of involving the patient himself cannot be overstressed, as cooperation is fundamental to nearly all physiotherapy treatment.

Long-term goals are generally directed at returning the patient to his maximum functional capacity. Specifically, goals may be simplified to functions that are important to the patient, e.g. to be able to walk home from the shops carrying one bag of shopping. When setting goals for an in-patient, consideration must be given to his discharge. If the home situation includes two flights of stairs to the bedroom then the goal of exercise tolerance should reflect this. If physiotherapy is to be continued at home after discharge, one of the goals must be to teach the patient or a relative how to perform the treatment effectively.

Short-term goals are the steps taken to achieve the long-term goals. In general these are small, simple activities that are more easily achieved. All goals, both short and long term, should state expected outcomes and time frames. The goals, especially the short-term goals, should be reviewed regularly as some patients may improve faster than others. If goals are not met within the agreed time frame, then revision is necessary. The time frame may have been too short, the goal inappropriate, or other problems need attention before this goal can be met.

The treatment plan includes the specifics of treatment, together with its frequency and equipment requirements. Patient education must not be omitted from the treatment plan as it is an important component of physiotherapy.

PROGRESS NOTES

These are written on a daily basis using the 'subjective, objective, analysis, plan' (SOAP) format:

- **S**ubjective — what the patient, doctors or nurses report
- **O**bjective — any change in physical examination or test, e.g. auscultation, chest radiograph
- **A**nalysis — the physiotherapist's professional opinion of any changes
- **P**lan — including changes in treatment and any further action.

Entries are made for each problem, signed and dated. If there have been no changes, nothing further needs to be written.

Progress notes may also include a graph or flow chart. Graphs are particularly useful in displaying the change in a parameter with time, for example an asthmatic's peak expiratory flow rates. Flow chart displays are useful if multiple factors are changing over a period of time, as may occur in the intensive care patient.

The short- and long-term goals provide a basis for evaluating the effectiveness of treatment in relation to the various problems. One of the best indicators of outcome is the change in objective findings after treatment. Although changes that occur immediately after a single treatment are related to physiotherapy intervention alone, changes over longer periods of time reflect treatment by the entire health team. Chest auscultation before and after a treatment may provide a simple indication of the effectiveness of that treatment. Similarly, the chest radiograph can demonstrate the effectiveness of physiotherapy treatment by showing diminution in the area of collapsed/consolidated lung. On a long-term basis, changes in lung function or exercise tolerance provide the most valuable measures of treatment outcome.

The analysis of outcome is then compared with that expected (i.e. the goals). If there are discrepancies between the actual and expected outcomes then the plan (P) documents the changes to the goals and/or treatment, as required.

DISCHARGE SUMMARY

Upon discharge or transfer elsewhere, a summary should be written of the patient's initial problems, treatment and outcomes. Instruction for home programmes and any other relevant information should also be included. Discharge summaries are helpful to other physiotherapists who may treat the patient in the future. The summary should always contain adequate information for future audit and studies of patient care.

AUDIT

'Audit' refers to the systematic and critical analysis of the quality of care. There are three main forms of audit: structure, process and outcome.

1. *Structural audit* examines the organization of resources within a certain area. This may address the availability of human and/or equipment resources, e.g. a hospital's requirements for transcutaneous electrical nerve stimulation (TENS) machines, batteries and electrodes.

2. *Process audit* investigates the system of delivery of care, e.g. studying the methods of patient referral.

3. *Outcome audit* is the most clinically based audit. It examines the results of physiotherapy care, e.g. assessing whether the goals of treatment have been met within the stated time frames.

The audit process is cyclical. Firstly, a standard of care is defined. The actual practice is then audited in comparison with the agreed standard. Discrepancies provoke further discussion. Changes are then made to eliminate these discrepancies. After an appropriate length of time the cycle begins again.

EDUCATIONAL PROGRAMME

By using a structured system of problem oriented medical records and audit, the problem oriented medical system allows identification of areas where goals are not being met within an appropriate time frame. Audit may also reveal situations where the agreed standards are not met. In both instances staff education programmes will improve patient care.

CONCLUSION

Accurate assessment should reveal the exact nature of the patient's problems and delineate those that physiotherapy can improve. Only then can the best treatment be chosen for that patient. Subsequent reassessment is essential to ensure that treatment is specific, effective and efficient. This process ensures high quality patient care.

REFERENCES

Ellis E 1985 Making a teaching stethoscope. Australian Journal of Physiotherapy 31: 244
Rubinstein I, Zamel N, DuBarry L, Hoffstein V 1990 Airflow limitation in mobidly obese, nonsmoking men. Annals of Internal Medicine 112: 828–832

Weed L 1968 Medical records that guide and teach. New England Journal of Medicine 279: 593–600

FURTHER READING

Bromley A I 1978 The patient care audit. Physiotherapy 64: 270–271
Forgacs P 1978 Lung sounds. Baillière Tindall, London

Heath J R 1978 Problem oriented medical systems. Physiotherapy 64: 269–270

2. Thoracic imaging

Conor D. Collins   David M. Hansell

CHEST RADIOGRAPHY AND OTHER TECHNIQUES

Different types of chest radiograph

Chest radiographs have been used as the main radiological investigation of the chest ever since the discovery of X-rays by Röntgen in 1895 and they comprise 25–40% of all radiological investigations. Chest radiographs are indicated in almost any condition in which a pulmonary abnormality is suspected.

The majority of chest radiographs are obtained in the main radiology department. The radiograph is obtained with the patient standing erect. Patients who are immobile or too ill to come to the main department have a chest radiograph performed using a mobile machine (portable film); the resulting chest radiograph differs from a departmental film in terms of projection, positioning, exposure and film used, and is therefore not strictly comparable with a conventional posteroanterior (PA) film. Other types of chest radiograph are the lateral, lordotic, apical and decubitus views; these are generally taken in the main department.

Departmental films are referred to as 'posteroanterior' (or PA) chest radiographs and describe the direction in which the X-ray beam traverses the patient. The patient is positioned with his anterior chest wall against the film cassette and his back to the X-ray tube. The arms are abducted to rotate the scapulae away from the posterior chest and the radiograph is taken during full inspiration. The tube is centred at the spinous process of the fourth thoracic vertebra. For portable films which are taken in an anteroposterior (AP) projection, the patient's back is against the film cassette and the X-ray tube is positioned at a variable distance from the patient. As the heart is anteriorly placed within the chest it is further from the cassette, and is therefore magnified in an AP radiograph. The degree of magnification depends on the distance between the patient and the X-ray tube.

For a lateral radiograph the patient is turned 90° and the side of interest placed against the film cassette. The arms are extended forwards and the radiograph is again taken in full inspiration.

Lateral decubitus views are sometimes useful for the demonstration of small pleural effusions. For this projection the patient lies horizontally with the side in question placed downwards. The film cassette is positioned at the back of the patient and the X-ray beam is horizontal, centred at midsternum. This provides a sensitive means of detecting small quantities of pleural fluid (50–100 ml) which cannot be identified on a frontal chest radiograph. However, ultrasonography is increasingly being used as a reliable means of confirming the presence of small pleural effusions.

Lordotic films are sometimes used to confirm middle lobe collapse and for demonstrating a questionable apical opacity otherwise obscured by the clavicle and ribs. For this AP projection the patient arches back so that the shoulders are touching the cassette with the centring point remaining the same. Linear tomography is another technique designed to reveal lesions otherwise hidden by the skeleton by blurring out everything over and under the lesion in question. This is achieved by having the X-ray tube and film cassette move at the same time but in opposite directions. These two techniques are less frequently used with the advent of computed tomography(CT).

Factors influencing the quality of a chest radiograph

The quality and thus diagnostic usefulness of a chest radiograph depends critically on the conditions under which it is obtained. Of particular importance are the radiographic exposure, the projection, the orientation of the patient relative to the film cassette, the X-ray tube to film distance, the depth of inspiration of the patient and the type of film–screen combination used.

The ideal chest radiograph provides an image of structures within the chest whilst exposing the patient to the lowest possible dose of radiation. Most radiology departments have a policy of obtaining either high kilovoltage (kVp) or low kilovoltage chest radiographs. Radiographs performed at a high kilovoltage (e.g. 140 kVp) have much to recommend them. Even at total lung capacity with the patient erect, nearly a third of the lungs is partially obscured by the mediastinal structures, diaphragm and ribs. With the low kilovoltage technique (80 kVp or less) these areas are often poorly visualized. This problem is partially overcome by using films exposed at 140 kVp. The normal vessel markings and subtle differences in soft tissue densities are better demonstrated and a further advantage is the better penetration of the mediastinum which improves visualization of the trachea and main bronchi. The disadvantage of high kilovoltage radiographs is the relatively poor demonstration of calcified structures so that rib fractures and calcified pulmonary nodules or pleural plaques are less conspicuous.

During exposure the X-ray beam is modified according to the structures through which it passes. The photons that have passed through the patient carry the information which then must be converted into a visual form. Some of the photons emerging from the patient are aligned in a virtually parallel direction and other photons are scattered. These scattered photons degrade the final image but can be absorbed by using lead strips embedded in an aluminium sheet positioned in front of the cassette. This device is known as a grid. Photons that are travelling in parallel pass through the grid to form the image on the film.

The sensitivity of film to direct X-ray exposure is very low, and if used alone as the image receptor would result in a prohibitively large X-ray dose to the patient. Intensifying screens made of a phosphorescent material are positioned on the inside of the cassettes and they convert the incident X-ray photons into visible light and it is this light which is recorded by the adjacent film. These phosphor screens are composed of either calcium tungstate or a rare earth containing compound. Rare earth phosphors emit more light in response to X-ray photons and, therefore, less radiation is necessary, compared with calcium tungstate screens, to produce the image. Similarly, improvements in the quality of X-ray film have also occurred over the years. Standard film emulsions tend to lack detail in the relatively under- or over-exposed areas of the radiograph and newer emulsions have been developed so that detail is similar in all areas of the chest radiograph. The choice of film–screen combination has a crucial influence on the quality and 'look' of the radiograph produced. Further variations may result from film processing problems.

Over the years much effort has been expended on producing radiographs which are less affected by these factors so that differences present in serial radiographs on the same patient represent real differences and not technical variations. Newer devices designed to expose accurately the various parts of the chest using automatic exposure devices are now being installed. One of these, the advanced multiple beam equalization radiography (AMBER) system, produces chest radiographs which greatly improve the demonstration of mediastinal abnormalities and pulmonary nodules which would otherwise be obscured by the overlying heart or diaphragm (Fig. 2.1).

In the intensive care setting, portable chest radiographs are often taken in less than ideal conditions. Multiple tubes, lines and dressings in conjunction with an immobile, supine patient and the use of a mobile low kilovoltage machine often result in suboptimal radiographs. One approach to this is the development of phosphor plate technology which is ultimately expected to replace conventional film–screen radiography.

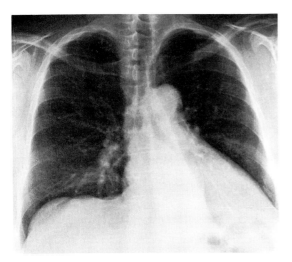

Fig. 2.1 Triangular opacity of left lower lobe collapse seen through the heart shadow on this AMBER chest radiograph.

The phosphor plate is placed inside a conventional cassette and stores some of the energy of the incident X-ray photons as a latent image (the image produced on a film or phosphor plate prior to development). The plate is scanned with a laser beam and the light emitted from the 'excited' latent image is detected by a photomultiplier. Thereafter this signal is processed in digital form. This digital image may be viewed either on a television monitor or on film (on which it has been laser printed). The great advantage of this system is that it can retrieve an image of diagnostic quality from a suboptimal exposure. Similar gross over- or under-exposure would result in a non-diagnostic conventional radiograph. Manipulation of the digital image, particularly 'edge enhancement' aids the detection of linear structures such as the edge of a pneumothorax. However, conventional film radiography retains two important advantages. It has an extremely high spatial resolution (ability to resolve small objects) and the necessary equipment is reliable and relatively inexpensive.

Other techniques

Fluoroscopy

The patient is positioned, either standing or lying, in a screening unit which allows immediate radiographic visualization of the area in question on a television monitor. The patient can be turned in any direction and this technique can help to distinguish pulmonary from extrapulmonary opacities. One of the main uses of fluoroscopy is to 'screen' the diaphragm to demonstrate paralysis or abnormal movement. It is also useful in needle placement during biopsy of lung masses.

Linear tomography

The principle of this technique is to 'blur out' over- and underlying structures. It is used to site lesions precisely within the chest and to determine whether there is cavitation or calcification within them. With the increasing availability of CT, linear tomography is rapidly becoming obsolete.

Ultrasonography

High frequency sound waves do not traverse air and the use of this technique is therefore limited in the chest. It is mainly used for cardiac work (echocardiography) and it has become an essential technique in the investigation of patients with valvular and ventricular function problems. Outside the heart, ultrasonography is very useful in distinguishing between fluid above the diaphragm (pleural effusion), fluid below the diaphragm (subphrenic collection), and pleural thickening. Chest radiography often cannot differentiate between pleural fluid and thickening with any certainty. Ultrasound can also be used to guide the placement of a drain into a pleural effusion.

Computed tomography

Computed tomography (CT) scanning depends on the same basic physical principle as conventional radiography, namely the absorption of X-rays by tissues of different densities. The basic components of a CT machine are a table on which the patient lies and a gantry through which the table slides. An X-ray tube and a series of detectors are housed within the gantry. The X-ray tube and detectors rotate around the patient. A computer is used to reconstruct the signals received by the detectors into an image. The images acquired are transverse (axial) cross-sections of the patient. In orientating the patient's right and left sides, it is now the convention to view all CT images as if from the patient's feet.

Because of the cross-sectional nature of CT it can accurately localize lesions seen on only one view on plain chest radiographs. The superior contrast resolution of CT allows superb demonstration of mediastinal anatomy (e.g. lymph nodes and individual vessels) as well as calcification within a pulmonary nodule. Its ability to produce highly detailed thin sections of the lung parenchyma allows the complex morphology of many interstitial lung diseases to be defined more clearly. Its disadvantages are its relatively high cost and increased radiation exposure to the patient compared with chest radiography.

Common indications for CT of the chest.

1. CT scanning is used to further evaluate hilar or mediastinal masses seen or suspected on a chest radiograph.

2. Within the lungs it can be used to further define the nature of a mass or cavitating lesion not clearly seen on the plain film.

3. In patients with normal chest radiographs but abnormal pulmonary function tests, thin section high resolution CT sections of the lung may provide the first radiological evidence of parenchymal disease. This type of scanning is also very useful for assessing patients with suspected bronchiectasis.

4. CT is useful in patients with neoplasms, both in assessing their operability and their response to treatment.

Magnetic resonance imaging

The physical principles of magnetic resonance imaging (MRI) are more complex and very different to those governing CT scanning. The equipment consists of a sliding table on which the patient lies within the bore of a large magnet. A combination of the intense magnetic field and a series of radiofrequency waves produce an alteration in the alignment of protons (mostly in water) resulting in the emission of different signals which are detected and subsequently analysed for

their intensity and position by a computer. The major advantages of MRI are that images may be obtained in any plane without the use of ionizing radiation. The disadvantages are its cost, limited availability and, in the chest, the images suffer from motion artefact due to breathing. As a result its application to chest imaging is as yet limited.

Interventional procedures

Percutaneous needle biopsy

Percutaneous needle biopsy of a pulmonary or mediastinal mass, to provide a histological specimen, is usually performed in patients in whom a bronchoscopic biopsy has failed or a thoracotomy is inappropriate. Different types of needle are used and the complication rate (pneumothorax and haemoptysis) bears some relation to the size of the needle. Contra-indications to the procedure include any patient with poor respiratory reserve unable to withstand a pneumothorax, pulmonary arterial hypertension, and a previous contralateral pneumonectomy.

Pulmonary and bronchial arteriography: superior vena cavography

Pulmonary arteriography. This is usually undertaken in the investigation of suspected pulmonary embolism and pulmonary arteriovenous malformations. It requires puncture of either the femoral vein in the groin or the antecubital vein in the elbow and the guiding of a catheter through the right side of the heart under fluoroscopy. The tip of the catheter is positioned in the main pulmonary artery or selectively placed in a smaller pulmonary artery. Contrast is then injected. Arteriography remains the most specific method of identifying pulmonary emboli; these are shown as filling defects which cause non-filling of branches of the arterial tree. It is also the best and most appropriate technique for the demonstration of pulmonary arteriovenous malformations. These can be treated at the time of the arteriogram by the injection of occlusive materials (embolization).

Bronchial arteriography. Demonstration of

the bronchial arteries requires catheterization of the femoral artery and passage of a catheter into the midthoracic aorta from where the bronchial arteries are selectively catheterized. The major indication for this procedure is recurrent or life-threatening haemoptysis in patients with a chronic inflammatory disease, usually bronchiectasis. Accurate placement of the catheter not only allows demonstration of the bleeding vessel but also allows embolization to be performed simultaneously.

Superior vena cavography. This is performed for the evaluation of superior vena caval (SVC) obstruction and the investigation of anatomical variants. More recently, patients with SVC compression due to tumour have been palliated by the insertion of an expandable metallic mesh wire stent at the site of the SVC narrowing, thus restoring flow and relieving symptoms.

THE NORMAL CHEST

Anatomy

On the normal posteroanterior radiograph (Fig. 2.2) the following structures can be identified:

- outline of the mediastinum and heart
- the hila
- pulmonary vessels and main bronchi
- diaphragm
- soft tissues and bones of the thoracic cage.

The heart and mediastinum

The mediastinum consists of the organs and soft tissues in the central part of the chest. These comprise the trachea, aortic arch and great vessels, superior vena cava and oesophagus. In children the thymus gland is a prominent component. On the two-dimensional chest radiograph these structures are superimposed and cannot be clearly distinguished from each other. The mediastinum is conventionally divided into superior, anterior, middle and posterior compartments. Whilst the boundaries of the latter three are arbitrary, it is usual to divide them into equal thirds. The superior mediastinum is that portion lying above the aortic arch and below the root of the neck.

The mediastinal border on the right is formed superiorly by the right brachiocephalic vein and superior vena cava. The mediastinal shadow to

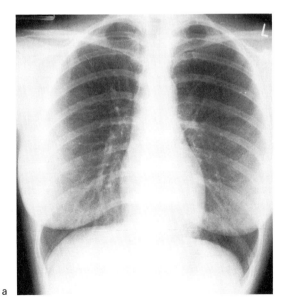

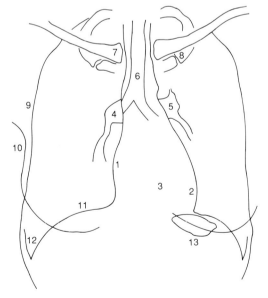

Fig. 2.2 **a** Normal PA chest radiograph. **b** Normal structures visible on a PA chest radiograph. 1, right atrium; 2, left ventricle; 3, right ventricle; 4, right pulmonary artery; 5, left pulmonary artery; 6, air within trachea; 7, clavicle; 8, first rib; 9, lateral border of hemithorax; 10, breast shadow; 11, right hemidiaphragm; 12, costophrenic angle; 13, gastric air bubble.

the left of the trachea above the aortic arch comprises the left carotid and left subclavian arteries together with the left brachiocephalic and jugular veins. On a correctly exposed chest radiograph, air in the trachea can be seen throughout its length as it descends downwards deviating slightly to the right above the carina where it is displaced by the aortic arch.

The heart lies eccentrically in the chest, with one-third of the cardiac shadow to the right of the spine and two-thirds to the left. The density of the cardiac shadow on the left and right of the spine should be identical. The right cardiac border on a chest radiograph is formed by the right atrium. The left cardiac border is composed of the apex of the left ventricle and superiorly the left atrial appendage. The outline of the right ventricle, which is superimposed on the left ventricle, cannot be identified on a frontal radiograph. The maximum transverse diameter of the heart should be less than half the maximum transverse diameter of the thorax, as measured from the inside border of the ribs (the so-called 'cardio-thoracic ratio').

The hila

Hilar shadows are a complex summation of the pulmonary arteries and veins with minor contributions from other components (the main bronchi and lymph nodes). In general, the hila are of equal density and are approximately the same size. Adjacent to the left hilum, the main pulmonary artery forms a localized bulge just above the left atrial appendage and just below the aortic arch. The area between the aortic arch and the main pulmonary artery is known as the 'aortopulmonary window.'

The superior pulmonary veins run vertically and converge on the upper and midhilum on both sides. It is not possible to distinguish arteries from veins in the outer two-thirds of the lungs. The inferior pulmonary veins run obliquely in a near horizontal plane below the lower lobe arteries to enter the left atrium beneath the carina (the division of the trachea into the right and left main stem bronchi). The hilar point is where the superior pulmonary vein on each side crosses the basal artery. This is more easily assessed on the

right than on the left. Using this as an index point, the left hilum is normally 0.5–1.5 cm higher than the right one.

Abnormalities of the hilar shadows in the form of increased density or abnormal configuration are usually the result of lymph node or pulmonary artery enlargement. The detection of subtle hilar abnormalities is difficult and requires experience and knowledge of the many outlines that the hila may assume in normal individuals.

Fissures, vessels and segmental bronchi within the lungs

Each lung is divided into lobes surrounded by visceral pleura. There are two lobes on the left (the upper and lower, separated by the major (oblique) fissure) and three on the right (the upper, middle and lower lobes which are separated by the major (oblique) and minor (horizontal or transverse) fissures). In the majority of normal subjects, some or all of the minor fissure is seen on a frontal radiograph. The major fissures are only identifiable on lateral projection. Each lobe of the lung contains a number of segments which have their own segmental bronchi. The walls of the segmental bronchi are invisible on the chest radiograph, except when seen end-on as ring shadows measuring up to 7 mm in diameter.

The pulmonary blood vessels are responsible for the branching and linear structures within the lungs. The diameter of the blood vessels beyond the hilum varies with the position of the patient and with haemodynamic factors. In the erect position there is a gradual increase in the diameter of the vessels, travelling from apex to base. This increase in size is seen in both the arteries and veins and is abolished if the patient lies supine.

The diaphragm

The interface between the lung and diaphragm should be sharp and, in general, the diaphragm is dome shaped with its highest point medial to the midclavicular line. The margin of the right hemidiaphragm at its highest point lies between the anterior ends of the fifth and seventh ribs. The right hemidiaphragm is higher than the left by up to 2 cm in the erect position. Laterally, the diaphragm dips downwards forming a sharp angle with the chest wall known as the 'costophrenic angle'. Filling in or blunting of these angles reflects pleural disease, either fluid or thickening.

Thoracic cage

On a high kilovoltage chest radiograph it should be possible to identify the edges of the vertebral bodies of the dorsal spine through the heart shadow. However, a high kilovoltage radiograph may 'burn out' the ribs, particularly the posterior portions. Because of this the chest radiograph may be an insensitive means of demonstrating rib abnormalities, particularly fractures.

Common anatomical variants

The trachea lies centrally, but in the elderly may deviate markedly to the right in its lower portion due to unfolding and dilatation of the aortic arch. A small ovoid soft tissue shadow just above the origin of the right main bronchus represents the azygos vein. This may be enlarged as a result of posture (supine position) or haemodynamic factors. It may be indistinguishable from an azygos lymph node.

Occasionally, extra fissures are seen in the lungs. The commonest of these is the azygos lobe fissure; this is seen as a fine white line running obliquely from the apex of the right lung to the azygos vein. Other accessory fissures are the superior and inferior accessory fissures, both of which are in the right lower lobe.

The surfaces of the two lungs abut each other anteriorly and posteriorly and give rise to two white lines projected over the vertebral column known as the 'anterior and posterior junction lines', respectively. Both of these may be seen overlying the trachea — the anterior line extending from the clavicles to the left main bronchus and the posterior line lying more medially and extending above the clavicles. The azygo-oesophageal recess line is a curved line projected over the vertebral column and extending from the azygos vein to the diaphragm. It represents the interface between the right lung and right oesophageal wall.

A small 'nipple' may occasionally be seen projecting laterally from the aortic knuckle due to the left superior intercostal vein. The term 'paraspinal line' refers to the line that parallels the left and right margins of the thoracic spine. The left is thicker than the right due to the adjacent aorta.

The lateral view

It is conventional to read the lateral film (Fig. 2.3) with the heart to the viewer's left and the dorsal spine to the right, irrespective of whether the film is labelled 'right' or 'left'. The chamber of the heart that touches the sternum is the right ventricle. Behind and above the heart lies lung, the density of which should be the same both behind the heart and behind the sternum. As the eye travels down the spine, the vertebral column should appear increasingly transradiant (Fig. 2.3a); the loss of this phenomenon suggests the presence of disease in the posterobasal segments of the lower lobes. In the middle of the lateral film lie the hilar structures with the main pulmonary artery anteriorly. The aortic arch should be easily identified, but only a variable proportion of the great vessels is visible depending on the degree of aortic unfolding. The brachiocephalic artery is most frequently identified arising anterior to the tracheal air column. The left and right brachio-cephalic vein forms an extrapleural bulge behind the upper sternum in about a third of individuals.

The course of the trachea is straight with a slight posterior angulation, but no visible indentation from adjacent vessels. The carina is not seen on the lateral view. The posterior wall of the trachea is always visible and is known as the 'posterior tracheal stripe'.

The oblique fissures are seen as fine diagonal lines running from the upper dorsal spine to the diaphragm anteriorly. The left is more vertically orientated and is visible just behind the right. The minor fissure extends forwards horizontally from the mid-right oblique fissure. Care must be taken not to confuse rib margins with fissure lines. As the fissures undulate, two distinct fissure lines may be generated by a single fissure. The fissures should be of no more than hairline width.

The scapulae are invariably seen in the lateral

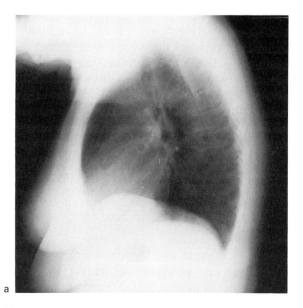
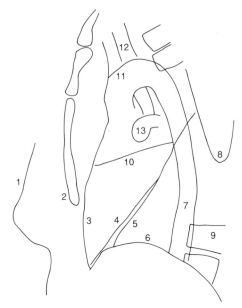

Fig. 2.3   a Normal lateral chest radiograph. **b** Normal structures visible on a lateral chest radiograph. 1, Breast shadow; 2, sternum; 3, position of right ventricle; 4, right oblique fissure; 5, left oblique fissure; 6, hemidiaphragm; 7, descending aorta; 8, inferior angle of scapula; 9, dorsal vertebrae; 10, horizontal fissure; 11, aortic arch; 12, trachea; 13, pulmonary artery.

view and since they are incompletely visualized, lines formed by the edge of the scapula can easily be confused with intrathoracic structures. The arms are held outstretched in front of the patient on a lateral view and these give rise to soft tissue shadows projected over the anterior and superior mediastinum. A band-like opacity simulating pleural disease is often seen along the lower half of the anterior chest wall immediately behind the sternum. The left lung does not contact the most anterior portion of the left thoracic cavity at these levels because the heart occupies the space. This band like opacity is known as the 'retrosternal line'.

Useful points in interpreting a chest radiograph

Documentary information. The name of the patient, and the time and date on which the radiograph was taken, particularly in relation to other films in a series, should all be noted. Often the film is annotated with the patient's date of birth. Of particular importance is the presence of the side marker ('right' or 'left'). The radiograph should also be marked 'AP' if the anteroposterior

projection was used; departmental posteroanterior (PA) films are generally not marked as such.

Radiographic projection. A judgement as to whether a radiograph is AP or PA can be made from the following evidence:

1. The position of the label (this varies from department to department and is open to error).
2. The relationship of the scapulae to the lung margins (in the PA projection the scapulae are projected clear of the lungs and in AP projection they overlie the lungs).
3. The appearances of the vertebral bodies in the cervicodorsal region. The vertebral end plates are seen more clearly in the AP projection and the laminae are more clearly seen in the PA projection.

Supine versus prone position. It is important to know whether a chest radiograph was taken in the erect or supine position. In the supine position, blood flow is more evenly distributed throughout the lungs, making the upper zone vessels equal in size to those in the lower zones. This has implications in assessing the chest radiograph of a patient suspected of being in cardiac failure. In addition, fluid is distributed throughout the dependent part of the pleural space and any air fluid levels that might be present on an erect film are impossible to detect. The position and contours of the heart, mediastinum and diaphragm are also different compared with an erect film. In the absence of any indication on the radiograph, one clue is the position of the gastric air bubble: if it is just under the left hemidiaphragm it is in the fundus and the patient is erect, whereas in the supine position air collects in the antrum of the stomach which lies centrally or slightly to the right of the vertebral column, well below the diaphragm.

Patient rotation. The patient may be rotated around one of three axes. Axial rotation is the commonest cause of unilateral transradiancy (one lung appearing darker than the other). It also distorts the mediastinal outline. The degree of rotation can be assessed by relating the medial ends of the clavicles to the spinous process of the vertebral body at the same level — they should be equidistant from the spinous processes.

Rotation about the horizontal coronal axis results in a more kyphotic or lordotic projection than normal. The main pulmonary artery and subclavian vessels may appear unduly prominent. Rotation around the horizontal sagittal axis usually leads to obvious tilt of the chest in relation to the edge of the radiograph which is assumed to be upright.

Physical attributes of the patient, such as a kyphoscoliosis or a depressed sternum (pectus excavatum), may also distort the appearance of the thoracic cage and its contents.

State of inspiration or expiration. The degree of inspiration is an important consideration for the correct interpretation of a chest radiograph. A poor inspiratory effort does not necessarily imply lack of patient cooperation and may as often be related to a pathological process. At full inspiration the midpoint of the right hemidiaphragm lies between the anterior end of ribs 5–7. A shallow inspiration affects the contour of the heart and mediastinum and may mimic the appearances of pulmonary congestion because the upper zone vessels will have the same diameter as the lower zone vessels.

Films taken deliberately with the patient in full expiration are invaluable in the investigation of air trapping. They are mandatory in any patient suspected of having inhaled a foreign body with consequent obstruction of a lobar bronchus. An expiratory film is also useful in accentuating a small pneumothorax.

Review areas. Several areas are difficult to assess on a frontal radiograph and should be scrutinized carefully. These review areas are:

- apices
- areas behind the heart
- hilar regions
- bones
- lung periphery just inside the chest wall.

Detection and description of radiographic abnormalities should then be undertaken and a differential diagnosis listed based on the abnormalities detected. With experience the structured search gives way to the rapid identification of abnormalities and a search for confirmatory radiological signs and associated abnormalities.

COMMON RADIOLOGICAL SIGNS

Consolidation

'Consolidation' is the term used to describe lung in which the air-filled spaces are replaced by the products of disease, e.g. water, pus or blood. The two most important radiological signs of consolidation are: (a) an air bronchogram, and (b) the silhouette sign. The causes of widespread consolidation may be divided into four categories (Table 2.1).

An air bronchogram is present when the airways contain air and appear as radiolucent (black) branching structures against a now white background of airless lung. The silhouette sign is present when the border of a structure is lost because the normally air-filled lung outlining the border is replaced by radio-opaque fluid or tissue. Recognition of this sign can help localize the affected area of abnormality within the chest. Thus, loss of a clear right heart border is due to right middle lobe consolidation or collapse.

Localized areas of consolidation are usually due to infection. In some cases the borders of the consolidation are clearly demarcated. This usually

Table 2.1   Causes of widespread pulmonary consolidation

Fluid transudation	Pulmonary oedema due to cardiac failure, renal failure, hepatic failure
Exudation	Infection, e.g. lobar pneumonia and bronchopneumonia, tuberculosis Adult respiratory distress syndrome (ARDS) Pulmonary haemorrhage due to contusion Pulmonary eosinophilia
Inhalation	Gastric contents Toxic fumes Oxygen toxicity
Infiltration	Lymphoma Alveolar cell carcinoma

corresponds to a fissure and the consolidation is confined to one lobe (lobar pneumonia) (Fig. 2.4). If consolidation is slow to clear with treatment, it may be secondary to partial obstruction of a lobar bronchus, such as carcinoma of the bronchus. Consolidation may also be widespread and affect both lungs (Fig. 2.5).

Collapse (atelectasis)

'Collapse' ('atelectasis') is the radiological term used when there is loss of aeration and, therefore, expansion in part or all of a lung. Collapse of a lobe or an entire lung is most frequently due to an endobronchial tumour, an inhaled foreign body, or a mucus plug.

Although collapse is most often thought of as occurring at a lobar level, focal areas of pulmonary collapse at a subsegmental level occur very commonly in postoperative patients. There are many signs of lobar collapse, but it is important to realize that not all these signs occur together. In addition, some non-specific signs may be present which indirectly point to the diagnosis and alert the observer to look for the more specific signs.

The most reliable and frequently present finding in lobar collapse is shift of the fissures, which invariably occurs to some extent. If air stays in the collapsed lobe, the contained blood vessels remain visible and appear crowded. If there is

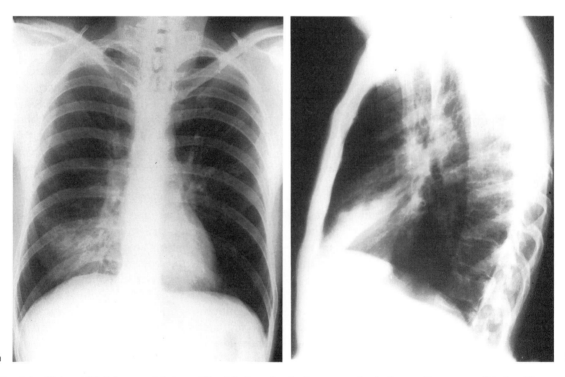

a   b

Fig. 2.4   Right middle lobe consolidation. **a** The right heart border is not seen clearly due to adjacent consolidation. Note that the right hemidiaphragm is clearly visible as far as the vertebral column. **b** The lateral view confirms the presence of consolidation in the right middle lobe with the posterior aspect well demarcated by the oblique fissure.

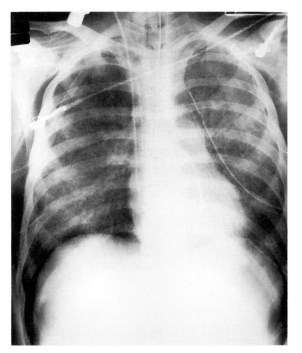

Fig. 2.5 Widespread air space consolidation in a patient with adult respiratory distress syndrome (ARDS). There are multiple chest drains for bilateral pneumothoraces.

marked volume loss the density of the collapsed and airless lobe increases. The hila may show two types of change consisting either of gross displacement upwards or downwards or of rearrangement of individual hilar components (i.e. vessels and airways) leading to changes in shape and prominence. Elevation of the hemidiaphragm, reflecting volume loss, is most marked in collapse of a lower lobe. 'Peaking' of the mid-portion of the hemidiaphragm occurs in upper lobe collapse due to displacement of the oblique fissure. The signs associated with collapse are listed in Table 2.2.

Table 2.2 Signs associated with a collapsed lobe

- Increased density of the collapsed lobe
- Shift of fissures
- Silhouette sign
- Hilar shift and distortion
- Crowding of vessels and airways
- Mediastinal shift
- Crowding of the ribs
- Elevation of hemidiaphragm

Collapse of individual lobes

Right upper lobe

On the posteroanterior (PA) radiograph there is elevation of the transverse fissure and of the right hilum. If the collapse is complete the non-aerated lobe is seen as an increased density alongside the superior mediastinum adjacent to the trachea (Fig. 2.6). On the lateral view the minor fissure moves upwards and the major fissure moves forwards. The retrosternal area becomes progressively more opaque and the anterior margin of the ascending aorta becomes effaced.

Right middle lobe

On the PA radiograph the lateral part of the minor fissure moves down and there is blurring of the normally sharp right heart border. This may be a subtle abnormality which is easily overlooked. On the lateral view the minor fissure moves downwards and lower half of the major fissure

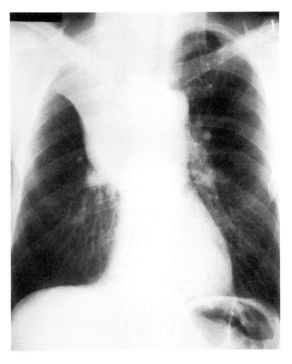

Fig. 2.6 Right upper lobe collapse. There is increased density medial to the elevated horizontal fissure. The cause was a large central tumour obstructing the right upper lobe bronchus.

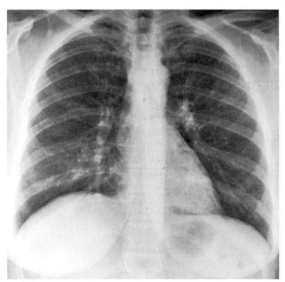

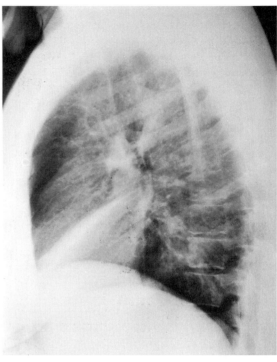

a
b

Fig. 2.7   Right middle lobe collapse. **a** Loss of the right heart border is the only definite radiographic evidence of right middle lobe collapse. **b** The lateral view shows the typical triangular opacity overlying the cardiac shadow.

moves forwards, giving rise to a triangular shadow visible behind the lower sternum (Fig. 2.7).

Right lower lobe

On the PA view there is an increase in density overlying the medial portion of the right hemidiaphragm and the right hilum is displaced inferiorly. The right heart border usually remains sharply defined since this is in contact with the aerated right middle lobe. On the lateral view the oblique fissure moves backwards, and with increasing collapse there is loss of definition of the right hemidiaphragm as well as increased density overlying the lower dorsal vertebrae (Fig. 2.8).

Left upper lobe

The main finding on the PA radiograph is of a veil-like increase in density, without a sharp margin, spreading outwards and upwards from the left hilum which is elevated. The aortic knuckle, left hilum and left heart border may have ill-defined outlines. As volume loss increases, the collapsed lobe moves closer to the midline and the lung apex may become lucent due to hyper-inflation of the apical segment of the left lower lobe. A sharp border may also return to the aortic arch. On the lateral view the oblique fissure moves upwards and forwards, remaining relatively straight and roughly parallel to the anterior chest wall. With marked collapse there is herniation of the right lung across the midline giving an anterior band lucency to the retrosternal region and making the ascending aorta and arch sharp once again (Fig. 2.9). On the PA projection collapse (or consolidation) of the lingular segment of the left upper lobe should be suspected when the left cardiac border is ill defined.

Left lower lobe

This is most commonly seen in patients following cardiac surgery and a thoracotomy due to the retention of secretions in the left lower lobe bronchus. On the PA view there is a triangular

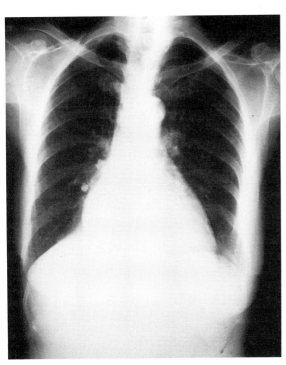

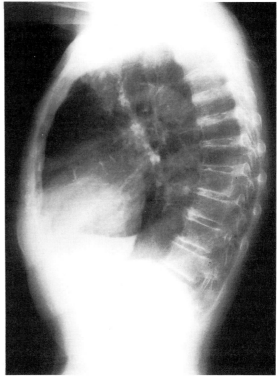

a

b

Fig. 2.8 Right lower lobe collapse. **a** The PA film shows loss of the outline of the medial portion of the right hemidiaphragm and there is increased density behind the right side of the heart. **b** On the lateral film the right hemidiaphragm is obscured posteriorly.

density behind the heart with loss of the medial portion of the left hemidiaphragm; if the PA radiograph is underexposed, it may be impossible to see this triangular opacity. On the lateral view there is displacement backwards of the oblique fissure and with increasing collapse there is increased density over the lower dorsal vertebrae. As non-aerated lung lies against the posterior hemidiaphragm this is now invisible (Fig. 2.1).

Pneumothorax

When air is introduced into the pleural space, the resulting pneumothorax can be recognized radiographically. There are numerous causes of a pneumothorax, but the commonest include penetrating injuries (e.g. stab wound, placement of a subclavian line) and breeches of the visceral pleura (e.g. spontaneous rupture of a subpleural bulla or mechanical ventilation with high

pressures) (see Fig. 2.5). The cardinal radiographic sign is the visceral pleural edge: lateral to this edge no vascular shadows are visible and medial to this the collapsed lung is of higher density than the contralateral lung (Fig. 2.10). It is important to remember that in the supine position, the air of a small pneumothorax will collect anteriorly in the pleural space; thus on a portable supine chest radiograph, the pneumothorax will be visible as an area of relative translucency without a visceral pleural edge necessarily being identifiable.

If air enters the pleural space during inspiration but cannot leave on expiration (usually because of a check-valve effect of the torn flap of the visceral pleura), pressure increases rapidly and this results in a life-threatening tension pneumothorax. This can be recognized by a shift of the mediastinum to the opposite side and straightening of the ipsilateral diaphragm (Fig. 2.11).

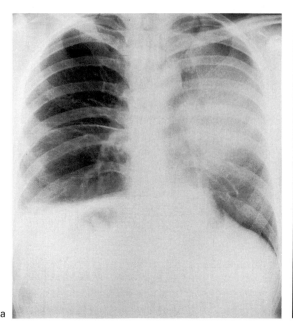
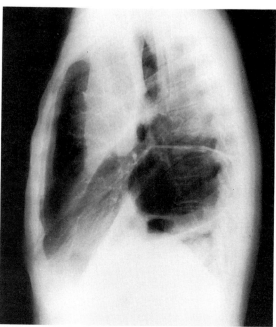

a

b

Fig. 2.9   Left upper lobe collapse: **a** There is a veil-like density in the left upper zone due to upper lobe collapse (the right hemidiaphragm is elevated due to previous trauma). **b** The lateral radiograph shows increased density anterior to the oblique fissure.

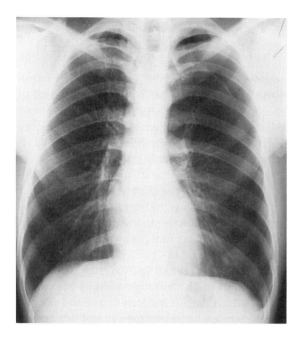

Fig. 2.10   Spontaneous pneumothorax: the visceral pleural edge is visible. There are no vascular shadows lateral to this edge and the partially collapsed left lung is of greater density than the right lung.

The opaque hemithorax

If one half of a chest is completely opaque (a white-out) it is due either to collapse of a lung or a large pleural effusion. If there is shift of the mediastinum to the affected side it implies that volume loss in the lung (i.e. collapse) on that side must have occurred. Where there is no shift of the mediastinum, or it is shifted slightly to the side of the white-out, this is usually due to constricting pleural disease (including pleural tumour). A pleural effusion which is large enough to cause complete opacification of a hemithorax will displace the mediastinum away from the side of the white-out. Whilst penetrated posteroanterior and lateral films may help, it is sometimes surprisingly difficult to differentiate between the causes of an opaque hemithorax. Ultrasound and computed tomography allow the distinction to be made with confidence, and the latter may give further information about the underlying disease.

Decreased density of hemithorax

The conditions outlined so far have all focused on

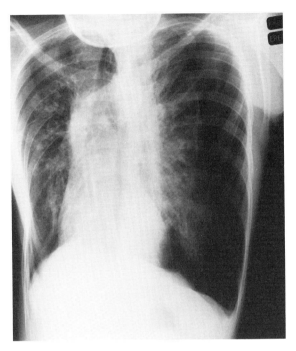

Fig. 2.11 Tension pneumothorax: this patient with cystic fibrosis has a left-sided tension pneumothorax. Note the shift of the mediastinum and straightening of the left dome of the diaphragm.

increased density of the lungs on plain radiographs. However, there are a number of causes where one lung appears less dense than the other side. When a chest radiograph demonstrates greater radiolucency of one lung compared with the other, it is necessary first to determine whether this appearance is due to a pulmonary abnormality; the radiograph should be checked for patient rotation and for soft tissue asymmetry, e.g. a mastectomy.

The pulmonary vessels are a helpful pointer to abnormalities causing a true decrease in density. In compensatory hyperinflation they are splayed apart. A search should also be made for a collapsed lobe. The vessels are considerably diminished or truncated in emphysema. Further radiological examination should include an expiration film if a pneumothorax is suspected. This will also demonstrate air trapping that occurs with bronchial obstruction. Computed tomography may also be useful in elucidating the cause of a hyperlucent lung. The lungs can be seen on computed tomography without the problem of overlying tissues, and any decrease in density is more readily apparent.

Elevation of the diaphragm

The right or left dome of the diaphragm may be elevated because it is paralysed, pushed up, or pulled up. However, there are a number of circumstances in which the diaphragm appears to be elevated without actually being so.

The radiographic evaluation of an apparently elevated diaphragm should begin with an assessment of the plain film, in particular evidence of prior surgery. Old radiographs are essential to determine whether the diaphragmatic elevation is long standing. A decubitus film is particularly useful in ruling out a suspected subpulmonary effusion; in this instance the pleural effusion is confined to the space between the lung base and the superior surface of the diaphragm. The radiograph will show what appears to be an elevated hemidiaphragm. Ultrasound will assist in determining if fluid is present above and/or below the diaphragm. If the hemidiaphragm is para- lysed, fluoroscopic examination is useful as it may demonstrate paradoxical movement on vigorous sniffing (instead of the diaphragm moving down it moves up). An important proviso is that a few normal individuals show this paradoxical movement of the diaphragm on sniffing. In congenital eventration part or all of the hemi- diaphragm muscle is made up of a thin layer of fibrous tissue and it may be difficult to distinguish from paralysis even on fluoroscopy.

Pleural disease

Because the chest radiograph is a two- dimensional image, abnormalities of the pleura and chest wall are often difficult to assess. Gross pleural abnormalities are usually obvious on a chest radiograph, but even when there is extensive pleural pathology it may be difficult to distinguish between pleural fluid, pleural thickening (e.g. secondary to a previous inflammatory process) and a neoplasm of the pleura. In such cases a lateral decubitus film or ultrasound scan is useful in identifying the presence of fluid. Computed tomography can readily identify the encasing and constricting nature of a mesothelioma. Ultrasound is often better than computed tomography in distinguishing between pleural fluid and pleural thickening.

The pulmonary mass

Most pulmonary nodules or masses are discovered by plain chest radiography. It is important that previous films are obtained if at all possible. If the mass was present on the previous films and has not changed over a number of years, it can be assumed that the lesion is benign and no further action needs to be taken. However, if the nodule was not previously present or has increased in size, then further investigation is warranted.

Computed tomography will detect or exclude the presence of other lesions within the lungs. The presence of calcification within the nodule, although often thought to be an indicator of benignity, will not exclude malignancy with complete certainty. In addition, computed tomography can be used to determine the presence of hilar or mediastinal lymph node enlargement as well as direct invasion of the adjacent mediastinum or chest wall. In patients in whom surgical resection of the pulmonary mass is not indicated, a cytological or histological specimen by percutaneous needle biopsy may be taken. This is usually reserved for small peripheral lesions that are not accessible by bronchoscopy. It can be performed under computed tomography guidance or fluoroscopy, but carries the complication of a pneumothorax (20%) or pulmonary haemorrhage (see other interventional techniques).

Pulmonary nodules

A large number of conditions are characterized by multiple pulmonary nodules (Fig. 2.12a). Combining the clinical information with an accurate description of the size and distribution of the nodules narrows down the list of differential diagnoses.

Metastatic deposits are by far the commonest cause of multiple pulmonary nodules of varying sizes in adult patients in the United Kingdom, but this is not the case world-wide. In some parts of the United States of America, histoplasmosis is

endemic and multiple lesions due to this condition may be more common than those due to malignancy. Making this important distinction may be difficult, and biopsy of one lesion may be the only reliable means of distinguishing a benign from a malignant cause for the multiple nodules.

Nodules are described as 'miliary' when they are less than 5 mm in diameter and are so numerous that they cannot be counted (Fig. 12b).

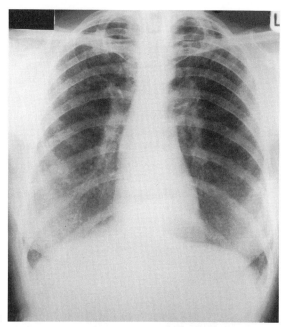

a

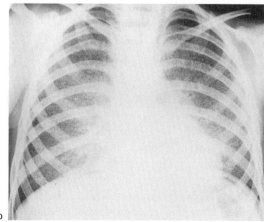

b

Fig. 2.12 **a** Multiple pulmonary nodules. The majority of these are greater than 5 mm in diameter. There is elevation of both hila secondary to fibrosis and volume loss in both upper lobes. The cause in this instance was sarcoidosis. **b** Multiple miliary nodules: these nodules are all less than 5 mm in diameter. The diagnosis was miliary tuberculosis.

The crucial diagnosis to consider, even if the patient is not particularly unwell, is miliary tuberculosis, since this life-threatening disease can be readily treated. If the patient is asymptomatic the differential diagnosis is more likely to lie between sarcoidosis, metastatic disease or a coal worker's pneumoconiosis. As ever, previous radiographs showing the rate of growth of the nodules may give valuable clues to the likely nature of the disease.

Cavitating pulmonary lesions

The radiological definition of cavitation is a lucency representing air within a mass or an area of consolidation. The cavity may or may not contain a fluid level, and is surrounded by a wall of variable thickness (Fig. 2.13).

The two most likely diagnoses in an adult presenting with a cavitating pulmonary lesion on a chest radiograph are a cancer or a lung abscess. In children, infection is the commonest cause. Cavitation secondary to necrosis is well recog-

nized in a variety of bacterial pneumonias, particularly those associated with tuberculosis, *Staphylococcus aureus*, anaerobes and *Klebsiella*. Diagnosis is usually by plain chest radiograph in the first instance, but computed tomography is also useful for localizing the abscess and sometimes to enable percutaneous aspiration to be undertaken. It also allows assessment of the relationship of the abscess to adjacent airways so that appropriate postural drainage can be planned.

In all age groups it is important to consider tuberculosis, especially if the cavitating lesions are in the lung apices. Linear or computed tomography may be necessary if the presence of cavitation is questionable; in addition computed tomography may show other features which help to narrow the differential diagnosis (e.g. pulmonary calcifications in tuberculosis, mediastinal lymph node enlargement in metastatic disease). In general, radiology alone cannot distinguish one cause of a cavitating mass from another.

SPECIFIC CONDITIONS

The postoperative and critically ill patient

In the context of intensive care medicine, the portable radiograph is one of the main means of monitoring critically ill patients. However, it is a far from perfect technique as the degree of inspiration is usually poor and may vary widely on serial radiographs. In addition, evaluation of cardiac size and the lung bases is, at best, difficult. This is often compounded by the rapidly changing haemodynamic state of the patient.

To some extent the advent of phosphor plate radiography has enabled more accurate assessments to be made because variations in exposure are not such a problem. Use of decubitus radiographs can be useful to evaluate the dependent side for fluid and the non-dependent side for small, but clinically important, pneumothoraces. For convenience it is useful to consider the various disease processes in the categories described below.

Support and monitoring apparatus

Careful radiographic monitoring of the position of

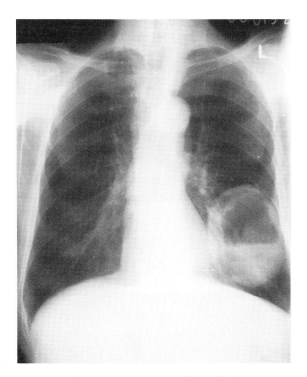

Fig. 2.13 Lung abscess: there is a thick-walled cavity containing a fluid level in the left lower lobe.

various tubes and catheters used in the postoperative and critically ill patient is essential to decrease
complications. Before evaluating the heart and
lungs it is good practice to check each of these
lines for proper positioning. The ideally placed
central venous line ends in the superior vena cava
(Fig. 2.14). Catheters terminating in the right
atrium or ventricle may cause arrhythmias or
perforation. Swan–Ganz catheters used to
monitor pulmonary capillary wedge pressure are
ideally sited in a main or lobar pulmonary artery.
Drugs inadvertently injected directly into the
wedged catheter may cause lobar pulmonary
oedema or necrosis. Both catheters (central
venous pressure line and Swan–Ganz) are
inserted percutaneously and, therefore, share
certain complications. The most frequent is a
pneumothorax due to puncture of the lung at the
time of subclavian vein insertion. If the catheter is
inserted into the mediastinum or perforates a vein
or artery, there may be dramatic widening of the
superior mediastinum due to haematoma. If the
catheter enters the pleural space, infused fluid
rapidly fills the pleural space. Catheter perforation
of the right atrium or ventricle may lead to cardiac
tamponade which may be manifested as progressive enlargement of the heart shadow on serial
radiographs.

The intra-aortic balloon pump is usually
inserted via the femoral artery and is used in
patients with intractable heart failure or in
weaning the patient from cardiopulmonary
bypass. On the frontal radiograph the tip of the
catheter should be seen lying in the aortic arch.

A cardiac pacemaker wire is usually inserted via
the external jugular, the cephalic or femoral vein
and passed under fluoroscopic control into the
apex of the right ventricle. Kinks or coils of wire
are undesirable and the wire should be examined
carefully along its entire length.

The tip of a correctly positioned endotracheal
tube (Fig. 2.14) lies in the midtrachea, approximately 5–7 cm above the carina. This distance is
needed to ensure that it does not descend into the
right main stem bronchus with flexion of the head
and neck or ascend into the pharynx when the
head and neck are extended. If the endotracheal
tube is inadvertently passed into the right main
stem bronchus (the more vertical of the two main

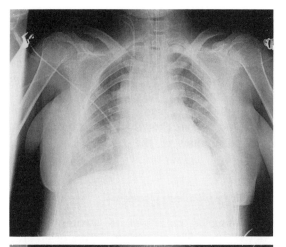

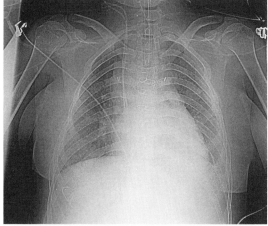

Fig. 2.14   Portable computed radiograph. This digital
radiograph taken in an intensive care unit demonstrates the
correct position of the tips of the two central venous lines and
endotracheal tube. The upper image resembles a conventional
radiograph and is used to examine the lungs; the lower image
(the same radiograph) has been manipulated to make
identification of lines easier.

bronchi), the left lung may collapse with a shift of
the mediastinum to the left and hyperinflation of
the right lung. If the endotracheal tube is
positioned just below the vocal cords, the tube
may retract into the pharynx, airway protection is
lost and aspiration may occur. If the tube remains
high in the trachea, inflation of the cuff may cause
vocal cord damage. Delayed complications
include focal tracheal necrosis leading ultimately
to a localized stricture. It is worth noting that,
even with correct positioning and cuff inflation,
an endotracheal tube is not an absolute guarantee

against aspiration of stomach contents into the airways.

Tracheostomy for long-term support has its own complications. A correctly placed tracheostomy tube should be parallel to the long axis of the trachea, approximately one-half to two-thirds the diameter of the trachea and end at least 5 cm from the carina. Marked subcutaneous or mediastinal emphysema may be due to tracheal injury or a large leak around the stoma. After prolonged intubation some tracheal scarring is inevitable. Symptomatic tracheal stenosis or collapse of a short length of the trachea is less common now due to use of low pressure occlusion cuffs on the endotracheal tubes. When positive end expiratory pressure (PEEP) is added, the patient's tidal volume and functional residual capacity increases. This is reflected in the radiograph as increased lung aeration. PEEP may open up areas of collapse and cause radiographic clearing. However, this may be spurious as any densities present will be less obvious due to the increased lung volume. Similarly, when weaned off PEEP the lung volume drops and the lungs may appear to be dramatically worse. Pulmonary barotrauma (air leakage due to elevated pressure) complicates approximately 10% of patients on positive pressure ventilation. If air continues to leak due to continued ventilation, a tension pneumothorax may develop. The chest radiograph is often the first indicator of this potentially fatal complication.

Collapse

Following laparotomy, at least half of all patients develop some postoperative pulmonary collapse. Volume loss is most often attributed to hypoventilation and retained secretions and it is most frequent in patients with chronic bronchitis, emphysema, obesity, prolonged anaesthesia or unusually heavy analgesia. The commonest radiographic manifestation is of linear densities which appear in the lower lung fields soon after surgery. Patchy, segmental or complete lobar consolidation is less common. When due to hypoventilation or large airway secretions, marked volume loss rather than dense consolidation is the usual appearance. Careful attention should be paid to unilateral elevation of the diaphragm and shifts of the minor fissure or hilar vessels. When collapse is due to multiple peripheral mucus plugs, the radiographic picture may be of pulmonary consolidation rather than volume loss. Areas of collapse tend to change rapidly and often clear with suction or physiotherapy. Postoperative collapse is not usually an infectious process, but if not treated promptly areas of collapse will usually become secondarily infected.

Aspiration pneumonia

Another frequent postoperative complication is the aspiration of gastric contents. A depressed state of consciousness and the presence of a nasogastric tube which disables the protective oesophagogastric sphincter are the most frequent predisposing factors. An endotracheal or tracheostomy tube does not always protect the patient from aspiration. The radiographic appearance of patchy, often bilateral, consolidation appears any time within the first 24 hours of aspiration and then progresses rapidly. In an uncomplicated case there is usually evidence of stability or regression by 72 hours, with complete clearing within 1–2 weeks. The infiltrates are usually patchy and diffuse and are most often seen at the lung bases, more commonly on the right. Complications include progression to adult respiratory distress syndrome (ARDS). Any worsening of the radiograph on the third day or thereafter should suggest the diagnosis of secondary infection.

Adult respiratory distress syndrome

Adult respiratory distress syndrome (ARDS) consists of progressive respiratory insufficiency following a major bodily insult and can be due to a large number of factors. Over the years it has been known as 'shock lung', 'stiff lung syndrome' and 'adult hyaline membrane disease'. At the pathophysiological level there is increased permeability by the pulmonary capillaries and the formation of platelet and fibrin microemboli. This results in alveolar oedema and haemorrhage which can affect the entire lung. After several days hyaline membranes form within the distal air spaces. As a general rule, symptoms occur on the second day after insult or injury, but the radiograph remains normal during the initial hours of clinical distress. Interstitial oedema is the first radiographic abnormality, which may be of a faint, hazy ground glass appearance (Fig. 2.5), and this is followed rapidly by patchy air-space oedema. By 36–72 hours after insult, diffuse global air-space consolidation is evident. It is the timing of the radiographic changes relative to the insult and the onset of symptoms, rather than the radiological appearance alone, that suggest the diagnosis of ARDS. The radiographic pattern of established ARDS is identical to that of pulmonary oedema, i.e. bilateral extensive consolidation. The radiology of patients with ARDS rarely allows a certain diagnosis of the underlying cause or supervening complications (e.g. aspiration or developing infections) to be made.

Pneumonia

Pulmonary infection may occur several days after surgery. Pneumonia may complicate collapse, but may result from aspiration or inhalation of infected secretions from the pharynx. The features of consolidation have already been covered, but the critically ill or postoperative patient frequently does not exhibit the expected features. Numerous factors, such as prior antibiotic therapy and coexistent heart or lung disease, conspire to modify the radiographic features. The radiographic appearance varies from a few ill-defined or discrete opacities to a pattern of coalescence and widespread patchy consolidation. Cavity or pneumatocele (a thin-walled air-filled space) formation is not infrequent.

Extrapulmonary air

The diagnosis of a pneumothorax is made by the identification of the thin line of the visceral pleura. Free air may also be found in the pulmonary interstitium, the mediastinum, the pericardial space and the subcutaneous tissues. In the intensive care setting, extrapulmonary air is most often due to barotrauma from mechanical ventilation or secondary to surgery or other iatrogenic procedures. Pulmonary interstitial emphysema is difficult to recognize radiographically and is

invariably due to ventilator-induced barotrauma. Unlike air bronchograms, the interstitial air is seen as black lines and streaks radiating from the hila; they do not branch or taper towards the periphery. Interstitial emphysema usually culminates in a pneumomediastinum, and this is shown on a frontal radiograph as a radiolucent band against the mediastinum bordered by the reflected mediastinal pleura. Air may outline specific structures such as the aortic arch, the descending aorta or the thymus.

Cardiac failure

The radiographic diagnosis of early left ventricular failure is largely dependent on changes in the calibre of the pulmonary vessels in the erect patient. As the left atrial pressure rises, blood is shunted to the upper zones. This is the first and most important radiographic sign of elevated left ventricular pressure (Fig. 2.15); it is important to remember that, because of redistribution of blood flow in the supine position, a supine radiograph does not allow this criterion to be used.

Interstitial pulmonary oedema then follows;

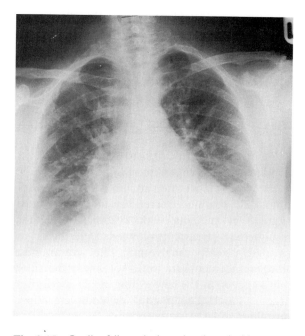

Fig. 2.15   Cardiac failure: the heart is enlarged with upper lobe blood diversion (prominent upper lobe vessels) and there are small basal pleural effusions.

this is manifested by blurring of the vessel margins, a perihilar haze and a vague increased density over the lower zones. When fluid fills and distends the interlobular septa, Kerley B lines (septal lines) may be visible. These are best visualized in the costophrenic angles as thin white lines arising from the lateral pleural surface. As the left ventricular pressure continues to rise, multiple, small, ill-defined opacities occur in the lower half of the lungs. These represent alveoli filling with fluid. Alveolar oedema may also appear as poorly defined bilateral 'butterfly' perihilar opacification. Increasing cardiac size usually accompanies cardiac failure but, if it occurs following acute myocardial infarction or an acute arrhythmia, cardiac failure may be present without an increase in cardiac size. Bilateral pleural effusions often accompany cardiac failure.

Pulmonary embolism

The postoperative or critically ill patient has numerous risk factors for the development of deep venous thrombosis and thus pulmonary embolism. In this group, where respiratory distress is often multifactorial, the diagnosis of pulmonary embolism is extremely difficult.

Conventional radiographic findings are non-specific and include elevation of the diaphragm, collapse or segmental consolidation. A small pleural effusion may appear during the first 2 days following the embolus. It is important to recognize that a normal chest radiograph does not exclude a major pulmonary embolus; indeed a normal radiograph in a patient with acute respiratory distress is suggestive of the diagnosis. A radionuclide perfusion scan is of use because if it is normal a pulmonary embolus can be excluded; however, this is not a practical test for a patient in an intensive care unit and the decision to treat with anticoagulants is often made clinically.

Kyphoscoliosis

Kyphoscoliosis makes assessment of the chest radiograph difficult and it is useful to reduce the distortion of thoracic contents due to the kyphoscoliosis by obtaining an oblique radiograph, positioning the patient in such a way that the spine appears at its straightest. Severe kyphoscoliosis may cause pulmonary arterial hypertension and cor pulmonale. Some congenital chest anomalies such as pulmonary agenesis (absence of a lung) and neurofibromatosis are associated with dorsal spine abnormalities. Because of the problems associated with getting a true posteroanterior and lateral view, computed tomography scanning is often the most satisfactory method of visualizing the lungs.

Bronchiectasis

This is a chronic condition characterized by local, irreversible dilatation of the bronchi, usually associated with inflammation. On a chest radiograph (Fig. 2.16a) the findings include: (a) the bronchial wall visible either as single thin lines or as parallel 'tram-lines'; (b) ring and curvilinear opacities which represent thickened airway walls seen end-on. These tend to range in size from 8 to 20 mm, have thin (hairline) walls, and may contain air–fluid levels; (c) dilated airways filled with secretions giving rise to broad band shadows some 5–10 mm wide and several centimetres long (seen end-on, these dilated fluid-filled airways produce rounded or oval nodular opacities); (d) overinflation throughout both lungs (particularly in cystic fibrosis); (e) volume loss where bronchiectasis is localized (this may give rise to crowding of bronchi or collapse due to mucus plugging that can be severe and result in complete collapse of a lobe); and (f) less specific signs include infective consolidation, scarring and pleural thickening.

The definitive diagnosis of bronchiectasis used to be made by bronchography (injection of contrast into the bronchial airway), but this is an invasive and unpleasant procedure and a viable alternative is high resolution computed tomography (Fig. 2.16b). With this technique, thin slices are taken throughout both lungs and the findings are similar to those on the plain film (thickened bronchial walls, bronchial dilatation, ring opacities containing air-fluid levels). Comparing the diameter of the bronchial wall with the adjacent vessel is helpful, as both should be approximately the same size. Computed tomography may also be helpful in determining

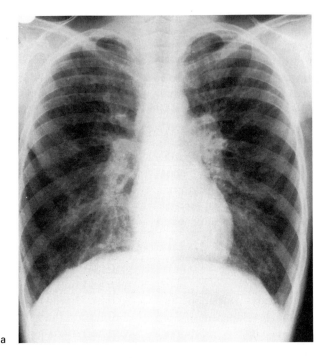

Fig. 2.16   a Cystic fibrosis: the lungs are over-inflated and there is widespread increased shadowing due to barely perceptible bronchial wall thickening and peribronchial consolidation. The proximal pulmonary arteries are enlarged due to a degree of pulmonary arterial hypertension. **b** Cystic fibrosis: computed tomography showing bronchial wall thickening and parallel bronchial dilatation (cylindrical bronchiectasis).

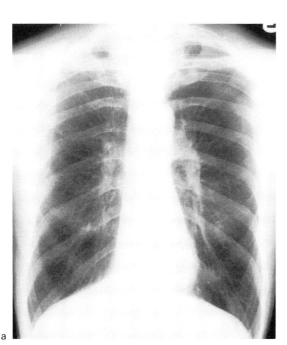
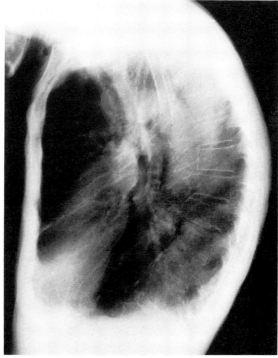

a   b

Fig. 2.17   Emphysema. **a** Both lungs are hyperinflated. There is dilatation of the proximal pulmonary arteries with pruning of the peripheral vasculature. **b** The retrosternal and retrocardiac areas are strikingly transradiant.

the optimum position for postural drainage. Upper lobe predominance is present in early cystic fibrosis, post tubercle infection and allergic bronchopulmonary aspergillosis. The remainder affect predominantly the middle and lower lobes.

Chronic airflow limitation

This comprises three conditions which are present simultaneously in a given patient to a greater or lesser degree: chronic bronchitis, asthma and emphysema. The first is diagnosed by the patient's history and, strictly speaking, does not have any characteristic radiological features. In asthma the chest radiograph is normal in the majority of patients between attacks, but as many as 40% reveal evidence of hyperinflation during an acute severe episode. In asthmatic children with recurrent infection, bronchial wall thickening occurs. Collapse of a lobe or an entire lung due to mucus plugging is another feature and may be recurrent affecting different lobes. Complications include a pneumomediastinum which arises

secondarily to pulmonary interstitial emphysema and pneumothorax due to rupture of a subpleural bulla. Expiratory radiographs will aid detection of this as well as demonstrating any air trapping secondary to bronchial occlusion.

Emphysema is a condition characterized by an increase in air spaces beyond the terminal bronchiole due to destruction of alveolar walls. Whilst it is strictly a pathological diagnosis, certain radiographic appearances are characteristic in more advanced cases. These include overinflation of the lungs, an alteration in the appearance of the pulmonary vessels, and the presence of bullae (Fig. 2.17). Overinflation results in flattening of the diaphragmatic dome and this results in an apparently small heart and a decreased cardiothoracic ratio. On the lateral chest radiograph the large retrosternal translucency caused by the hyperinflated lungs is particularly striking (Fig. 2.17b). The pulmonary vessels are abnormal: the smooth gradation in size of vessels from the hilum outwards is lost, with the hilar vessels being larger than normal and tapering abruptly, so-called 'pruning' of the vessels. However, the lungs are usually unevenly involved and this is mirrored by the uneven distribution of pulmonary vessels. When emphysema is predominantly basal in distribution, there is prominent upper lobe blood diversion which should not be mistaken for evidence of left-heart failure. Bullae are recognized by their transradiancy, their hairline walls and a distortion of adjacent pulmonary vessels. They vary greatly in size and are occasionally big enough to occupy an entire hemithorax. When large they are an important cause of respiratory distress. Complications of bullae formation are infection and haemorrhage, which are usually manifested as the presence of an air–fluid level. Pneumothorax is another complication and can on occasions be difficult to distinguish from a large bulla.

FURTHER READING

Armstrong P, Wilson A G, Dee P 1990 Imaging of diseases of the chest. Year Book Medical Publishers, Chicago

Goodman L R, Putman C E 1991 Intensive care radiology: imaging of the critically ill, 3rd edn. W B Saunders, Philadelphia

Grainger R G, Allison D J 1989 Diagnostic radiology. An Anglo American textbook of imaging, 2nd edn. Churchill Livingstone, Edinburgh

Kattan K R, Wiot J F 1973 How was this chest Röentgenogram taken, AP or PA? American Journal of Roentgenology 117: 843–845

Keats T E 1988 Atlas of normal roentgen variants that may simulate disease, 4th edn. Year Book Medical Publishers, Chicago

Lipscomb D J, Flower C D R, Hadfield J W 1981 Ultrasound of the pleura: an assessment of its clinical value. Clinical Radiology 32: 289–290

Reed J C 1987 Chest radiology: plain film patterns and differential diagnosis, 2nd edn. Year Book Medical Publishers, Chicago

Sagel S S, Aronberg D J 1982 Thoracic anatomy and mediastinum. In: Lee J K T, Sagel S S, Stanley R J (eds) Computed body tomography. Raven Press, New York

Simon G 1975 The anterior view chest radiograph — criteria for normality derived from a basic analysis of the shadows. Clinical Radiology 26: 429–437

Trapnell D H 1973 The differential diagnosis of linear shadows in chest radiographs. Radiological Clinics of North America 11: 77–92

Vix V A, Klatte E C 1970 The lateral chest radiograph in the diagnosis of hilar and mediastinal masses. Radiology 96: 307–316

3. Cardiopulmonary function testing

Michael D. L. Morgan   Sally J. Singh

INTRODUCTION

In health the human cardiopulmonary system has enormous reserve capacity to cope with the demands of exercise or illness. We are not normally aware of breathlessness or fatigue as a feature of resting activity. Furthermore, unless we harbour athletic ambitions we are unlikely to explore the boundaries of our physiological limitations, and assure ourselves that spare capacity would be present if it ever became necessary. The measurement of physiological capacity in health is, therefore, a matter of relevance only to the curious or the serious competitor who wishes to improve his performance. In patients with heart or lung disease the erosion of physiological reserve eventually imposes limitations upon the activities of daily life. Under these circumstances the measurement of cardiopulmonary function allows the accurate assessment of disability and of the effect of therapeutic intervention. This chapter examines the scientific basis of clinical measurement and its relevance to physiotherapy. In the current climate of clinical audit, the physiotherapist must understand the need for objective demonstration of the effectiveness of the treatment given.

The human body is an infinitely complex structure, the secrets of which are gradually being exposed by scientific investigation. Certain aspects of cardiopulmonary function can be assessed with some accuracy, but it must be remembered that such measurements are only a snapshot of a component of an organism which is constantly changing and may be influenced by the making of the measurement. It is therefore important to understand exactly what measurement is being made and under what circumstances it is valid before assessing its importance. Given this limitation, carefully made measurements are a valuable addition to clinical practice.

The cellular basis of respiration depends primarily on the production of energy and function from the aerobic metabolism of food. The requirements of an individual cell are simply the regular provision of oxygen and nutrients and the disposal of the acidic waste products of carbon dioxide and water. In a unicellular organism these requirements need only an environment for diffusion. By contrast, man requires a complex collection, distribution and disposal system to service the needs of the body. This system itself requires energy to function, and its capacity imposes a limit on the function of the whole organism. In man oxygen is extracted from the atmosphere by the lungs and delivered to the tissues via the blood. Cardiac function ensures the internal cellular delivery of oxygen and the removal of carbon dioxide back to the lungs for exhalation. The examination of the components of this system can be seen to be somewhat artificial in view of the interdependence of the activities. However, it is reasonable and conventional to consider the process in terms of three compartments. Firstly the lungs themselves, secondly the effectiveness of the integrated activity of gas exchange and acid–base balance, and finally the capacity of the circulatory system to deliver.

LUNG FUNCTION

The apparently simple function of the lung is to deliver oxygen to the gas exchanging surface and exhaust carbon dioxide to the atmosphere. To

47

achieve this, air is drawn by conductive flow into the alveoli and presented to the gas exchanging surface where diffusion effects the process of exchange. The carriage of air through the airways depends on the patency of the tubes as well as on the consistency of the lung and the power of the respiratory muscles. These aspects of pulmonary function are commonly measured in lung function laboratories.

General principles of measurement

Lung function measurements may be made for several reasons. They are useful in describing the lung for diagnostic purposes and subsequently in monitoring change. Accuracy and consistency are therefore very important, and conventions exist for the procedures of measurement and expression of results. In general, a measurement will only be accepted after multiple attempts have been scrutinized and expressed under standard conditions. These are usually body temperature and atmospheric pressure (BTPS). To guarantee accuracy, laboratory practice should include regular physical and biological calibration of the equipment. In health there are several factors which influence the magnitude of lung function. These include height, sex and age, and to a lesser degree weight and ethnic origin (Cotes 1979, Anthonisen 1986). As a result, assessment of normality can only be made by comparison with reference values. The latter are obtained from the study of large numbers of normal people from the relevant population (European Community for Coal and Steel 1983). Once obtained, results can be expressed as percentage predicted or, more correctly, by comparison with the 95% confidence interval for that value.

Airway function

For the purposes of measurement the lung has only one portal of entry and exit, i.e. through the mouth, and airway function is assessed by quantification of gas flow or volume. The calibre of the airways reduce through their generations and the major resistance to gas flow is normally in the upper airway. The larger airways are supported by cartilage, while the smaller airways are held patent by the radial traction of the surrounding lung so that their calibre increases with the volume of the lung. The diameter of these airways is also controlled by neural tone which is predominantly parasympathetic. The disruption of airway function can occur through physical or rigid obstruction to a large airway by, for example, a tracheal tumour. It may also occur due to more widespread disease in asthma, when large numbers of smaller airways are affected by episodic alteration of their calibre by smooth muscle contraction, mucosal oedema and intra-luminal secretions. In chronic bronchitis obstruction occurs by mucosal thickening and mucous secretion, but in emphysema the mechanism is different. Though seldom occurring in isolation from other forms of airway obstruction, the result of parenchymal emphysema is to weaken the elastic structure which maintains radial traction on the airways and allows them to close too early in expiration. Tests of airway function measure airway calibre and are now well established in clinical practice. Most tests of airway patency examine expiratory function. There are three common methods:

- Spirometry (FEV_1 and FVC)
- Flow–volume curves
- Peak expiratory flow (PEF).

Production of the spirogram from a maximal forced expiration following a full inspiration is reliable and provides the forced expiratory volume in one second (FEV_1) and the forced vital capacity (FVC) (Fig. 3.1). The measurement is usually made using a spirometer which measures volume, or derived from a flow signal obtained from a pneumotachograph. Most commonly, the FEV_1 and FVC are measured during the same manoeuvre, but a greater vital capacity may be obtained in patients with airway disease if it is performed slowly. Reduction in FEV_1 with relative preservation of FVC or vital capacity (VC) is known as an 'obstructive' pattern, which indicates and grades airway obstruction: $FEV_1/FVC < 75\%$ is graded as mild, $< 60\%$ as moderate, and $< 40\%$ as severe impairment (American Thoracic Society 1986). Simultaneous reduction in both FEV_1 and FVC with an increase

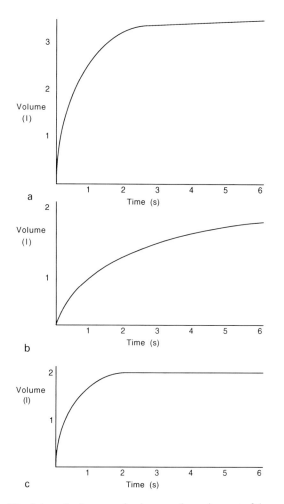

Fig. 3.1   a In the normal spirogram the major part of the vital capacity (FVC) is expelled in 1 s (FEV_1). **b** In patients with airway obstruction the FEV_1 is reduced to a greater degree than the FVC. This pattern is known as 'obstructive'. **c** When the lungs are small and empty quickly the pattern is known as 'restrictive'.

in the FEV_1/FVC ratio is called a 'restrictive' defect and is usually associated with a reduction in lung volume. Abnormal values are defined as those recognized to be outside the normal range of two standard deviations for sex, height and age. This usually requires a reduction of about 15% from predicted values. Thus simple spirometry can detect and quantify airway obstruction, but gives no indication of the cause.

Measurement of the flow–volume curve is now commonplace in most hospitals and can provide information about the nature of airway obstruc-

tion. In this test the gas flow from a full maximum expiration is plotted against the expired volume as the lung empties (Fig. 3.2). The flow of gas from the lung reaches a peak (the PEF) after about 100 milliseconds and then declines linearly as the lung empties. If the measurement is continued into the subsequent full inspiration, a flow volume 'loop' is produced and inspiratory flow rates can be measured. The shape of the expiratory and inspiratory portions are different, since in expiration the active expulsion is assisted by the elastic recoil of the lung while inspiratory flow rates are a reflection of airway calibre and inspiratory muscle strength only. Something of the nature of the airway obstruction can be learnt from consideration of the actual and relative values of PEF, Peak inspiratory flow (PIF) and the values of expiratory flow at 50% and 75% vital capacity (MEF_{50} and MEF_{75}). Simple inspection of the loop is often sufficient to distinguish between rigid upper airway obstruction, intraluminal obstruction in chronic bronchitis and asthma, and the 'pressure-dependent' collapse seen in pure emphysema with relative preservation of inspiratory flow rates.

The PEF is one component of the flow–volume manoeuvre which has been used with increasing popularity. This has been encouraged by the availability of simple devices for its measurement. Provided that the patient does not have weak respiratory muscles and has made a maximum effort, the PEF will reflect airway calibre. The absolute values obtained are not particularly helpful unless they are extremely low, but the easily repeated measurements can be used to obtain valuable insight into the mechanisms of variable airway obstruction in asthma. There is a normal diurnal variation in airway calibre of about 50 l/min which is exaggerated in patients with poorly controlled asthma (Fig. 3.3) (Benson 1983). Wider variation will be seen approaching or recovering from an attack and following exposure to trigger factors. The real value of the PEF lies in its repeatability and its portability. The issue of meters to patients with asthma allows domiciliary and occupational investigation of asthma. It also provides a tool for patients to use to monitor their asthma objectively as part of a self-management plan. In past years, the PEF chart has been used during hospital admissions to

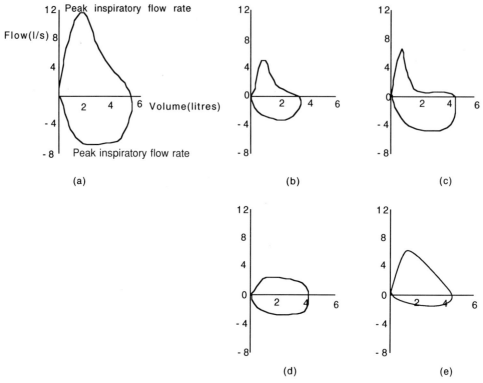

Fig. 3.2   a The normal flow–volume loop has a characteristic shape. **b** Airway obstruction from asthma or chronic bronchitis appears as a concave expiratory limb and reduced inspiratory flows. **c** In emphysema the expiratory flows are suddenly attenuated, but the inspiratory flows are relatively well preserved. **d** A rigid obstruction to a major airway can produce an oval loop. **e** Inspiratory flows are reduced in diaphragm weakness or extrathoracic tracheal obstruction.

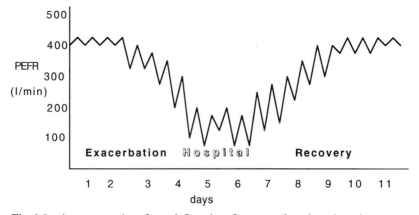

**Fig. 3.3   ** A reconstruction of a peak flow chart from an asthmatic patient. As an attack develops, the normal diurnal variation increases and the mean values drop until treatment reverses the pattern in recovery. The decline and recovery may take several days.

record the progress and predict the discharge of patients with airway disease. Although this is valuable in asthma where the airway obstruction is variable, it can show no change at all in patients with chronic airflow limitation in spite of a clinical improvement. In this case the twice weekly measurement of FEV_1 and FVC is more likely to mirror progress than will the slavish recording of the PEF chart (Gibson 1990).

The physical properties of the lung

The two lungs contain millions of alveoli within a fibroelastic matrix. They do not have a very rigid structure and are held in contact with the rib cage by surface-tension forces at the apposition of the two pleural surfaces. The resting volume of the lung (the functional residual capacity (FRC)) is thus determined by the outward spring of the rib cage and the inward elastic recoil of the lung matrix. Expansion and contraction of the lung therefore involves the controlled stretching or relaxation of the lung by the respiratory muscles away from FRC. The position of FRC can be influenced if the lung is stiffer than usual (as in interstitial disease), or if it is more compliant (as when damaged by emphysema). The measurement of the lung's volume can therefore give some insight into these conditions.

The actual volume of the lung must be measured indirectly in life since the lungs obviously cannot be removed for the measurement. There are several techniques which measure slightly different aspects of volume. The most familiar method is helium dilution, which involves rebreathing through a closed circuit a mixture of gas containing a known concentration of helium which is not absorbed into the circulation. The measurement of the final concentration of helium is used to calculate the gas dilution, or the 'accessible' volume, of the lung. An alternative method uses the Boyle's law principle — gas in the chest is compressed and the change in pressure is used to calculate the volume of gas within the chest. This method requires a large airtight box or plethysmograph. In both methods the actual volume that is estimated is the FRC, and total lung capacity (TLC) and residual volume (RV) are obtained from an additional spirometric trace. A further method involves the calculation of the total volume of the lung from the dimensions of a chest radiograph. This volume includes the gas, and also the tissue and blood volume. Since the techniques do measure different aspects of volume, consistency in sequential measurements is important. In normal lungs the results are very similar, but where there is airway obstruction the values may be disparate. Such disparity can be used to advantage, e.g. in calculating the degree of trapped gas as the difference between the plethysmographic and helium dilution lung volumes.

The chest wall and the respiratory muscles

To maintain their shape the lungs depend on the support of the rib cage and the patency of the airways and alveoli. The expansion of the rib cage by the respiratory muscles is responsible for the tidal flow of gas into and out of the lungs. Over the past few years there has been increasing awareness of the importance of disease of the respiratory muscles and the bony rib cage in contributing to respiratory failure. Such conditions include myopathies and polio as well as skeletal malformations such as scoliosis which decrease rib cage compliance and reduce the effectiveness of the musculature. The respiratory muscles include the diaphragm as the major muscle of inspiration and the intercostal muscles and scalenes. The latter together with the sternomastoids are known as the 'accessory muscles', but actually have a stabilizing role in tidal breathing. The combination of the respiratory muscles and the bony rib cage is called the 'chest wall' and conceptually is considered as the organ which inflates the lungs. Weakness of the respiratory muscles will eventually lead to ventilatory failure which may first become apparent during the night as an exaggeration of the normal nocturnal hypoventilation (Shneerson 1988) (Fig. 3.4).

The function of the respiratory muscles is difficult to study directly since the muscles have complex origins and insertions. Furthermore, their product, which is the pressure generated within the thoracic cavity, depends on the coordinated action of many muscles the individual

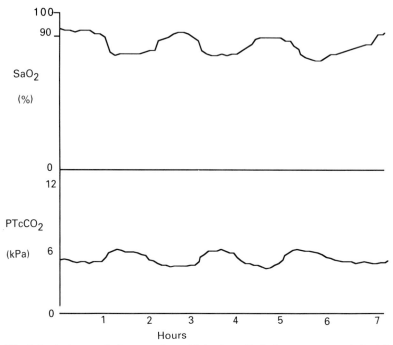

Fig. 3.4   A sleep study from a patient with kyphoscoliosis demonstrates periodic falls in SaO$_2$ associated with rapid eye movement (REM) sleep. The lower panel shows the simultaneous rises in transcutaneous carbon dioxide (PTcCO$_2$) associated with the episodes of hypoventilation.

functions of which may be difficult to distinguish in life. It is possible to make some assessment of both the strength and endurance of the muscles and also to separate the diaphragm from the other muscles. The simple strength that the inspiratory and expiratory muscles can generate as pressure is easy to measure. The maximum inspiratory pressure (PiMax) and expiratory pressure (PeMax) are easy to measure with a manometer or electronic gauge. The normal values of approximately -100 cmH$_2$O and $+120$ cmH$_2$O (Black & Hyatt 1971) are well in excess of that needed to inflate the lungs (5–10 cmH$_2$O) and, therefore, provide a sensitive measure of developing muscle weakness. These measurements do have a learning requirement and are not suitable for monitoring of patients with rapidly developing muscle weakness such as Guillain–Barré syndrome. Under these circumstances the sequential measurement of the vital capacity is much more reliable, since a failure to maintain it will predict ventilatory failure.

The strength of the diaphragm can be separated from the other muscles by measuring the pressure gradient across it. This is achieved by using balloons attached to pressure transducers to estimate the pressure in the oesophagus and the stomach. The gradient across the diaphragm during a maximum inspiration or sniff is an indirect measure of the strength of the diaphragm. If required, a value free of volition can be obtained by electrical stimulation of the phrenic nerve in the neck, or even by magnetic stimulation of the cerebral cortex. Fortunately, measurements of separate diaphragm strength are seldom required in clinical practice. A simple guide to diaphragm function can be obtained by observation of the change in vital capacity with posture. When supine, the vital capacity normally falls by 8–10%, but when diaphragm weakness is present it may fall by more than 30%. The measurement of the supine vital capacity is, therefore, a good screening test of diaphragm function (Green & Laroche 1990).

The respiratory muscles are duty bound to contract regularly through life to sustain it.

Consequently, the prediction of fatigue or the measurement of endurance capacity would have more relevance to clinical practice. The identification of fatigue is not very reliable and there is no simple test that can be applied at the bedside. There are, however, several ways of estimating respiratory muscle endurance capacity. The simplest is the maximum voluntary ventilation (MVV), while other methods include breathing through resistances. One of the more interesting examples of the latter is incremental threshold loading, where increasing resistances are added until they can no longer be sustained. This makes a test for the respiratory muscles which is similar to the exercise tests used for the systemic musculature (Martyn et al 1987).

Gas exchange and oxygen delivery

The requirements of the average cell for oxygen are quite modest, and a mitochondrion may need a PO_2 of as little as 1 kPa to function effectively. At sea level the atmospheric PO_2 is 20 kPa (Fio_2=0.21) and in the process of delivering oxygen to the cell there is a loss along this gradient. This is illustrated in Figure 3.5. The first step is the dilution of inspired air with expired air within the alveolus. Each tidal breath (V_T) contains a portion of gas which will remain within the airways and not come into contact with the alveoli. This is known as the 'dead space ventilation' (V_D) and must be achieved before any effective alveolar ventilation (V_A) can taken place:

$$V_T = V_D + V_A$$

Alveolar gas therefore contains a mixture of fresh gas and some expired CO_2, and the alveolar PO_2 is reduced to about 16 kPa before gas exchange begins.

At the alveolar level, gas exchange involves the transfer across the alveolar–capillary membrane of oxygen molecules to the blood and the reverse transfer of carbon dioxide. This is achieved by simple diffusion, which is amplified in the case of oxygen by the affinity of haemoglobin. It normally takes mixed venous blood about 300 ms to traverse a capillary, and complete equilibrium usually occurs in about 100 ms. This aspect of oxygen transfer from the lung to the blood can be

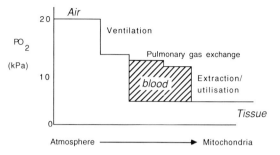

Fig. 3.5 A gradient of PO_2 from the air to the tissues is determined by losses in the initial ventilation of the lungs, circulation in the blood and transfer across the interstitial fluid. Fortunately, the mitochondrial oxygen requirements are very small.

tested using carbon monoxide. Carbon monoxide has a very strong affinity for haemoglobin, follows the same path into the blood and can be measured easily. This principle forms the basis of the carbon monoxide transfer test which measures the amount of carbon monoxide which can be transferred to the blood in the course of a single breath (TLCO). This gives a rough indication of the gas transferring ability of the lung as a whole and is reduced in conditions like fibrosing alveolitis, emphysema and pneumonectomy where the quality or quantity of the gas exchanging surface is reduced. If the total TLCO is corrected for lung volume then the subsequent value is known as the 'coefficient of gas transfer' (KCO) and describes the gas exchanging quality of the lung that is available for ventilation. For example, a very large normal man and small child should have different TLCOs but their KCO values should be identical.

The carbon monoxide transfer test can give some information about the ability of the lung to transfer gas, but there is not a direct relationship between the TLCO and arterial oxygenation. The lung contains millions of alveolar capillary units, and adequate oxygenation depends on the coordinated, satisfactory function of the whole unit. The pulmonary causes of arterial hypoxaemia have four major origins:

- Hypoventilation
- Interference with pulmonary diffusion
- Ventilation/perfusion imbalance
- True shunt.

Hypoventilation is fairly easy to recognize because the fall in arterial PO_2 is associated with a rise in arterial PCO_2. This occurs in ventilatory failure associated with airway obstruction, chest wall disease and drug intoxication. Interference with pulmonary diffusion is quite rare because the process is very efficient. However, the system may be stretched at altitude or in the presence of disease such as fibrosing alveolitis. Even in this disease the hypoxia is related to increased pulmonary capillary transit time rather than to diffusion failure. The most common contribution to hypoxaemia in many diseases is ventilation/perfusion imbalance $(\dot{V}/\dot{Q})$. Since effective lung function depends on the coordination of equivalent ventilation and perfusion to all units, it is not surprising that failure of the local matching mechanisms can cause trouble. The most extreme example would be a pulmonary embolus where ventilation continues in an area with no circulation. In other conditions such as asthma, the patchy distribution of airway obstruction will have similar but less dramatic effects. Some blood passes through the lung without coming into contact with the gas exchanging surface. Normally this is a very small quantity ($<5\%$), but effective shunts can be considerable in pneumonia and other conditions where the alveoli are blocked by inflammatory exudate although the circulation continues through the ineffective portion of the lung. This results in extreme hypoxia which cannot easily be corrected by additional oxygen.

Oxygen carriage and arterial blood gases

Oxygen and carbon dioxide are carried in the blood in different ways. Oxygen is immediately bound to haemoglobin and released in the tissues under conditions of low oxygen tension or acidosis. Very little oxygen is carried in solution in the blood under conditions of normal pressure, although this can be increased in a hyperbaric chamber. By contrast, carbon dioxide is carried in the blood entirely in solution, mostly as bicarbonate. The difference between the two forms of carriage of the metabolic gases is fundamental to the interpretation of the measurement of arterial blood gases. The individual cell requires oxygen to survive, but the carriage of oxygen in the blood will have no effect on the body other than the delivery. By contrast, the chemistry involved in the carriage of carbon dioxide controls the short-term acid–base state of the body. When considering blood gas measurements, it is best to examine these functions separately.

The normal atmospheric PO_2 is 20 kPa falling to 16 kPa within the alveolus. The arterial PO_2 (PaO_2) is usually about 14 kPa in a healthy subject. Although we are used to these values they are only true at sea level and really only have relevance because the partial pressure is easy to measure. What matters to the individual cell is the quantity of oxygen that it receives, not the pressure. Oxygen delivery to the tissues depends on other factors which include the amount of haemoglobin, the degree of saturation of haemoglobin with oxygen and the rate at which oxygenated blood is delivered to the tissues. Assuming that the haemoglobin and the cardiac output is normal, then the measurement of oxygen saturation of haemoglobin is more relevant to oxygen delivery than is the PaO_2. The PaO_2 is related to oxygen saturation in a complex manner determined by the properties of haemoglobin and known as the 'oxygen dissociation curve' (Fig. 3.6). This relationship demonstrates that, under most conditions, once PaO_2 reaches 8 kPa, haemoglobin is fully saturated and cannot carry more oxygen. Thus an arterial PO_2 above that value is only an insurance measure. Recently, the availability of pulse oximeters has made the non-invasive measurement of oxygen saturation (SaO_2) commonplace. Pulse oximeters work by transcutaneous examination of the colour spectrum of haemoglobin which changes with its degree of saturation. These instruments are reasonably accurate over the top range of saturation, but become unreliable below about 50% (Tremper & Barker 1989). The measurement of SaO_2 is an extremely valuable tool for monitoring patients' safety. There are, however, some important aspects of interpretation of their use which may be potentially hazardous. Oximetry provides information about oxygen saturation and this will relate to ventilation only if the inspired oxygen level is normal. Monitoring oxygen saturation will not detect underventilation and a rising $PaCO_2$. In patients who are breathing additional oxygen, a

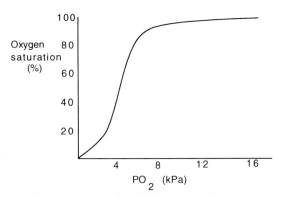

Fig. 3.6 The oxygen dissociation curve relates oxygen saturation to ambient PO_2. In lung disease it is important to recognize that oxygen delivery is assured if PaO_2 is in excess of 8 kPa.

bicarbonate, standard bicarbonate and base excess. The appreciation of the acid–base state requires examination of $PaCO_2$ and pH. Abnormalities are usually described in terms of their generation (Fig. 3.7). For example, a respiratory acidosis resulting from underventilation will display a low pH and an elevated $PaCO_2$. If this has been present for any length of time the serum bicarbonate will have become elevated and acid is excreted by the kidneys to compensate. In cases of nocturnal hypoventilation the daytime PaO_2 may be normal, but the elevation of the base excess gives a clue to the ventilatory history. If an alkalosis (high pH) is associated with a low $PaCO_2$, then this could be due to voluntary hyperventilation and is termed a 'respiratory alkalosis'. The build up of acid products in diabetes or renal failure will result in a low pH and bicarbonate together with a low $PaCO_2$ in an attempt to compensate for a metabolic acidosis. Finally, the loss of acid from the stomach in prolonged vomiting can produce a metabolic alkalosis which is characterized by high pH, high bicarbonate and normal $PaCO_2$. These sketches of blood gas disturbance are superficial interpretations, but they provide a useful framework for clinical management under most circumstances.

false sense of security can be given by a normal SaO_2 even though the $PaCO_2$ is rising. Furthermore, accurate recording of SaO_2 requires a good peripheral circulation which may often be compromised in patients who are hypovolaemic.

The assessment of acid–base status requires the measurement of arterial blood gas tensions. The average blood gas analyser measures PO_2, PCO_2 and pH. It subsequently calculates from the Henderson–Hasselbalch equation the values of

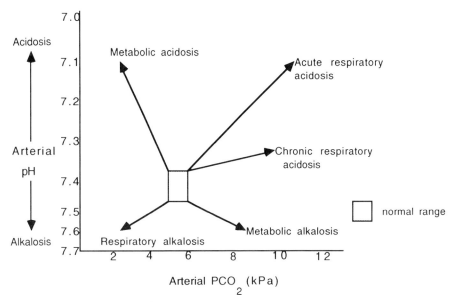

Fig. 3.7 Acid–base relationships

Respiratory failure

Respiratory failure is defined as inadequate oxygen delivery. As we have seen, this can be due to a variety of circumstances and may or may not be accompanied by a disturbance of the CO_2 level. The critical PaO_2 level is about 8 kPa, since a lower pressure than this will prejudice oxygen saturation and delivery. Therefore, respiratory failure is defined as PaO_2 <8 kPa. If $PaCo_2$ is elevated above 6.5 kPa, this is termed 'ventilatory failure' and is associated with chronic airflow limitation or other forms of hypoventilation. The understanding of respiratory failure has changed in recent years with the recognition that it is seldom due to a single malfunction of the respiratory system (Fig. 3.8). For example, the rise in $PaCO_2$ and hyperinflation associated with worsening airway obstruction may adversely affect the respiratory muscles and introduce a chest wall contribution to failure. Conversely, the loss of lung volume associated with muscle weakness may lead to atelectasis and decreased pulmonary compliance, which will in turn put a greater load on the lung. Understanding of the complexities of chronic respiratory failure has helped to improve the outlook for some groups of patients, e.g. patients with ventilatory failure due to chest wall disease or obstructive sleep apnoea. In these conditions there are abnormalities of breathing during sleep which may result in nocturnal hypoventilation or transient apnoea that produce periods of oxygen desaturation which may spill over to the day time. Recognition of this by oximetry and other more detailed somnography may result in effective treatment by nocturnal nasal intermittent positive pressure ventilation (NIPPV) or continuous positive airway pressure (CPAP) (Bott et al 1992, Keilty & Bott 1992).

Posture and thoracic surgery

A knowledge of the effect of posture and thoracic surgery on pulmonary function is obviously very important to the physiotherapist. The circumstances of treatment make this knowledge of practical benefit. Lung function measurements are usually made sitting or standing, but the major postural effect occurs due to gravity in the supine position. There is a small fall in vital capacity (VC) (8%) and a reduction in functional residual capacity (FRC) while lying down which results from repositioning of the diaphragm and pooling of blood in the chest. This change can be used to advantage to identify patients with covert diaphragm weakness where the VC may drop by more than 30%. Gravity also produces a change in the distribution of ventilation and perfusion within the lungs. In the supine posture ventilation

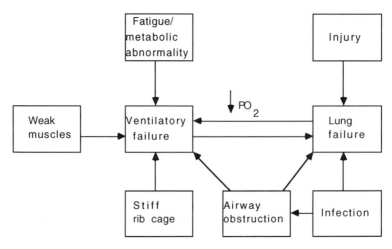

Fig. 3.8 Respiratory failure results from damage to the lung or inability to ventilate it. However, most situations have contributions from several mechanisms which result in a fall in PaO_2.

and perfusion is preferentially directed to the dependent zones (Kaneko et al 1966). This is important in adults if the lung disease is unilateral since oxygenation will be better if the good lung is dependent.

Physiotherapists are often involved in the assessment of patients for cardiothoracic surgery and their subsequent management. Some thoracic surgery such as bullectomy or decortication improves lung function, but most procedures impair the lung. The mechanisms of impairment include the anaesthetic, the thoracotomy and pulmonary resection. Following anaesthesia there is an immediate loss of FRC and subsequently VC which reaches a trough of about 40% at 24 hours and may take up to 2 weeks to recover (Jenkins et al 1988). This immediate loss of volume is associated with a widened gradient across the lung (A–aDO$_2$) and potential hypoxia which is worsened by obesity, age and smoking. The effect of the thoracotomy itself is to reduce the VC by approximately 10%, which recovers over a period of 3 months. There are no strong arguments for the benefit of median sternotomy over thoracotomy as far as recovery of long-term lung function is concerned. In the short term the physiotherapist should be cautious during treatment when gas exchange will be impaired if the patient is lying on the thoracotomy side.

The surgical removal of lung tissue does not necessarily have the predictable effects on function that might be imagined. Following pneumonectomy the functional state of the patient is remarkably stable, and in the long term the VC and total lung capacity (TLC) become slightly larger than expected for one lung. The TLCO eventually settles to 80% predicted and the KCO may be high since the whole pulmonary blood flow now travels through one lung. The changes after lobectomy are surprisingly different. The long-term effects may be small but in the postoperative phase the disruption may be unexpectedly large. The contusion of lung adjacent to the lobectomy sets up $\dot{V}/\dot{Q}$ disturbances which may in the short term be as significant as removal of the whole lung.

The physiological assessment of patients for thoracic surgery is not really very straightforward (Zibrak et al 1990, Olsen 1992). There is no single test which allows a distinction to be made between success and failure. It is important to consider the nature of the operation and the preoperative function as well as general health, weight and smoking habit. If there is any doubt about the suitability of a candidate from their spirometry and history (particularly cough, sputum and breathlessness) then some assessment of exercise capacity is advisable.

The effect of growth and ageing on lung function

The respiratory system reaches its peak in the third decade of life. Development of the lung continues from birth until the end of adolescence and starts to deteriorate after the age of 25 years. Fortunately, in the absence of disease there is sufficient reserve capacity to see out old age without discomfort!

The actual measurement of pulmonary function in childhood is problematic because of the obvious lack of cooperation. It is possible to measure lung volume and partial flow volume curves in infancy by using an adapted plethysmograph. This is possible in the sedated child by producing a pneumatic 'hug' as an alternative to active expiration. In older children it is difficult to obtain cooperation for measurements until they are about 8 years old. After this age lung function can be measured easily, but there are difficulties in interpretation and production of reference values. The inconsistency of the timing of puberty and rapid growth spurts make comparisons difficult, but normal ranges have been produced for these age groups (Polgar & Promadhat 1971).

The most obvious differences between children and adults lie in the development of airway function. The airways develop faster than the alveoli which may not reach maturity until about the seventh year. As the lung matrix develops, the airway walls remain strong and relatively patent. As a result expiratory flow rates, although lower than in adulthood, are relatively high. For example, the FEV$_1$/FVC ratio may be greater than 90% and the expiratory flow volume curve may have a flat or convex appearance. In addition to airway patency there are also developments in the behaviour of the chest wall with growth. In childhood the musculoskeletal structures are immature and flexible. Rib cage distortion is often seen in childhood during illness, but disappears with growth and muscularization. The combination of airway patency and plasticity of the chest wall allows an interesting experiment. In childhood the residual volume (RV) is not determined by airway closure but by the strength of the expiratory muscles. Thus if children or young adults are hugged at the end of a forced expiration more air can be expelled. After the age of 25 years, RV is determined by premature airway closure and the lungs cannot be emptied further.

Life after 25 years is all downhill for the respiratory system. As with general ageing, the tissues become less elastic and the lung elastic recoil diminishes. TLC tends to remain static but RV rises as the FEV_1 and FVC fall with age. Arterial PO_2 and A–aDO_2 worsen but do not reach critically low values. Exercise capacity, as judged by oxygen consumption, shows a decline with age but can be retarded by regular activity. As general levels of activity reduce with age, these effects are not usually important, but the changes may be accelerated by smoking or disease.

Interpretation of lung function tests

The value of lung function tests lies in the description of pathophysiology which may give a guide to diagnosis. Once a baseline has been established, changes in function can be used to assess progress with natural history or treatment. Although there may be some investigations which are specific to various diseases it is seldom possible to rely on a single investigation for the purpose. The usual description of disease requires the combination of spirometry, lung volume and gas transfer measurement. The addition of bronchodilator response, a flow–volume loop and blood gases would provide further information, while additional specific tests are requested as indicated. The additional tests may include an exercise study or respiratory muscle function test to examine the relevant

aspect. Interpretation of the tests involves the comparison of the values to the reference population and a description of the pattern of abnormality if present. A helpful report will also give some guidance on the accuracy of the clinical diagnosis and suggest confirmatory investigations if the diagnosis is unclear. Some examples of clinical cases and the patterns of abnormal lung function are given in Table 3.1.

Table 3.1 Conclusions from pulmonary function tests are best derived from the examination of several measurements. **a** A 66-year-old man with chronic airflow limitation. There is an increase in lung volumes, or hyperinflation of TLC and RV. The spirometry is obstructive but there is good bronchodilator reversibility, especially in the vital capacity. TLCO is slightly reduced but not as low as would be found in severe emphysema. The picture is one of smoking-related airflow obstruction, with the potential for some improvement. **b** A 49-year-old man with cryptogenic fibrosing alveolitis. There is a 'restrictive' defect with loss of lung volumes. Spirometry is not restrictive because of coexisting smoking-related airway obstruction. After treatment with prednisolone (10 March 1992) all values improved. **c** A 40-year-old woman with severe muscle weakness. There is a 'restrictive' picture, but the KCO is elevated because gas exchange is relatively normal. Respiratory muscle strength is reduced.

a

	Predicted	Observed	Post bronchodilator
FEV_1 (L)	2.86	1.15	1.30
FVC (L)	4.11	2.80	3.55
FEV_1/FVC (%)	70	41	37
TLC (L)	6.98	7.47	
RV (L)	2.54	4.24	
TLCO mmol min^{-1} kPa^{-1}	8.80	6.72	
KCO mmol min^{-1} kPa^{-1} L^{-1}	1.33	1.06	
VA (L)		6.33	

b

	Predicted	23 April 1991	10 March 1992
FEV_1 (L)	3.75	1.70	2.45
FVC (L)	4.94	2.40	3.30
FEV_1/FVC (%)	75	71	74
TLC (L)	7.59	4.34	5.55
RV (L)	2.41	1.67	2.10
TLCO mmol min^{-1} kPa^{-1}	10.97	5.82	7.36
KCO mmol min^{-1} kPa^{-1} L^{-1}	1.57	1.38	1.77
VA (L)		4.06	4.20

Table 3.1 (cont'd)

c

	Predicted	Observed
FRV$_1$ (L)	2.27	0.8
FVC (L)	2.83	1.10
FEV$_1$/FVC (%)	77	73
TLC (L)	4.25	1.89
RV (L)	1.22	0.85
TLCO (mmol/min. kPa. 1)	7.49	3.84
KCO (mmol/min. kPa. 1)	1.79	2.44
VA (L)	4.15	1.58
P_eMax (cmH$_2$O)	59–127	50
P_iMax (cmH$_2$O)	29–117	40

The measurement of disability and exercise testing

Static lung function tests can describe the physical properties of the lungs, but do not always reflect the performance of the cardiopulmonary system in action. The relationship between disability and, for example, spirometry is only a general one and individual predictions about exercise performance cannot be made. To assess disability it must generally be measured by some form of exercise test or inferred from questioning the patient. Exercise tests are valuable in making an objective assessment of disability and in observing the physiological response to exercise in order to assist diagnosis. Tests of exercise performance can either be performed in a complex manner in the laboratory or simply by observation of walking achievement down a hospital corridor. The former generally examine the detailed physiological response while walking tests can give a useful and reproducible assessment of disability.

Questionnaires

One of the difficulties in assessing lung disease through interview is the problem of silent deterioration. As disease affects the lung its impact on daily life may go unnoticed until there has been considerable loss of physiological capacity. Most people simply do not ordinarily stress the lungs to the extent of disclosure. Furthermore, patients with exercise limitation adopt a restricted lifestyle which my hide their disability. Sometimes simple questions can identify the disruption of normal activity. The more useful questions include inquiry about exercise tolerance in terms of walking distance on the flat before stopping for a rest, and ability to cope with hills and stairs. A more subtle approach is to ask whether a patient can keep up with their spouse or continue a conversation while walking.

Human performance and quality of life are heavily influenced by mood and other psychological influences. An overall picture of disability can be judged by application of a detailed questionnaire designed to cover either general features of disability or those which relate to specific examples. In patients with lung disease the Chronic Respiratory Questionnaire (CRQ) and St George's Questionnaire have been validated for patients with COPD and asthma, respectively (Guyatt et al 1987, Jones 1991). These questionnaires are quite good at distinguishing change after an intervention but not so good at comparisons between patients or absolute assessment. This is particularly true of the CRQ which uses individualized questions to obtain sensitivity.

Laboratory estimation of exercise capacity

Observation of the physiological response to exercise is the gold standard measurement of disability. This is usually performed during a progressive maximal test which is completed when the subject is unable to continue. Sometimes, more detailed information about endurance or the pathophysiology can be obtained from a steady-state performance at a fixed workload. The vehicle for exercise is usually a treadmill or a cycle ergometer. The latter provides a stable platform and more accurate assessment of workload, while the walking action on the treadmill will be more familiar to most patients. The choice is often determined by local circumstances. While the exercise is progressing the basic physiological response is observed by measuring ventilation, heart rate and oxygen uptake and carbon dioxide production. Other measurements such as oxygen saturation or cardiac output can be made if necessary. The test is conducted in such a fashion as to obtain a symptom-limited duration of about 10 min with the increments of work-load increased every minute by about 50 W. During this period the heart rate will rise linearly with work load. Ventilation also rises linearly until about 60% of maximum work load when it increases disproportionately. Oxygen uptake ($\dot{V}O_2$) will also rise linearly until the same point above which the rate of uptake slows and eventually reaches a plateau at the maximum oxygen uptake ($\dot{V}O_2$ max) (Fig. 3.9). The $\dot{V}O_2$ max is determined in health by the cardiovascular delivery of oxygen to the muscles and is a crude estimate of capacity and cardiopulmonary fitness. The point of inflection of pulmonary ventilation, the $\dot{V}E$ versus $\dot{V}O_2$ slope, is known as the anaerobic threshold and is thought to represent the ability to use the potential capacity and can be improved with physical training. In very unfit people the $\dot{V}O_2$ max can be improved with training, but this soon reaches a ceiling and further fitness is achieved by improvement of anaerobic threshold or endurance capacity (Astrand & Rodahl 1986).

The value of exercise testing in lung disease lies in the measurement of the degree of disability by assessment of the maximal work load and $\dot{V}O_2$ max in comparison with reference values. If a patient fails to achieve his predicted performance the mode of failure can help to identify the mechanism. For example, in patients with lung disease the early rise of $\dot{V}E$ may be characteristically in excess of expected but reach a premature limit imposed by the physical constraints of damaged lungs. Concurrently the heart rate response may be attenuated, in contrast to patients with cardiac disease where the test may have to be terminated because of early attainment of maximum predicted heart rate. It is always important to determine why the subject stops at the end of a test. This is best achieved by the visual presentation of a scale of breathlessness or fatigue at regular intervals. In health, maximum performance is limited by oxygen uptake or motivation, while in lung disease the limit may be ventilatory and in cardiac disease it may be due to inadequate cardiac output. Usually these mechanisms can be distinguished, although it must be remembered that patients with cardiac or pulmonary disease become inactive and unfit.

Field exercise tests

Laboratory tests of performance are the most accurate but are not always available and require expensive equipment. As an alternative, several field tests have been developed which can measure performance; the results of such tests relate quite well to laboratory estimates. Such tests are popular with physiotherapists, athletic coaches and the military since they can be applied easily to large numbers of subjects and do not need dedicated equipment or training. There are two main categories of field test — those which are unpaced and those where the speed of activity is imposed.

One of the first unpaced tests was the 12 min running test which was developed to assess the fitness of military personnel. This concept was adapted to the needs of the respiratory patient by downgrading the activity to a walk along a hospital corridor. Later, a reduction of the time to 6 min appeared to have no disadvantages. The 12 and 6 min walks have become familiar forms of assessment for respiratory patients (McGavin et al 1976, Butland et at 1982). The test procedure is extremely simple, with a course marked out along the corridor and the patient given the simple instruction to cover as much ground as possible in the time permitted. These tests have proven value but also have some limitations. There is quite a large learning effect and the reproducibility only becomes acceptable after two or more attempts

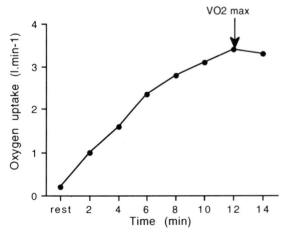

Fig. 3.9   The relationship between work and oxygen uptake during progressive exercise.

(Mungall & Hainsworth 1979, Knox et al 1988). In addition, no two patients will attack the test in the same way and the relative stresses may not allow direct comparison. Lastly, the lack of pace constraint makes the test performance vulnerable to mood and encouragement. Nevertheless, these simple tests require no equipment and, within their limitations, provide valuable information about general exercise capacity and major therapeutic changes.

The second type of field exercise test imposes a pace on the patient which reduces the effect of motivation and encouragement. An endurance walking test instructs the patient to walk at a fast pace for an unlimited distance and measures the time and distance travelled. Another form of constrained exercise is the step test where the subject steps up and down a couple of steps in time to a metronome signal. Inability to continue signals the end of the test and could be due to fatigue or breathlessness. This test has the capacity for incremental progression by increasing the pacing rate, but is a rather unnatural form of exercise.

An attempt to combine the comprehensive nature of incremental laboratory tests and the flexibility of the 6 min walk has been made in the shuttle walk test. This is an adaptation of the 20 m shuttle running test where a subject runs between two cones 20 m apart with the pace determined by a series of audio signals (Léger & Lambert 1982). At intervals the pace increases until the subject can continue no longer. For patients with lung disease the shuttle distance is reduced to 10 m and the pace increments altered to provide a comfortable start and reasonable range (Fig. 3.10) (Singh et al 1992). Under these circumstances the test provides a similar physiological stimulus and can be combined with measurements of heart rate and breathlessness to obtain almost as much information as provided by the laboratory standard.

CARDIAC FUNCTION

In many respects the heart is a more simple organ than the lung and much of its function is accessible to measurement. It is, however, a less forgiving organ and minor abnormalities of

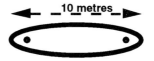

Level	Shuttles /level	Speed (mph)
1	3	1.12
2	4	1.50
3	5	1.88
4	6	2.26
5	7	2.64
6	8	3.02
7	9	3.40
8	10	3.78
9	11	4.16
10	12	4.54
11	13	4.92
12	14	5.30

a

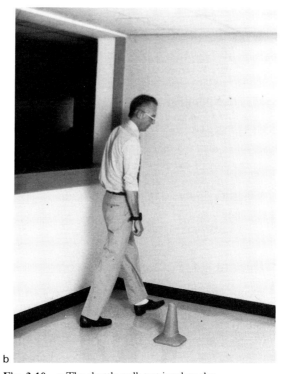

b

Fig. 3.10 **a** The shuttle walk test involves the perambulation of an oval 10 m course. The walking speeds are increased every minute and thereby increase the number of shuttles per level. **b** The subject turns around the cone in the shuttle walk in time with an audio signal. This subject is wearing a heart rate telemeter on his wrist.

coronary artery or cardiac muscle function may have dramatic effects. The major components of the heart include the myocardial muscle pump, the electrical conduction pathways, the internal valvular system and the coronary vasculature which supplies the muscle. Apart from congenital defects in the structure of the heart, disease can affect any of these components. Like the lung, the heart has a relatively limited symptomatic response to injury, and disease will present as chest pain, breathlessness, disturbance of heart rhythm or overt peripheral oedema. Cardiac failure occurs when the heart is unable to supply the expected demand of cardiac output. This may occur naturally at extremes of vigorous exercise when the cardiovascular delivery of oxygen cannot be maintained. When cardiac function cannot be maintained on moderate exercise or at rest then cardiac failure is present.

Although the two sides of the heart must be in overall balance, the pattern of failure will depend on the site of pathology. Left ventricular failure occurs when that ventricle cannot empty effectively and the resulting pulmonary venous hypertension may lead to pulmonary oedema. By contrast, the relative failure of the right ventricle leads to engorgement of the systemic venous system, resulting in peripheral oedema, ascites and elevated neck veins. The combination of left and right ventricular disorder is known as 'biventricular' or 'congestive' cardiac failure. Investigation of cardiac function includes examination of its structural, electrical and haemodynamic aspects. As for the lung, these features can be examined at rest or during exercise in order to uncover cardiac reserve.

Cardiac imaging

In recent years there have been advances in the technology available for the functional study of the heart. Apart from conventional radiology the heart is accessible to imaging by ultrasound, radionuclide and magnetic resonance techniques which complement each other. The simple chest radiograph can still provide valuable functional information about the presence of failure and is probably the most useful clinical tool for monitoring its progress (Fig. 3.11). Enlargement of the heart on a radiograph either represents increased muscle bulk or, more commonly, dilatation resulting from increased fibre length in failure. Pulmonary venous pooling will fill the upper lobe vessels as the first sign of trouble, followed by definition of the interlobular lymphatics which become visible as Kerley B lines. If the pulmonary venous pressure rises above about 25 mmHg there is a risk of interstitial oedema. This is first visible as loss of definition of the hilum, but subsequently may produce widespread shadowing. If congestive failure is present the picture may be complicated by pleural effusions. The radiograph can therefore provide a useful picture of dysfunction.

Ultrasound examination of the heart has become an invaluable asset to cardiac investigation and has superseded many invasive techniques. Standard echocardiography provides a sound image of the structure of the heart, while Doppler echo is able to identify flow patterns and pressure gradients within the chambers. The conventional echocardiogram is performed in M mode ('Motion' mode) and two-dimensional imaging. The original M mode technique uses a narrow single beam of sound to image a portion of the heart. It remains valuable in the examination of mitral and aortic valve function where the rapid movements of the leaflets can be scanned. Indirect estimates of function can be obtained by measurement of valve closure rates and patterns. In a significant proportion of patients, particularly those with coexistent lung disease, it is impossible to obtain a satisfactory picture. Two dimensional or cross sectional echocardiography uses a fan array of transducers to obtain a cross sectional image of the heart. This provides much clearer pictures of the relationships between the heart's structures. It can also use the dimensional changes through the cardiac cycle to calculate the ejection fraction and estimate the cardiac output. Such measurements are not extremely accurate because they are based on stable geometric assumptions, but they can be useful. It may be difficult to guarantee images in some patients, but the recent development of transoesophageal probes has improved the scope of cross sectional imaging. Doppler echocardiography has added a new dimension to functional imaging. The

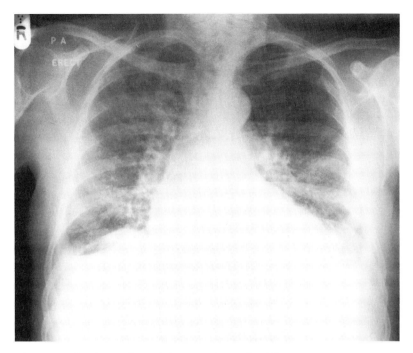

Fig. 3.11   The chest radiograph in congestive cardiac failure.

Doppler principle uses the flow of blood through the heart to calculate its velocity. It is able to detect turbulent flow and use its presence to estimate the pressure gradient across the valves. Sometimes it is also possible to measure pulmonary artery pressure. As confidence is growing with this technique the requirement for direct invasive measurement of cardiac function is less common.

Imaging of the heart and its circulation by using nuclear isotopes is a well developed technique. Two main techniques are in regular use. Injection of thallium 201 into the bloodstream leads to rapid distribution of the isotope through the tissues in proportion to the local blood flow. The coronary circulation is no different and the isotope is distributed within the heart. If the isotope is injected during exercise, areas of under-perfusion relating to coronary artery disease are highlighted. This technique is more sensitive than exercise cardiography, but cannot be specific about the site of arterial disease. Another use of nuclear isotopes in the assessment of cardiac function involves the labelling of the red blood

cell with technetium 99m. The radioactivity contained within the circulation allows examination of passage through the heart and calculation of the ejection fractions of both ventricles. The images are obtained with a conventional gamma camera, but the timing of the capture is determined by gating to the electrocardiogram (ECG). This technique is called a 'MUGA scan' (multi-gated acquisition scan) and is one of the most accurate, non-invasive methods of measuring ejection fraction. An alternative radionuclide method of obtaining ejection fraction depends on a more complex capture of first pass isotope, but this is not widely used.

Magnetic resonance imaging (MRI) is a developing field which holds promise for the functional exploration of the heart. The images of the heart and great blood vessels are often striking in their clarity. The magnetic properties of oxygen in blood promise the possibility of detailed, non-invasive measurement of function. At present the technique is still held back from its potential by the necessity for long scan times and ECG gating, but advances in this field are likely to be rapid.

The electrical function of the heart

The electrocardiogram (ECG) is the most established of the modern cardiological investigations.
In fact, it has become so familiar that it could be
considered as an extension of the clinical examination. The ECG can provide information about
the function of the intracardiac conducting tissue.
In most instances it reflects the presence of
cardiac disease on its electrical properties. Some
conditions produce characteristic patterns of ECG
abnormality. Examples include myocardial infarction and ischaemia, pericarditis and pulmonary
embolism. In diseases which affect the conducting
tissue the arrhythmias that they produce can be
identified. The presence of heart failure cannot be
determined from the ECG alone. However, infer-
ences can be made from the presence of large
complexes due to ventricular hypertrophy or very
small complexes in pericardial effusion.

The standard ECG is not always helpful in
patients with palpitations, particularly if it does not
capture the arrhythmia. In these circumstances the
provision of 24 or 48 hour recording may be
helpful. If the problem is likely to occur with even
less frequency, the ECG can be recorded at home
during an event and 'phoned in'.

The exercise ECG has developed an importance of its own in the assessment of ischaemic
heart disease. In this investigation the ECG is
recorded during a progressive exercise test. This is
usually a treadmill test, but cycle and step tests
have been used. In the UK the most popular
treadmill protocol is the Bruce (p. 326) variety
where both the speed and the gradient of the
treadmill are increased every 3 min. Other protocols such as the Balke or Naughton (Jones 1988)
are just as acceptable for producing the stimulus.
The indications for exercise electrocardiography
include the investigation of angina and post-
myocardial infarction assessment as well as the
postoperative examination of bypass surgery. The
most common abnormalities associated with
ischaemic heart disease on exercise are ST
segment changes. False positive changes are quite
common, but the exercise ECG has become quite
a sensitive guide to the presence of ischaemic
heart disease and a good predictor of prognosis
after myocardial infarction.

Haemodynamic function

Access to the chambers and blood vessels of the
heart is available through cardiac catheterization.
This technique was originally developed as a
research tool to examine the physiology of the
circulation by measuring intracardiac pressures.
The passage of catheters into the heart is now
commonplace in cardiological investigation and
on intensive care units. Its value no longer lies
solely in the measurement of function, but can also
provide a vehicle for therapeutic intervention in
the form of balloon valvuloplasty or angioplasty.

The assessment of function during cardiac
catheterization employs the measurement of
pressure, the injection of contrast media or the
sampling of blood. These objectives are achieved
by insertion of the catheter into the left or right
heart via a femoral or brachial blood vessel. A
right heart catheter is passed into the right
ventricle from a peripheral vein and can be guided
further into the pulmonary artery. The left
ventricle is accessible from the femoral artery by
crossing the aortic valve. Both coronary arteries
are also entered by this route. The pressure in the
left atrium may be difficult to obtain directly
unless there is a perforation in the atrial septum.
An approximation to the left atrial pressure can be
obtained by wedging the right heart catheter in a
small pulmonary artery. A special flow directed
catheter, the Swan–Ganz catheter, with a balloon
attached to the tip has been developed to facilitate
the passage into the pulmonary circulation.

Knowledge of the pressures within the heart is
useful to assess the need for surgery in patients
with valvular disease. The demonstration of a
significant gradient across the mitral or aortic
valve will confirm the clinical or ultrasound
impression. The pulmonary artery wedge pressure
(PawP) is a guide to the left atrial pressure and
can predict the likelihood of pulmonary oedema
or guide complex fluid replacement in intensive
care units or operating theatres.

Injection of radiological contrast can either
outline the coronary blood vessels (angiogram) or
the cavity of the ventricle. The former is the
standard assessment in ischaemic heart disease,
while the latter is the most informative method for
describing the motion of the heart and for calcu-

lating the ejection fraction. In general, angiography is more descriptive of the structure rather than the function of the heart.

The estimation of cardiac output can be made non-invasively by a variety of, sometimes inventive, methods. However, to be of value the estimate should be accurate and is obtained by catheterization. The classical method is called the 'Fick principle' where the result is computed from the total oxygen uptake and the arteriovenous oxygen difference. Although this method is accurate it is unacceptably invasive. The most popular method now uses a modified pulmonary artery catheter to measure output by thermodilu-

tion. In this case a known bolus of cold saline is injected into the superior vena cava and the temperature drop is recorded in the pulmonary artery. The cardiac output is calculated by using a bedside computer. Knowledge of the cardiac output and its changes can be a very powerful clinical tool. It is especially useful in the management of very sick patients where the manipulation of cardiac output by combination of inotrope drugs and vasodilators can ensure optimal oxygen delivery for the tissues. Another example of its value is the exploration of cardiac reserve of output during exercise or electrical pacing or pharmacological stimulation.

REFERENCES

American Thoracic Society 1986 Evaluation of impairment/disability secondary to respiratory disorders. American Review of Respiratory Disease 133: 1205–1209

Anthonisen N R 1986 Tests of mechanical function. In: Fishman AP (ed) Handbook of respiratory physiology, The respiratory system III. American Physiological Society, Bethesda

Astrand P-O, Rodahl K 1986 Textbook of work physiology, 3rd edn. McGraw-Hill, New York, p 753–784

Benson M K 1983 Diseases of the airways. In: Weatherall D J, Ledingham J G G, Warrel D A (eds) Oxford textbook of medicine. Oxford University Press, Oxford, vol 2, p 15.60–15.70

Black L F, Hyatt R E 1971 Maximal static respiratory pressures in generalised neuromuscular disease. American Review of Respiratory Disease 103: 641–650

Bott J, Keilty S E J, Brown A, Ward E M 1992 Nasal intermittent positive pressure ventilation. Physiotherapy 78:93–96

Butland R J A, Gross E R, Pang J et al 1982 Two-, six-, and twelve-minute walking test in respiratory diseases. British Medical Journal 284:1607–1608

Cotes J E 1979 Lung function, 4th edn. Blackwell Scientific, Oxford

European Community for Coal and Steel 1983 Standardized lung function testing. Bulletin Europeén de Physiopathologie Respiratoire 19 (suppl 5):1–95

Gibson G J 1990 Respiratory function tests. In: Brewis R A L, Gibson G J, Geddes D M (eds) Respiratory medicine. Baillière Tindall, London, p 229–244

Green M, Laroche C M 1990 Respiratory muscle weakness. In: Brewis R A L, Gibson G J, Geddes D M (eds) Respiratory medicine. Baillière Tindall, London, p 1373–1387

Guyatt G H, Berman L B, Townsend M et al 1987 A measure of the quality of life for clinical trials in chronic lung disease. Thorax 42:773–778

Jenkins S C, Soutar S A, Moxham J 1988 The effects of posture on lung volumes in normal subjects and in patients pre- and post-coronary artery surgery. Physiotherapy 74:492–496

Jones N L 1988 Clinical exercise testing, 3rd edn. W B Saunders, Philadelphia

Jones P W 1991 Quality of life measurement for patients with

disease of the airway. Thorax 46:676–682

Kaneko K M, Milic-Emili J, Dolovich M B et al 1966 Regional distribution of ventilation and perfusion as a function of body position. Journal of Applied Physiology 21:767–777

Keilty S E J, Bott J 1992 Continuous positive airways pressure. Physiotherapy 78:90–92

Knox A J, Morrison J F J, Muers M F 1988 Reproducibility of walking test results in chronic obstructive airways disease. Thorax 43:388–392

Léger L A, Lambert J 1982 A multi-stage 20-m shuttle run test to predict VO_2 max. European Journal of Applied Physiology 49:1–12

McGavin C R, Gupta S P, McHardy G J R 1976 Twelve-minute walking test for assessing disability in chronic bronchitis. British Medical Journal 1:822–823

Martyn J B, Moreno R H, Pare P D, Pardy R L 1987 Measurement of inspiratory muscle performance with incremental threshold loading. American Review of Respiratory Disease 135:919–923

Mungall I P F, Hainsworth R 1979 Assessment of respiratory function in patients with chronic obstructive airways disease. Thorax 34:254–258

Olsen G N 1992 Pre-operative physiology and lung resection. Chest 101:300–301

Polgar G, Promadhat V 1971 Pulmonary function testing in children: techniques and standards. W B Saunders, Philadelphia

Pride N B 1983 The function of lungs and its investigations. In: Weatherall D J, Ledingham J G G, Warrel D A (eds) Oxford textbook of medicine. Oxford University Press, Oxford, vol 2, p 15.21–15.30

Shneerson J 1988 Disorders of ventilation. Blackwell Scientific, Oxford, p 78–85

Singh S J, Morgan M D L, Scott S et al 1992 The development of the shuttle walking test of disability in patients with chronic airways obstruction. Thorax 47: 1019–1024

Tremper K K, Barker S J 1989 Pulse oximetry. Anesthesiology 70: 98–108

Zibrak D J, O'Donnell C R, Marton K 1990 Indications for pulmonary function testing. Annals of Internal Medicine 112: 763–771

FURTHER READING

American College of Sports Medicine 1991 Guidelines for exercise testing and prescription, 4th edn. Lea & Febiger, Philadelphia

Cotes J E 1979 Lung function, 4th edn. Blackwell Scientific, Oxford

Jones N L 1988 Clinical exercise testing, 3rd edn. W B Saunders, Philadelphia

Muller W F, Scacci R, Gast L R 1987 Laboratory evaluation of pulmonary function. J B Lippincott, Philadelphia

Nunn J F 1987 Applied respiratory physiology, 3rd edn. Butterworths, London

West J B 1992 Pulmonary pathophysiology, 4th edn. Williams & Wilkins, Baltimore

West J B 1990 Respiratory physiology, 4th edn. Williams & Wilkins, Baltimore

4. Monitoring and interpreting medical investigations

John S. Turner

MONITORING

Introduction

There has been an explosion of computer and video technology in recent years, and patient monitoring has benefited from this in no small way. The ability to detect and rapidly react to changes in physiology is now possible, and it is this that has become the essence of modern intensive care.

The ideal monitoring system is not yet a reality (although several major manufacturers would deny this), but it is coming closer all the time. This system would need to be accurate, precise, and reliable. It would be sensitive to small changes in the parameters it monitors, yet able to distinguish and eliminate artefacts. It would preferably be non-invasive for the sake of safety. It would function on a real-time rather than an intermittent basis. It would have a memory for previous data and would be able to show trends. Its memory module would be moveable to allow it to capture data in the ward, in transport, and in another environment such as an operating theatre. It would also almost certainly be extremely expensive!

Conventional observations

Back to reality. Nursing observations have for many years included the taking of the patient's temperature, pulse, respiratory rate, and blood pressure. These are performed manually and carefully charted at intervals varying from quarter-hourly to six-hourly to daily, being performed more frequently in high-care areas. These practices are quite adequate for general ward situations where patients are not critically ill, and are even useful in intensive care units (ICUs), both for making physical contact with the patient and for checking the invasively monitored observations.

The major limitation of intermittently performed observations is that they may only establish the presence of an abnormality some time after it has developed. Thus the ability to react immediately at the development of an abnormality is lost. More frequently performed observations are obviously superior in this regard, but real-time continuous monitoring is the ultimate goal of monitoring.

Non-invasive monitoring

Non-invasive monitoring of a variety of parameters is now routinely practised in many areas, especially ICUs and operating theatres. Commonly monitored parameters include temperature, heart rate, blood pressure and oxygen saturation. Respiratory rate may be measured by some monitoring systems, and in certain circumstances end-tidal CO_2 and transcutaneous PO_2 and PCO_2 monitoring may be performed. These may all be displayed on a single monitor screen. Technical problems and artefacts can occur with the display of any of these parameters, so the patient's clinical status must be checked before acting on a monitor display abnormality.

Temperature

Temperature is continuously monitored by means of an oesophageal or rectal probe. Problems are rarely encountered with this method. The oesophageal temperature may be lower if the gases for respiratory support are unwarmed and the rectal probe may occasionally fall out without being noticed, leading to an erroneously low temperature being displayed. A rectum full of faeces may also lead to a lower temperature being recorded.

Heart rate

Heart rate is measured from the electrocardiogram (ECG) trace. Artefacts are common. Interference (usually from patient movement or a warming blanket) may confuse the monitor into showing the presence of a tachycardia or arrhythmia, while small complexes may be interpreted as asystole. Physiotherapy may also cause movement artefacts. On the ECG trace, large T waves (and occasionally P waves or a pacemaker spike) may be interpreted as QRS complexes, leading to the displayed heart rate being double the actual rate. Detached or dried-out electrodes will lead to asystole being displayed. Sinus tachycardia, sinus bradycardia, and atrial fibrillation are described below.

Respiratory rate

Respiratory rate may be measured by making use of the changing impedance across the chest wall as it moves with respiration. In systems which offer this parameter, the sensors are built into the ECG leads. The heart rate and other movements of the chest can cause overreading of respiratory rate, while electrodes placed too far apart may not give a reading at all.

Appropriate physiotherapy treatment (e.g. for lobar lung collapse) may reduce a rapid respiratory rate, but it must be emphasized that an already tachypnoeic patient should not be allowed to become exhausted during treatment as he may rapidly decompensate. This may even necessitate emergency intubation. Close contact with the medical and nursing staff should therefore be maintained in such cases.

Blood pressure

Blood pressure is monitored with a pressure cuff around the upper arm. An oscillometric method is used to measure blood pressure, with automatic cuff inflation and deflation. The accuracy of such systems is generally good, but the cuff needs to be applied correctly and be of the appropriate size for the arm. The system also needs to be calibrated correctly against a mercury column. Non-invasive blood pressure monitoring is performed intermittently, but the interval between readings may be as short as 1 minute.

Physiotherapy treatment may cause a patient to become hypertensive, especially if the treatment causes pain or anxiety. The hypotensive patient may occasionally become more unstable, and here the risks and benefits of treatment need to be carefully balanced.

Oxygen saturation

Oxygen saturation (Clark et al 1992) is continuously measured by a pulse oximeter with a probe on a finger or ear lobe. There are two methods: the functional method which measures the difference between oxyhaemoglobin and deoxyhaemoglobin, and the fractional method which measures all types of haemoglobin over a wide spectrum of light absorption. The former method may record erroneously high saturations if there is a high concentration of carboxyhaemoglobin (the combination of carbon monoxide and haemoglobin) in the blood, while the latter method will be inaccurate if a light emitting diode (LED) or ultraviolet light (including sunlight) is close to the probe. Saturations are generally accurate between 100% and 80%, but may be inaccurate at lower levels. The saturation trace must be observed to correspond with the heart rate; if this is not so the reading may be erroneous. Low saturations with either method may be due to poor peripheral perfusion, painted or nicotine-stained fingernails, pierced ears, intravenous contrast medium, or injected dyes.

Hypoxaemia has been shown to occur both during and after chest physiotherapy (Tyler 1982); awareness and careful monitoring are therefore important. A patient on a ventilator and on high inspired oxygen concentrations or positive end-expiratory pressure may become dangerously hypoxaemic during tracheal suctioning. Strategies to limit this risk include preoxygenation and use of a sealed suction port (as used for fibreoptic bronchoscopy).

End-tidal CO₂

End-tidal CO_2 ($ETCO_2$) may be measured on an intubated patient. The method works by the principle of absorption of infra-red light. A probe from the monitor is inserted into the ventilator circuit close to the end of the endotracheal tube. $ETCO_2$ correlates well with PCO_2 in normal lungs, but less well in diseased lungs (Clark et al 1992). It is used widely in anaesthesia and for the ventilation of head-injured patients, but its use in other contexts is less well defined.

In paediatric (especially neonatal) patients, transcutaneous PO_2 and PCO_2 measurements are practised in many centres. The transcutaneous electrode is fixed to the skin which it heats and makes permeable to gas transport. Local hyperaemia arterializes the capillary blood. Good correlation between transcutaneous and arterial measurements has been shown. However, transcutaneous measurements have been shown to be sensitive but not specific indicators of blood gas status as they may be influenced not only by the partial pressure of the gas but also by a reduction in cardiac output or local blood flow. They have not gained acceptance in adult critical care practice.

Invasive monitoring

This requires the use of an invasive catheter, which is inserted into an artery, a central vein, the pulmonary artery or, in some neurosurgical centres, the extradural space (for intracranial pressure (ICP) monitoring). The catheter is connected to a transducer which is in turn connected to a pressure monitor (Fig. 4.1). The monitor displays pressure wave-forms and values on a real-time basis (Fig. 4.2). We have become accustomed to seeing these displays (often in a variety of bright colours), and usually blindly accept that each component of the system is working correctly and accurately; this is unhappily not always the case and we may be lulled into a false and dangerous sense of security.

Inaccuracies may (and commonly do) occur from any one (or a combination) of the following:

- The catheter may be incorrectly positioned.
- The catheter may be partially blocked or kinked.
- The connecting tubing may be partially blocked or kinked, or it may allow too much resonance in the system leading to exaggerated pressure wave forms (under-damping).
- The transducer may be faulty or incompatible with the other equipment.
- The monitor may be incorrectly calibrated.
- The pressure bag (which pressurizes the system.

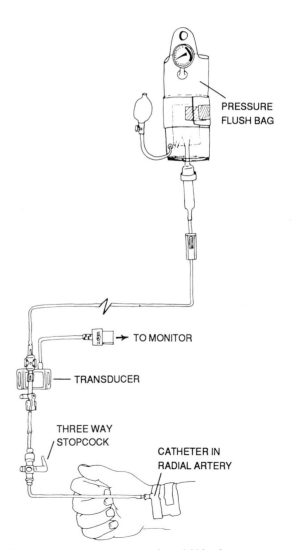

PRESSURE FLUSH BAG

TO MONITOR

TRANSDUCER

THREE WAY STOPCOCK

CATHETER IN RADIAL ARTERY

Fig. 4.1 Invasive monitoring of arterial blood pressure.

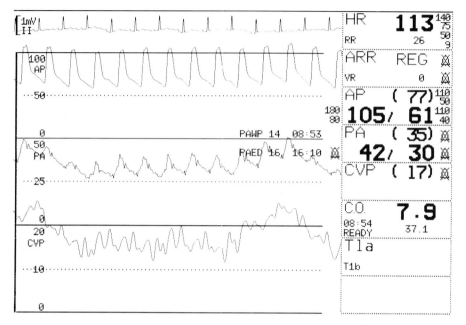

Fig. 4.2   Display of pressure wave forms and ECG trace on monitor screen. HR, heart rate; ARR, arrhythmia monitoring; REG, regular; AP, arterial pressure; PA, pulmonary artery pressure; CVP, central venous pressure; CO, cardiac output.

for flushing and to prevent backflow) may not be properly inflated.

All these aspects of invasive pressure monitoring need to be checked regularly, especially if the readings do not correlate with the clinical appearance of the patient. In many cases, potentially harmful treatment has been instituted on the basis of totally incorrect information.

Common invasively monitored parameters include arterial blood pressure and central venous pressure (CVP). *Arterial cannulation* allows continuous monitoring of blood pressure as well as easy access for blood gas analysis. The radial artery on the non-dominant side is the most common site of insertion; other sites include brachial, dorsalis pedis, and femoral arteries. The femoral artery is especially useful in states of shock, when peripheral pulses may be impalpable. The catheter is usually inserted percutaneously, but may be introduced by surgical cut-down. Complications of arterial cannulation are uncommon and include infection and, rarely, thrombosis. Disconnection of the catheter from the line can easily occur with movement of the

patient; vigorous bleeding will follow and exsanguination is a real risk. These lines should always therefore remain visible and care should be taken when moving the patient.

CVP measurement involves placement of a catheter into a central vein (generally the superior vena cava), usually via the subclavian or internal jugular vein. The basilic, external jugular, and femoral veins may also be used for access; the advantage of these sites is that there is no risk of pneumothorax and that bleeding is easier to control. Disadvantages of these routes include difficulty with accurate placement and a higher incidence of thrombosis. The CVP represents the state of filling of the vasculature and heart, more specifically the right side of the heart. If correctly interpreted, it can yield valuable diagnostic information and guide fluid therapy. The complications associated with all central venous catheters are not insubstantial: they include vascular erosion, air embolism, bleeding, thrombosis, and infection. Again, disconnection can occur with movement. Bleeding will occur if the end of the catheter is below the level of the heart, while air may be sucked into the system and air embolism may result if the end of the catheter is above that level. Air embolism is a very serious event and can result in immediate collapse and death.

With a *pulmonary artery catheter*, pulmonary capillary wedge pressure (PCWP) may be monitored and cardiac output (CO) may be measured by means of the thermodilution technique. Systemic vascular resistance (SVR), pulmonary vascular resistance (PVR), oxygen delivery, and oxygen consumption may also be calculated.

The pulmonary artery catheter is inserted via a central vein through the right side of the heart into the pulmonary artery. At its tip it has a balloon which is inflated when the catheter is in the heart and this allows the catheter to be carried through the heart chambers by the flow of blood (Fig. 4.3). When the inflated balloon occludes the pulmonary artery, the catheter no longer measures pulmonary artery pressure but PCWP. By a series of extrapolations, left atrial pressure and, therefore, left ventricular preload can be gauged (Fig. 4.4). This gives valuable information over and above CVP measurement when the left

and right sides of the heart are not functioning equally. The left heart alone may fail in anterior myocardial infarction and the right heart alone may fail in pulmonary embolism, cor pulmonale, pericardial constriction, and right ventricular infarction. In all these settings, measurement of CVP alone may give totally misleading information about left ventricular filling. The interpretation of the PCWP is not always straightforward and has many pitfalls for the unwary (Raper & Sibbald 1986).

Measurement of cardiac output is an integral part of pulmonary artery catheterization. The resultant calculations of SVR, oxygen delivery, and oxygen consumption give an enormous amount of information about the state of the heart and circulation. Manipulation of these variables by vasoactive drugs is useful in a variety of disease states, including sepsis, pulmonary oedema, adult respiratory distress syndrome, and cardiogenic shock.

Left atrial pressure may be measured directly by means of a catheter inserted into the left atrium at the time of cardiac surgery. The catheter is

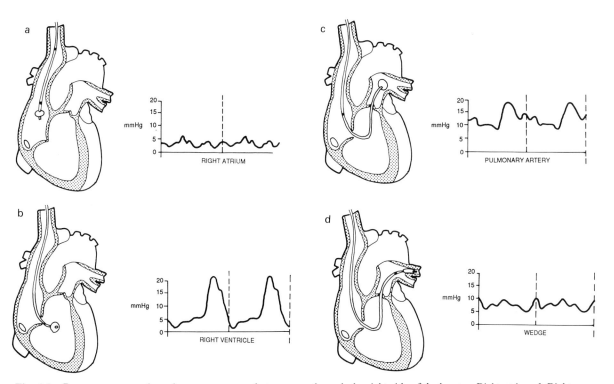

Fig. 4.3   Pressure traces as the pulmonary artery catheter passes through the right side of the heart. **a** Right atrium. **b** Right ventricle. **c** Pulmonary artery. **d** Pulmonary capillary wedge pressure.

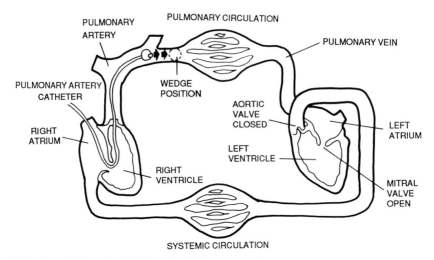

Fig. 4.4   In diastole, with the mitral valve open, pulmonary capillary wedge pressure corresponds to left atrial pressure.

brought out through the chest wall and monitoring takes place in the conventional way. All the above mentioned complications may occur; in addition, displacement may occasionally result in pericardial tamponade.

Intracranial pressure monitoring may be performed in patients with head injuries, brain surgery, intracranial and subarachnoid haemorrhage, and cerebral oedema from other causes. However, the frequency of use of this technique depends on the enthusiasm of individual units. Such monitoring may give an indication of a rise in ICP before it becomes clinically evident, thus allowing therapeutic manoeuvres (hyperventilation, mannitol, surgery) to be initiated before cerebral damage occurs. The importance of ICP measurement is that it provides an estimate of cerebral perfusion pressure (cerebral perfusion pressure = mean arterial pressure − ICP) which in turn relates to cerebral blood flow (CBF). Raised ICP causes reduced CBF which leads to tissue hypoxia and acidosis, raised PCO_2, cerebral vasodilation, and oedema, all of which cause a further rise in ICP.

ICP may be measured by means of an extradural or subarachnoid bolt, an intraventricular catheter (inserted through the skull into the lateral ventricle), or an epidural catheter. The former methods are the most widely used (Fig 4.5). The intraventricular catheter has the additional advantage of being able to drain cerebrospinal fluid, thereby relieving raised ICP. All these methods are invasive and the potential complications are not insignificant, the most serious being infection.

Physiotherapy procedures have been shown to cause a rise in ICP, especially in patients whose ICP is already raised. Major factors are prolonged treatment time, manual chest hyperinflation, and suctioning (Garradd & Bullock 1986). These authors recommend careful observation of ICP when it is monitored, shorter and more frequent treatments, brief application of manual hyperinflation, and additional sedation prior to suctioning. Avoidance of head-down positioning is also helpful. In practice, however, ICP monitoring may not be available, and the benefits of treatment need to be carefully balanced against the known risks.

ECG monitoring

It is beyond the scope of this chapter to cover arrhythmia recognition and management, but the more common arrhythmias are discussed and examples of ECG traces given (Fig. 4.6). Physiotherapy procedures may both cause arrhythmias (Hammon et al 1992) and may worsen those already present. Great awareness and care is needed, especially in those patients at risk of developing arrhythmias.

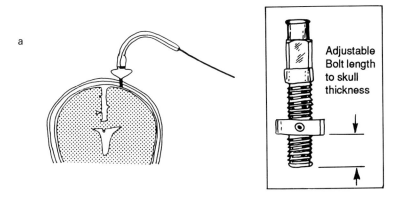

Adjustable Bolt length to skull thickness

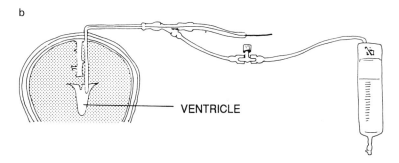

VENTRICLE

Fig. 4.5 Intracerebral pressure monitoring. **a** Extradural or subarachnoid bolt. **b** Intraventricular catheter with cerebrospinal fluid drainage bag.

1. *Sinus bradycardia* is a sinus rhythm below 60 beats/min. The common causes are drugs (e.g. beta blockers) and hypoxaemia; bradycardia may be a warning sign that the latter is occurring and, as such, should be taken very seriously. Vagal stimuli from tracheal suctioning may also be implicated. Care with suctioning and generous preoxygenation may be necessary; occasionally it is reassuring to have atropine drawn up and ready to inject.

2. *Sinus tachycardia* is a sinus rhythm above 100 beats/min. Pain and anxiety are common causes, but occasionally it may be precipitated by haemodynamic instability or respiratory distress. Procedures should be carefully explained to the patient, and adequate analgesia should be given before physiotherapy begins.

3. *Atrial fibrillation* is a common arrhythmia in critically ill patients. It is a totally irregular rhythm that may reach a ventricular rate of up to 200 beats/min and cause haemodynamic instability. It may be paroxysmal. The cause is usually multifactorial, but common precipitating factors include hypokalaemia, hypoxaemia, dehydration or overhydration, ischaemic heart disease, and cardiac surgery.

Patients at risk of developing arrhythmias often have ischaemic heart disease or a history of arrhythmias. However, critically ill patients may suddenly develop a rhythm disturbance, the cause of which is usually multifactorial. A patient may have recently had an arrhythmia (often of short duration) so it is vital to check the charts and to communicate with the doctors and nurses looking after the patient.

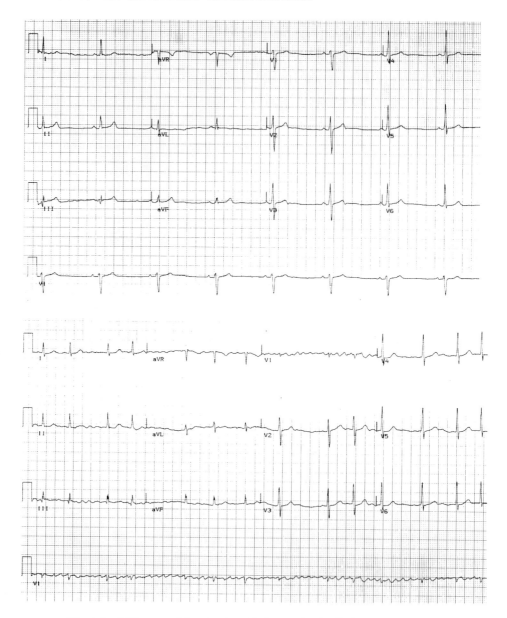

Fig. 4.6   ECG traces of sinus bradycardia (top) and atrial fibrillation (bottom).

The present state of development is that most good monitoring systems today have memory capacity and can display past values on a minute-to-minute basis. Trends can be graphically displayed and analysed. A printer link may allow ECG or pressure traces to be printed and retained. Already in use in some centres are systems that utilize a specialized software package which enables the rapid recording, storage, display and reporting of a wide range of clinical data. Data are either downloaded directly from the patient monitors or entered manually. Hard copies of relevant data are produced using a printer. This system totally replaces nursing charts and is an extremely attractive option in terms of labour saving, accuracy, convenience and immediacy.

INTERPRETING MEDICAL INVESTIGATIONS

A number of blood and microbiological tests are regularly performed on patients in hospital, leading to an enormous amount of data which needs to be responsibly interpreted (even when it is sometimes irresponsibly requested!). It is clearly vital to know the normal values for these tests, which abnormalities are important and which are not, and how to respond to any abnormalities which need treatment. The more commonly performed haematological, biochemical, and microbiological tests are discussed with these issues in mind. Normal values depend on the test technique, the units in which the result is given, and the local reference values.

Haematology

Full blood count

This is usually performed in an automated blood analyser which produces a printout of results. Included in most analysers are the following (the abbreviations given are commonly used).

Haemoglobin (Hb). Haemoglobin is the red oxygen-carrying pigment in red blood cells (RBCs). Its primary function is the transport of oxygen. Hb is easy to measure (it can be measured in the ward with a Spencer haemoglobinometer) and is an indirect measure of the number of RBCs in the circulation and, therefore, of the total red cell mass. In states of dehydration or overhydration Hb may be falsely raised or lowered.

A reduced red cell mass is referred to as 'anaemia', while an increased red cell mass is known as 'polycythaemia' or 'erythrocytosis'. There are many causes of anaemia, but those most commonly seen are acute or chronic blood loss, iron deficiency, and chronic illness or inflammation. Polycythaemia may be primary (from a disorder of the bone marrow) or secondary (due to chronic hypoxaemic lung disease or cyanotic heart disease, renal carcinoma, cerebellar haemangioblastoma, or uterine fibroids).

Mean corpuscular volume (MCV). This is a measure of the size of the RBCs. A low MCV (small RBCs) is referred to as 'microcytosis': the most common cause is iron deficiency. A high MCV is referred to as 'macrocytosis', and is most often caused by vitamin B_{12} or folate deficiency. The MCV is useful in narrowing down the differential diagnosis of anaemia and other blood disorders.

Mean corpuscular haemoglobin (MCH). This is calculated by dividing the Hb by the total red cell count. It reflects the amount of Hb in the RBCs.

White cell count (WCC). The white blood cells, or leukocytes, perform a variety of functions in the body. Their major role is to defend the body against infection, and their interaction in achieving this goal is remarkable. The neutrophils (the predominant type of leukocyte) perform the immediate response to infection by phagocytosing offending organisms. Lymphocytes are involved in the production of antibodies, and play a pivotal role in both cell-mediated and humoral immunity. The monocyte–macrophage cell line is also involved in immunity, primarily by processing antigens and presenting them to immunocompetent lymphocytes. They also have an important phagocytosing and scavenging function, and incidentally play a role in the regulation of haematopoiesis.

The functions of eosinophils and basophils are poorly understood, but eosinophils seem to be important in the defence against parasitic infections and in allergic disorders.

Platelet count (Plt). Platelets circulate in the bloodstream as tiny discs less than half the size of RBCs and are an essential component in blood clotting. They are part of the first-line reaction to a breach in the vascular endothelium. A reduction in the platelet count is known as 'thrombocytopenia' while an increase is called 'thrombocytosis'. There are many causes for thrombocytopenia, but the common ones seen in critically ill patients include sepsis, disseminated intravascular coagulopathy (see below), drug-related causes, and consumption by dialysis machines or other extracorporeal circuits.

Differential count

This looks primarily at the white cells in the blood, but at the same time the morphology of the red blood cells and the platelets may be commented upon. A drop of blood is smeared smoothly across a glass slide; this is then stained and examined under a microscope. The different cells are counted in a high power field and the numbers are given as a percentage. Absolute numbers of calls will thus depend upon the total white cell count. The differential count may be useful in diagnosis of specific infections or infiltrations, allergic or parasitic disorders, and assessing immune status.

Clotting profile

This is generally performed in a patient who is either bleeding or is at high risk of developing a bleeding problem. Indices measured include prothrombin time, partial thromboplastin time (PTT), platelets, fibrinogen, and fibrin degradation products (FDPs). There is a wide variety of bleeding disorders with an even wider variety of causes; patients may be at risk for spontaneous haemorrhage or haemorrhage caused by minor trauma (such as physiotherapy procedures).

Prothrombin time and partial thromboplastin time measure the integrity of different limbs of the clotting cascade. The prothrombin time is now usually given as the ratio of measured time over control time, with international standardization of the reagents used: it is thus referred to as the 'international normalized ratio' (INR).

In acutely ill patients, there are two commonly found disorders of coagulation. Firstly, a dilutional coagulopathy may occur from massive blood transfusions without the addition of clotting factors. The INR and PTT are prolonged, and platelets and fibrinogen are reduced. Secondly, disseminated intravascular coagulopathy (DIC) may be caused by a wide variety of precipitating events, including sepsis, trauma, and incompatible blood transfusions (Bick 1988). Clotting factors are consumed by inappropriate intravascular coagulation, and there is thus a deficiency of them which leads to bleeding. Again INR and PTT are prolonged, platelets and fibrinogen are low (they may be extremely low), and FDPs are present in large amounts, representing the fibrinolysis (clot breakdown) that is taking place intravascularly.

Patients with a DIC or thrombocytopenia (especially when the platelet count is less than 20) may be at risk of pulmonary haemorrhage. Great care should be taken during suctioning and physiotherapy, and the potential benefits should be weighed against this risk.

Biochemistry

Arterial blood gases

These not only give an indication of oxygenation and carbon dioxide clearance, but also of acid–base status. Most automated blood gas machines measure only pH, PO_2 and PCO_2, and extrapolate from these values the bicarbonate and oxygen saturation. These extrapolations are accurate under most circumstances, but oxygen saturation may be fallacious in the presence of carboxyhaemoglobin. Hypoxaemia (PaO_2 of less than 8 kPa or 60 mm Hg at sea level) and hypercarbia ($PaCO_2$ of more than 6 kPa or 45 mmHg) are easy to recognize and their causes are not discussed here. The metabolic and respiratory causes of acidosis and alkalosis are a little more complex and may cause confusion.

In simple terms, in acidosis the pH is always low (normal pH is 7.36–7.44) and in alkalosis the pH is always high (remember that pH is an inverse and logarithmic expression of hydrogen ion concentration). Metabolic causes of acidosis and alkalosis involve a primary change of the bicarbonate concentration, and respiratory causes involve a change of $PaCO_2$. The different disorders are discussed further below and some rather simplistic examples are given in Table 4.1.

Metabolic acidosis. This is probably the most serious acid–base disorder. It may be caused by either an excess of acid (lactate, ketoacids, metabolites, or poisons) or a loss of bicarbonate by the small intestine or the kidneys. Lactate accumulates in states of inadequate oxygen delivery to the tissues; this is usually seen in shock of any cause. Ketoacids accumulate in diabetic ketoacidosis which is always associated with a

Table 4.1 Examples of acid–base disturbances and the compensatory mechanisms

Disorder	pH	P_aCO_2	Bicarbonate	Compensation
Metabolic acidosis	7.2	5	18	CO_2
Compensation	7.4	3	18	
Respiratory acidosis	7.2	8	26	Bicarbonate
Compensation	7.4	8	36	
Metabolic alkalosis	7.5	5	34	CO_2
Compensation	7.4	7	34	
Respiratory alkalosis	7.5	3	26	Bicarbonate
Compensation	7.4	3	20	

raised blood glucose. Both lactate and ketoacids may be measured in the laboratory. In renal failure, tubular dysfunction reduces bicarbonate generation; in addition, there are unmeasured acidic anions in the blood, and glomerular dysfunction leads to a reduction in the amount of sodium available for exchange with hydrogen ions. Poisons or drugs in overdose may be acidic, e.g. ethylene glycol and aspirin.

Compensation for the acidosis occurs by hyperventilation with a resultant fall in $PaCO_2$. This accounts for the deep sighing respiration (Kussmaul breathing) often seen in metabolic acidosis.

Treatment of metabolic acidosis is controversial. For many years bicarbonate was the mainstay of treatment, but recent evidence is now accumulating that its effects are mainly cosmetic and may be harmful (Cooper et al 1990). These include shifting the oxygen dissociation curve thereby inhibiting the release of oxygen, causing hypernatraemia and hyperosmolarity, and provoking an intracellular acidosis (Ritter et al 1990). It would seem that treatment of the cause of the acidosis should be the primary objective.

Respiratory acidosis. The primary problem is a raised $PaCO_2$. This is the result of alveolar hypoventilation, the cause of which may be inadequate minute volume (as in a weak or tired patient) or increased dead space (as in severe chronic obstructive airways disease). Often these occur in combination. Compensation occurs by an increase in plasma bicarbonate; this is done mainly by the kidneys, which increase bicarbonate reabsorption in the tubules.

The plasma bicarbonate level may be useful in differentiating acute from chronic respiratory

acidosis. In the acute state bicarbonate is normal, while in the chronic state it is raised due to the aforementioned compensatory mechanisms. This distinction may have important clinical consequences, for example in differentiating severe asthma from chronic lung disease.

Metabolic alkalosis. This may be caused by an excess of bicarbonate (always iatrogenic) or a loss of acid (either from the stomach or the kidneys). Acid may be lost from the stomach in cases of upper gastrointestinal tract obstruction or ileus; litres of fluid may be lost daily. The most common cause of acid loss by the kidneys is hypokalaemia. Here there is an inadequate amount of potassium ions available for exchange with sodium ions; hydrogen ions are sacrificed in their place.

Respiratory alkalosis. Here the primary problem is a low $PaCO_2$, which is always a result of hyperventilation. This may occur in a spontaneously breathing person who is anxious, in pain, or has a respiratory disorder (causes include asthma, pneumonia, pulmonary embolus, and adult respiratory distress syndrome). Rarely, neurological disorders (affecting the respiratory centre) will cause hyperventilation. It may also be seen in a mechanically ventilated patient who is being given too large a minute volume or who is tachypnoeic for any of the reasons mentioned above.

Electrolytes

Sodium and potassium are often measured as part of an automated biochemistry run, although many ICUs will have a separate electrolyte analyser that works on the principle of ion-selective electrodes.

These analysers may be more accurate for potassium measurements than for sodium. Their advantage is obviously their immediacy.

Hyponatraemia has a variety of causes (Jamieson 1985), but is more commonly caused by relative excess of water than deficiency of sodium. This is often iatrogenic, following excessive administration of hypotonic fluids. Another common cause is the syndrome of inappropriate antidiuretic hormone (ADH) secretion, in which ADH is secreted despite hypotonicity of the serum. The result is water retention and, thereby, hyponatraemia. The causes of this syndrome are numerous and include malignancies, pulmonary disorders, and disturbances of central nervous system function.

Hypernatraemia is most often caused by water depletion. A true sodium excess is uncommon and is always iatrogenic. Both hyponatraemia and hypernatraemia may cause neurological signs ranging from confusion to coma.

Hypokalaemia, on the other hand, is potentially far more dangerous. It may predispose to cardiac arrhythmias, especially if combined with hypoxaemia. Hyperkalaemia may predispose to ventricular tachycardia and fibrillation. Physiotherapy treatment may have to be postponed until these abnormalities have been corrected.

Glucose

This needs to be regularly monitored in diabetics and in all critically ill patients. Blood glucose can easily be measured in the ward by means of reagent strips. A very high blood glucose level is almost always caused by diabetes mellitus or an intravenous infusion of high glucose content, while a slightly raised value may be caused by stress. The causes of a low blood glucose include starvation, liver failure (failure to produce glucose), insulin therapy, or an insulin-secreting tumour.

Renal function tests

These include urea and creatinine. Urea is formed mainly from protein breakdown and creatinine mainly from muscle breakdown; there are obligatory amounts of both of these that need to be handled by the kidneys daily. If formation

increases or excretion decreases, serum levels will rise. Renal failure causes both urea and creatinine to rise, though often at different rates. In hypovolaemic or low cardiac output states, urea rises more than creatinine, whilst in rhabdomyolysis (breakdown of skeletal muscle) creatinine rises faster than urea.

Liver function tests

Very few so-called 'liver function tests' actually measure liver function. Instead they simply represent the result of liver damage: raised enzymes reflect damage to cells and raised bilirubin may reflect a variety of abnormalities, not all of which actually occur in the liver.

Enzymes such as lactate dehydrogenase (LDH) and aspartate aminotransferase (AST) are not specific to liver tissue, and even when they are produced by damaged liver cells give little clue to the underlying pathology. Gamma glutamyl transferase (GGT) and alanine aminotransferase (ALT) are found in few other tissues, but again do not reflect causation. Alkaline phosphatase (ALP) is also not specific to liver cells, but that fraction which comes from the liver is concentrated in bile ducts and, as such, gives a clue to biliary disease or obstruction.

Bilirubin is a pigment that is produced from the breakdown of haem (from the haemoglobin in red blood cells). The liver takes up circulating bilirubin, conjugates it and excretes it in bile via the biliary tract. The clinical manifestation of a raised plasma bilirubin level is jaundice. In most hepatic disorders, both the conjugated and unconjugated fractions of bilirubin are raised. However, a predominantly unconjugated hyperbilirubinaemia (raised levels of unconjugated bilirubin in the blood) is often due to massive breakdown of red blood cells as in haemolysis or haematoma. Conjugated hyperbilirubinaemia is commonly seen in hepatitis or biliary tract obstruction; in the latter the classical clinical triad of dark urine, pale stools, and pruritis is seen.

In critical illness, two distinct syndromes of liver dysfunction have been described (Hawker 1991). These are ischaemic hepatitis, occurring early and characterized by a massive rise in AST and ALT with only a slight rise in bilirubin, and ICU jaundice which develops later, is part of the syndrome of multiple organ failure, and is characterized by a massive rise in bilirubin with only a slight enzyme rise.

Tests that reflect the synthetic capacity of the liver are more useful in determining actual liver function. Protein synthesis is one of the major functions of the liver; these proteins include clotting factors, albumin, and globulins. Thus, measuring the INR (see above) and serum albumin can give a good idea of the synthetic function of the liver, provided there are no other reasons for these tests to be abnormal.

Cardiac enzymes

Enzymes are released by all damaged muscle cells. Cardiac enzyme estimations are therefore performed to confirm myocardial damage, usually caused by a myocardial infarct but occasionally caused by chest trauma. There is a characteristic pattern of enzyme rise, with creatine kinase (CK) rising first, followed by AST and then LDH. For more specificity, isoenzymes (specific fractions of the enzymes) of CK and LDH may be measured. CK is also present in skeletal muscle, so the myocardial fraction (MB fraction) is measured to exclude skeletal muscle damage (from surgery, trauma, or intramuscular injections) as a source. LDH is present in many other tissues, including skeletal muscle, red blood cells, liver, and lung. The LD1 and LD2 fractions are specific for cardiac muscle or red blood cells (the distinction is easily made clinically).

Electrical cardioversion has been said to cause CK (and specifically the MB fraction) to rise. This may be important in determining whether a patient has had a myocardial infarct. The evidence is that measurable myocardial damage rarely follows cardioversion, and that when CK MB is raised, the elevation is small (Ehsani et al 1976).

Microbiology

Blood cultures

These are usually taken when the patient is pyrexial, in an attempt to isolate microorganisms which may be present in the bloodstream. The blood is drawn (usually from a forearm vein) in strictly aseptic conditions, placed in a special culture medium, incubated at 37°C, and then cultured in the laboratory. A positive result is almost always of serious consequence, although contaminants may occur, usually from poor aseptic technique. A positive blood culture does not identify the site of sepsis, although the type of organism cultured may give a clue. The source of the sepsis needs to be found and dealt with in its own right.

Sputum/tracheal aspirate

Sputum is produced when a non-intubated patient coughs up pulmonary secretions, while a tracheal aspirate is a suctioned specimen from an endotracheal tube or tracheostomy. There is always a risk that a sputum specimen may contain mainly saliva, and that it may be contaminated by oral organisms. Tracheal aspirates, on the other hand, represent the microflora of the lower airways, and are much less likely to be contaminated, although after prolonged mechanical ventilation the tracheobronchial tree is often colonized by oral organisms. Physiotherapists are often requested to obtain these specimens, upon which future treatment may be based, and great care should be taken to get adequate and representative samples.

Newer methods of obtaining uncontaminated specimens which accurately reflect the microbiology of a specific lung segment include protected specimen brushing with quantitative colony counts (Fagon et al 1988) and bronchoalveolar lavage (Kahn & Jones 1987).

A sputum or tracheal aspirate specimen is stained with Gram's stain, examined under a microscope, and cultured. Antibiotic sensitivities are performed on a positive culture. One must be aware that the presence of organisms on tracheal aspirate may not be indicative of pulmonary infection, but may simply represent colonization. To make the diagnosis of pulmonary infection (and, therefore, to start antibiotics) one needs to have most of the following criteria: purulent secretions, white blood cells on Gram's stain of tracheal aspirate, organisms on culture of tracheal aspirate, fever, raised white blood cell count, infiltrates on the chest radiograph, and a reduction in PaO_2.

Community acquired pneumonia has been well studied in many countries and the organisms accounting for most cases have been established. *Streptococcus pneumoniae* is the commonest organism by far, followed by *Mycoplasma pneumoniae* (in epidemics) and influenza virus. The logical antibiotic management of community acquired pneumonia has been described (Harrison et al 1987).

Diagnosis of pneumonia in a patient already on a ventilator is often much more difficult, although some of the newer diagnostic methods mentioned above are useful (Meduri 1990). Clinical judgement may still be necessary to differentiate colonization from infection.

Swabs and specimens from other sites

These may be taken from superficial wounds or from deep sites. Positive superficial cultures may represent skin colonization, so it is important to look for local (redness, pus) and systemic (pyrexia, raised white blood cell count) evidence of sepsis before starting antibiotic therapy. Local therapy with frequent cleaning and dressings is usually all that is required for superficial sepsis. Specimens obtained from needle aspiration or during operative procedures (i.e. from the abdominal cavity or chest) are not likely to represent colonization, and such infections cannot be treated topically—surgical drainage and antibiotic therapy are needed.

Urine

Urine specimens may be contaminated with perineal flora, so they are either taken by a midstream urine collection with strict attention to aseptic technique or from a urinary catheter. The urine is spun down in a centrifuge, and then stained, examined, and cultured in the same way as sputum. Although patients with long-term indwelling urinary catheters may develop bacterial bladder colonization with no clinical consequence, in other patients urinary tract infections may be a considerable source of morbidity.

REFERENCES

Bick R L 1988 Disseminated intravascular coagulation and related syndromes: a clinical review. Seminars in Thrombosis and Haemostasis 14: 299–338

Clark J S, Votteri B, Ariagno R L et al 1992 State of the art. Noninvasive assessment of blood gases. American Review of Respiratory Disease 145: 220–232

Cooper D J, Walley K R, Wiggs B R, Russell J A 1990 Bicarbonate does not improve haemodynamics in critically ill patients who have lactic acidosis. Annals of Internal Medicine 112: 492–498

Ehsani A, Ewy G A, Sobel B E 1976 Effects of electrical countershock on serum creatine phosphokinase (CPK) isoenzyme activity. American Journal of Cardiology 37: 12–18

Fagon J Y, Chastre J, Hance A J et al 1988 Detection of nosocomial lung infection in ventilated patients: use of a protected specimen brush and quantitative culture techniques in 147 patients. American Review of Respiratory Disease 138: 110–116

Garradd J, Bullock M 1986 The effect of respiratory therapy on intracranial pressure in ventilated neurosurgical patients. The Australian Journal of Physiotherapy 32: 107–111

Hammon W E, Connors A F, McCaffree 1992 Cardiac arrhythmias during postural drainage and chest percussion of critically ill patients. Chest 102: 1836–1841

Harrison B D W, Farr B M, Connolly C K et al 1987 The hospital management of community-acquired pneumonia. Recommendations of the British Thoracic Society. Journal of the Royal College of Physicians of London 21: 267–269

Hawker F 1991 Liver dysfunction in critical illness. Anaesthesia and Intensive Care 19: 165–181

Jamieson M J 1985 Clinical algorithms. Hyponatremia. British Medical Journal 290: 1723–1728

Kahn F W, Jones J M 1987 Diagnosing bacterial respiratory infection by bronchoalveolar lavage. Journal of lnfectious Disease 155: 855–861

Meduri G U 1990 Ventilator-associated pneumonia in patients with respiratory failure. A diagnostic approach. Chest 97: 1208–1219

Raper R, Sibbald W J 1986 Misled by the wedge? The Swan–Ganz catheter and left ventricular preload. Chest 89: 427–434

Ritter J M, Doktor H S, Benjamin N 1990 Paradoxical effect of bicarbonate on cytoplasmic pH. Lancet 335: 1243–1246

Tyler M L 1982 Complications of positioning and chest physiotherapy. Respiratory Care 27: 458–466

FURTHER READING

Hampton J R 1986 The ECG in practice. Churchill
  Livingstone, Edinburgh
Rapaport S I 1987 Introduction to haematology, 2nd edn.
  Lippincott, Philadelphia
Sherlock S 1988 Diseases of the liver and biliary system.
  Blackwell Scientific, Oxford

Volk W A, Benjamin D C, Kadner R J, Parsons J T 1991
  Essentials of medical microbiology, 4th edn. Lippincott,
  Philadelphia
Zilva J F, Pannall P R, Mayne P D 1988 Clinical chemistry
  in diagnosis and treatment, 5th edn. Edward Arnold,
  London

5. Mechanical support

John S. Turner

INTRODUCTION

Medical technology has advanced in quantum leaps over the last 40–50 years and efficient mechanical support of lungs, heart, and kidneys is now available. The gastrointestinal tract may be supported by means of total parenteral nutrition and the haemopoeietic system by cell transfusion and colony-stimulating factors (such as granulocyte-macrophage colony-stimulating factor). There is as yet no effective form of hepatic support, although liver transplantation is being performed in the acute setting as is heart and lung transplantation. The indications for these dramatic and heroic measures are however limited.

This chapter covers respiratory, cardiac, and renal support, with most of the emphasis being placed on respiratory support including newer forms of ventilation and weaning.

RESPIRATORY SUPPORT

Respiratory failure is usually defined as the inability to maintain a PaO_2 of more than 8 kPa (60 mmHg) or a $PaCO_2$ of less than 6 kPa (45 mmHg). The causes are numerous and some of the more common ones are listed below in the section on indications for mechanical ventilation. Respiratory support aims to correct these biochemical abnormalities. This can be performed in a number of ways.

Oxygen therapy

Oxygen is delivered by means of face mask or nasal cannulae. Oxygen therapy will correct the majority of less severe cases of hypoxia, but obviously cannot correct hypercarbia.

Continuous positive airway pressure

In the technique of continuous positive airway pressure (CPAP), oxygen is delivered by a system that maintains a positive pressure in the circuitry and airways throughout inspiration and expiration. CPAP is useful in cases where lung volumes are reduced, in particular the functional residual capacity (Fig. 5.1). Examples of this include subsegmental lung collapse, pneumonia, and adult respiratory distress syndrome. Again hypercarbia cannot be corrected and may be worsened as dead-space ventilation may be increased. CPAP usually improves ventilation–perfusion (V/Q) mismatch and, by improving lung compliance, it may reduce the work of breathing.

There are two basic methods of providing

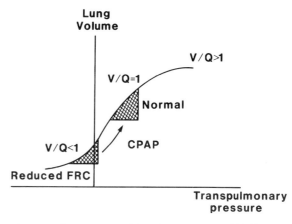

Fig. 5.1 Continuous positive airway pressure (CPAP) increases a reduced functional residual capacity (FRC).

83

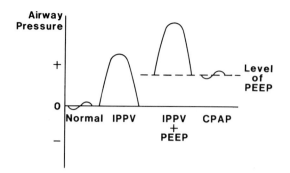

Fig. 5.2   Pressure–time curves of various modes of ventilation.

CPAP: continuous-flow or demand-flow. Continuous-flow systems have gas flowing through the circuit throughout the respiratory cycle. A high gas flow (50–100 l/min) is necessary to maintain this flow during the initial phase of inspiration. There is no demand valve to open, but the system is noisy and uses large volumes of oxygen and air. On the other hand, demand-flow systems (including the CPAP mode on ventilators) allow gas to flow only when inspiration is initiated and a demand valve is thereby opened. This is a quieter system and uses less gas, but a certain amount of work is required of the patient in order to open the demand valve. Some systems are worse than others in this regard (Bersten et al 1989), although a modification of the demand-flow system known as 'flow-by' seems to present the patient with little additional work. This system is not widely available at present. When CPAP is combined with positive pressure ventilation, it is generally known as 'positive end expiratory pressure' (PEEP) (Fig. 5.2).

Conventional mechanical ventilation

Mechanical ventilation has evolved from negative pressure ventilators used in the polio epidemic of the 1950s. Positive pressure ventilators that followed are now controlled by sophisticated microprocessor technology. The physiology, principles and practice of mechanical ventilation have recently been reviewed (Hubmayr et al 1990, Schuster 1990).

The basic principles of how a ventilator works remain unchanged. Very simply, *inspiration* may be generated by application of either a constant pressure or a constant flow of gas to the lungs, and *expiration* may be allowed when either a set pressure has been reached, a set volume has been delivered, or a set time has passed. Modern ventilators have a variety of ventilation modes which allow for comfortable patient–ventilator interaction. Ventilation modes commonly employed and available on most modern ventilators include the following:

1. *Controlled mandatory ventilation (CMV)* — here the patient has no control over ventilation. Breaths are delivered at a rate and volume that are determined by adjusting the ventilator controls, regardless of the patient's attempts to breathe. If the patient is not unconscious or paralysed, CMV may be extremely uncomfortable.

2. *Intermittent mandatory ventilation (IMV)* — here respiratory rate and tidal volume are set as above, but the patient may breathe spontaneously between the mandatory breaths, which still are delivered at the preset regular intervals.

3. *Synchronized intermittent mandatory ventilation (SIMV)* — the mandatory breaths are delivered in synchrony with the patient's breathing. Again the patient may breathe on his own, but the mandatory breaths will be delivered at a time in the ventilatory cycle that is convenient for the patient (a breath will therefore not be delivered while the patient is breathing out). Patient comfort is improved.

4. *Inspiratory pressure support (IPS)* — this is a relatively new ventilatory technique, introduced in 1981. Its use and application have not yet been fully evaluated, and remain controversial (Kacmarek 1989). It is a pressure-limited form of ventilation, with each breath being triggered by the patient. Once a breath is triggered, a flow of gas enters the circuit, with the pressure rapidly reaching the preset level. This pressure is maintained until the flow decreases to a ventilator-specific level, at which time expiration is allowed. The patient has full control over the respiratory rate. IPS can deliver the same level of ventilation (as assessed by gas exchange) as SIMV, often with lower peak airway pressures, as long as the patient has an adequate respiratory drive. Alone or in combination with SIMV, it can make ventilation more comfortable for the

patient. Theoretically, by allowing some degree of muscle training without permitting fatigue, IPS would be helpful in weaning patients from mechanical ventilation. To date, clinical trials addressing this issue have shown conflicting results.

Non-invasive ventilation

Non-invasive ventilation (ventilation without an endotracheal tube or tracheostomy) can be delivered by negative or positive pressure techniques. Negative pressure ventilation is epitomized in the large and frightening 'iron lung', used in the 1950s for the ventilation of patients with poliomyelitis. Newer and much more compact and comfortable negative pressure ventilators are now available (Shneerson 1991), and domiciliary ventilation with them is feasible.

Nasal intermittent positive pressure ventilation (NIPPV) was originally used for nocturnal ventilation of patients with advanced chronic lung disease (usually with hypercarbia). A number of patients were well enough to be treated at home, so ventilators were designed for domiciliary use. These are compact, simple to use, and run off an air compressor. More recently, NIPPV has been used in acute respiratory failure from various causes, but mainly in patients with chronic obstructive airways disease (COAD) (Elliott et al 1990). A recent review (Branthwaite 1991) covers the practical aspects of this form of ventilation. Although the purpose-built machines are the most popular, almost any mechanical ventilator can be used for NIPPV. All that is needed is the ability to deliver a tidal volume at a rate that may also allow spontaneous respiration. Alarms for low pressure (caused by disconnection) and apnoea are useful. Indications are being reviewed and revised all the time. The majority of patients selected for NIPPV only require ventilatory assistance at night (often at home) and include those with chronic respiratory failure from thoracic deformity, COAD, and static or slowly progressive neuromuscular disease. Patients with high spinal cord lesions may be ventilated for most if not all of the day. Patients with acute respiratory failure in COAD may also be candidates for NIPPV.

Indications for mechanical ventilation

The indications for ventilation vary for different disorders and are rarely absolute. In practical (and somewhat simplistic) terms they include the following.

Adult respiratory distress syndrome. A patient who has a PaO_2 of less than 8 kPa (60 mmHg) on oxygen and CPAP.

Pneumonia. A patient who is unable to clear secretions or who has a PaO_2 of less than 8 kPa (60 mmHg) on oxygen and CPAP.

Asthma. A patient who is becoming exhausted or confused, usually with a rising $PaCO_2$.

Chronic obstructive airways disease. Similar to asthma, but a higher $PaCO_2$ may be normal for the patient.

Respiratory muscle weakness. A patient who is unable to clear secretions, who has lost bulbar function, or who cannot produce a vital capacity of more than 15 ml/kg.

Blunt chest trauma. A patient who, despite adequate analgesia, cannot produce a vital capacity of more than 15 ml/kg, or is unable to clear secretions, or who has a PaO_2 of less than 8 kPa (60 mmHg) on oxygen and CPAP.

Pulmonary oedema. This is largely a clinical decision, as pulmonary oedema tends to improve very quickly with appropriate medical treatment. Patients who are moribund or not responding to treatment will need ventilation, as will patients who have had a large myocardial infarct.

Other system involvement. Patients may be ventilated simply to support the respiratory system when they have a life-threatening disorder of another system, e.g. multiple trauma or septic shock.

Elective postoperative ventilation. Some patients may be electively ventilated postoperatively, either because of the magnitude of the surgery or because they have impaired pulmonary function.

Aims and complications of respiratory support

The first and most important aim of respiratory support is to oxygenate the patient. This is initially done by increasing the inspired oxygen concentration. Oxygen concentrations of above 50% are toxic to the lungs if used for any length of time, with toxicity increasing exponentially as the concentration rises further. Positive end expiratory pressure (PEEP) may be added to improve oxygenation. Once levels of PEEP above 10 cmH$_2$O are used, a pulmonary artery catheter may be needed to measure oxygen delivery. PEEP may depress cardiac output more than it improves oxygenation, and oxygen delivery may therefore be compromised. Increasing the inspiratory time to allow for higher mean airway pressures but lower peak inspiratory pressure (PIP) may improve oxygenation. Sedation and occasionally muscle relaxants may be necessary to ventilate a critically ill patient.

Barotrauma, which is related to PIP, needs to be avoided. There is no pressure which is absolutely safe, but barotrauma occurs with significant frequency once the PIP exceeds 50 cmH$_2$O, and increases exponentially as pressures rise above this level. Manoeuvres to lower PIP include reducing the tidal volume, reducing PEEP, and allowing a longer inspiratory time.

The importance of carbon dioxide removal has decreased recently. Patients with severe respiratory failure have been ventilated in a way that allows the $PaCO_2$ to rise to up to 8 kPa (60 mmHg) or more (Hickling et al 1990). This concept of 'permissive hypercapnia' has been used in a variety of situations and generally allows a smaller tidal volume and minute volume to be used, reducing the incidence of barotrauma and oxygen toxicity.

Patient comfort and acceptability can be achieved by carefully matching patient and ventilator. Tidal volume, rate, and inspiratory time can be manipulated to make the patient comfortable. This is an art, and demands patience and understanding. Occasionally, sedation is needed, but this should be a last resort.

Respiratory support is not without complications, some of which are minor and some of which may be lethal. The more commonly occurring complications include barotrauma, haemodynamic disturbances, nosocomial infections, alteration in gastrointestinal motility, and a positive fluid balance (Pingleton 1988).

Weaning from respiratory support

Criteria for weaning from mechanical ventilation were first described in the 1970s. They are adequate in most cases, but their relatively high failure rate has led investigators to look at other predictors of a successful wean. These include work of breathing (Fiastro et al 1988), and more recently the 'CROP index' and rapid shallow breathing index (Yang & Tobin 1991). The latter is simple to perform and is by far the most practically useful of the above. It is calculated by allowing the patient to breathe room air through a spirometer for 1 minute while the respiratory rate is counted. The minute volume (measured on the spirometer) is divided by the respiratory rate to give an average tidal volume. The index is calculated by dividing the respiratory rate by the tidal volume (in litres). Weaning is unlikely with an index above 100, and likely with an index below 100.

Conventional weaning criteria involve clinical, mechanical, and biochemical parameters:

Clinical

- The clinical condition of the patient is improving.
- The patient is cooperative and alert and able to clear secretions.
- There is no abdominal distension, cardiovascular instability, or likelihood of prolonged immobility.
- The respiratory rate is less than 30 breaths/min.

Mechanical

- Vital capacity is more than 15 ml/kg.
- Maximal inspiratory mouth pressure is more than 20 cmH$_2$O.
- Minute volume is less than 10L/min.

Biochemical

- Normal pH and $PaCO_2$.
- PaO_2 more than 8 kPa (60 mmHg) on no more than 40% oxygen and 5 cm PEEP.

Once the above criteria are satisfied, weaning may be started. Before and during the weaning period, meticulous attention needs to be paid to nutrition, electrolyte status, control of infection and bronchospasm, and mobilization of the patient. The last factor is probably the most important, and the physiotherapist will be very involved in sitting and then standing and walking the patient. Even patients with many lines, tubes, and catheters can be mobilized with a little ingenuity. Weaning can be performed in two different ways. Either the proportion of breathing performed by the ventilator can be gradually reduced, letting the patient perform a greater and greater amount of breathing until he is independent of the ventilator (IMV was the first ventilatory mode to allow this), or the patient can be allowed to breathe spontaneously for progressively longer periods with full ventilation between them (the so-called 'T-piece method'). Both methods have their proponents, although there is probably little to choose between them. The latter method is commonly used in difficult weans.

Common problems which may cause difficulties with weaning (Branthwaite 1988) include the following:

- Impaired ventilatory drive.
- Upper and lower airway incompetence, obstruction, or secretions.
- Lung parenchymal fluid or infection.
- Pleural effusion or pneumothorax.
- Chest wall abnormality, instability, or respiratory muscle weakness.
- Electrolyte or nutritional problems.
- Cardiovascular insufficiency.

Unconventional respiratory support

Less conventional modes of respiratory support include extracorporeal membrane oxygenation (ECMO), extracorporeal carbon dioxide removal (ECCO$_2$R), intravenacaval oxygenation (IVOX) and high frequency jet ventilation (HFJV). These modes are only available in major centres, are costly and extremely labour intensive, and have not yet been shown in controlled studies to hold any advantage over conventional ventilation (Evans & Keogh 1991). They have their enthusiasts however, and in their hands the results are impressive.

Extracorporeal membrane oxygenation

This is a well established and useful technique in neonatal respiratory distress syndrome, but has not shown advantages over conventional ventilation in controlled trials in adults. However, it may still be a useful technique for short periods, especially as a bridge to transplantation, an indication for which it has been used successfully. The technique involves a high-flow extracorporeal circuit from the inferior vena cava to the aorta using cannulae in the femoral vein and artery. A membrane oxygenator is used in the circuit to provide oxygenation and carbon dioxide removal. The extracorporeal blood flow is up to 80% of the cardiac output, and vital organs may be poorly perfused with non-pulsatile blood flow.

Extracorporeal carbon dioxide removal

An uncontrolled trial has shown startling results with the ECCO$_2$R technique (Gattinoni et al 1986), with a survival rate of 47% in 55 patients with adult respiratory distress syndrome in whom the mortality was predicted to be more than 90%. A low flow venovenous circuit is used with a membrane oxygenator and the patient is ventilated at a slow rate with very small tidal volumes. Complications are less common than with ECMO. A controlled trial comparing ECCO$_2$R with conventional ventilation is currently being performed.

Complications of extracorporeal gas exchange (ECMO and ECCO$_2$R) include haemorrhage, thrombosis and thromboembolism, sepsis, and multiple organ failure, although the latter complication may merely reflect the organ failure associated with the respiratory failure for which the technique is used.

Intravenacaval oxygenation

Intravenacaval oxygenation (IVOX) has been recently developed (Conrad et al 1993) and clinical trials still need to be performed. A catheter with multiple fine tubes within it is placed in the inferior vena cava. Oxygen is passed through these at subatmospheric pressure and gas exchange takes place by passive diffusion.

High frequency jet ventilation

In high frequency jet ventilation (HFJV), small

pulses of gas at a rate of 60–600 per minute are delivered from a jet nozzle at the proximal end of the endotracheal tube, with humidified warmed air being entrained from a bias gas source. Lung volume is maintained with a higher mean airway pressure, thereby improving oxygenation. There are several theories as to how gas exchange can occur with such an unphysiological method of ventilation. Diffusion of gas and regional convective currents seem to play a major role. Although a controlled clinical trial has shown no advantage over conventional ventilation (Carlon et al 1983), the technique has been shown to be safe, and newer computer controlled prototypes are showing promise.

CARDIAC SUPPORT

Even before heart transplantation was pioneered in 1967, the need for an artificial heart had been identified. This could be used for short-term support of the heart while waiting for it to recover from an acute insult (such as myocardial infarction or cardiac surgery) or for a donor heart to become available for transplantation, or for long-term cardiac support. There are modalities available which provide partial to complete support, but they are expensive and may have significant side-effects.

Intra-aortic balloon pump

The intra-aortic balloon pump (IABP) comprises a sausage-shaped balloon (15 mm × 280 mm and inflated by 40 ml of gas) mounted on a dual-lumen catheter. The balloon is introduced via the femoral artery, either percutaneously or by surgical dissection and direct vision, to the thoracic aorta (Fig. 5.3). Correct positioning of the catheter is confirmed by fluoroscopy or chest radiography. The catheter is attached to a console with a helium gas source for balloon inflation. The IABP is triggered by the electrocardiogram (ECG) to deflate during ventricular systole and to inflate during diastole. By so doing it improves cardiac performance (the left ventricle ejects into an 'empty' aorta) and improves myocardial perfusion (which occurs during diastole and is

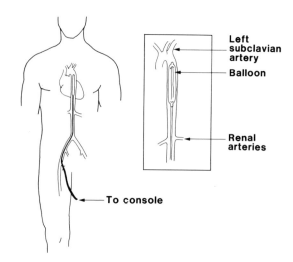

Fig. 5.3   Placement of the intra-aortic balloon pump.

enhanced by the blood not running off into the aorta).

Indications for the use of the IABP include cardiogenic shock (after myocardial infarction), unstable angina, weaning from cardiopulmonary bypass, and stabilization of patients with acute mitral regurgitation or ventricular septal defect following myocardial infarction. In these cases it is used as a bridge to definitive surgery, although the mortality for these defects remains in the region of 50%. The IABP cannot generate a cardiac output independent of the heart, and a minimum cardiac output of about 1.5 L/min is needed for it to be effective.

The IABP is clearly a major invasive device, and complications may be serious. They include aortic dissection, arterial perforation, limb ischaemia, thrombocytopenia, and dislodgement of atherosclerotic emboli. Air embolism may occur if the balloon bursts. Major bleeding may occur following removal of the IABP.

Ventricular assist device

A ventricular assist device (VAD) is simply a pump that functions in parallel with the heart. Blood is withdrawn from the venous side of the circulation and returned to the arterial side, usually with a catheter in the left atrium and the left ventricle (left ventricular assist device or LVAD). Occasionally, both sides of the heart need support and this is achieved with a biventricular assist device (BIVAD). The VAD can provide most of the cardiac output, but the flow it delivers is not pulsatile, which may adversely affect vital organs such as the kidneys. Indications for its use include failure to wean from cardiopulmonary bypass (Adamson et al 1989) and bridging to heart transplantation (Hill 1989). It is not without significant complications, with haemorrhage, thromboembolism, and septicaemia being the most common.

RENAL SUPPORT

Before the advent of dialysis and transplantation, chronic renal failure (CRF) was invariably fatal and acute renal failure (ARF) usually fatal. Today, although ARF still carries a high mortality rate, especially when part of the complex of multiple organ failure, CRF can be effectively managed in dialysis and renal transplantation programmes.

The aims of renal support are very simple. They include control of fluid, electrolytes, and acid–base status, and elimination of uraemic toxins and drugs. These aims can be carried out in a number of ways which are detailed below.

General principles of dialysis

All forms of dialysis involve diffusion of solute across a semipermeable membrane and down a concentration gradient. In peritoneal dialysis the membrane is the peritoneum and the blood flow is provided by the capillaries supplying it. In all forms of haemodialysis, the membrane is composed of cellophane or cuprophane and blood flow is provided by an extracorporeal circuit.

Conventional haemodialysis

Haemodialysis (HD) was first described in 1960 and is now the most commonly used dialysis therapy for both ARF and CRF. Blood is pumped through an extracorporeal system which includes a filter with a semipermeable membrane, and dialysate (usually water mixed with predetermined concentrations of electrolyes and buffer)

flows in a countercurrent direction through the filter, on the other side of the membrane. A gradient is thus created for electrolytes and metabolic waste products to diffuse across the membrane, and fluid is driven across by hydrostatic pressure.

Vascular access is obtained by intravenous catheters or by the surgical creation of arteriovenous fistulae or shunts. HD is generally performed for 4–6 hours at a time, either daily or on alternate days. Although HD allows rapid correction of fluid and electrolyte abnormalities, it may not be well tolerated in critically ill, haemodynamically unstable patients. Hypotension may develop and cause further ischaemic insult to the kidney. Hypoxaemia almost invariably occurs; it is caused by neutrophil aggregation in the lungs and complement activation in the filter membrane.

Continuous forms of renal support

Conventional haemodialysis is not well tolerated in critically ill patients as it may produce rapid changes in intravascular volume, blood pressure, PaO_2, and pH. Slower but continuous forms of haemodialysis were developed to address this problem. The terminology is confusing; terms such as CAVH, CAVHD, CVVH, and CVVHD (see below) perplex the uninitiated. The treatment choices differ in several ways (Schetz et al 1989). Access to the circulation may be by both arterial and venous cannulae (arteriovenous) or by venous cannulae (venovenous). The blood flow through the circuit may be pumped by an external pump or by the patient's own arterial pressure as in arteriovenous systems. Pure haemofiltration may be performed, or may be combined with dialysis (Fig. 5.4). Whatever the method, the extracorporeal circuit needs to be anticoagulated to prevent the blood from clotting.

Continuous haemofiltration

In continuous haemofiltration (Paradiso 1989), blood flow in the extracorporeal circuit may be driven by a pump with vascular access provided by venous catheters (continuous venovenous

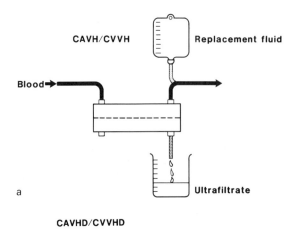

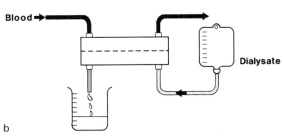

Fig. 5.4 Continuous renal support: the concepts of filtration and dialysis. **a** Haemofiltration alone. **b** Haemofiltration with dialysis.

haemofiltration or CVVH) or may be driven by the patient's own arterial pressure with an arterial and a venous catheter (continuous arteriovenous haemofiltration or CAVH). The hydrostatic pressure created in either system drives filtrate through the semipermeable membrane. This filtrate is essentially plasma water, but as it moves across the membrane it drags solutes with it by the process of convection. Large amounts of filtrate may be removed (up to 1 L/hour), and this fluid (the ultrafiltrate) is replaced with a fluid that has an electrolyte composition similar to plasma.

Continuous haemofiltration with dialysis

The terminology for continuous haemofiltration with dialysis (Miller et al 1990) is similar to the above, with the variants being continuous veno-venous haemofiltration with dialysis (CVVHD) and continuous arteriovenous haemofiltration with dialysis (CAVHD). Here dialysis fluid is pumped through the filter in a countercurrent

direction to the blood flow (similar to HD outlined above). Greater solute clearance can be achieved, and as the hydrostatic pressure does not need to be as high as in CVVH, less ultrafiltrate is formed and less replacement fluid is needed. As CAVHD does not involve actively pumping blood into the extracorporeal circuit, it can be used in haemodynamically very unstable patients and is probably the technique of choice in that situation.

Peritoneal dialysis

The peritoneum is an excellent semi-permeable membrane and is used as such in peritoneal dialysis (PD). A catheter is inserted percutaneously into the peritoneal cavity and dialysate (usually 1–2 L) is allowed to run in, remain in the peritoneal cavity for a period of time, and then run out. Dialysate comes in premixed bags and its composition allows for the removal of electrolytes and uraemic waste products. Solute clearance is determined by dialysate flow rate, peritoneal permeability, peritoneal vascularity, and blood flow. Dialysate with a high glucose concentration allows large amounts of fluid to be removed by osmosis.

The most common complication of PD is abdominal discomfort caused by raised intra-abdominal pressure and splinting of the diaphragm; this may result in basal subsegmental lung collapse and hypoxaemia. Peritonitis is a more serious problem, and usually relates to contamination of the dialysate at the time of bag changes. Prompt recognition and the instillation of intraperitoneal antibiotics are the mainstays of treatment. Other complications include bowel perforation (usually at the time of catheter insertion) and hyperglycaemia.

The main advantage of PD is that correction of fluid and metabolic abnormalities is gradual and there is minimal haemodynamic disturbance (although ventilation may be compromised by the intra-abdominal fluid). However, clearance of uraemic toxins is generally less efficient than with HD, and this may be a problem in critically ill hypermetabolic patients. In addition, PD cannot be used in patients with acute intra-abdominal pathology or recent abdominal surgery.

Indications for renal support

Acute renal failure

The indications for renal support in acute renal failure are generally based on clinical parameters rather than on biochemistry alone. They include the speed of deterioration of renal function, the general clinical scenario, and the likely rapidity of recovery. Absolute indications for urgent renal support are fluid overload, hyperkalaemia, or acidosis unresponsive to conventional treatment. The urea and creatinine values are useful as a guide to starting renal support, but absolute values are controversial. As a rough rule, dialysis is often started when urea is greater than 40 mmol/l, creatinine is greater than 500 μmol/l, or when potassium is greater than 6 mmol/l.

Chronic renal failure

The decision to initiate renal support in a patient with chronic renal failure is usually made by the renal unit in a major hospital. It is almost always coupled with entering the patient onto a waiting list for renal transplantation, using renal support as a bridge until a live-related or cadaver transplant can be performed. Patients are fully assessed for their suitability to enter such a programme by a team that generally includes physicians, nurses, a social worker, and a psychiatrist.

Potential hazards for physiotherapists

Mechanical problems

These include kinking of support lines, disconnection of different parts of the circuit and, worst of all, displacement of catheters from artery or vein. The former will cause the system to stop functioning or to function less well, but the latter can cause spectacular haemorrhage which may be fatal if not noticed immediately. Disconnection may also cause air embolism. Great care should therefore be taken when moving patients on dialysis.

Haemodynamic

Patients on renal support may be relatively intravascularly fluid depleted and changes in posture may produce hypotension and, occasionally, cardiac arrhythmias.

Infection

Renal failure produces a state of relative immunosuppression with patients being more susceptible to infection. Meticulous care therefore needs to be taken with sterile techniques such as suctioning and even manual hyperinflation.

Respiratory

Patients on dialysis are prone to hypoxaemia (for the reasons mentioned above) and may desaturate rapidly during suctioning or turning.

REFERENCES

Adamson R M, Dembitsky W P, Reichman R T et al 1989 Mechanical support: assist or nemesis? Journal of Thoracic and Cardiovascular Surgery 98: 915–921

Bersten A D, Rutten A J, Vedig A E, Skowronski G A 1989 Additional work of breathing imposed by endotracheal tubes, breathing circuits, and intensive care ventilators. Critical Care Medicine 17: 671–677

Branthwaite M A 1988 Problems in practice. Getting a patient off the ventilator. British Journal of Diseases of the Chest 82: 16–22

Branthwaite M A 1991 Non-invasive and domiciliary ventilation: positive pressure techniques. Thorax 46: 208–212

Carlon G C, Howland W S, Ray C et al 1983 High frequency jet ventilation. A prospective randomised evaluation. Chest 84: 551–559

Conrad S A, Eggerstede J M, Morris V F, Romero M D 1993 Prolonged intracorporeal support of gas exchange with an intravenacaval oxygenator. Chest 103: 158–161

Elliott M W, Steven M H, Phillips G D, Branthwaite M A 1990 Non-invasive mechanical ventilation for acute respiratory failure. British Medical Journal 300: 358–360

Evans T W, Keogh B F 1991 Extracorporeal membrane oxygenation: a breath of fresh air or yesterday's treatment. Thorax 46: 692–694

Fiastro J F, Habib M P, Shon B Y, Campbell S C 1988 Comparison of standard weaning parameters and the mechanical work of breathing in mechanically ventilated patients. Chest 94: 232–238

Gattinoni L, Pesenti A, Mascheroni D et al 1986 Low frequency positive pressure ventilation with extracorporeal

CO_2 removal in severe acute respiratory failure. Journal of the American Medical Association 256: 881–886

Hickling K G, Henderson S J, Jackson R 1990 Low mortality associated with low volume pressure limited ventilation with permissive hypercapnia in severe adult respiratory distress syndrome. Intensive Care Medicine 16: 372–377

Hill J D 1989 Bridging to cardiac transplantation. Annals of Thoracic Surgery 47: 167–171

Hubmayr R D, Abel M D, Rehder K 1990 Physiologic approach to mechanical ventilation. Critical Care Medicine 18: 103–113

Kacmarek R M 1989 Inspiratory pressure support: does it make a clinical difference? Intensive Care Medicine 15: 337–339

Miller R, Kingswood C, Bullen C, Cohen S 1990 Renal replacement therapy in the ICU: the role of continuous arteriovenous haemodialysis. British Journal of Hospital Medicine 43: 354–362

Paradiso C 1989 Hemofiltration: an alternative to dialysis. Heart & Lung 18: 282–290

Pingleton S K 1988 State of the art. Complications of acute respiratory failure. American Review of Respiratory Disease 137: 1463–1493

Schetz M, Lauwers P M, Ferdinande P 1989 Extracorporeal treatment of acute renal failure in the intensive care unit: a critical view. Intensive Care Medicine 15: 349–357

Schuster D P 1990 A physiologic approach to initiating, maintaining, and withdrawing ventilatory support during acute respiratory failure. The American Journal of Medicine 88: 268–278

Shneerson J M 1991 Non-invasive and domiciliary ventilation: negative pressure techniques. Thorax 46: 131–135

Yang K L, Tobin M J 1991 A prospective study of indexes predicting the outcome of trials of weaning from mechanical ventilation. New England Journal of Medicine 324: 1445–1450

6. Cardiopulmonary resuscitation

John S. Turner

INTRODUCTION

Cardiac or respiratory arrest, whether it occurs in the street, in hospital, or in the intensive care unit (ICU), has a dramatic impact on both the victim and the rescuers. It is common, being the leading cause of sudden death in the community, and is also potentially treatable in a large number of cases, as a review of several community-based studies has shown (Safar 1988). An estimated 100 000 deaths may be prevented annually in the USA by the swift application of cardiopulmonary resuscitation (CPR). For this to become a reality, intensive education amongst medical, nursing and paramedical personnel as well as the general public would be necessary. This sort of training is not unrealistic in developed countries: in Belgium, for example, more than 100 000 citizens were recently trained in CPR over a 2-year period.

Cardiopulmonary resuscitation is a relatively modern concept, with the first report on closed-chest cardiac massage being published over three decades ago (Kouwenhoven et al 1960). Techniques have been refined since then and standards and guidelines have been laid down (American Heart Association 1986). Although our understanding of the mechanics of CPR and the pathophysiology of cardiorespiratory arrest has improved (Krause et al 1986, Safar 1988, Pepe 1990), the basic principles remain the same. More recent guidelines show some differences (Holmberg et al 1992, Chamberlain et al 1992).

There is, however, a negative side to CPR. Many long-term survivors of out-of-hospital cardiac arrest suffer some degree of permanent brain damage (Abramson et al 1985, Levy et al 1985), which may be devastating and lead to enormous economic and emotional costs. Before the advent of CPR, none of these unfortunate victims would have survived.

RISK SITUATIONS

One scenario that every physiotherapist dreads is that of a patient having a cardiac or respiratory arrest during treatment. This is fortunately very rare, but it is vital to be aware of situations (most of which are specific to the ICU) where the risk is high. They include:

1. The patient who has had a recent myocardial infarct. The risk of arrhythmia, reinfarction or pulmonary oedema declines with time.

2. Any hypoxaemic patient, especially those needing high inspired oxygen concentrations and positive end expiratory pressure (PEEP). Procedures that may worsen hypoxaemia or precipitate arrhythmias include suctioning and turning the patient.

3. Patients with neuromuscular disorders, e.g. Guillain–Barré syndrome or tetanus. These patients are at high risk of autonomic instability and may develop sudden and dramatic hypotension and arrhythmias.

4. Mobilization of patients who have had a period of prolonged immobility or who are obese. These patients carry a high risk of deep venous thrombosis of the leg veins which may result in acute pulmonary embolism.

5. Patients with severe chronic obstructive pulmonary disease receiving nebulizer therapy. The high inspired oxygen concentration blunts hypoxic respiratory drive.

SUSPICION OF CARDIAC OR RESPIRATORY ARREST

Most cardiac arrests are unpredictable, especially when they occur out of the hospital. The following signs are suggestive, but not diagnostic, of cardiac or respiratory arrest. Recognition and confirmation are described in the next section.

- Sudden loss of consciousness or decrease in level of consciousness.
- Sudden loss of muscle tone.
- Change in patient's colour to a blue or grey hue.
- Gasping respiration or complete cessation of breathing.

RECOGNITION

Pulseless

Cardiac arrest may be recognized by pulselessness in any large artery. The carotid artery is usually the most reliable and accessible vessel. It can best be palpated just lateral to the trachea at about the level of the thyroid cartilage. Five to ten seconds should be allowed for palpation as the pulse may be weak, slow or irregular.

No respiration

Respiration may be detected by observing movement of the chest wall, hearing air moving out of the mouth and nose, and feeling flow of air from the mouth and nose. The absence of these signs indicates respiratory arrest.

Upper airway obstruction should always be excluded. After cardiopulmonary arrest the upper airway usually becomes obstructed by the tongue falling backwards into the pharynx, but upper airway obstruction by a foreign body may in fact be the cause of respiratory and then cardiac arrest. This is usually clearly evident as the victim makes vigorous and frantic respiratory efforts to no avail. Complete airway obstruction leaves the victim unable to speak, breathe or cough. He may clutch his neck and his face will become red and then blue. Without prompt management, unconsciousness and death will follow. This syndrome usually occurs during eating and has been termed 'the steakhouse syndrome' (as meat is the most common foreign body) or 'the café coronary' (as it is often mistaken for a heart attack).

The Heimlich manoeuvre (Heimlich 1975) may be life-saving in cases of upper airway obstruction. The rescuer gets behind the victim (who is usually in a sitting position), makes a fist with one hand and places it against the victim's abdomen just below the xiphisternum. The fist is then grasped by the other hand and pressed inwards with a quick upward thrust. The forced expiration so caused usually dislodges the foreign body.

RESUSCITATION

This may be divided into basic life support (BLS), as taught to civilians and paramedical personnel and practised in out-of-hospital cardiac arrests, and advanced life support (ALS) which is taught to doctors and specialized nurses, involves sophisticated ancillary equipment and techniques, and can only be performed in a hospital setting. The basic principles are summarized in Table 6.1.

Basic life support

The ABC of BLS is well known and represents the mainstay of treatment. CPR should be initiated immediately cardiac or respiratory arrest is recognized, as the brain cells begin suffering irreversible hypoxic damage within minutes of cessation of effective circulation. CPR should therefore be carried out at the site of collapse unless this is technically impossible, e.g. in a car, in a bath or swimming pool, or on a flight of stairs. CPR is exhausting, so help should be summoned as quickly as possible.

CPR should be taught and practised on one of the many manikins available specifically for this purpose. The following basic principles serve as an introduction.

A Airway

In the unconscious patient the airway may be blocked by the tongue or a foreign body such as food, vomitus, blood or false teeth. It is essential to check manually and by direct vision for such foreign bodies and to remove them with a finger

Table 6.1   Basic principles of cardiopulmonary resuscitation

Basic life support (BLS)

	Without equipment	With equipment
Airway	Manual airway clearance Head-tilt/chin-lift	Airway suction Guedel airway Endotracheal tube
Breathing	Mouth-to-mouth	Bag ventilation Ventilator
Circulation	Chest compression	Chest compression

Advanced life support (ALS)

Drugs		IV line Adrenaline
ECG		ECG monitoring
Fibrillation		Defibrillation

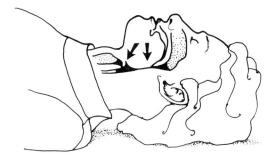

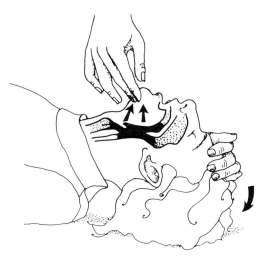

Fig. 6.1   The head-tilt/chin-lift manoeuvre.

or piece of clothing before resuscitation is started. The airway should then be opened by applying the head-tilt/chin-lift manoeuvre (Fig. 6.1). The head is tilted backwards and the chin lifted upwards. This causes the epiglottis and tongue to be pulled forward and airway patency is thereby established. An artificial (Guedel) airway may be inserted.

Although tracheal intubation provides the ideal airway, time should not be wasted trying to intubate the victim. It is vital to note that air entry is the goal of establishing an airway, and effective artificial respiration can be performed using the simple manoeuvre outlined above.

B *Breathing*

No apparatus or sophisticated equipment is needed for artificial respiration. The rescuer's exhaled air provides enough oxygen and a large enough tidal volume for the victim. Mouth-to-mouth respiration (the 'kiss of life') is performed as follows. Maintaining a patent airway with the head-tilt/chin-lift manoeuvre, the rescuer pinches the victim's nose closed between finger and thumb, takes a deep breath, seals his lips around the victim's mouth, and breathes out slowly. The victim's chest should be seen to move and exhalation takes place passively. This manoeuvre should be performed 12–15 times per minute (American Heart Association 1986). Mouth-to-mouth respiration is performed together with closed-chest cardiac massage (see below) and the two are inseparable in CPR.

C Circulation

Closed-chest cardiac massage has traditionally been thought to compress the heart between sternum and spine and thereby pump blood into the circulation. This view has been challenged and studies using echocardiography during CPR have shown that the mitral and tricuspid valves remain open during cardiac massage, with the heart therefore acting as a passive conduit rather than a pump (Werner et al 1981, Peters & Ihle 1990). Probably both mechanisms play a role.

Cardiac compression is hard work. To make it both easier and more effective, the rescuer should get his weight firmly above the victim. This is easy if the victim is on the ground, but if on a bed the rescuer should either stand on a platform or kneel on the bed itself. The heel of one hand is placed on the lower half of the sternum, covered with the other hand, and the sternum is depressed 3–5 cm with short thrusts of the arms. A firm surface below the patient is essential. The chest should be compressed 80–100 times per minute (American Heart Association 1986). CPR may be performed by one or two rescuers.

One-rescuer CPR. This is the technique that should be primarily taught to lay persons. Fifteen chest compressions are performed at a rate of 80–100 per minute. The airway is then opened and two breaths given. Chest compression is then recommended and the cycle continues. After 4–6 cycles, the victim should be reassessed for the return of breathing or pulse. If these are absent, CPR should continue, with pauses for reassessment (and rest for the rescuer) every few minutes. CPR should not be interrupted for periods of more than 7–10 seconds.

Two-rescuer CPR. When another rescuer arrives, it is advised that he calls for help and relieves the first rescuer, continuing with one-rescuer CPR (American Heart Association 1986).

CPR can, however, be performed in a coordinated technique by two rescuers. One rescuer performs the cardiac compressions and every five compressions allows a pause for the other to open the airway and provide breathing. The rescuers should take turns at providing the cardiac compressions as this is the most tiring role.

Advanced life support

Full details of ALS are beyond the scope of this chapter. The basic principles are described below in alphabetical order. Adjunctive equipment and special skills are needed, and these include oxygen, oropharyngeal airways, endotracheal tubes, intravenous lines, emergency drugs, and an electrical defibrillator. It should be emphasized that BLS should not be delayed while awaiting the arrival of this equipment.

ALS initially continues the basic principles of BLS by establishing the airway with endotracheal intubation, maintaining breathing with an Ambu bag and oxygen, and continuing circulatory support.

Drugs

Before any drugs can be administered, a secure intravenous line needs to be established, usually by catheterizing a central vein. However, it should be noted that both adrenaline and atropine are well absorbed from the tracheobronchial tree and may be administered via the endotracheal tube before intravenous access has been established. Many of the drugs traditionally used in CPR have not been shown to be of benefit in well performed studies, and drug protocols are in a constant state of flux.

Adrenaline is the drug of choice for all cardiac rhythms as it has both an inotropic effect and causes peripheral vasoconstriction, promoting blood flow to the central circulation and vital organs. It is recommended that 0.5–1.0 mg be given every 5 min during CPR (American Heart Association 1986). This dose may be inadequate, as animal studies suggest, and an infusion may be required (Krause et al 1986).

Sodium bicarbonate has traditionally been given to counter metabolic acidosis. However, more and more evidence is now accumulating that its effects are mainly cosmetic and may be harmful. The effects include shifting the oxygen dissociation curve, thereby inhibiting the release of oxygen, causing hypernatraemia and hyperosmolarity, and provoking an intracellular acidosis. It may be helpful in hyperkalaemia.

Calcium chloride's traditional role in CPR (to strengthen cardiac contractility) has not been proven in clinical studies. In fact, high levels of calcium may be detrimental. It should only be used in hyperkalaemia.

Lignocaine hydrochloride is the antiarrhythmic agent of choice for ventricular ectopy and tachycardia. It is usually given as a loading dose of 1 mg/kg and followed by an infusion of 1–4 mg/min.

Newer agents which are showing promise in clinical studies include new calcium antagonists like nimodipine (which has a cerebral protective effect) and beta blockers (to reduce the incidence of reperfusion arrhythmias), and desferrioxamine (an iron chelator which may reduce iron-dependent lipid peroxidative membrane injury). Interest in free oxygen radicals has prompted the suggestion that radical scavengers such as vitamin C, vitamin E, n-acetylcysteine, and selenium may be useful in preventing the damage caused by them.

Electrocardiograph

The three main mechanisms of cardiac arrest, namely ventricular fibrillation, asystole, and electromechanical dissociation, respond to different forms of therapy and may be identified by the electrocardiography. Monitoring of the electrocardiogram (ECG) should therefore be started as soon as the basic resuscitation steps have been carried out. Ventricular fibrillation carries a far better prognosis than the other rhythms.

Fibrillation

Early defibrillation is critical in the treatment and successful outcome of patients with ventricular fibrillation. If no ECG monitoring is available, it is recommended that defibrillation should be carried out 'blind' as soon as a defibrillator is available (American Heart Association 1986). If initially it is unsuccessful, it should be repeated at higher power. It should rapidly convert ventricular fibrillation or tachycardia to sinus rhythm, and may convert asystole into a cardiac rhythm.

Sternal thump. A precordial thump or a cough (in the conscious patient) has been known to convert ventricular tachycardia or fibrillation to sinus rhythm. However, it can also convert stable ventricular tachycardia into ventricular fibrillation. For this reason it is advised that it be used in patients with monitored ventricular fibrillation and in witnessed cardiac arrest where a defibrillator is unavailable (American Heart Association 1986).

CONTROVERSIAL ISSUES

Withholding CPR

In practice there are few reliable and definitive signs of death that can be quickly and easily applied to the collapsed victim. Clearly, rigor mortis, extreme lividity, decapitation or tissue decomposition is irrefutable evidence of death. On the other hand, a witnessed recent collapse is useful evidence for potential resuscitation. Absence of a pulse or breathing for more than 5–10 minutes (in the absence of hypothermia) will lead to irreversible brain damage, and resuscitation probably should not be initiated.

When to stop CPR

Immediately it is realized that CPR has been inappropriately initiated, it should be stopped. CPR for longer than 15 minutes leads to significantly poorer neurological outcome (Abramson et al 1985), and CPR for longer than 30 minutes is only very rarely successful (Gauthier & Lacroix 1990). Once involved in CPR, one may lose all sense of time, and it is useful to make a point of looking at one's watch at the outset (although this is very difficult to do in practice) and at intervals thereafter. In the hypothermic patient it is important to note that the victim is not dead until he is 'warm and dead'. In other words, CPR should continue until the body temperature reaches 35°C. Patients whose brain and other organs are not protected by hypothermia will suffer irreversible organ damage much sooner.

Ethical matters

CPR should not be initiated if the patient has made an express wish not to be resuscitated or the medical staff have issued a do-not-resuscitate (DNR) order. The latter often causes difficulty both from within the medical team and when viewed from outside. There are three rationales for a DNR order (Tomlinson & Brody 1988): no medical benefit from CPR, a poor quality of life before CPR, and a poor quality of life after CPR. In these situations CPR would cause further suffering for the patient and family as well as further expense and inappropriate use of often limited facilities. In general, good communication between patients, their families, and the attending medical staff will prevent major problems from arising.

REFERENCES

Abramson N S, Safar P, Detre K M et al 1985 Neurologic recovery after cardiac arrest: effect of duration of ischemia. Critical Care Medicine 13: 930–931

American Heart Association 1986 Standards and guidelines for cardiopulmonary resuscitation and emergency cardiac care. Journal of the American Medical Association 255: 2841–3044

Chamberlain D, Bossaert L, Carli P et al 1992 Guidelines for advanced life support. Resuscitation 24: 111–121

Gauthier M, Lacroix J 1990 When to stop CPR? In: Vincent J L (ed) Update in intensive care and emergency medicine. Springer-Verlag, Berlin, p 632–642

Heimlich H J 1975 A life-saving manoeuvre to prevent food-choking. Journal of the American Medical Association 234: 398–401

Holmberg S, Handley A, Baht J et al 1992 Guidelines for basic life support. Resuscitation 24: 103–110

Kouwenhoven W B, Jude J R, Knickerbocker G G 1960 Closed-chest cardiac massage. Journal of the American Medical Association 173: 1064–1067

Krause G S, Kumar K, White B C 1986 Ischemia, resuscitation, and reperfusion: mechanisms of tissue injury and prospects for protection. American Heart Journal 111: 768–777

Levy D E, Bates D, Caronna J J et al 1985 Predicting outcome from hypoxic-ischemic coma. Journal of the American Medical Association 253: 1420–1426

Pepe P E 1990 Current standards and future directions of basic and advanced cardiopulmonary resuscitation. In: Vincent J L (ed) Update in intensive care and emergency medicine. Springer-Verlag, Berlin, p 565–585

Peters J, Ihle P 1990 Mechanics of the circulation during cardiopulmonary resuscitation. Intensive Care Medicine 16: 11–27

Safar P 1988 Resuscitation from clinical death: pathophysiologic limits and therapeutic potentials. Critical Care Medicine 16: 923–941

Tomlinson T, Brody H 1988 Ethics and communication in do-not-resuscitate orders. New England Journal of Medicine 318: 43–46

Werner J A, Greene H L, Janko C L et al 1981 Visualisation of cardiac valve motion in man during external chest compression using two-dimensional echocardiography. Circulation 63: 1417–1421

FURTHER READING

Evans T R (ed) 1991 ABC of resuscitation, 2nd edn. British Medical Journal, London

7. Physiotherapy skills: positioning and mobilization of the patient

Elizabeth Dean

INTRODUCTION

The purpose of this chapter is to provide a framework for clinical decision making with respect to positioning and mobilizing patients with cardiopulmonary dysfunction. 'Cardiopulmonary dysfunction' refers to impairment of one or more steps in the oxygen transport pathway. First, the oxygen transport pathway and the factors that contribute to impairment of oxygen transport are described. Second, three clinically significant effects of positioning and mobilization are distinguished:

1. To improve oxygen transport in acute cardiopulmonary dysfunction.
2. To improve oxygen transport in the post-acute and chronic stages of cardiopulmonary dysfunction.
3. To prevent the negative effects of immobility, particularly those that adversely affect oxygen transport.

In addition, the physiological and scientific rationale for use of positioning and mobilization for each of the above effects is described. Conceptualizing cardiopulmonary dysfunction as impairment of the steps in the oxygen transport pathway and exploiting positioning and mobilization as primary interventions in remediating this impairment will maximize physiotherapy efficacy.

The following terms (Ross and Dean 1989) have been adopted in this chapter:

1. *Body positioning* refers to the application of positioning to optimize oxygen transport, primarily by manipulating the effect of gravity on cardiopulmonary and cardiovascular function.
2. *Mobilization and exercise* refer to the application of progressive exercise to elicit cardiopulmonary and cardiovascular responses to enhance oxygen transport. In the context of cardiopulmonary physiotherapy, 'mobilization' refers to low-intensity exercise for acutely ill patients.

3. *Optimizing oxygen transport* is the goal of positioning and mobilization. The 'adaptation' or 'training-sensitive' zone defines the upper and lower limits of the various indices of oxygen transport needed to elicit the optimal adaptation of the steps in the oxygen transport pathway. This zone is based on an analysis of the factors that contribute to cardiopulmonary dysfunction, and thus is specific for each patient.

CONCEPTUAL FRAMEWORK FOR CLINICAL DECISION MAKING

The oxygen transport pathway

Optimal cardiopulmonary function and gas exchange reflect the optimal matching of oxygen demand and supply (Dantzker 1983, Weber et al 1983). The efficiency with which oxygen is transported from the atmosphere along the steps of the oxygen transport pathway to the tissues determines the efficiency of oxygen transport overall (Fig. 7.1). The steps in the oxygen transport pathway include ventilation of the alveoli, diffusion of oxygen across the alveolar capillary membrane, perfusion of the lungs, biochemical reaction of oxygen with the blood, affinity of oxygen with haemoglobin, cardiac output, integrity of the peripheral circulation, and oxygen extraction at the tissue level (Johnson 1973). At rest, the demand for oxygen reflects basal metabolic requirements. Metabolic demand normally changes in response to positional,

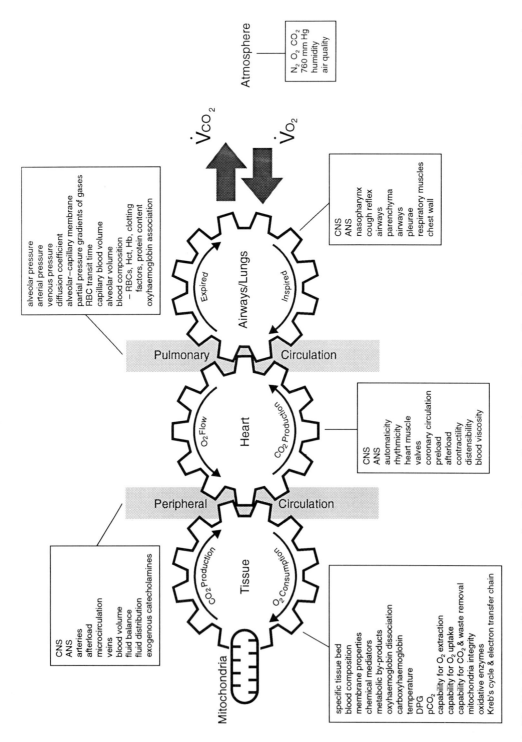

Fig. 7.1   A scheme of the components of ventilatory–cardiovascular–metabolic coupling underlying oxygen transport. Modified from Wasserman et al (1987). CNS, central nervous system; ANS, autonomic nervous system; DPG, diphosphoglycerate; RBC, red blood cell; Hct, haematocrit; Hb, haemoglobin.

exercise, and psychological stressors. When one or more steps in the oxygen transport pathway is impaired secondary to cardiopulmonary dysfunction, oxygen demand at rest and in response to stressors can be increased significantly. Impairment of one step in the pathway may be compensated by other steps, thereby maintaining normal gas exchange and arterial oxygenation. However, with more severe impairment involving several steps, arterial oxygenation may be reduced, the work of the heart and lungs increased, tissue oxygenation impaired and, in the most extreme situation, multisystem organ failure may ensue.

While the oxygen transport pathway ensures that an adequate supply of oxygen meets the demands of the working tissues, the carbon dioxide pathway ensures that carbon dioxide, a primary by-product of metabolism, is eliminated. This pathway is basically the reverse of the oxygen transport pathway in that carbon dioxide is transported from the tissues via the circulation to the lungs for elimination. Carbon dioxide is a highly diffusible gas and is readily eliminated from the body. However, carbon dioxide retention is a hallmark of diseases in which the ventilatory muscle pump is operating inefficiently or the normal elastic recoil of the lung parenchyma is lost.

Factors contributing to cardiopulmonary dysfunction

Cardiopulmonary dysfunction, in which oxygen transport is threatened or impaired, results from four principal factors, namely, the underlying disease pathophysiology, bed rest/recumbency and immobility, extrinsic factors imposed by the patient's medical care, and intrinsic factors relating to the patient (Table 7.1) (Dean 1993, Dean & Ross 1992b). An analysis of those factors that contribute to cardiopulmonary dysfunction provides the basis for positioning and mobilization to enhance oxygen transport for a given patient. The treatment is then directed at the specific underlying contributing factors. In some cases, e.g. low haemoglobin, the underlying impairment of oxygen transport cannot be affected by physical intervention. However, because such factors influence treatment

Table 7.1 Factors contributing to cardiopulmonary dysfunction, i.e. factors that compromise or threaten oxygen transport*

I.	**Cardiopulmonary pathophysiology**
	Acute
	Chronic—primary
	—secondary
	Acute and chronic
II.	**Bed rest/recumbency and immobility**
III.	**Extrinsic factors**
	Fever
	Malaise
	Reduced arousal
	Surgical procedures
	Dressings and bindings
	Casts/splinting devices/traction
	Incisions
	Invasive lines/catheters
	Monitoring equipment
	Medications
	Intubation
	Mechanical ventilation
	Suctioning
	Pain
	Anxiety
	Multisystem complications
	Hospital admission
IV.	**Intrinsic factors**
	Age
	Gender
	Ethnicity
	Congenital abnormalities
	Smoking history
	Occupation
	Air quality
	Obesity
	Nutritional deficits
	Deformity
	Fluid and electrolyte balance
	Impaired immunity
	Anaemia/polycythaemia
	Thyroid abnormalities
	Previous medical and surgical history

* Adapted from Dean (1993), Dean & Ross (1992b) and Ross & Dean (1992)

outcome, they need to be considered when planning, modifying and progressing treatment.

THERAPEUTIC EFFECTS OF POSITIONING AND MOBILIZATION

To improve oxygen transport in acute cardiopulmonary dysfunction

Positioning and mobilization have profound acute effects on cardiopulmonary and cardiovascular function, and hence on oxygen transport (Table 7.2). These effects translate into improved gas exchange overall: reduction in the fraction of inspired oxygen, pharmacologic and ventilatory support (Burns & Jones 1975, Dean 1985, Svanberg 1957). Such effects need to be exploited in the management of acute cardiopulmonary dysfunction with the use of positioning and mobilization as primary treatment interventions to enhance oxygen transport and as between-treatment interventions (Dean & Ross 1992a, Ross & Dean 1992).

Positioning

Physiological and scientific rationale. The distributions of ventilation (V_A), perfusion (Q), and ventilation and perfusion matching in the lungs are primarily influenced by gravity, and hence by body position (Clauss et al 1968, West 1962, 1977). The intrapleural pressure becomes less negative down the upright lung. Thus, the apices have a greater initial volume and reduced compliance than do the bases. Because the bases are more compliant, they exhibit greater volume changes during ventilation. In addition to these gravity-dependent interregional differences in lung volume, ventilation is influenced by intraregional differences which are dependent on regional mechanical differences in the compliance of the lung parenchyma and the resistance to air flow in the airways. Perfusion increases down the upright lung such that the V_A/Q ratio in the apices is disproportionately high compared with that in the bases. Ventilation and perfusion matching is optimal in the mid-lung region. Manipulating body position, however, alters both interregional and intraregional determinants of ventilation and perfusion and their matching. When considering specific positions to enhance arterial oxygenation

Table 7.2   Acute effects of upright positioning and mobilization on oxygen transport*

	Stimulus	
Systemic response	Positioning (supine to upright)	Mobilization
Cardiopulmonary	↑ Total lung capacity ↑ Tidal volume ↑ Vital capacity ↑ Functional residual capacity ↑ Residual volume ↑ Expiratory reserve volume ↑ Forced expiratory volumes ↑ Forced expiratory flows ↑ Lung compliance ↓ Airway closure ↑ PaO_2 ↑ AP diameter of chest ↓ Lateral diameter of rib cage and abdomen Altered pulmonary blood flow distribution ↓ Work of breathing	↑ Alveolar ventilation ↑ Tidal volume ↑ Breathing frequency ↑ A–a0$_2$ gradient ↓ Pulmonary arteriovenous shunt ↑ Functional residual capacity ↑ Distension and recruitment of lung units with low ventilation and low perfusion
Cardiovascular	↑ Total blood volume ↓ Central blood volume ↓ Central venous pressure ↓ Pulmonary vascular congestion ↑ Lymphatic drainage ↓ Work of the heart	↑ Cardiac output ↑ Stroke volume and heart rate ↑ Oxygen binding in blood ↑ Oxygen dissociation and extraction at the tissue level

* Adapted from Dean & Ross (1992b) and Imle & Klemic (1989).

AP, anteroposterior. ↑, increases; ↓, decreases.

for a given patient, one needs to consider the underlying pathophysiology impairing cardiopulmonary function, the effects of bed rest/recumbency and immobility, and aspects of the patient's care, in addition to physiological considerations.

Although the negative effects of the supine position have been well documented for several decades (Dripps & Waters 1941, Dean & Ross 1992a), supine or recumbent positions are frequently assumed by patients in hospital. These positions are associated with significant reductions in lung volumes and flow rate, and increased work of breathing (Craig et al 1971, Hsu & Hickey 1976). The decrease in functional residual capacity (FRC) contributes to closure of the dependent airways and reduced arterial oxygenation (Ray et al 1974). This effect is accentuated in older persons (Leblanc et al 1970) and patients with cardiopulmonary disease (Fowler 1949).

The haemodynamic consequences of the supine position are also remarkable. The gravity-dependent increase in central blood volume may precipitate vascular congestion, reduced compliance and pulmonary oedema (Sjostrand 1951, Blomqvist & Stone 1983), and the commensurate increase in stroke volume increases the work of the heart (Levine & Lown 1952). Within 6 hours, a compensatory diuresis can lead to a loss of circulating blood volume and orthostatic intolerance, i.e. haemodynamic intolerance to the upright position. Bed rest deconditioning has been attributed to this reduction in blood volume and the impairment of the volume-regulating mechanisms rather than physical conditioning per se (Hahn-Winslow 1985). Thus, the upright position is essential to maximize lung volumes and flow rates, and this position is the only means of optimizing fluid shifts such that the circulating blood volume and the volume-regulating mechanisms are maintained. The upright position coupled with movement is necessary to promote normal fluid regulation and balance (Lamb et al 1964).

Side-to-side positioning is frequently used in the clinical setting. If applied in response to assessment rather than routinely (Chuley et al 1982), the benefits derived from such positioning could be enhanced. Adult patients with unilateral lung disease may derive greater benefit when the affected lung is uppermost (Remolina et al 1981). Arterial oxygen tension is increased secondary to improved ventilation of the unaffected lung when this lung is dependent. Patients with uniformly distributed bilateral lung disease may derive greater benefit when the right lung is lowermost (Zack et al 1974). In this case, arterial oxygen tension is increased secondary to improved ventilation of the right lung which may reflect the increased size of the right lung compared with the left, and that in this position, the heart is subjected to less compression. Although various studies have shown beneficial effects of side lying, positioning should be based on multiple considerations including the distribution of disease if optimal results are to be obtained.

The prone position has considerable physiological justification in patients with cardiopulmonary compromise (Douglas et al 1977). The beneficial effects of the prone position on arterial oxygenation may reflect improved lung compliance, tidal ventilation, diaphragmatic excursion and FRC, and reduced airway closure (Dean 1985). A variant of the prone position, prone abdomen free, has shown additional benefits over prone abdomen restricted. In the prone abdomen free position, the patient is positioned such that the movement of the abdomen is unencumbered by the bed. This can be achieved either by raising the patient's body in relation to the bed so that the abdomen falls free, or by using a bed with a hole cut out at the level of the abdomen. Despite compelling evidence to support the prone position, this position may be poorly tolerated in some patients, or may be contraindicated in haemodynamically unstable patients. In these situations, intermediate positions approximating prone may produce many of the beneficial effects and minimize any potential hazard.

Positioning for drainage of pulmonary secretions may be indicated in some patients (Kirilloff et al 1985). Historically, these positions have been based on the anatomical arrangement of the bronchopulmonary segments to facilitate drainage of a particular segment. The bronchiole to the segment of interest is positioned perpendicularly to facilitate drainage with the use of gravity. The efficacy of postural drainage compared with deep breathing and coughing induced with mobilization/exercise and repositioning of the patient has not been established.

Assessment and treatment planning. Body positioning, i.e. the specific positions selected, the duration of time spent in each position, and the frequency the position is assumed, is based on a consideration of the factors that contribute to cardiopulmonary dysfunction. Understanding of the physiology of cardiopulmonary and cardiovascular function and the effects of disease, highlight certain positions that are theoretically ideal. However, these positions need to be modified or may be contraindicated for a given patient, based on other considerations (Table 7.1). For example, if extreme positional changes are contraindicated, small degrees of positional rotation performed frequently can have significant benefit on gas exchange and arterial oxygenation. A three-quarter prone position may produce favourable results when the full prone position is contraindicated or is not feasible. This modification may simulate the prone abdomen free position which has been shown to augment the effect of the traditional prone abdomen restricted position

(Douglas et al 1977). Furthermore, a three-quarter prone position may be particularly beneficial in patients with obese or swollen abdomens who may not tolerate other variations of the prone position. With attention to the patient's condition, invasive lines and leads, and appropriate monitoring, a patient can be aggressively positioned (Fig. 7.2).

The time which a patient spends in a position and the frequency with which that position is assumed over a period of time are based on the indications for the position and treatment outcome. Objective measures of the various steps that are compromised in the oxygen transport pathway as well as indices of oxygen transport overall, are used in making these decisions. Subjective evaluation based on clinical judgement also has a place. A specific position can be justified, provided there is objective and subjective evidence of improvement. Signs and symptoms of deterioration need to be monitored so that deleterious positions can be avoided and that deterioration secondary to excessive time in any one position can be detected. Prolonged duration in any single position will inevitably lead

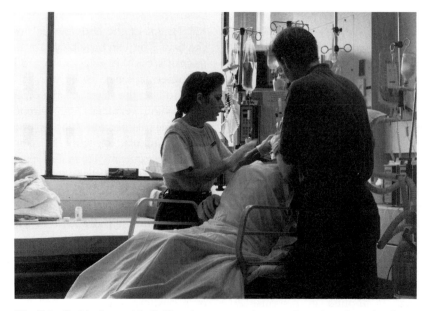

Fig. 7.2 Positioning a critically ill patient may require several people and continual monitoring of the patient's response. Even though a position (particularly an upright position) may only be tolerated for a short period of time, the physiological benefits are considerable.

to compromise of the function of dependent lung zones.

The ratio of treatment to between-treatment time is low. Typically, between-treatment time consists of some combination of positioning and mobilization. Positioning and mobilizing patients between treatments may be incorporated as an extension of treatment. Patients require monitoring and observation during these periods, as well as treatments. Between-treatment time may incorporate the use of maximally restful positions that do not compromise oxygen transport. Lastly, patients are positioned and mobilized between treatments to prevent the negative effects of immobility and recumbency.

Special consideration (e.g. with respect to specific positioning and the use of supports) needs to be given to positioning patients who are comatose or paralysed in that their joints and muscles are relatively unprotected and prone to trauma.

Progression. Progression of positioning involves decision making to incorporate new positions or modify previous positions, to modify the duration spent in each position and the frequency with which each position is assumed over a period of time. These decisions are also based on the factors that contribute to cardiopulmonary dysfunction and objective and subjective indices of change in the patient's cardiopulmonary status. With improvement in cardiopulmonary status, the patient spends more time in erect positions and is mobilized more frequently and independently.

Mobilization

Physiological and scientific rationale. The acute response to mobilization/exercise reflects a commensurate increase in oxygen transport to provide oxygen to the working muscles. The increase is dependent on the intensity of the mobilization/exercise stimulus. The demand for oxygen and oxygen consumption ($\dot{V}O_2$) increases as exercise continues, with commensurate increases in minute ventilation ($\dot{V}E$), i.e. the amount of air inhaled per minute, cardiac output, and oxygen extraction at the tissue level. Relatively low intensities of mobilization can have

a direct and profound effect on oxygen transport in patients with acute cardiopulmonary dysfunction (Lewis 1980, Dull & Dull 1983, Dean & Ross 1992b) and need to be instituted early after the initial pathological insult (Orlava 1959, Wenger 1982). The resulting exercise hyperpnoea, i.e. the increase in $\dot{V}E$, is effected by an increase in tidal volume and breathing frequency. In addition, ventilation and perfusion matching is augmented by the distension and recruitment of lung zones with low ventilation and low perfusion. Spontaneous exercise-induced deep breaths are associated with improved flow rates, and mobilization of pulmonary secretions (Wolff et al 1977). In clinical populations, these effects elicit spontaneous coughing. When mobilization is performed in the upright position, the anteroposterior diameter of the chest wall assumes a normal configuration compared with the recumbent position in which the anteroposterior diameter is reduced and the transverse diameter is increased. In addition, diaphragmatic excursion is favoured, flow rates augmented and coughing is mechanically facilitated. The work of breathing may be reduced with caudal displacement of the diaphragm and the work of the heart is minimized by the displacement of fluid away from the central circulation to the legs.

Although passive movement of the limbs has been promoted by some clinicians as a means of enhancing gas exchange and various facilitation techniques have been promulgated (Bethune 1975), there is little scientific evidence to support their use. Thus, time allocated to the use of passive movement may compete with time for positioning and mobilization, i.e. interventions with demonstrated clinical efficacy. Although passive movement may have a dubious effect on cardiopulmonary function, passive movement has several other important benefits on neuromuscular and musculoskeletal function which support their use provided they do not replace active movement.

Assessment and treatment planning. For practical and ethical considerations, the mobilization plan for the patient with acute cardiopulmonary dysfunction cannot be based on a standardized exercise test, as is the case for patients with chronic illness. However, response to a mobilization/exercise stimulus can be assessed during a patient's routine activities, such as turning or moving in bed, activities of daily living or responding to routine medical procedures. Comparable to prescribing exercise for the patient with chronic cardiopulmonary dysfunction, the parameters are specifically defined so that the stimulus is optimally therapeutic. The optimal stimulus is that which stresses the oxygen transport capacity of the patient and effects the greatest adaptation without deterioration or excessive distress.

To promote adaptation of the steps in the oxygen transport pathway to the stimulation of acute mobilization, the stimulus is administered in a comparable manner to that in an exercise programme prescribed for chronic cardiopulmonary dysfunction. The components include a pre-exercise period, a warm-up period, a steady-state period, a cool-down period and a recovery period (Blair et al 1988). These components optimize the response to exercise by preparing the cardiopulmonary and cardiovascular systems for steady-state exercise, and by permitting these systems to re-establish resting conditions following exercise. The cool-down period, in conjunction with the recovery period, ensures that exercise does not stop abruptly and allows for biochemical degradation and removal of the by-products of metabolism. Mobilization consists of discrete warm-up, steady-state and cool-down periods; the components need to be identified, even in the patient with a very low functional capacity, i.e. a critically ill patient who may be only able to sit up over the edge of the bed. In such cases, preparing to sit up constitutes a warm-up period for the patient; the stimulus of sitting unsupported for several minutes while being aroused and encouraged to talk, constitutes a steady-state period. Returning to bed constitutes the cool-down period. In the recovery period, the patient continues to be observed to ensure that mobilization was tolerated well and that the indices of oxygen transport return to resting levels. This information is then used as the basis for mobilization in the next treatment.

Valid and reliable monitoring practices provide the basis for the parameters of mobilization, assessing the need for progression, and defining the adaptation or training-sensitive zone. Monitoring is also essential given that subjecting patients to mobilization/exercise stimulation is inherently risky, particularly for patients with cardiopulmonary dysfunction. Indices of overall oxygen transport in addition to indices of the function of the individual steps in the oxygen transport pathway provide a detailed profile of the patient's cardiopulmonary status. In critical care settings, the physiotherapist has access to a wide range of measures to assess gas exchange. Minimally, in the general ward setting, measures of breathing frequency, arterial blood gases, arterial saturation, heart rate, blood pressure and clinical observation provide the basis for ongoing assessment, mobilization/exercise, and progression. With appropriate attention to the patient's condition, invasive lines and leads, and appropriate monitoring, a patient can be aggressively mobilized and ambulated (Fig. 7.3).

A fundamental requirement in defining the parameters for mobilization is that the patient's oxygen transport system is capable of increasing the oxygen supply to meet an increasing metabolic demand. If not, mobilization is absolutely contraindicated and the treatment of choice to optimize oxygen transport is body positioning. However, in the case of a patient being severely haemodynamically unstable, even the stress of positioning may be excessive. Thus, although critically ill patients may be treated aggressively, every patient has to be considered individually, otherwise the patient may deteriorate or be seriously endangered.

Progression. Progression and modification of the mobilization stimulus occur more frequently in the management of the patient with acute cardiopulmonary dysfunction compared with the progression of the exercise stimulus for the patient with chronic illness. The status of acutely ill patients can vary considerably within minutes or hours. Whether the mobilization stimulus is increased or decreased in intensity depends on the patient's status and altered responses to mobilization. The mobilization stimulus is adjusted such that it remains optimal despite the patient's changing metabolic needs. Capitalizing on narrow windows of opportunity for therapeutic interven-

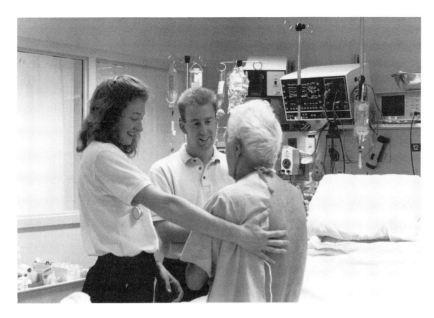

Fig. 7.3 Example of mobilizing a patient to a self-supported upright sitting position. Mobilizing a critically ill patient needs to be a priority wherever possible. Short frequent sessions to the erect position (sitting or standing if possible) with continual monitoring of the patient's response should be the goal.

tion must be exploited 24 hours a day with respect to the type of mobilization stimulus, its intensity, duration and frequency, particularly in the critically ill patient.

The 'immovable' patient. Given the well-documented negative effects of immobility, the 'immovable' patient deserves special consideration. Although bed rest is ordered for patients frequently without reservation, the risks need to be weighed against the benefits. Immobility coupled with recumbency constitutes a death knell for many severely compromised patients. Thus, an order for bed rest needs to be evaluated and challenged to ensure that this order can be physiologically justified.

Kinetic beds and chairs. Advances in furniture technology to facilitate positioning and mobilizing patients have lagged behind advances in clinical medicine, particularly in the critical care area. Conventional hospital beds are designed to be stationary, and their widths and heights are often non-adjustable, making them difficult for the patient to get in and out of bed. Kinetic beds and chairs have become increasingly available over the past decade; however, they are not widely used clinically. These devices were originally designed to facilitate positioning and moving heavy and comatose patients. Some beds are designed to rotate on their long axis from side to side over several minutes. Other beds simulate a side to side movement with inflation and deflation of the two sides of an air-filled mattress. Although these beds have potential cardiopulmonary benefit (Glavis et al 1985, Kyle et al 1992), they do not replace active positioning and movement. Mechanically adjustable bedside chairs constitute an important advance. These chairs adjust to a flat horizontal surface that can be adjusted to bed height and positioned beneath the patient lying on the bed. The device with the patient on top is then wheeled parallel to the bed where it can be adjusted back into a chair, and thus the patient assumes a seated position. The degree of recline can be adjusted to meet the patient's needs and for comfort. This chair also facilitates returning the patient to bed. The disadvantages of kinetic beds and chairs include the expense, and the potential for overreliance on them. Without these devices, a heavy patient may require several people and several minutes to position in a chair which may be only tolerated for a few minutes. However, the cardiopulmonary benefits of the stimulation of preparing to be moved, the reflex attempts of the patient to assist, as well as actually sitting upright in a chair, are not reproduced by bed positioning alone or by a kinetic bed. Research is needed to determine the indications and potential benefits of kinetic beds and chairs so that they can be judiciously used in the clinical setting.

To improve oxygen transport in post-acute and chronic cardiopulmonary dysfunction

In post-acute and chronic cardiopulmonary dysfunction, a primary consequence of impaired oxygen transport is reduced functional work capacity (Wasserman & Whipp 1975, Belman & Wasserman 1981). Work capacity can be improved with long-term exercise which improves the efficiency of the steps in the oxygen transport pathway, promotes compensation within the pathway as well as by other mechanisms. To optimize the patient's response, exercise can be carried out in judicious body positions in which oxygen transport is favoured.

Exercise is the treatment of choice for patients whose impaired oxygen transport has resulted from chronic cardiopulmonary dysfunction. Body positioning, however, may have some role in severe patients in optimizing oxygen transport at rest. Barach and Beck (1954), for example, reported that emphysematous patients were less breathless, had reduced accessory muscle activity and had a significant reduction in ventilation when positioned in a 16° head-down position. Some patients exhibited greater symptomatic improvement than in the upright position with supplemental oxygen. Classic relaxation positions, e.g. leaning forward with the forearms supported, can also be supported physiologically.

Physiological and scientific rationale. Although the physiological responses to long-term exercise in patients with chronic cardiopulmonary disease may differ from those in healthy persons, patients can significantly improve their functional work capacity (Table 7.3). In healthy persons, an improvement in aerobic capacity reflects

Table 7.3 Chronic effects of mobilization/exercise on oxygen transport

Systemic response	
Cardiopulmonary	↑ Capacity for gas exchange ↑ Cardiopulmonary efficiency ↓ Submaximal minute ventilation ↓ Work of breathing
Cardiovascular	Exercise-induced bradycardia ↑ Maximum VO_2 ↓ Submaximal heart rate, blood pressure, myocardial oxygen demand, stroke volume, cardiac output, work of the heart, perceived exertion ↑ Plasma volume Cardiac hypertrophy ↑ Vascularity of the myocardium
Tissue level	↑ Vascularity of working muscle ↑ Myoglobin content and oxidative enzymes in muscle ↑ Oxygen extraction capacity

↑, increases; ↓, decreases.

improved efficiency of the steps in the oxygen transport pathway to adapt to increased oxygen demands imposed by exercise stress. This adaptation is effected by both central (cardiopulmonary) and peripheral (at the tissue level) changes (Wasserman & Whipp 1975, Dean & Ross 1992b). Such aerobic conditioning is characterized by a training-induced bradycardia secondary to an increased stroke volume and increased oxygen extraction capacity of the working muscle. These adaptation or training responses result in an increased maximal oxygen uptake and maximal voluntary ventilation, and reduced submaximal $\dot{V}E$, cardiac output, heart rate, blood pressure and perceived exertion. Patients with chronic lung disease, however, are often unable to exercise at the intensity required to elicit an aerobic training response. Their functional work capacity is improved by other mechanisms, e.g. desensitization to breathlessness, improved motivation, improved biomechanical efficiency, increased ventilatory muscle strength and endurance or some combination (Belman & Wasserman 1981, Loke et al 1984). Patients with chronic heart disease such as patients with infarcted left ventricles may be able to train aerobically; however, training adaptation primarily results from peripheral rather than central factors (Bydgman & Wahren 1974, Hossack 1987, Ward et al 1987).

Planning an exercise programme. The exercise programme is based on the principle that oxygen delivery and uptake is enhanced in response to an exercise stimulus which is precisely defined for an individual in terms of the type of exercise, its intensity, duration, frequency and the course of the training programme. These parameters are based on an exercise test in conjunction with assessment findings. Exercise tests are performed on a cycle ergometer, treadmill or with a walk test. The general procedures and protocols are standardized to maximize the validity and reliability of the results (Blair et al 1988, Dean et al 1989). The principles of and guidelines for exercise testing and training patients with chronic lung and heart disease have been well documented (Dean 1993). The training-sensitive zone is defined by objective and subjective measures of oxygen transport determined from the exercise test. The components of each exercise training session include baseline, warm-up, steady-state portion, cool-down and recovery periods (Blair et al 1988, Dean 1993). The cardiopulmonary and cardiovascular systems are gradually primed for sustaining a given level of exercise stress, whilst in addition the musculoskeletal system adapts correspondingly. Following the steady-state portion of the training session, the cool-down period permits a return to the resting physiological state. Cool-down and recovery periods are essential for the biochemical degradation and elimination of the metabolic by-products of exercise.

Progression. Progression of the exercise programme is based on a repeated exercise test. This is indicated when the exercise prescription no longer elicits the desired physiological responses — specifically, when the steady-state work rate consistently elicits responses at the low end or below the lower limit of the training-sensitive zone for the given indices of oxygen transport. This reflects that maximal adaptation of the steps in the oxygen transport pathway to the given exercise stimulus has occurred. The degree of conditioning achieved is precisely matched to the demands of the exercise stimulus imposed.

To prevent the negative effects of immobility

Although physiologically distinct, the effects of immobility are frequently confounded by the effects of recumbency in the hospitalized patient. Immobility and the concomitant reduction in exercise stress affect virtually every organ system in the body with profound effects on the cardiovascular and neuromuscular systems. Recumbency and the elimination of the vertical gravitational stress exerts its effects primarily on the cardiovascular and cardiopulmonary systems (Dock 1944, Harrison 1944, Blomqvist & Stone 1983). The most serious consequences of immobility and recumbency are those resulting from the effects on the cardiopulmonary and cardiovascular systems, and hence on oxygen transport. Although other consequences of immobility, e.g. increased risk of infection, skin breakdown, deformity and thromboemboli, may not constitute the same immediate threat to oxygen transport and tissue oxygenation, they can have significant implications with respect to morbidity and mortality (Rubin 1988). Thus, immobility and recumbency need to be minimized, and mobility and the upright position maximized to avert the negative consequences of immobility, the risk of morbidity associated with these effects, and the direct and indirect cardiopulmonary and cardiovascular effects. These negative consequences are preventable with frequent repositioning and mobilizing of the patient (Table 7.4). The prevention of these effects is a primary goal of positioning and mobilizing patients between treatments.

SUMMARY AND CONCLUSION

Cardiopulmonary dysfunction refers to impairment of one or more steps in the oxygen transport pathway which can impair oxygen transport overall. Factors that can impair the transport of oxygen from the atmosphere to the tissues include cardiopulmonary pathology, bed rest and recumbency, extrinsic factors related to the patient's medical care, intrinsic factors related to the patient or some combination of these factors. Positioning and mobilization are two interventions that have potent and direct effects on several

Table 7.4 Effects of positioning and mobilization that prevent the negative effects of immobility and recumbency*

Systemic response	
Cardiopulmonary	Increases alveolar ventilation
	Decreases airways closure
	Alters the distributions of ventilation, perfusion and ventilation and perfusion matching
	Alters pulmonary blood volume
	Alters distending forces on uppermost lung fields
	Decreases secretion pooling
	Secretion mobilization and redistribution
	Alters chest wall configuration and pulmonary mechanics
	Varies work of breathing
Cardiovascular	Alters cardiac compression (positioning), wall tensions, filling pressures
	Alters preload, afterload, and myocardial contraction
	Alters lymphatic drainage
	Varies work of the heart
	Stimulates pressure and volume-regulating mechanisms of the circulation
	Stimulates vasomotor activity
	Maintains normal fluid balance and distribution
Tissue level	Alters hydrostatic pressure and tissue perfusion
	Maintains oxygen extraction capacity (mobilization)

* Many of the preventive effects of body positioning and mobilization are comparable; however, the magnitude of these effects in response to mobilization tends to be greater than with body positioning.

of the steps in the oxygen transport pathway. These interventions have a primary role in improving oxygen transport in acute and chronic cardiopulmonary dysfunction, and in averting the negative effects of immobility and recumbency particularly those related to cardiopulmonary and cardiovascular function.

The principal goal of physiotherapy in the management of cardiopulmonary dysfunction is to optimize oxygen transport. A systematic approach to achieving this goal consists of:

1. Distinguishing the specific steps in the oxygen transport pathway which are impaired or threatened.

2. Establishing which factors contribute to this impairment.

3. Distinguishing which factors are (a) amenable to positioning and mobilization and (b) not directly amenable to positioning and mobilization, as these factors will modify treatment.

4. Specifying the parameters for positioning and mobilization so that they directly address the factors responsible for the cardiopulmonary dysfunction wherever possible, i.e. to elicit the acute effects of these interventions to enhance oxygen transport, or to elicit the long-term effects on oxygen transport, i.e. training responses and improved functional work capacity.

5. Avoiding the multisystem consequences of immobility and recumbency, particularly those that impair or threaten oxygen transport.

6. Recognizing when the risk of positioning or mobilizing a patient exceeds the benefits of these interventions.

Conceptualizing cardiopulmonary dysfunction as impairment of the steps in the oxygen transport pathway, and identifying the factors responsible for each impaired step provides a systematic approach to clinical decision making in cardiopulmonary physiotherapy. Positioning and mobilization can then be specifically directed at the mechanisms underlying cardiopulmonary dysfunction wherever possible. Such an approach will maximize the efficacy of positioning and mobilizing patients with cardiopulmonary dysfunction and enhance the outcome of medical management overall.

REFERENCES

Barach A L, Beck G J 1954 Ventilatory effect of head-down position in pulmonary emphysema. American Journal of Medicine 16: 55–60

Belman M J, Wasserman K 1981 Exercise training and testing in patients with chronic obstructive pulmonary disease. Basics of Respiratory Disease 10: 1–6

Bethune D D 1975 Neurophysiological facilitation of respiration in the unconscious patient. Physiotherapy Canada 27: 241–245

Blair S N, Painter P, Pate R R et al 1988 Resource manual for guidelines for exercise testing and prescription. Lea & Febiger, Philadelphia

Blomqvist C G, Stone H L 1983 Cardiovascular adjustments to gravitational stress. In: Shepherd J T, Abboud F M (eds) Handbook of physiology. Section 2: circulation. American Physiological Society, Bethesda, vol 2, p 1025–1063

Burns J R, Jones F L 1975 Early ambulation of patients requiring ventilatory assistance. Chest 68: 608

Bydgman S, Wahren J 1974 Influence of body position on the anginal threshold during leg exercise. European Journal of Clinical Investigation 4: 201–206

Chuley M, Brown J, Summer W 1982 Effect of postoperative immobilization after coronary artery bypass surgery. Critical Care Medicine 10: 176–178

Clauss R H, Scalabrini B Y, Ray R F, Reed G E 1968 Effects of changing body position upon improved ventilation–perfusion relationships. Circulation 37 (suppl 2): 214–217

Craig D B, Wahba W M, Don H F 1971 'Closing volume' and its relationship to gas exchange in seated and supine positions. Journal of Applied Physiology 31: 717–721

Dantzker D R 1983 The influence of cardiovascular function on gas exchange. Clinics in Chest Medicine 4: 149–159

Dean E 1985 Effect of body position on pulmonary function. Physical Therapy 65: 613–618

Dean E 1993 Bedrest and deconditioning. Neurology Report (in press)

Dean E 1993 Advances in rehabilitation for older persons with cardiopulmonary dysfunction. In: Katz P R, Kane R L, Mezey M D (eds) Advances in long-term care. Springer-Verlag, New York Ch.1 p. 1–271

Dean E, Ross J 1992a Discordance between cardiopulmonary physiology and physical therapy: toward a rational basis for practice. Chest 101: 1694–1698

Dean E, Ross J 1992b Mobilization and exercise conditioning. In: Zadai C (ed) Pulmonary management in physical therapy. Churchill Livingstone, New York

Dean E, Ross J, Bartz J, Purves S 1989 Improving the validity of exercise testing: the effect of practice on performance. Archives of Physical Medicine and Rehabilitation 70: 599–604

Dock W 1944 The evil sequelae of complete bed rest. Journal of the American Medical Association 125: 1083–1085

Douglas W W, Rehder K, Froukje B M 1977 Improved oxygenation in patients with acute respiratory failure: the prone position. American Review of Respiratory Disease 115: 559–566

Dripps R D, Waters R M 1941 Nursing care of surgical patients. I. The 'stir-up'. American Journal of Nursing 41: 530–534

Dull J L, Dull W L 1983 Are maximal inspiratory breathing exercises or incentive spirometry better than early mobilization after cardiopulmonary bypass? Physical Therapy 63: 655–659

Fowler W S 1949 Lung function studies. III. Uneven pulmonary ventilation in normal subjects and patients with pulmonary disease. Journal of Applied Physiology 2: 283–299

Glavis C, Sparacino P, Holzemer W, Skov P 1985 Effect of a rotating bed on mechanically ventilated critically ill patients. Presented at the Third kinetic therapy seminar, San Antonio

Hahn-Winslow E 1985 Cardiovascular consequences of bed rest. Heart & Lung 14: 236–246

Harrison T R 1944 The abuse of rest as a therapeutic measure for patients with cardiovascular disease. Journal of

the American Medical Association 125: 1075–1078

Hossack K F 1987 Cardiovascular responses to dynamic exercise. In: Hanson P (ed). Exercise and the heart. W B Saunders, Philadelphia, p 147–156

Hsu H O, Hickey R F 1976 Effect of posture on functional residual capacity postoperatively. Anesthesiology 44: 520–521

Imle P C, Klemic N 1989 Changes with immobility and methods of mobilization. In: Mackenzie C F (ed) Chest physiotherapy in the intensive care unit, 2nd edn. Williams & Wilkins, Bethesda, p 188–214

Johnson R L 1973 The lung as an organ of oxygen transport. Basics of Respiratory Disease 2: 1–6

Kirilloff L H, Owens H R, Rogers R M, Mazzocco M C 1985 Does chest physical therapy work? Chest 88: 436–444

Kyle K, Jackiw A, Schroeder S et al 1992 Cardiopulmonary effects of kinetic bed therapy in mechanically ventilated patients. Presented at the American Thoracic Society meeting, San Antonio

Lamb L E, Johnson R L, Stevens P M 1964 Cardiovascular deconditioning during chair rest. Aerospace Medicine 23: 646–649

Leblanc P, Ruff F, Milic-Emili J 1970 Effects of age and body position on airway closure in man. Journal of Applied Physiology 28: 448–451

Levine S A, Lown B 1952 'Armchair' treatment of acute coronary thrombosis. Journal of the American Medical Association 148: 1365–1369

Lewis F R 1980 Management of atelectasis and pneumonia. Surgical Clinics of North America 60: 1391–1401

Loke J, Mahler D A, Man S F P 1984 Exercise improvement in chronic obstructive pulmonary disease. Clinics in Chest Medicine 5: 121–143

Orlava O E 1959 Therapeutic physical culture in the complex treatment of pneumonia. Physical Therapy Review 39: 153–160

Ray J F, Yost L, Moallem S et al 1974 Immobility, hypoxemia, and pulmonary arteriovenous shunting. Archives of Surgery 109: 537–541

Remolina C, Khan A V, Santiago T V, Edelman N H 1981 Positional hypoxemia in unilateral lung disease. New England Journal of Medicine 304: 523–525

Ross J, Dean E 1989 Integrating physiological principles into the comprehensive management of cardiopulmonary dysfunction. Physical Therapy 69: 255–259

Ross J, Dean E 1992 Body positioning. In: Zadai C (ed) Pulmonary management in physical therapy. Churchill Livingstone, New York

Rubin M 1988 The physiology of bed rest. American Journal of Nursing 88: 50–56

Sjostrand T 1951 Determination of changes in the intrathoracic blood volume in man. Acta Physiologica Scandinavica 22: 116–128

Svanberg L 1957 Influence of position on the lung volumes, ventilation and circulation in normals. Scandinavian Journal of Laboratory Investigation 25 (suppl): 7–175

Ward A, Malloy P, Rippe J 1987 Exercise prescription guidelines for normal and cardiac populations. Cardiology Clinics 5: 197–210

Wasserman K, Whipp B J 1975 Exercise physiology in health and disease. American Review of Respiratory Disease 112: 219–249

Wasserman K, Hansen J E, Sue D Y, Whipp B J 1987 Principles of exercise testing and interpretation. Lea & Febiger, Philadelphia

Weber K T, Janicki J S, Shroff S G, Likoff M J 1983 The cardiopulmonary unit: the body's gas transport system. Clinics in Chest Medicine 4: 101–110

Wenger N K 1982 Early ambulation: the physiologic basis revisited. Advances in Cardiology 31: 138–141

West J B 1962 Regional differences in gas exchange in the lung of erect man. Journal of Applied Physiology 17: 893–898

West J B 1977 Ventilation and perfusion relationships. American Review of Respiratory Disease 116: 919–943

Wolff R K, Dolovich M B, Obminski G, Newhouse M T 1977 Effects of exercise and eucapnic hyperventilation on bronchial clearance in man. Journal of Applied Physiology 43: 46–50

Zack M B, Pontoppidan H, Kazemi H 1974 The effect of lateral positions on gas exchange in pulmonary disease. American Review of Respiratory Disease 110: 49–55

FURTHER READING

American College of Sports Medicine 1991 Guidelines for exercise testing and prescription, 4th edn. Lea & Febiger, Philadelphia

Bates D V 1989 Normal pulmonary function. Respiratory function in disease, 3rd edn. W B Saunders, Toronto

Convertino V A 1987 Aerobic fitness, endurance training, and orthostatic intolerance. Exercise and Sports Sciences Review 15: 223–259

Dantzker D R 1991 Cardiopulmonary critical care, 2nd edn. W B Saunders, Philadelphia

McArdle W D, Katch F I, Katch V L 1991 Exercise physiology. Energy, nutrition, and human performance, 3rd edn. Lea & Febiger, Philadelphia

Pollack M L, Wilmore J H 1990 Exercise in health and disease, 2nd edn. W B Saunders, Philadelphia

Reinhart K, Eyrich K (eds) 1989 Clinical aspects of oxygen transport and tissue oxygenation. Springer-Verlag, London

West J B 1990 Respiratory physiology: the essentials, 4th edn. Williams & Wilkins, Baltimore

West J B 1990 Ventilation, blood flow and gas exchange, 5th edn. Blackwell Scientific, Oxford

8. Physiotherapy skills: techniques and adjuncts

Barbara A. Webber   Jennifer A. Pryor

This chapter discusses many of the physiotherapy techniques and adjuncts available to the cardiorespiratory physiotherapist. Breathing techniques can be divided into normal breathing, known as 'breathing control', where minimal effort is expended and breathing exercises where either the inspiratory phase is emphasized as in thoracic expansion exercises or expiration is emphasized as in the huff of the forced expiration technique.

BREATHING CONTROL

Breathing control is normal tidal breathing using the lower chest with relaxation of the upper chest and shoulders. This used to be known as 'diaphragmatic breathing', but this term is a misnomer as during normal tidal breathing there is activity not only in the diaphragm but also in the internal and external intercostal muscles, the abdominal and scalene muscles (Green & Moxham 1985).

To teach breathing control the patient should be in a comfortable well-supported position either sitting (Fig. 8.1) or in high side lying (Fig. 8.2). The patient is encouraged to relax his upper chest, shoulders and arms while using the lower chest. One hand, which may be either the patient's or the physiotherapist's, or one hand of each, can be positioned lightly on the upper abdomen. As the patient breathes in, the hand should be felt to rise up and out, as the patient breathes out, the hand sinks down and in. Inspiration is the active phase, expiration should

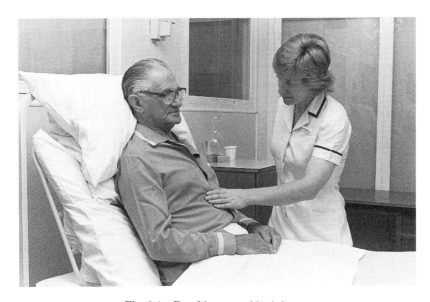

Fig. 8.1 Breathing control in sitting.

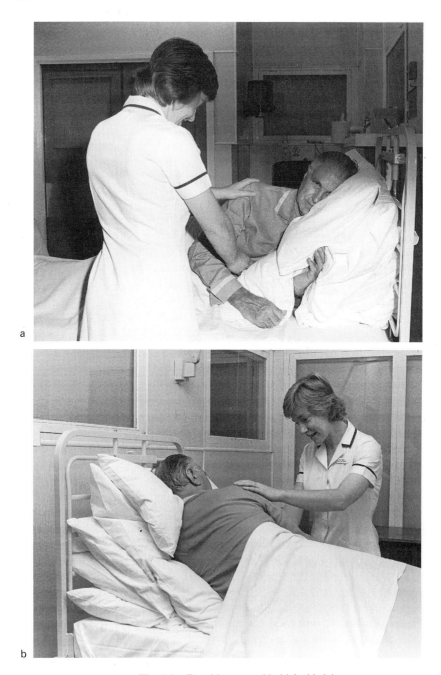

Fig. 8.2 Breathing control in high side lying.

be relaxed and passive and both inspiration and expiration should be barely audible. Inspiration through the nose allows the air to be warmed, humidified and filtered before it reaches the upper airways. If the nose is blocked, breathing through the mouth will reduce the resistance to the flow of air and will reduce the work of breathing. If the patient is very breathless breathing through the mouth will reduce the anatomical dead space.

Some patients reflexly use pursed-lip breathing.

Breathing through pursed lips has the effect of generating a small positive pressure during expiration which may reduce to some extent the collapse of unstable airways, for example in emphysema. This technique increases the work of breathing, particularly if it has become a forced noisy manoeuvre, and many patients no longer need to use pursed-lip breathing when they have relearned breathing control (normal breathing), which minimizes the work of breathing.

There are positions which optimize the length tension status of the diaphragm (Sharp et al 1980, Dean 1985). By sitting or standing leaning forward, the abdominal contents raise the anterior part of the diaphragm, possibly facilitating its contraction during inspiration. A similar effect can be seen in the side lying and high side lying positions where the curvature of the dependent part of the diaphragm is increased. This effect combined with relaxation of the head, neck and shoulders clinically promotes the pattern of breathing control.

Any breathless patient, for example patients with emphysema, asthma, pulmonary fibrosis or lung cancer, will benefit from using breathing control in positions which encourage relaxation of the upper chest and shoulders and allow movement of the lower chest and abdomen. One of the most useful positions is high side lying (Fig. 8.2). For maximal relaxation of the head, neck and upper chest, the neck should be slightly flexed and the top pillow should be above the shoulder supporting only the head and neck. Other useful positions are:

- Relaxed sitting (Fig. 8.3)
- Forward lean standing (Fig. 8.4)
- Relaxed standing (Fig. 8.5)
- Forward lean sitting (Fig. 8.6)
- Breathless children may prefer a kneeling position (Fig. 8.7).

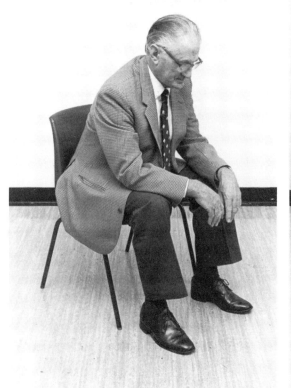
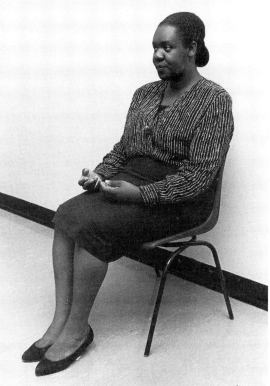

a   b

Fig. 8.3   Relaxed sitting.

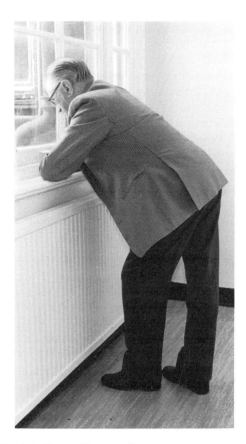

Fig. 8.4   Forward lean standing.

These positions discourage the tendency of breathless patients to push down or grip with their hands, which causes elevation of the shoulders and overuse of the accessory muscles of breathing. Figure 8.3b shows a position that is often preferred by patients who are overweight.

Breathing control is also used to improve exercise tolerance in breathless patients when walking up slopes, hills and stairs (Fig. 8.8). Breathless patients tend to hold their breath on exertion and rush, for example up a flight of stairs, arriving at the top extremely breathless and unable to speak. The simple technique of relaxing the arms and shoulders, reducing the walking speed a little and using the pattern of breathing *in* on climbing one step and breathing *out* on climbing the next step can lead to a marked reduction in breathlessness and the ability to converse on arrival at the top of the flight of stairs (Webber 1991). When this technique has been mastered

some patients, on days when they are less breathless, may find breathing *in* for *one* step and *out* for *two* steps more comfortable.

The severely breathless patient may find the combination of breathing control with walking also helpful when walking on level ground. A respiratory walking frame (Fig. 8.9) with or without portable oxygen can be used to assist ambulation in the severely breathless patient.

Breathing control is an integral part of the active cycle of breathing techniques and is also used to control a bout or paroxysm of coughing.

THE ACTIVE CYCLE OF BREATHING TECHNIQUES

The active cycle of breathing techniques is used to mobilize and clear excess bronchial secretions. It has been shown to be effective in the clearance of bronchial secretions (Pryor et al 1979), to improve lung function (Webber et al 1986) and it does not increase airflow obstruction (Thompson & Thompson 1968, Pryor & Webber 1979, Pryor et al 1993). It is a flexible method of treatment which can be adapted for use in any patient, young or old, medical or surgical, where there is a problem of excess bronchial secretions. It can be used with or without an assistant.

It is a cycle of breathing control, thoracic expansion exercises and the forced expiration technique (Webber 1990).

Thoracic expansion exercises

Thoracic expansion exercises are deep-breathing exercises emphasizing inspiration. Inspiration is active and may be combined with a 3 second hold before the passive relaxed expiration. The postoperative manoeuvre of a 3 second hold at full inspiration has been said to decrease collapse of lung tissue (Ward et al 1966). This 'hold' may also be of value in some patients with medical chest conditions, but it is probably unnecessary in the presence of hyperinflation, and cannot be achieved in the very breathless patient.

In the normal lung the resistance to airflow via the collateral ventilatory system is high, but with increasing lung volume and in the presence of lung pathology the resistance decreases, allowing

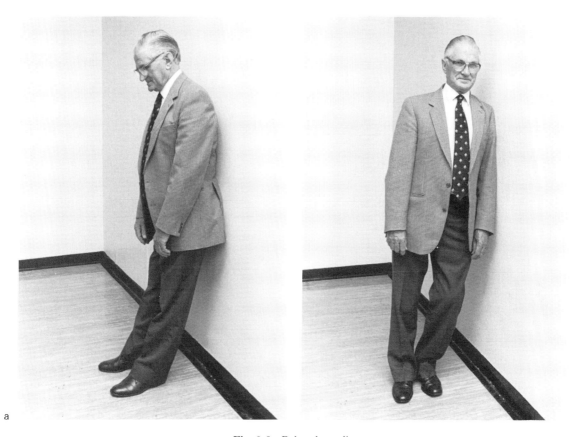

a   b

Fig. 8.5   Relaxed standing.

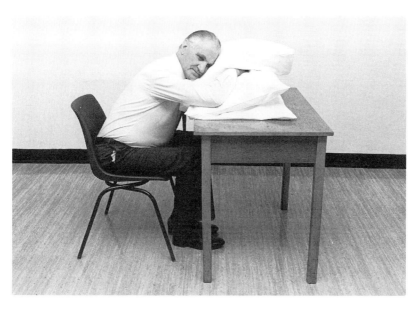

Fig. 8.6   Forward lean sitting.

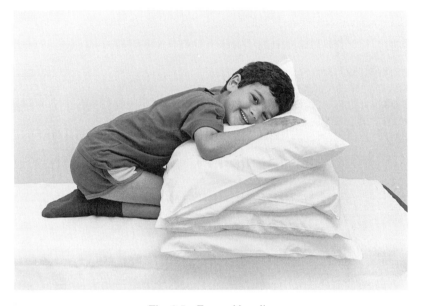

Fig. 8.7   Forward kneeling.

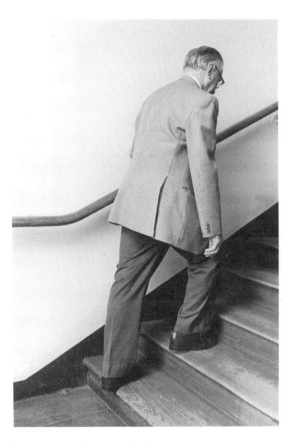

Fig. 8.8   Breathing control while stair climbing.

air to flow via the collateral channels—the pores of Kohn, canals of Lambert and channels of Martin (Menkes & Traystman 1977) (Fig. 8.10). When air can move behind secretions it can assist in mobilizing them.

The effectiveness of thoracic expansion exercises in re-expanding lung tissue and in mobilizing and clearing excess bronchial secretions can also be explained by the phenomenon of interdependence (Mead et al 1970). This is the effect of expanding forces exerted between adjacent alveoli. At high lung volume the expanding forces between alveoli are greater than at tidal volume and assist in re-expansion of lung tissue.

Three or four expansion exercises are usually appropriate before pausing for a few seconds for a period of breathing control. Any more deep breaths could produce the effects of hyperventilation or could tire the patient.

Thoracic expansion exercises can be encouraged with proprioceptive stimulation by placing a hand, either the patient's or the physiotherapist's, over the part of the chest wall where movement of the chest is to be encouraged. There is no evidence to support an increase in ventilation to the lung underlying the hand (Martin et al 1976), but there is an increase in chest wall movement and an increase in lung volume.

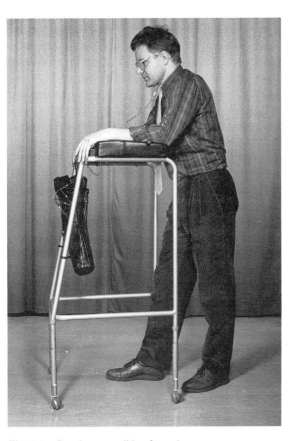

Fig. 8.9 Respiratory walking frame in use.

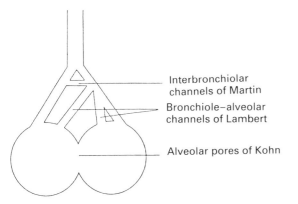

Interbronchiolar
channels of Martin

Bronchiole–alveolar
channels of Lambert

Alveolar pores of Kohn

Fig. 8.10 Collateral ventilation pathways.

Sometimes an additional increase in lung volume can be achieved by using a 'sniff' manoeuvre at the end of a deep inspiration. This manoeuvre may not be appropriate in patients who are hyperinflated, but for surgical patients who need further motivation to increase their lung volume it can be a useful technique.

Thoracic expansion exercises may be combined with chest shaking, vibrations, and/or chest clapping. These techniques may further assist in the clearance of secretions (pp. 122–126).

The forced expiration technique

The forced expiration technique is a combination of one or two forced expirations (huffs) and periods of breathing control. A huff to low lung volume will move the more peripherally situated secretions and a huff from a high lung volume will clear secretions that have reached the more proximal airways.

With any forced expiratory manoeuvre there is dynamic compression and collapse of the airways downstream (towards the mouth) of the equal pressure point (West 1992). This is an important part of the clearance mechanism of either a huff or a cough.

As lung volume decreases during a forced expiratory manoeuvre the equal pressure points move more peripherally, and below functional residual capacity they move towards the alveoli. At lung volumes above functional residual capacity the equal pressure points are located in lobar or segmental bronchi (Macklem 1974). A series of coughs without intervening inspirations was advocated by Mead et al (1967) to clear bronchial secretions, but clinically a single continuous huff down to the same lung volume is as effective and less exhausting.

The mean transpulmonary pressure during voluntary coughing is greater than during a forced expiration. This results in greater compression and narrowing of the airways which limits airflow and reduces the efficiency of bronchial clearance (Langlands 1967). In 1989, Freitag et al demonstrated an oscillatory movement of the airway walls in addition to the squeezing action produced by the forced expiratory manoeuvre.

When mobilizing and clearing peripheral secretions it is an unnecessary expenditure of energy to start the huff from a high lung volume. A huff from mid-lung volume is more efficient and probably more effective. To huff from mid-lung

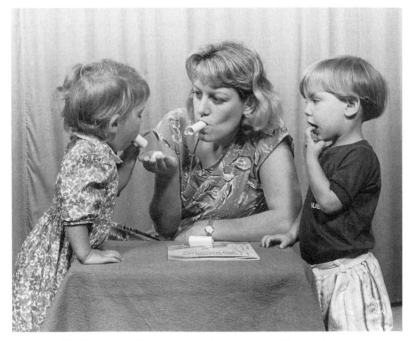

Fig. 8.11   Huffing games. (Reproduced with permission of the Royal Brompton Hospital)

volume a medium-sized breath should be taken in, and with the mouth and glottis open, the air is squeezed out using the chest wall and abdominal muscles. It should be long enough to loosen secretions from the more peripherally situated airways and should not just be a clearing noise in the back of the throat. However, if the huff is continued for too long it may lead to unnecessary paroxysmal coughing. Too short a huff may be ineffective (Partridge et al 1989), but when the secretions have reached the upper airways, a shorter huff or a cough from a high lung volume is used to clear them.

The huff is a forced but not violent manoeuvre. The length of the huff and force of contraction of the expiratory muscles can be altered to maximize airflow from the periphery and to minimize airway collapse.

A peak flow mouthpiece, or similar piece of tubing, may improve the effectiveness of the huff as it helps to keep the glottis open. In some people huffing through a tube at a tissue or cotton-wool balls may help to perfect the technique.

The huff can be introduced to children as blowing games (Thompson 1978) and from about

the age of 2 years they are usually able to copy others doing a huff (Fig. 8.11).

An essential part of the forced expiration technique is the pause for breathing control after one or two huffs which prevents any increase in air flow obstruction. The length of the pause will vary from patient to patient. In a patient with bronchospasm or unstable airways, or in one who is debilitated and fatigues easily, longer pauses (perhaps 10–20 seconds) may be appropriate. In patients with no bronchospasm the periods of breathing control may be considerably shorter (perhaps two or three breaths or 5–10 seconds).

Zach et al (1985) have expressed concern that airway instability in patients with cystic fibrosis may be increased by bronchodilator drugs, and this airway instability could lead to an increase in airflow obstruction during a forced expiratory manoeuvre. However, there is no evidence to support this concern with the use of the forced expiration technique in patients with cystic fibrosis (Pryor et al 1993).

In the tetraplegic patient, clearance of secretions from the upper airways is difficult because maximum lung volume cannot be achieved and the equal pressure points will therefore never reach the largest airways (Morgan et al 1986). Secretions can be cleared from the smaller airways, but accumulate in the larger upper airways.

Application of the active cycle of breathing techniques

The cycle of breathing control, thoracic expansion exercises and the forced expiration technique (Fig. 8.12) is adapted for each patient. Sometimes one set of thoracic expansion exercises will be followed by the forced expiration technique, but if secretions loosen slowly it may be more appropriate to use two sets of thoracic expansion exercises, as shown in Figure 8.12. The surgical patient will probably benefit from the 3 second hold with the thoracic expansion exercises (Fig. 8.13), but there is probably no indication for the use of chest clapping, and wound support may be more suitable than chest compression during huffing and coughing (Fig. 8.14).

In many patients the active cycle of breathing techniques will effectively clear secretions in the sitting position, but in others gravity-assisted positions will be required.

For patients with a moderate amount of bronchial secretions, for example with bronchiectasis or cystic fibrosis, a minimum of 10 minutes in any productive position is usually necessary. For patients with minimal secretions, for example some asthmatics, some chronic bronchitics or following surgery, less time is required. The 'endpoint' of a treatment session can be recognized, either by the physiotherapist or the patient treating himself, when an effective huff to low lung volume in two consecutive cycles has been dry sounding and non-productive. The sicker patient may not reach this end-point before tiring and should stop when fatigue is recognized.

It is important to introduce the concept of self-treatment at an early stage. Patients in hospital should be encouraged to take some responsibility for their treatment (Fig. 8.15). Surgical patients should continue with their breathing exercises in between the treatment sessions with the physiotherapist. Medical patients can perhaps start by doing their own evening treatment. If the patient takes responsibility for his treatment before discharge home, both the patient and physiotherapist will have the confidence that treatment will be continued effectively at home.

Revision of techniques at appropriate intervals is necessary to assess the effectiveness of the treat-

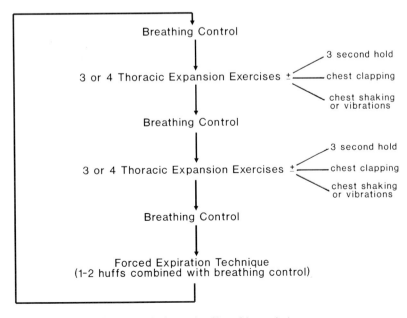

Fig. 8.12   Active cycle of breathing techniques.

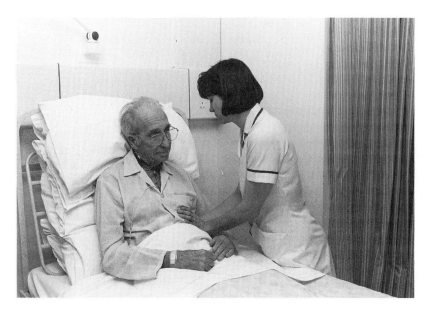

Fig. 8.13   Thoracic expansion exercises.

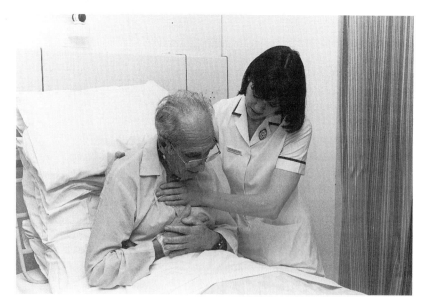

Fig. 8.14   Huffing with wound support.

ment regimen, and to correct and update techniques as necessary. Currie et al (1986) recognized the importance of reassessment to maintain patient compliance.

Chest clapping

Chest clapping is performed using a cupped hand with a rhythmical flexion and extension action of the wrist. The technique is often done with two hands (Fig. 8.16) but, depending on the area of the chest, it may be more appropriate to use one hand. For the infant chest clapping is performed using two or three fingers of one hand. Single-handed chest clapping is probably the technique of choice for self-chest clapping.

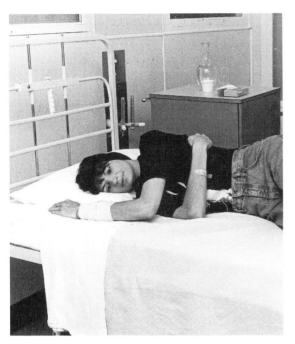

Fig. 8.15 Self-treatment—thoracic expansion exercises.

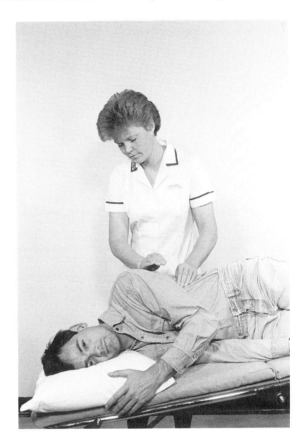

Fig. 8.16 Chest clapping.

Chest clapping should never be uncomfortable and should be done over a layer of clothing to avoid sensory stimulation of the skin. It should not be necessary to use extra layers of clothing or towelling as the force of the chest clapping should be adapted to suit the individual.

Using an oesophageal balloon mechanical percussion has been shown to increase intrathoracic pressure (Flower et al 1979) and this same effect has been demonstrated with chest clapping (Flower 1980), but this change in intrathoracic pressure has not been correlated with an increase in the clearance of bronchial secretions. Andersen (1987) hypothesized that the air-filled alveoli would buffer increases in intrathoracic pressure and markedly reduce the mechanical effect of chest clapping.

Some studies (Campbell et al 1975, Wollmer et al 1985) have demonstrated an increase in airflow obstruction when chest clapping is included in the treatment regimen, but other studies (Pryor & Webber 1979, Gallon 1991) have shown no increase in airflow obstruction with chest clapping.

In infants and small children not yet old enough to do voluntary breathing techniques, and in paralysed patients chest clapping appears to stimulate coughing, probably by the mobilization of secretions.

Chest clapping has been shown to cause an increase in hypoxaemia (Falk et al 1984, McDonnell et al 1986), but when short periods of chest clapping (less than 30 seconds) have been combined with three to four thoracic expansion exercises no fall was seen in oxygen saturation (Pryor et al 1990).

In a group of clinically stable patients with cystic fibrosis no advantage was shown when chest clapping was used in addition to thoracic expansion exercises (Webber et al 1985), but this cannot be extrapolated to either all medical chest conditions or to acute chest problems. Single-handed chest clapping (Fig. 8.17) is advocated in self-treatment as it is difficult to coordinate two-handed clapping at the same time as using thoracic expansion exercises.

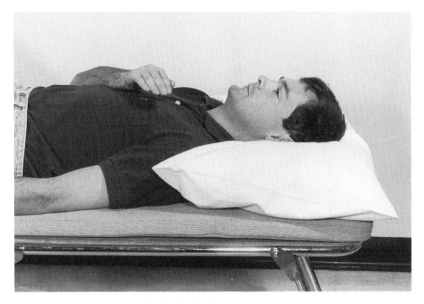

Fig. 8.17   Self-chest clapping.

If a patient feels that self-chest clapping is beneficial, but the physiotherapist thinks that it is tiring and may be causing hypoxaemia, the patient could be monitored using an oximeter. If oxygen desaturation occurs during the self-chest clapping the patient should be persuaded to omit the clapping, but to continue with the thoracic expansion exercises.

The benefits of chest clapping remain uncertain, but if chest clapping is considered to be clinically beneficial for an individual it should be continued, provided there are no harmful effects.

There is probably no indication for chest clapping in postoperative patients and in patients following chest injury, but it may be a necessary technique in the infant and young child to stimulate coughing. Severe osteoporosis and frank haemoptysis are contraindications, although chest clapping is unlikely to increase bleeding when bronchial secretions are lightly streaked with blood.

Vigorous and rapid chest clapping may lead to breath holding and may induce bronchospasm in a patient with hyperreactive airways. There is no evidence that alteration in the rate of chest clapping increases or decreases the mobilization of bronchial secretions. A rhythmical comfortable rate for both patient and physiotherapist is probably the most appropriate.

Chest shaking, vibrations and compression

The hands are placed on the chest wall and, during expiration, a vibratory action in the direction of the normal movement of the ribs is transmitted through the chest using body weight. This action augments the expiratory flow and may help to mobilize secretions. It is unknown whether airway closure will be increased if the vibratory action is continued into the expiratory reserve volume, but the techniques are frequently combined with thoracic expansion exercises which would counteract any resulting airway closure.

The vibratory action may be either a coarse movement (chest shaking) or a fine movement (chest vibrations). Little work has been done on the effects of either coarse or fine vibrations and physiotherapists have tended to adopt the techniques that they find the most helpful clinically.

In infants, vibrations are performed using two fingers in contact with the chest wall. Chest vibrations and shaking should never be uncomfortable and should be adapted to suit the individual patient. Patients doing their own chest physio-therapy may find self-chest vibrations helpful. One hand is placed on top of the other on the appropriate part of the chest wall and vibrations or shaking are carried out during expiration. With the hands in a similar position chest compression throughout expiration is often helpful (Fig. 8.18) to augment the forced expiratory manoeuvre of the huff. When lying on the side, self-compression can be given over the side of the chest with the upper arm and elbow and the hand of the other arm (Fig. 8.19).

The physiotherapist or other carer may give compression during huffing or coughing. Some patients find this helpful, but others prefer to be unsupported. Postoperative patients usually find

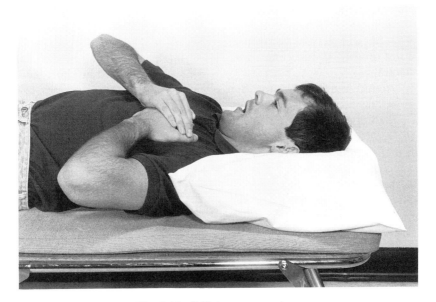

Fig. 8.18   Self-chest compression.

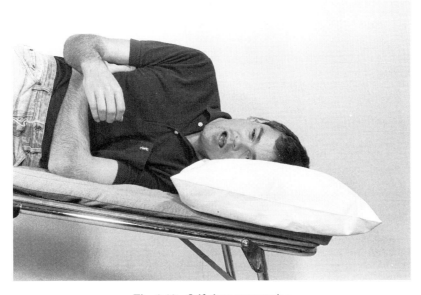

Fig. 8.19   Self-chest compression.

that supporting the wound facilitates both huffing and coughing. With fractured ribs and other chest injuries shaking of the chest wall would be inappropriate, but compressive support may assist the clearance of secretions.

In the paralysed patient the technique of rib springing may be used where compression of the chest wall is continued throughout expiration and overpressure is applied at the end of the breath out. By releasing the hands quickly inspiration is encouraged. This technique is inappropriate in the non-paralysed patient and may be harmful as compression against a reflexly splinted chest wall may produce rib fractures.

In the drowsy, semicomatose patient (for example, the chronic bronchitic in respiratory failure with sputum retention), chest compression similar to, but less vigorous than, rib springing may stimulate a deeper inspiration.

Chest shaking or chest vibrations can also be used during the expiratory phase of a manual hyperinflation treatment (p. 157) to assist the clearance of secretions.

Care must be taken when using the techniques of chest shaking, vibrations and compression if there are signs of osteoporosis or metastatic deposits affecting the ribs or vertebral column.

Gravity-assisted positions

Gravity, combined with the active cycle of breathing techniques, can be used to assist the clearance of bronchial secretions (Sutton et al 1983, Hofmeyr et al 1986). Nelson (1934) described the use of positioning for draining secretions based on the anatomy of the bronchial tree. The recognized positions (Thoracic Society 1950) (Fig. 8.20) are shown in Figures 8.21 to 8.31 and described in Table 8.1.

Many patients cannot tolerate some of the recognized positions and high side lying (Fig. 8.32) or side lying (Fig. 8.15) may be more appropriate. At school, college, work or when on holiday modified positions may be easier, more convenient and likely to encourage patient compliance (Figs 8.15 and 8.33).

The necessity for gravity assisted positions will depend on the quality and quantity of the bronchial secretions. Clinical evidence suggests that gravity will assist the clearance of more fluid secretions.

Table 8.1   Gravity-assisted positions (numbers refer to Fig. 8.20 and patient position is shown in Figs 8.21 to 8.31)

	Lobe	Position
Upper lobe	1 Apical bronchus	1 Sitting upright
	2 Posterior bronchus	
	(a) Right	**2a** Lying on the left side horizontally turned 45° on to the face, resting against a pillow, with another supporting the head
	(b) Left	**2b** Lying on the right side turned 45° on to the face, with three pillows arranged to lift the shoulders 30 cm (12 in.) from the horizontal
	3 Anterior bronchus	3 Lying supine with the knees flexed
Lingula	4 Superior bronchus	**4 & 5** Lying supine with the body a quarter turned to the right maintained by a pillow under the left side from shoulder to hip.
	5 Inferior bronchus	The chest is tilted downwards to an angle of 15°
Middle lobe	4 Lateral bronchus	**4 & 5** Lying supine with the body a quarter turned to the left maintained by a pillow under the right side from shoulder to hip. The chest is tilted
	5 Medial bronchus	downwards to an angle of 15°
Lower lobe	6 Apical bronchus	6 Lying prone with a pillow under the abdomen
	7 Medial basal (cardiac) bronchus	7 Lying on the right side with the chest tilted downwards to an angle of 20°
	8 Anterior basal bronchus	8 Lying supine with the knees flexed and the chest tilted downwards to an angle of 20°
	9 Lateral basal bronchus	9 Lying on the opposite side with the chest tilted downwards to an angle of 20°
	10 Posterior basal bronchus	10 Lying prone with a pillow under the hips and the chest tilted downwards to an angle of 20°

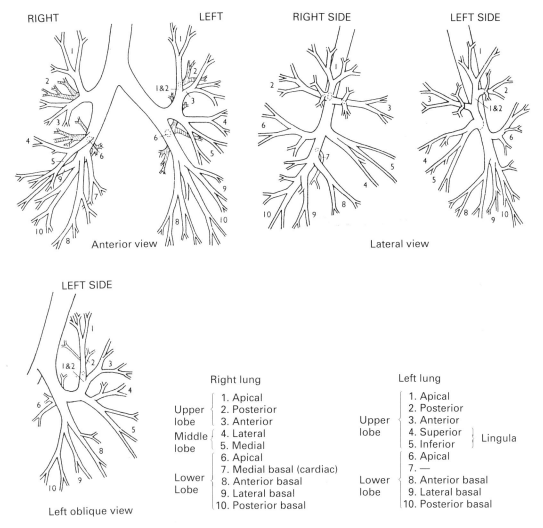

Fig. 8.20 Diagram illustrating the bronchopulmonary nomenclature approved by the Thoracic Society (1950). Reproduced by permission of the Editor of *Thorax*.

It is inappropriate to use the downward chest tilted positions immediately following meals and in the following conditions: cardiac failure, severe hypertension, cerebral oedema, aortic and cerebral aneurysms, severe haemoptysis, abdominal distension, gastro-oesophageal reflux, and after recent surgery or trauma to the head or neck.

MECHANICAL PERCUSSION

Mechanical percussors have been shown to increase intrathoracic pressure (Flower et al 1979), but Pryor et al (1981) could not demonstrate any increase in sputum clearance or improvement in lung function with mechanical percussion. Vibratory jackets utilize the principle of mechanical percussion, but the apparatus is cumbersome and most people prefer simple but effective techniques which can be carried out without equipment or assistance.

GLOSSOPHARYNGEAL BREATHING

Glossopharyngeal breathing (GPB) is a technique useful in patients with a reduced vital capacity due

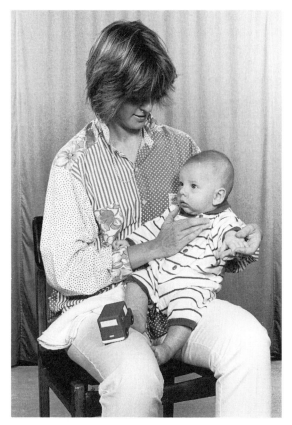

Fig. 8.21   Apical segments upper lobes.

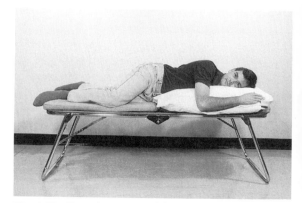

Fig. 8.22   Posterior segment right upper lobe.

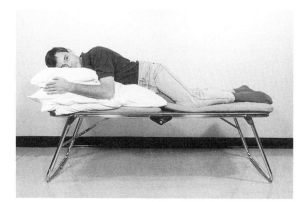

Fig. 8.23   Posterior segment left upper lobe.

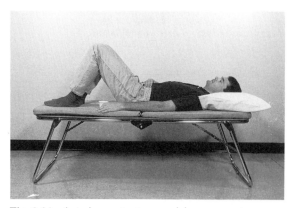

Fig. 8.24   Anterior segments upper lobes.

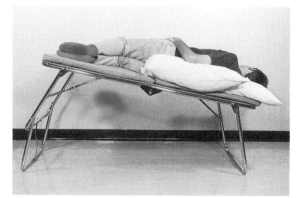

Fig. 8.25   Lingula.

to respiratory muscle paralysis, for example following poliomyelitis or in tetraplegics. It is a trick movement that was first described by Dail (1951) when patients with poliomyelitis were observed to be gulping air into their lungs. It was this gulping action that gave the technique the name 'frog breathing'.

GPB is a form of positive pressure ventilation produced by the patient's voluntary muscles where boluses of air are forced into the lungs.

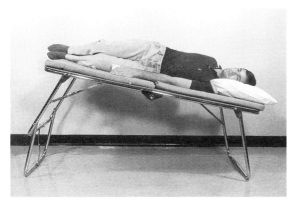

Fig. 8.26 Right middle lobe.

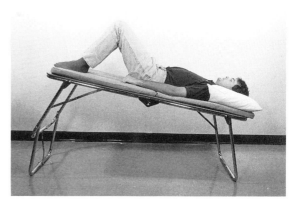

Fig. 8.29 Anterior basal segments.

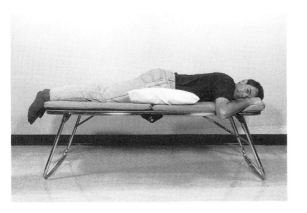

Fig. 8.27 Apical segments lower lobes.

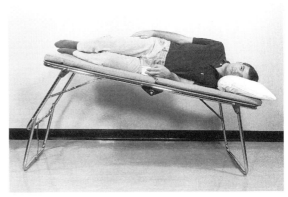

Fig. 8.30 Lateral basal segment right lower lobe.

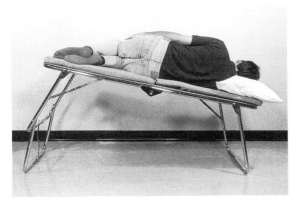

Fig. 8.28 Right medial basal and left lateral basal segments lower lobes.

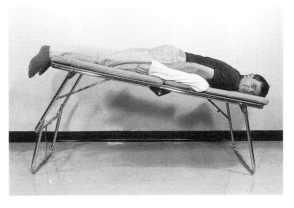

Fig. 8.31 Posterior basal segments lower lobes.

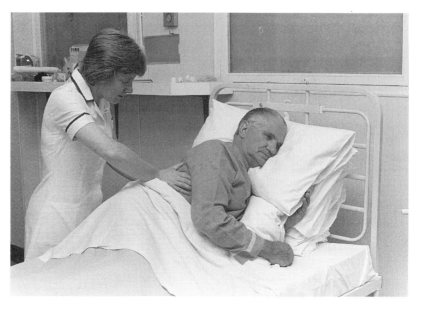

Fig. 8.32   Assisted treatment in high side lying.

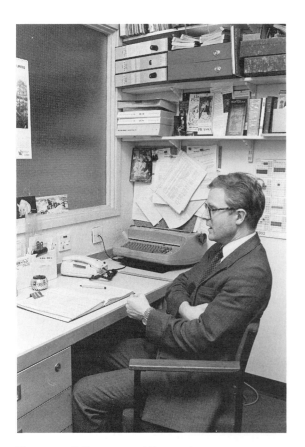

Fig. 8.33   Self-treatment while at work.

Paralysed patients dependent on a mechanical ventilator may be able to use GPB continuously, other than during sleep, to substitute the mechanical ventilation. The most common use of GPB is in patients who are able to breathe spontaneously but whose power to cough and clear secretions is inadequate. The technique may enable these patients to shout to attract attention and it may help to maintain or improve lung and chest wall compliance (Dail et al 1955).

To breathe in, a series of pumping strokes is produced by action of the lips, tongue, soft palate, pharynx and larynx. Air is held in the chest by the larynx which acts as a valve as the mouth is opened for the next gulp.

Before starting to teach a patient GPB it is helpful for him to inflate his chest using an intermittent positive pressure ventilator with a mouthpiece. He can practise holding the breath while removing the mouthpiece and avoiding escape of air through the larynx or nose. The most important step in learning GPB is the up and down movement of the cricoid cartilage while keeping the jaw still. The patient can practise by watching the movement in a mirror and feeling the cartilage with his fingers.

When this movement has been achieved a cycle of three steps is practised:

1. The mouth and pharynx are filled with air by depressing the cricoid cartilage and tongue (Fig. 8.34a).

2. While maintaining this position the lips are closed, trapping the air (Fig. 8.34b).

3. The floor of the mouth and cricoid cartilage are allowed to rise to their normal position while air is pumped through the larynx into the trachea (Fig. 8.34c).

This sequence should be practised slowly at first and then gradually speeded up until the movement flows. A leak of air may occur through the nose and, until it is prevented by the soft palate, a nose clip may be required.

The next stage is to take a maximum breath in and, while holding this breath, to add several glossopharyngeal gulps, to augment the vital capacity. When correct the patient will feel his chest filling with air, and the physiotherapist can test the 'GPB vital capacity' by putting a mouthpiece attached to the expiratory limb of a Wright's respirometer in the patient's mouth before he exhales.

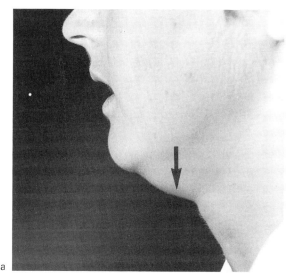

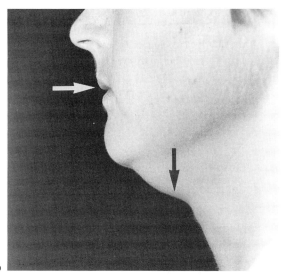

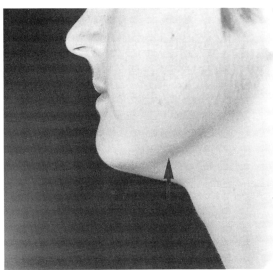

Fig. 8.34   The stages of glossopharyngeal breathing.

The respirometer can be used to measure the volume per gulp, the patient will require less effort and reach his maximum capacity more quickly if he develops a bigger volume per gulp. A study by Kelleher and Parida (1957) reported a group of patients in whom the average volume per gulp varied from 25 to 120 ml, and when teaching GPB an attempt should be made to achieve at least 60 ml per gulp. When used for clearance of secretions, 10–20 gulps may be required to obtain a maximal vital capacity, but if GPB is being used continuously as a substitute for normal tidal breathing approximately 6–8 gulps may be taken before breathing out.

GPB would normally be taught with the patient in a comfortable sitting position, but when mastered should be practised in positions useful for the patient to clear his bronchial secretions. After filling his chest to capacity he signals to the physiotherapist who compresses his chest as he lets the air out. The patient may have sufficient muscle power to apply compression himself or carers can be taught to give assistance.

GPB is learnt easily by some patients, but others need time and patience to acquire this skill and must be motivated to practise frequently during the learning period. It is a valuable technique to consider when treating tetraplegic or poliomyelitis patients with a vital capacity of less than 2 litres. Instruction can begin when the patient has reached a stable condition, but it is inappropriate in the acute phase or during an acute chest infection. When successfully learnt it is invaluable during a period of chest infection to assist in the clearance of secretions. For a patient with a chest infection nursed in a 'tank' ventilator ('iron lung'), assisted coughing (Higgens 1966) may be more effective if the patient uses GPB to augment the inspiratory volume received from the ventilator before chest compression is applied.

It is possible to teach GPB to patients with an uncuffed tracheostomy tube, provided there is an effective seal round the tube to avoid air leaks.

GPB should not be attempted in patients with neuromuscular disorders affecting swallowing, and in patients with a progressive disorder intermittent positive pressure breathing (IPPB) may be more appropriate than GPB. The technique is contraindicated in patients with airflow obstruction or pulmonary disease.

AUTOGENIC DRAINAGE

Autogenic drainage aims to maximize airflow within the airways and by this to improve the clearance of mucus and to improve ventilation (David 1991). Jean Chevaillier developed this concept in Belgium in the late 1960s, but little was published in English until 1979 (Dab & Alexander 1979). Autogenic drainage is a combination of breathing control and breaths at various lung volumes.

Chevaillier described three phrases: 'unstick', 'collect' and 'evacuate' (Schöni 1989). Breathing at low lung volumes is said to mobilize peripheral mucus. This is the first or 'unstick' phase. It is followed by a period of tidal breathing which is said to 'collect' mucus in the middle airways. Then, by breathing at higher lung volumes, the 'evacuate' phase, expectoration of secretions from the central airways is promoted. Coughing is discouraged until the 'evacuate' phase is reached.

The Germans have simplified this (David 1991) and do not split autogenic drainage into three phases. They found that patients were uncomfortable breathing at low lung volumes and recommended breathing around tidal volume while breath holding for 2–3 seconds at the end of each inspiration. Expectoration is encouraged when the patient is ready.

The flow volume curve is frequently used to support an increase in airflow with the unforced expiratory manoeuvre of autogenic drainage (Schöni 1989). However, it must be remembered that it is only possible to go outside the flow–volume curve if pressure-dependent collapse exists.

Autogenic drainage is usually practised in the sitting position. It takes 10–20 hours to teach the main principles and sessions of 30–45 minutes twice a day are necessary (David 1991). It is unsuitable for children under the age of about 8 years.

POSITIVE EXPIRATORY PRESSURE

The positive expiratory pressure (PEP) mask was first described by Falk et al (1984) who found an increase in sputum yield and an improvement in transcutaneous oxygen tension when compared with postural drainage, percussion and breathing exercises as practised at that time in Denmark. It was suggested that the increase in sputum yield was produced by the effect of PEP on peripheral airways and collateral channels.

The PEP apparatus consists of a face mask and a one-way valve to which expiratory resistances can be attached. A manometer is inserted into the system between the valve and resistance to monitor the pressure which should be between 10 and 20 cm H_2O during mid-expiration (Falk & Andersen 1991).

The patient sits leaning forward with his elbows supported on a table and holding the mask firmly over the nose and mouth (Fig. 8.35). A mouthpiece can be used in place of the mask if this is preferred. The patient breathes at tidal volume with a slightly active expiration for about six to ten breaths and the lung volume should be kept up by avoiding complete expiration. This is followed by the forced expiration technique to clear the secretions that have been mobilized. The duration and frequency of treatment is adapted to each individual, but treatment is usually performed for 15 minutes twice a day in patients with stable chest disease with excess bronchial secretions (Falk & Andersen 1991). In postoperative patients short periods of PEP used every hour as a prophylactic treatment have been described by Ricksten et al (1986).

The study by Falk et al (1984) in patients with cystic fibrosis compared an assisted 'conventional' postural drainage treatment with an unassisted PEP mask regimen and found that the PEP mask regimen was more effective and the one preferred by the patients. In order to reduce the variables studied, Hofmeyr et al (1986) compared the unassisted treatment of PEP combined with the forced expiration technique and thoracic expansion exercises combined with the forced expiration technique (the active cycle of breathing techniques). This study could not show any advantage in using the PEP mask, more sputum being produced when the active cycle of breathing techniques was used.

Falk and Andersen (1991) suggest that with the PEP treatment the increase in lung volume may

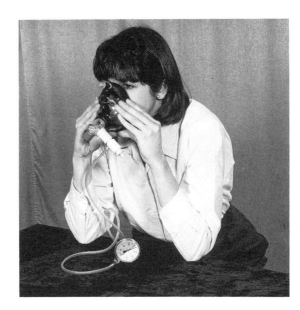

Fig. 8.35 Using the PEP mask.

allow air to get behind secretions blocking small airways and assist in mobilizing them. This effect may also be achieved by the thoracic expansion exercises.

van der Schans et al (1991) studied mucus clearance with PEP using a radio-aerosol technique in patients with cystic fibrosis. They showed that PEP temporarily increased lung volume, but did not lead to an improvement in mucus transport.

If a patient is in a non-compliant phase and unwilling to carry out the active cycle of breathing techniques regularly, PEP could be introduced as an alternative method of treatment for a period of time.

High-pressure PEP is a modified form of PEP mask treatment described for the treatment of patients with cystic fibrosis by Oberwaldner et al (1986). By using high pressures of PEP (50–120 cm H_2O), secretions may be mobilized more easily in patients with unstable airways. While sitting upright the patient holds the mask firmly against the face. Six to ten rhythmical breaths at tidal volume are followed by an inspiration to total lung capacity and then a forced expiratory manoeuvre against the resistance to low lung volume which usually results in the expectoration of sputum (Oberwaldner et al 1991).

An individual optimum expiratory resistance is carefully determined by spirometry. It is the resistance that allows the patient to expire to a volume greater than his usual forced vital capacity. The technique is only recommended for use where full lung function equipment is available for regular reassessment of the appropriate expiratory resistance for each individual. Meticulous care must be taken as an incorrect resistance can lead to a deterioration in lung function.

FLUTTER VRP1

The Flutter VRP1 (Flutter) is a small, simple portable device (Fig. 8.36) claimed to increase the expectoration of bronchial secretions, improve lung function and improve oxygenation (Liardet 1990). It is pipe-shaped with a single opening at the mouthpiece and a series of small outlet holes at the top of the bowl. The bowl contains a high density stainless steel ball-bearing enclosed in a small cone.

The Flutter is placed in the mouth and inspiration is either through the nose or through the mouth by breathing around the Flutter (it is not possible to breathe in through the Flutter). A 2–3 second hold is recommended at the end of a full inspiration and then, with the lips sealed

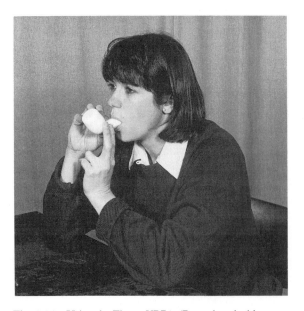

Fig. 8.36 Using the Flutter VRP1. (Reproduced with permission of the Royal Brompton Hospital.)

around the mouthpiece, the breath out should be slow and complete. The device is held horizontally and tilted slightly downwards until a maximal oscillatory effect can be felt (Liardet 1990).

During expiration the movement of the ball along the surface of the cone creates a positive expiratory pressure (PEP) and an oscillatory vibration of the air within the airways. The Flutter combines the techniques of oral high frequency oscillation (OHFO) and PEP. It can be used in the sitting position or in the position of supine lying.

Early studies on the Flutter were on laboratory models, computer-assisted experiments and uncontrolled clinical trials (Girard 1989). Althaus and Leuenberger (1988) compared the Flutter with autogenic drainage and concluded that lung function improved and that the expectoration of sputum was easier when the Flutter was used, although there is no statistical analysis of their data available. Kieselmann et al (1991) also compared autogenic drainage and the Flutter, and concluded that both regimens were equally effective, but the Flutter was easier to teach.

Clinical trials were undertaken in subjects following thoracotomy and in subjects with cystic fibrosis (Lyons et al 1992, Pryor & Webber 1992, Chatham et al 1993). These studies used the active cycle of breathing techniques as the control and none of them could support the claims of an increase in sputum clearance, lung function or oxygen saturation when the Flutter was used. In patients with cystic fibrosis less sputum is produced during treatment with the Flutter than with the active cycle of breathing techniques alone (Lyons et al 1992, Pryor et al).

ORAL HIGH FREQUENCY OSCILLATION

Oral high frequency oscillation (OHFO) has developed from high frequency jet ventilation and is for use in the spontaneously breathing patient.

Sine wave oscillations can be produced in a column of air by an eccentric cam piston or the diaphragm of a loudspeaker (George & Geddes 1985) and these can be superimposed on normal tidal breathing. A positive pressure is produced when gas flows into a subject and an equal negative pressure when the gas flow is reversed.

Low volumes (approximately 48 ml) and pressures (approximately 0.2–2.0 cm H_2O with a mean pressure of zero) allow the subject to breathe spontaneously.

In 'normal' subjects (i.e. subjects without pulmonary pathology), mucociliary clearance has been shown to increase and minute volume to decrease (George et al 1985a, 1985b).

During a 6 minute walking test in patients with chronic respiratory disease, an increase in exercise tolerance and a slight reduction in breathlessness was demonstrated (George et al 1984). However, when Pryor et al (1989) studied the use of OHFO as an adjunct to the active cycle of breathing techniques in patients with chronic bronchitis, they could not demonstrate an increase in mucociliary clearance as measured by the weight of sputum expectorated during treatment, an increase in exercise tolerance or any alteration in the forced expiratory volume in one second (FEV_1), forced vital capacity (FVC) or oxygen saturation. A reduction in breathlessness was observed when OHFO was not used.

van Hengstum et al (1990) measured tracheo-bronchial clearance using radio-aerosol techniques in patients with chronic bronchitis. Thirty minutes of OHFO in sitting, 30 minutes of the forced expiration technique in gravity assisted positions and 30 minutes of huffing alone in sitting, as a control, were compared. Tracheobronchial clear-ance using the regimen of the forced expiration technique was significantly greater than either OHFO or the control.

In a group of subjects with cystic fibrosis an increase in tracheobronchial clearance was demonstrated with OHFO and the forced expiration technique in gravity-assisted positions, but the increase was small and the weight of sputum expectorated favoured the use of the forced expiration technique alone, without OHFO, in gravity-assisted positions (George et al 1986).

There would seem to be differences in the effects of OHFO in normal subjects, in subjects with chronic airflow limitation and in those with cystic fibrosis. OHFO has been used in some countries where the active cycle of breathing techniques is not taught.

INTERMITTENT POSITIVE PRESSURE BREATHING AND PERIODIC CONTINUOUS POSITIVE AIRWAY PRESSURE

Intermittent positive pressure breathing

Intermittent positive pressure breathing (IPPB) is the maintenance of a positive airway pressure throughout inspiration, with airway pressure returning to atmospheric pressure during expira-tion. The Bird Mark 7 ventilator (Fig. 8.37) is a

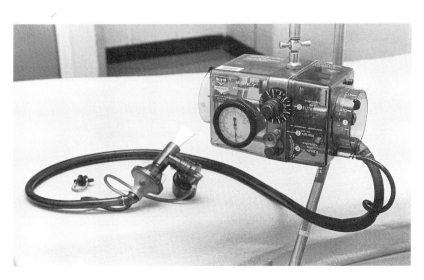

Fig. 8.37 The Bird Mark 7 ventilator.

pressure cycled device convenient to use for providing IPPB as an adjunct to physiotherapy in the spontaneously breathing patient.

IPPB has been shown to augment tidal volume (Sukumalchantra et al 1965), and using an IPPB device in the completely relaxed subject the work of breathing during inspiration approaches zero (Ayres et al 1963). These two effects support the use of IPPB to help in the clearance of bronchial secretions when the use of the active cycle of breathing techniques alone is not maximally effective, for example in the semicomatose patient with chronic bronchitis and sputum retention (Pavia et al 1988), or in a patient with neuromuscular disease and a chest infection. The reduction in the work of breathing can be used with effect in the acute severe exhausted asthmatic, but there is no evidence that the effect of bronchodilators delivered by IPPB is greater than from a nebulizer alone (Webber et al 1974).

An ideal IPPB device for use with physiotherapy should be portable and have simple controls. Other important features are:

Positive pressure. The range of pressures is 0–35 cm H_2O.

Sensitivity. The patient should be able to 'trigger' the inspiratory phase with minimal effort. Fully automatic control is unpleasant for most patients and unnecessary for physiotherapy. A hand triggering device is useful to test the ventilator and nebulizer.

Flow control. With ventilators such as the Bird Mark 7 the inspiratory gas is delivered at a flow rate which can be preset by means of a control knob. Optimal distribution of gas to the more peripheral airways is achieved at relatively slow flow rates, but if the patient is very short of breath and has a fast respiratory rate, a slow inspiratory phase may be unacceptable. It is often useful to alter the flow control several times during a single treatment session, providing slow breaths during the periods attempting to mobilize peripheral secretions and a faster flow rate when a patient is recovering his breath after expectoration. The Bennett PR-1 and AP-5 do not require flow-rate adjustment because automatic variable flow is provided with each breath. This feature is known as 'flow sensitivity' and means that the flow of the inspired gas

adapts to the resistance of the individual's airways.

Nebulizer. An efficient nebulizer in the circuit is necessary to humidify the driving gas and, when appropriate, to deliver bronchodilator drugs. The nebulizer in the Bird circuit is driven automatically with the inspiratory phase of the ventilator, but the Bennett has a separate control knob for the nebulizer.

Air-mix control. When driven by oxygen, air must be entrained by the apparatus to provide an air/oxygen mixture for the patient. Some Bird and Bennett devices have a control which should be set to give a mixture, while others have no control but automatically entrain air. The use of 100% oxygen for a patient is very rare, and when it is indicated an IPPB device with an air-mix control will be needed. When air is not entrained through the apparatus the flow rate control must be regulated to provide an adequate flow to the patient.

When IPPB is driven by oxygen and the air-mix control is in use, the percentage of oxygen delivered to the patient is approximately 45% (Starke et al 1979). This percentage will be considerably higher than the controlled percentage delivered by an appropriate venturi mask, for example to a patient with chronic bronchitis. This higher percentage is rarely dangerous during treatment because the patient's ventilation is assisted and the removal of secretions as a result of treatment is likely to lead subsequently to an improvement in arterial blood gas tensions (Gormezano & Branthwaite 1972).

It has been suggested that a few patients become more drowsy during or after IPPB as a result of the high percentage of oxygen received. Starke et al (1979) showed that increased drowsiness caused by hypercapnia occurred whether oxygen or air was the driving gas for IPPB and that the deterioration was dependent on inappropriate settings of the ventilator. The pressure and flow controls must be set to provide an adequate tidal volume, this being particularly important when treating patients with a rigid thoracic cage (Starke et al 1979).

Occasionally, IPPB may be powered by Entonox (p. 162) and in this case the air-mix control would need to be in the position to provide 100% of the driving gas with no additional air entrained.

Breathing circuit. To prevent cross infection it is essential for each patient to have his own breathing circuit which consists of tubing, nebulizer, exhalation valve and a mouthpiece or mask. The majority of patients prefer to use a mouthpiece, but a face mask is required when treating confused patients. A flange mouthpiece (Fig. 8.38) is useful for patients who have difficulty making an airtight seal around the mouthpiece.

The type of breathing circuit used will depend on the local means of sterilization. They can be autoclavable, non-disposable but non-autoclavable, or disposable.

Preparation of the apparatus

1. Normal saline solution or a combination of a bronchodilator drug and normal saline (3–4 ml in total) is inserted into the nebulizer.

2. The breathing circuit is connected to the IPPB ventilator, and the ventilator connected to the driving gas source. It can be used from an oxygen or air cylinder if piped compressed gas is unavailable.

3. If there is an air-mix control, this should be in the position for entrainment of air.

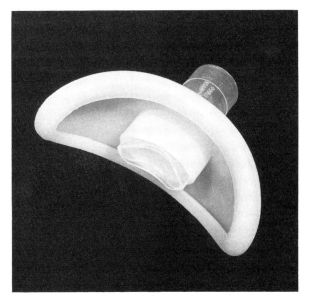

Fig. 8.38   Flange mouthpiece for use with IPPB.

4. If there is an automatic control (expiratory timer) this should be turned off to allow the patient to 'trigger' the machine at his desired rate.

5. The sensitivity, flow and pressure controls are set appropriately for the individual. With the Bird Mark 7 the sensitivity control is usually adjusted to a low number (5–7) where minimal inspiratory effort is required. The pressure and flow controls are adjusted to provide regular assisted ventilation without discomfort. A patient with a rigid rib cage will require a higher pressure setting to obtain an adequate tidal volume than someone with a more mobile rib cage.

When adjusting the settings for a new patient it may be easiest to start with the pressure at 12 cm H_2O and the flow at 10, then gradually increase the pressure and reduce the flow until the pattern of breathing is the most appropriate for the individual. Some IPPB devices do not have numbered markings, but after finding the most effective settings for a patient during one treatment, it is useful to note the positions of the controls in order to use these as a starting point at the next treatment. The controls to be set on the Bennett PR-1 are the nebulizer, sensitivity and pressure.

6. Before starting a treatment the hand triggering device is operated to check that there are no leaks in the breathing circuit and that the nebulizer is functioning well.

Treatment of the patient

The position in which IPPB is used depends on the indication for treatment. It may be used in side lying (Fig. 8.39), high side lying (Fig. 19.4, p. 395) or in the sitting position. The patient should be positioned comfortably and encouraged to relax the upper chest and shoulder girdle.

After explaining the purpose of the IPPB treatment the patient is asked to close his lips firmly around the mouthpiece and then to make a slight inspiratory effort which will trigger the device into inspiratory flow. He should then relax throughout inspiration allowing his lungs to be inflated. When the preset pressure is reached at the mouth the ventilator cycles into expiration, the patient should remain relaxed and let the air out quietly.

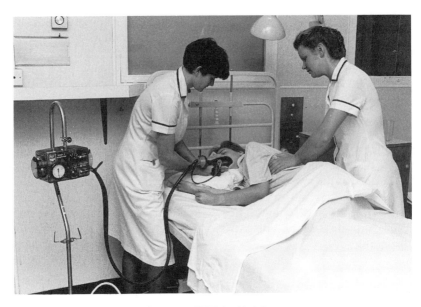

Fig. 8.39 IPPB in side lying.

If the patient attempts to assist inspiration there will be a delay in reaching the cycling pressure. A delay will also occur if there is a leak around the mouthpiece, at any of the circuit connections, or from the patient's nose. A nose clip may be required until he becomes familiar with the technique.

The physiotherapist will find it useful to watch the manometer on the ventilator in order to detect any faults in the patient's technique. At the start of inspiration the needle should swing minimally to a negative pressure and then swing smoothly up to the positive pressure set, before cutting out into expiration and returning to zero. A larger negative swing at the beginning of inspiration shows that the patient is making an unnecessary effort in triggering the device. If the patient makes an active effort throughout inspiration the needle will rise very slowly to the inspiratory set pressure, and if he attempts to start expiration before the preset pressure is reached the needle will rise sharply above the set pressure and then cut out into expiration.

When IPPB is taught correctly the work of breathing is relieved, but if the patient is allowed to assist either inspiration or expiration there will be an increase in the work of breathing.

The patient should pause momentarily after expiration, before the next inspiration to avoid hyperventilation and possible dizziness. Occasionally children using IPPB tend to swallow air during treatment. It is important to observe the size of the abdomen before and during IPPB to recognize signs of abdominal distension and discontinue IPPB if this occurs.

When IPPB is used to relieve the work of breathing while delivering bronchodilator drugs, e.g. in the acute severe asthmatic patient, it is often helpful for the physiotherapist to hold the breathing circuit to allow the patient to relax his shoulders and arms as much as possible.

A face mask for IPPB is used in the drowsy or confused patient, and in those with facial weakness unable to make an airtight seal at the mouth. When using IPPB to assist in mobilizing secretions the patient would be positioned to assist drainage of secretions, for example in side lying. The patient's jaw should be elevated and the mask held firmly over the face ensuring an airtight fit. Chest shaking during the expiratory phase may be used to assist in mobilizing secretions. In a drowsy patient it may be necessary to stimulate coughing using nasotracheal suction (p. 161) if spontaneous coughing is not stimulated by IPPB and chest shaking.

In medical patients with retained secretions and poor respiratory reserve IPPB may be useful both to mobilize secretions, and to relieve the effort of breathing following expectoration. The flow control on a Bird ventilator should be adjusted to give a slow but comfortable breath to mobilize secretions, but the patient's increased respiratory requirements following the exertion of expectoration necessitate speeding up the flow control and possibly reducing the pressure until he has returned to his normal breathing pattern.

IPPB may be used in patients with chest wall deformity, for example kyphoscoliosis, when they have difficulty clearing secretions during an infective episode. To achieve an adequate increase in ventilation in patients with a rigid rib cage, the pressure setting needs to be higher than for a more mobile rib cage. Long-term domiciliary IPPB may be considered in patients with severe restrictive chest wall deformity in an attempt to increase lung compliance. A volume-preset IPPB device, for example the Cape Minor ventilator, has been shown to be more effective than a pressure-cycled device in these patients. A greater improvement in vital capacity was obtained and this was maintained for several months (Simonds et al 1989). The volume is set to give a slight stretch to the chest and the patient is encouraged to use the IPPB device for 5–10 minutes two or three times a day.

Occasionally, in postoperative patients IPPB is the adjunct of choice when the patient is unable to augment his tidal volume adequately during treatment. In these patients in contrast to the relaxed technique normally used with IPPB, thoracic expansion may be actively encouraged during the inspiratory phase.

Bott et al (1992) have reviewed the literature on IPPB and concluded that IPPB is an important adjunct to chest physiotherapy.

Periodic continuous positive airway pressure

Continuous positive airway pressure (CPAP) is the maintenance of a positive pressure throughout inspiration and expiration during spontaneous breathing. Periodic continuous positive airway pressure (PCPAP) is the application of this on a periodic or intermittent basis.

One way of producing CPAP is to use a commercially available high-flow (50–80 l/min generator. Wide-bore tubing transmits the high flow to the patient who breathes in and out using a mouthpiece and nose clip (Fig. 8.40) or a mask (Fig. 8.41). On the expiratory limb of the circuit is a threshold resistor valve and in clinical practice a resistance of 5–10 cm H_2O is used. Both fixed inspired oxygen (FiO_2) generators and variable FiO_2 generators are available. Care must be taken when a fixed FiO_2 generator (providing approximately 33% oxygen) is used in a hypercapnic patient. It may be necessary to drive the high-flow generator from an air supply with added oxygen entrained through the air supply inlet to provide the appropriate FiO_2. As large volumes of room air are entrained, additional humidification is only occasionally required with PCPAP. If humidification is indicated, as in a patient with very tenacious secretions, a large volume vapour humidifier is recommended to humidify the high flow adequately (Fig. 8.48, p. 151).

In order to maintain a positive pressure within the airways throughout inspiration and expiration, the patient's peak inspiratory flow rate must be exceeded at all times. This can be detected by a continuous flow of air through the expiratory resistor. This can either be felt or monitored using a respirometer or other flow-sensitive device.

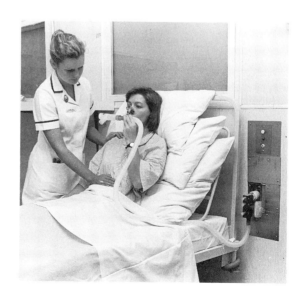

Fig. 8.40 PCPAP using a mouthpiece.

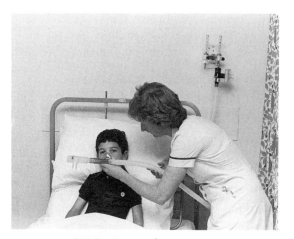

Fig. 8.41   PCPAP using a mask.

PCPAP has been shown to increase functional residual capacity (FRC) (Gherini et al 1979, Stock et al 1985, Lindner et al 1987) and to reduce the work of breathing (Gherini et al 1979). The reduction in the work of breathing is probably due to an increase in lung compliance with the patient breathing at a higher lung volume (Hinds 1987a). These two effects support the use of PCPAP in restrictive lung problems, for example in the treatment of postoperative subsegmental lung collapse.

In normal lungs the resistance to collateral flow via the interalveolar pores of Kohn, bronchiole–alveolar channels of Lambert, and probably the interbronchiolar channels of Martin, is high (Menkes & Traystman 1977), but this alters in disease and may also change at high lung volumes. Andersen et al (1980) have proposed that CPAP increases collateral flow to poorly ventilated or non-ventilated air spaces to aid the resolution of lung collapse. Interdependence (Mead et al 1970) may also be important and Menkes and Britt (1980) state that an increase in lung volume is the simplest and most effective way of reducing the resistance within the airways.

There are as yet no guidelines for treatment based on rigorous clinical studies. This is probably because there are so many variables to consider—the underlying pathology, the optimal pressure within the airways, the optimal time for treatment and the position of the patient.

A treatment regimen may be outlined as follows: after positioning the patient, a period of PCPAP (10–15 minutes) using breathing control is followed by the active cycle of breathing techniques—thoracic expansion exercises and the forced expiration technique. Chest clapping is omitted as some of the literature (Falk et al 1984) suggests a reduction in FRC with chest clapping and this would negate the effects of the PCPAP.

The periods of PCPAP are discontinued only to allow for expectoration of secretions mobilized to the upper airways and it may be appropriate to repeat the regimen more than once during the same treatment session. Treatment sessions are repeated as necessary, but when the active cycle of breathing techniques alone is as effective, PCPAP should be discontinued.

When deciding on the position of the patient during PCPAP, consideration should be given to the optimal position for increasing FRC (i.e. sitting upright) and the effect of gravity on bronchial secretions (which may indicate a tipped position). More than one position may be appropriate; for example, with a left lower lobe collapse, sitting upright should improve FRC (Hinds 1987a), and right side lying with the foot of the bed raised should assist drainage of secretions from the left lower lobe.

When PCPAP is used in children it is important to observe the size of the abdomen before and during PCPAP. Some children swallow air during treatment which may cause abdominal distension and PCPAP should be discontinued if this occurs.

The description of PCPAP outlined must not be confused with CPAP used for weaning a patient from a ventilator or as a means of avoiding intubation and mechanical ventilation. It should also not be confused with positive expiratory pressure (PEP) where a positive pressure is present only during expiration and the work of breathing is increased.

The efficacy of PCPAP as an adjunct to chest physiotherapy has yet to be validated, but it would appear to be effective in restrictive lung problems, particularly in postoperative lung collapse.

Contraindications for IPPB and PCPAP

- Pneumothorax
- Large bullae

- Lung abscess as the size of the air space may increase
- Severe haemoptysis as treatment is inappropriate until the bleeding has lessened
- Postoperative air leak unless the advantages of IPPB or PCPAP will outweigh the possibility of increasing the air leak during treatment
- Bronchial tumour in the proximal airways would contraindicate the use of IPPB or PCPAP to assist in the clearance of secretions. (Air may flow past the tumour during inspiration and may be trapped on expiration as the airways narrow. There would be no contraindication if the tumour were situated peripherally.)

IPPB or PCPAP?

The effects of IPPB and PCPAP are outlined in Table 8.2. In clinical practice the decision of when to use IPPB and when to use PCPAP is often not straightforward. The patient with asthma (an obstructive lung problem) who is exhausted may benefit from IPPB to reduce the work of breathing while receiving nebulized bronchodilators, and in the presence of hyperinflation it would be disadvantageous to consider a modality which would increase FRC. The patient with controlled asthma and subsegmental lung collapse presents with a predominantly restrictive problem and PCPAP would be the modality of choice to aid re-expansion of the lung collapse.

Table 8.2   The effects of IPPB and PCPAP

IPPB	PCPAP
10–20 cm H_2O pressure during inspiration	5–10 cm H_2O pressure during inspiration and expiration
No change in FRC	Increase in FRC
Reduction in work of breathing	Reduction in work of breathing
Augmented tidal volume	No change in tidal volume
Increase in collateral ventilation(?)	Increase in collateral ventilation (?)

The patient with steroid rib fractures complicating cystic fibrosis presents with a predominantly obstructive problem. PCPAP would not augment tidal volume, but would assist in the mobilization of bronchial secretions probably by increasing collateral ventilation owing to an increase in lung volume. An augmented tidal volume would cause an unnecessary increase in chest wall discomfort.

An adjunct to treatment should be considered when a maximal effect is not being achieved by simpler means. Conversely, when an equivalent effect can be achieved without an adjunct its use should be discontinued.

INCENTIVE SPIROMETRY

Incentive spirometers are mechanical devices introduced in an attempt to reduce postoperative pulmonary complications. The patient takes a slow deep breath in, with his lips sealed around the mouthpiece (Fig. 13.11, p. 308) and is motivated by visual feedback, for example a ball rising to a preset marker. The patient aims to generate a predetermined flow or to achieve a preset volume and he is encouraged to hold his breath for 2–3 seconds at full inspiration. A short, sharp inspiration can activate the flow generated incentive spirometry devices with little increase in tidal volume, but with a volume-dependent device an increase in tidal volume must be achieved before the preset level can be reached.

The pattern of breathing while using an incentive spirometer is important. Expansion of the lower chest should be emphasized rather than the use of the accessory muscles of respiration which would encourage expansion of the upper chest.

Diaphragmatic movement (Chuter et al 1990) is now thought to be an important factor in the prevention of postoperative pulmonary complications. Incentive spirometry has been shown to increase abdominal movement in normal subjects, but not in subjects following abdominal surgery (Chuter et al 1989). Postoperatively an increase in diaphragmatic movement has been observed by encouraging an increase in lung volume while using the pattern of breathing control without the resistive loading of an incentive spirometer (Chuter 1990). This may help to reduce postoperative pulmonary complications by increasing ventilation to the dependent parts of the lungs.

Incentive spirometry has been compared with intermittent positive pressure breathing (Oikkonen et al 1991), continuous positive airway pressure (Stock et al 1985) and chest physiotherapy (Hall et al 1991) in patients following surgery. Few differences between the regimens have been reported.

There may be a place for the use of incentive spirometry in children and in some adolescents to provide motivation to increase lung volume following surgery, but the use of breathing control and thoracic expansion exercises with an inspiratory hold should be encouraged, and combined with ambulation may be more effective in the prevention of postoperative pulmonary complications.

INHALED DRUGS

An understanding of the aerosol particle and its pattern of deposition within the airways is essential when considering the delivery of drugs by the inhaled route. A suspension of fine liquid or solid particles in air is known as an 'aerosol'. The pattern of deposition of aerosol particles within the bronchial tree depends on particle size, method of inhalation and on the degree of airflow obstruction (Newman et al 1986).

Large particles in the size range $5–10\,\mu m$ deposit by impaction in the oropharynx and upper airways where the cross-sectional diameter of the airway is small and the airflow high. The total cross-section of the airway increases rapidly beyond the tenth generation of bronchi, airflow slows significantly and particles of $0.5–5\,\mu m$, known as the 'respirable particles', deposit in the small airways and alveoli by gravitational sedimentation. It is the particles of less than $2\,\mu m$ that reach the alveoli. Gravitational sedimentation is time dependent and enhanced by breath holding. A more central patchy deposition is seen in patients with airflow obstruction (Clarke 1988).

The topical deposition of a drug by inhalation allows a smaller dose to be given than when other routes are used, the onset of action is often more rapid, and with minimal systemic absorption the side-effects are lessened.

Pressurized aerosol and dry powder inhalers

Numerous devices are available for the inhalation of drugs, ranging from the simple pressurized aerosol or powder inhalers to a variety of nebulizers. The physiotherapist should be aware of the range of possibilities to enable the patient to gain maximum benefit from the prescribed drugs. Choice of device may be dependent on the patient's age, coordination and dexterity in addition to severity of the respiratory condition.

Practice with placebo inhalers may be necessary to perfect the technique. Even if a patient has been using an inhalation device for a long time, it is always worth observing his technique as it may not be effective.

To gain maximum effect from a pressurized aerosol (metered dose inhaler (MDI)) it should first be shaken to ensure that the drug is evenly distributed in the propellent gases. The inhaler is held upright and the cap is removed. The patient breathes out gently, but not fully, and then with the mouth around the mouthpiece of the inhaler, the device is pressed to release the drug as soon as inspiration has begun. The breath in should be slow and deep and inspiration should be held for 10 seconds, if possible, before breathing out gently through the nose (Burge 1986, Clarke 1988). Effective technique is essential as it is known that only about 10% of the drug reaches the lungs (Clarke 1988).

Frequently, the prescribed dose will involve the inhalation of more than one 'puff'. It is recommended that puffs be taken one after the other. If the inhalation technique described above is used, the length of time between inhalations will be 15–20 seconds which allows sufficient time to overcome the problem of cooling of the metering chamber as the gas evaporates. Compliance is improved when doses are taken one after the other (Burge 1986).

Patients with arthritic hands may find the 'Haleraid' (Fig. 8.42) a useful gadget. By altering the direction of pressure required for releasing the drug it becomes an easier action to perform.

Large volume spacers (Fig. 13.10, p. 302) can be used to improve the deposition of the drug in the lungs to approximately 15% (Clarke 1988)

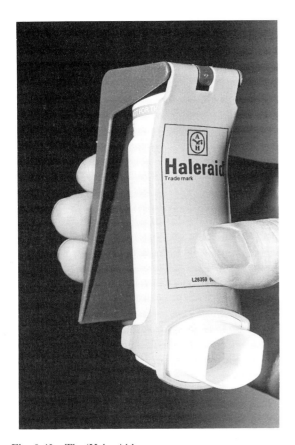

Fig. 8.42 The 'Haleraid.'

and to reduce the deposition in the oropharynx as the larger particles drop out in the spacer rather than the oropharynx. This helps to minimize any adverse side-effects.

Spacers may be cone or pear shaped, the shape of a 'puff' from a pressurized aerosol. The patient is encouraged to take a slow deep breath with a hold, but if this is difficult tidal breathing can be used. Gleeson and Price (1988) showed that a bronchodilator was equally as effective when a child breathed several times at tidal volume through a spacer when compared with a deep breath and inspiratory hold.

In patients with a good pressurized aerosol technique there may be no additional advantage in using a spacer, but in patients with a poor technique, in severely breathless patients and in those with candidiasis or dysphonia from inhaled steroids a spacer should be considered (Clarke 1988, Keeley 1992). The addition of a piece

of corrugated tubing (approximately 15 cm in length) attached to the mouthpiece of a pressurized aerosol may act as a cheap and effective spacer. Oral candidiasis can be minimized by rinsing the mouth thoroughly following inhalation.

For people with poor coordination a breath-actuated pressurized inhaler (e.g. Autohaler) may be considered (Newman et al 1991) or a dry powder device. The dry powder inhalers are breath actuated, releasing the drugs on inspiration, and require a faster inspiratory flow rate than a pressurized inhaler. The inspiratory flow required depends on the resistance within the device.

It is not only important that the patient can use the device effectively, but also that the patient or parent can easily recall whether a dose of the drug has been taken. The pierced numbered blisters on the Diskhaler have this advantage over the multi-dose reservoir powder devices which are simple to use, but where it is not so obvious that a dose has been taken.

For inhalation therapy to be effective in infants and children, the appropriate device for the age and ability of the child (p. 302) must be selected (Reiser & Warner 1986). It may be necessary to use a domiciliary nebulizer system in early childhood.

For each inhalation device the individual instructions should be carefully read and followed.

Nebulizers

A nebulizer may be used for the inhalation of drugs if a more simple method cannot produce the optimal effect. A nebulizer breaks up the solution to be inhaled into fine droplets which are suspended in a stream of gas.

Jet nebulizers

The majority of nebulizers are jet nebulizers which operate on the venturi principle. As the driving gas is forced through a narrow orifice, a negative pressure is created around the orifice causing suction of the liquid up a feed tube. The liquid mixed with the gas is blown out as a cloud of particles. As this hits a baffle the large particles adhere to the baffle and then fall back into the reservoir of the liquid drug. The small particles suspended in the stream of gas are inhaled by the patient.

The performance of an individual nebulizer may be described by the mass median aerodynamic diameter (MMAD) of the particles or by the respirable output. The MMAD indicates the range of size of particles leaving the nebulizer. Half of the aerosol mass from the nebulizer is of particles smaller than the MMAD and half of the aerosol mass of particles is larger than the MMAD. The respirable output of a nebulizer provides a better indication of performance. It reflects the percentage of respirable particles delivered in one minute:

[(percentage of particles of 1–5 μm) × (mass output per minute)] g/min.

The efficiency of a jet nebulizer and the size of particles depend on several factors which include the construction of the jet, the baffle, the shape of the chamber and the power of the driving gas. When selecting a nebulizer, consideration should be given to the optimal particle sizes of the drug to be delivered. Inhaled pentamidine or antibiotics need to be delivered to the more peripheral airways (requiring a high percentage of particles of less than 2 μm), whereas bronchodilator drugs probably have their effect in the more central airways.

The dose of a prescribed nebulized bronchodilator may seem large compared with that from a pressurized aerosol, but only 10–20% of the initial dose is received by the patient and only 50% of this reaches the lungs. The drug which does not reach the patient is lost in the equipment and exhaled gas (Lewis & Fleming 1985).

The design and technology of nebulizers has been changing rapidly. It used to be essential to have a minimum flow of 6 l/min to produce particles within the respirable range (Clay et al 1983), but some nebulizers now produce a similar range of particles at lower flow rates. Another development is the design which allows entrainment of air by the venturi effect into the chamber of the nebulizer, giving a higher respirable output and

thus a shorter time required for delivery of the drug.

With all jet nebulizers there is a volume of solution (0.5–1 ml) which remains in the nebulizer after it has been run to 'dryness'. This is known as the 'dead volume'. The patient should be encouraged to tap the side of the nebulizer to allow as much solution as possible to be delivered. A minimum of 3 ml of solution should be used to deliver an adequate percentage of the prescribed drug. Clay et al (1983) found that when a 2 ml solution was used only 50% of the dose was released as aerosol, but with a volume of 4 ml 60–80% was released.

Jet nebulizers can be powered by either piped compressed air or oxygen, or a portable air compressor. For patients in hospital it is often convenient to use approximately 6 l/min from the piped oxygen supply, and in hypoxic patients without carbon dioxide retention oxygen should be used. For patients retaining carbon dioxide who are dependent on their hypoxic drive to stimulate breathing, compressed air should be the driving gas (Gunawardena et al 1984). A higher flow rate (more than 8 l/min) is required to nebulize viscous solutions within an acceptable period of time.

A face mask is necessary for the infant and child (Fig. 8.43), but as soon as the child will cooperate a mouthpiece should be used to minimize deposition of the drug on the face and in the nasal passages (Wolfsdorf et al 1969). Other disadvantages of a mask are facial skin irritation from nebulized antibiotics and steroids, and nebulized ipratropium bromide and salbutamol by mask have been associated with glaucoma in a group of adults with chronic airflow limitation (Shah et al 1992). A mouthpiece should have an opening for entrainment of air during inspiration, and through which expiration can occur.

When inhaling from a nebulizer the patient should be in a comfortable and well-supported position. The optimal pattern of breathing has not yet been ascertained, but a recommended one is to intersperse deep breathing with breathing at tidal volume. The deep breathing will increase peripheral deposition of the drug and the periods of breathing control will prevent hyperventilation.

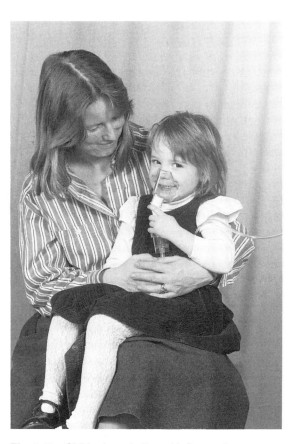

Fig. 8.43   Child using nebulizer with face mask.

Ultrasonic nebulizers

An aerosol can also be created by high frequency (1–2 MHz) sound waves. An electric current applied to a piezo-electric crystal causes ultrasonic vibrations. The sound waves will travel through a liquid to the surface where they produce an aerosol. The MMAD is influenced by the frequency of oscillation of the crystal. Ultrasonic nebulizers can produce a higher output than jet nebulizers, but most of the particles are larger being in the range 3.7–10.5 μm (Clarke 1988). An advantage of ultrasonic nebulizers is that they operate quietly. A small volume of drug can be nebulized in a large volume ultrasonic nebulizer by the insertion of a drug chamber.

The majority of ultrasonic nebulizers are fan assisted (Fig. 21.2, p. 424), but a few models require the patient to breathe in actively to open a valve to the nebulizing chamber. Patients with very poor respiratory reserve, and children, may find this additional effort difficult.

Indications for the use of nebulizers

Bronchodilator drugs. Infants and children not yet able to manage the more simple inhalation devices benefit from nebulized bronchodilators, but it has been shown that parents need written instruction in addition to verbal instruction to act appropriately in an acute situation (Bendefy 1991).

Some patients demonstrate a more significant response to nebulized bronchodilators than to bronchodilators via a simple inhaler. This includes those with asthma and chronic airflow limitation. Patients admitted to hospital with an acute attack of asthma and a few severe asthmatic patients who have life-threatening falls in peak expiratory flow in the night or early morning when at home, may respond better to nebulized bronchodilator drugs than to other methods of delivery during these episodes. If nebulized bronchodilators are not producing their usual effect the patient must seek medical advice, as further treatment is probably indicated. A common side-effect associated with β_2 agonists is muscle tremor, especially of the hands. Bronchodilator solutions should be isotonic and free of preservatives in order to prevent paradoxical bronchoconstriction (Editorial 1988).

Corticosteroids and prophylactic drugs. Nebulized corticosteroids are occasionally used in the treatment of asthma, especially in children, if airflow obstruction is not controlled by β_2 agonists and sodium cromoglycate. The incidence of attacks of asthma may be reduced by the inhalation of sodium cromoglycate and related drugs. They are not of value in the treatment of acute attacks of asthma and are more effective in children than in adults.

Antibiotics, antifungal drugs and pentamidine. Nebulized *antibiotic drugs* may be used in some cases of resistant chest infection in patients with deteriorating lung function and persistent pseudomonal infection (Hodson et al 1981). The nebulizer should be fitted with a one-way valve system and either wide-bore tubing to allow the exhaled gas to be vented out through a window (Fig. 8.44) or an effective filter. This is necessary to prevent small quantities of antibiotics from remaining in the atmosphere which could lead to neighbouring patients, family members and medical personnel receiving a subtherapeutic dose (Smaldone et al 1991) and to environmental organisms becoming resistant to the antibiotic. A nose clip is necessary if the patient is breathing partially through the nose.

Occasionally, inhaled antibiotics are prescribed for a pseudomonal infection in the upper respiratory tract, for example a patient with cystic fibrosis following lung transplantation. For this treatment a mask should be used and the patient encouraged to breathe through his nose.

More than one antibiotic may be prescribed. A few antibiotics are compatible when mixed, but others must be inhaled separately. Either normal saline or sterile water is used to reconstitute a powdered antibiotic or to make a prescribed solution up to the necessary volume for nebulization. The diluent should be that which will make the solution as near as possible to isotonic. Information on the correct solution for dilution and the advisability of mixing drugs should be obtained from a pharmacist.

Nebulized antibiotics may be hypo- or hypertonic solutions and may cause airflow obstruction.

The first dose of a nebulized antibiotic should be monitored by recording the FEV_1 and FVC before, immediately after, 15 minutes after and, if evidence of airflow obstruction persists, 30 minutes after the inhalation. Airflow obstruction can usually be controlled by the inhalation of a bronchodilator taken before physiotherapy for the clearance of secretions, preceding the inhalation of the antibiotic.

Viscous solutions of antibiotic drugs (e.g. carbenicillin, ticarcillin and ceftazidime) require either a driving gas with a flow of more than 8 l/min or a specifically designed nebulizer.

Antifungal agents are occasionally inhaled in the treatment of pulmonary fungal infections. A one-way valve system is not necessary as there is no evidence of resistance to these drugs.

Pentamidine isothianate is an antiprotozoal drug and is sometimes used in the treatment of *Pneumocystis carinii* pneumonia (p. 424). A one-way valve system is necessary (Smaldone et al 1991).

Analgesic drugs. Marcain and lignocaine (Howard et al 1977) can be inhaled by nebulizer in the treatment of intractable cough which may occur after a viral infection. The analgesic effect of Marcain is of longer duration and it is usually used in preference to lignocaine. A 3–4 ml dose of 0.5% Marcain is inhaled up to three times per

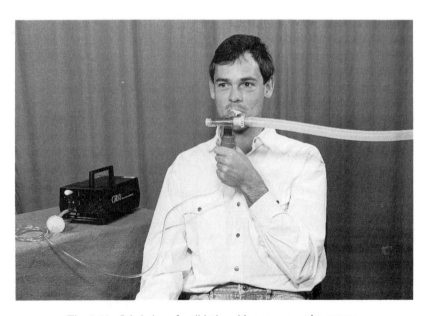

Fig. 8.44 Inhalation of antibiotics with a one-way valve system.

day. The patient should not eat or drink for $1\frac{1}{2}$ hours after the inhalation.

Clinically, morphine has been shown to relieve breathlessness in some patients with severe chronic lung disease. A study (Young et al 1989) has demonstrated an increase in exercise endurance in patients with severe breathlessness on exertion.

Mucolytic agents. Hypertonic saline (3–7%) (Pavia et al 1978) may assist in the clearance of secretions if it is inhaled before physiotherapy. It may also be used in sputum induction (p. 423), but its mode of action is unclear. Hypertonic saline (Schoeffel et al 1981) may cause an increase in airflow obstruction and a test dose using spirometry is necessary.

Acetylcysteine should be used with caution. A reduction in sputum viscosity does not necessarily produce an increase in expectoration of sputum and bronchospasm may be induced. A test dose using spirometry is also necessary with this drug. Acetylcysteine is inactivated by oxygen and, if nebulized, the driving gas should be air.

The development of recombinant human deoxyribonuclease (DNase) which acts on the deoxyribonucleic acid (DNA) in purulent lung secretions may be an important drug for inhalation in the future. Early studies in patients with cystic fibrosis indicate an improvement in lung function with DNase (Ranasinha et al 1993).

Domiciliary nebulization

If there is an indication for domiciliary nebulization in either children or adults, careful instructions are essential, both verbal and written, and equipment should be appropriately selected.

Ideally, the air compressor should be portable, lightweight and quiet when in operation. The flow rate required for most drugs is 6–7 l/min, but viscous antibiotics may require a higher powered compressor producing a minimum of a 8 l/min or a nebulizer specifically designed for antibiotics. Some patients may benefit from a compressor that can be used when travelling, either by using a 12 volt adaptor in a socket in the car, 'crocodile clips' fitted on to a battery, or more conveniently a compact battery pack supplied with the compressor (Fig. 8.45). Those travelling to a country using a different voltage may require a transformer or a dual-voltage compressor. Some compressors incorporate a universal power pack which adapts to voltages throughout the world. An international travel plug adaptor is an accessory required for all who travel abroad. A foot pump may be useful to power a nebulizer where no electricity is available, but it

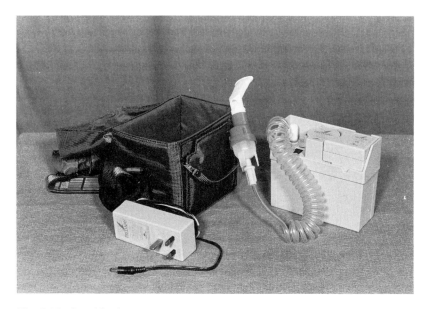

Fig. 8.45 Portable air compressor with battery pack (Freeway Lite, Medic-Aid Ltd).

requires considerable energy to operate. It is advisable to take a letter from a doctor explaining the need to travel with drugs, and possibly syringes and needles, when travelling abroad.

The standard flow head supplied for the domiciliary use of oxygen is unsuitable for driving a nebulizer as the maximum output is only 4 l/min. Flow meters capable of providing higher flows of oxygen could be used, but this system is less economic and more restricting to the patient's lifestyle than a portable compressor. An oxygen concentrator does not produce a high enough flow to drive a nebulizer.

Practical and written instructions in the care and cleaning of the equipment must be given. A spare jet nebulizer and inlet filter should be available. The nebulizer must be washed and dried after each treatment to keep the jets clear, and once a week the nebulizer should be disinfected using a disinfecting agent (e.g. Milton). The transducer of an ultrasonic nebulizer should be cleaned regularly with acetic acid (white vinegar) to maintain its efficiency. An annual check of output, and general and electrical safety should be undertaken, and there should be provision for servicing as required.

Bronchodilator response studies

The value of bronchodilator response studies in the assessment of patients for nebulized bronchodilators is controversial (Mestitz et al 1989, O'Driscoll et al 1990, Goldman et al 1992). Short-term responses may not reflect a long-term response. A peak flow meter (Fig. 19.2, p. 393) is often used to assess bronchodilator response. This will be suitable in a patient with asthma, but will not detect the more subtle response of a change in FVC which can occur in those with more irreversible airflow obstruction (Fig. 8.46). For these patients the response to a bronchodilator, detected by a change in FVC, may lead to an increase in exercise ability and improved quality of life.

The unnecessary use of nebulized bronchodilators can restrict activities of daily living. A nebulizer and air compressor system should only be prescribed if a simple device used correctly is not as effective.

Objective measurements of bronchodilator response can be made by serial recordings of FEV_1 and FVC. Preceding the study the drugs to be tested should be withheld for 4–6 hours, but all other drugs should be continued as prescribed. 'Stable baseline readings, with correct technique, must first be obtained. The best result of two or three attempts is taken, allowing a pause of at least 30 seconds between each attempt. Baseline readings are repeated at 5 min intervals until the maximum pretreatment level is known. Some patients will continue to improve over several minutes, while others will soon reach a plateau or decrease their FEV_1 or FVC.

Having ensured a correct technique, the bronchodilator is then inhaled and spirometry is repeated at the appropriate time interval for the particular drug. After salbutamol (Ventolin), or terbutaline (Bricanyl), readings can be made at 15 and 30 min intervals (Ruffin et al 1977), whereas with the slower acting ipratropium bromide (Atrovent), recordings are made 40 and 60 min from the time of inhalation (Loddenkemper 1975). In each case recordings should be continued until the maximum response is achieved, for example if the response to salbutamol is greater at 30 min than at 15 min the spirometry is repeated at 10 min intervals until a plateau or fall in FEV_1 or FVC is recorded. If time is limited, this outline can be modified, recordings being taken at the expected times of maximal improvement (30 min following Ventolin and Bricanyl and 60 min following Atrovent).

The same principle can be applied when comparing different methods of delivery of the same drug or when comparing the response to two different bronchodilators. If comparing the response of a patient to Ventolin by pressurized aerosol and a nebulized solution of Ventolin, measurements are made until maximum response is reached after inhalation by pressurized aerosol and then the nebulized solution is given immediately. Any additional response is determined by the postnebulizer recordings. If response to one method of delivery is determined on one occasion and to the other method on a separate occasion, the results are unlikely to be comparable because the baseline readings and other factors such as the time of testing and dose of

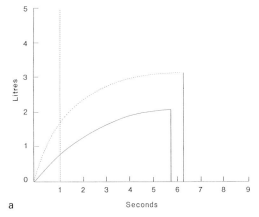

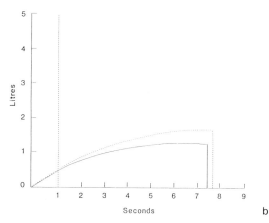

Fig. 8.46 **a** Increase in FEV_1 and FVC. **b** Increase in FVC only.
Spirometry before bronchodilator. --------- Spirometry after bronchodilator. . . .

steroid drugs may be different. Similarly, when comparing the response to two different drugs (for example, Ventolin and Atrovent) the second should be given as soon as maximum response has been achieved with the first' (Webber 1988).

McGavin et al (1976) demonstrated that the inhalation of a bronchodilator preceding exercise can improve exercise tolerance, but the improvement does not correlate with changes in FEV_1 and FVC.

O'Driscoll et al (1990) in their study on home nebulizers could not demonstrate a correlation between formal lung function testing and the domiciliary use of a nebulizer system. They recommended that patients who are referred for consideration of home nebulizer therapy be given the equipment to try under supervision for several weeks at home and that the patient's subjective assessment should be considered.

An objective study which demonstrates to the patient a positive response to a simple inhalation device with no further response to nebulized drugs, often relieves the patient who has felt that a compressor system would be necessary.

Many patients with asthma keep a diary card at home which will include recordings of peak expiratory flow before and after bronchodilator drugs. These will only be valid if the technique when using the meter is correct. Points to emphasize are:

- the patient should take a maximum breath in (in his haste to carry out the manoeuvre the patient may not take a full deep breath)
- expiration should be short and sharp
- sufficient rests (at least 15 seconds) should be allowed between 'blows' to prevent any increase in airflow obstruction with the forced expiratory manoeuvre
- the same position, sitting or standing, should be used for taking the readings.

HUMIDIFICATION

A device to provide humidification of the airways may be considered if either the normal means of humidifying the airway or the mucociliary escalator are not functioning effectively.

The mucous membranes of the upper airway normally provide warmth and humidification of the inspired air. The temperature and humidity of the inspired air varies, but the gas in the alveoli is fully saturated with water vapour at body temperature. There is a temperature and humidity gradient from the nose to the point where the gas reaches 37°C and 100% relative humidity (Shelly et al 1988). This point is normally just below the carina in the adult, but varies depending on the temperature and water content of the inspired gas, and the tidal volume. The upper airway acts as a heat and moisture exchanger with the fully saturated expired gas giving up some heat and water to the mucosa (Chatburn 1987).

The epithelial lining of the airway, from the trachea to the respiratory bronchioles, contains ciliated cells which are responsible for moving mucus and other particulate matter proximally to the level of the larynx.

The optimal temperature for cilial activity is normal body temperature with reduced activity occurring below 20°C and above 40°C (Wanner 1977). The cilia beat within a watery fluid known as the 'periciliary' or 'sol' layer. A mucus layer 'gel' covers the periciliary layer and interacts with the tips of the cilia.

The efficiency of mucus transport is dependent on correctly functioning cilia, and the composition of the periciliary and mucus layers. If the periciliary layer becomes too shallow, as with dehydration, the cilia become enmeshed in the viscous mucus layer and cannot function effectively. If the periciliary layer is too deep the tips of the cilia are not in contact with the mucus layer and propulsion of the mucus is inefficient.

The viscosity of mucus is increased during bacterial infection due to an increase in the DNA content of the mucus (Wilson & Cole 1988), and with the hypersecretory disorders of, for example, bronchiectasis, cystic fibrosis and chronic airflow limitation, there is an increase in both quantity and viscosity of mucus secretions. Bacteria directly affect cilial beating and coordination, disrupt the epithelium, stimulate mucus secretion and alter periciliary fluid composition (Cole 1990). Humidification has been shown to enhance tracheobronchial clearance when used as an adjunct to physiotherapy in a group of patients with bronchiectasis (Conway et al 1992).

Clarke (1990) has suggested that the efficiency of cough increases with a decrease in viscosity of mucus and an increase in the periciliary layer of the airway. Conway (1992) hypothesizes that humidification of water or saline aerosol produces an increase in depth of the periciliary and mucus layers, thereby decreasing viscosity and enhancing the shearing of secretions by huffing or coughing.

High humidification may be indicated to assist clearance of secretions when the clearance mechanism is not optimally effective and when the upper airway heat and moisture exchange system is bypassed by an endotracheal or tracheostomy tube. Patients with a long-term tracheostomy develop metaplasia of the tracheal epithelium and adequate humidification of the inspired gas

occurs spontaneously, but additional humidification may be required during an episode of respiratory infection (Oh 1990).

Methods of humidification

Systemic hydration

Adequate humidification may be obtained by increasing the oral or intravenous fluid intake of a patient. Breathless patients find drinking fluids an effort, but need encouragement to avoid dehydration. Patients with chronic sputum production should be reminded to maintain an adequate fluid intake to lessen the viscosity of the mucus. During periods of infection and fever a higher fluid intake is required.

Heated water bath humidifiers

Gas is blown over a reservoir of heated sterile water and absorbs water vapour which is then inhaled by the patient. If the delivery tube is cold there is a temperature drop as the gas passes along the tube and condensation occurs. The humidifier should be positioned below the level of the patient's airway to avoid flooding of the airway by condensed water. There should be a water trap in the circuit and care is needed to empty the tubes regularly. A heated delivery tube eliminates the problem of condensation.

The Fisher & Paykel humidifier (Fig. 8.47) consists of a heater base and a water filled chamber. The inspired gas passes through an aluminium spiral scroll within the chamber which increases the vaporizing area. A heated delivery tube is incorporated to deliver the gas near to 37°C. This humidifier can be used for the spontaneously breathing patient or can be incorporated into a ventilator circuit, continuous positive airway pressure circuit (Fig. 8.48) and is suitable for use with a nasal intermittent positive pressure ventilator. Sterile water must be used in these devices. If saline is used, it is the water only which vaporizes and the sodium chloride crystalizes out.

Heat and moisture exchangers

A heat and moisture exchanger is a lightweight

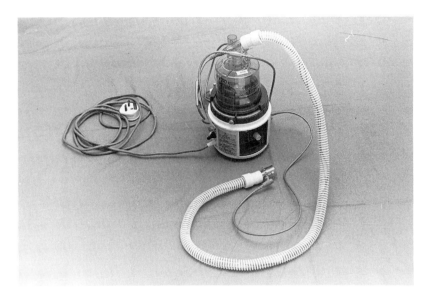

Fig. 8.47   The Fisher & Paykel heated humidifier.

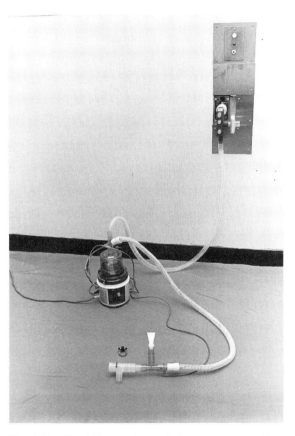

Fig. 8.48   Humidification in a periodic continuous positive airway pressure circuit.

disposable device often used in the intubated patient either mechanically ventilated or breathing spontaneously and is convenient for use in the ambulant patient. The humidifier acts in a similar way to the nasopharynx. The heat and moisture of the exhaled gas are retained either by condensation (condenser humidifier) or by absorption, and returned in the inhaled gas as it passes through the device. A variety of hygroscopic materials and chemicals is used for absorption within heat and moisture exchangers.

Heat and moisture exchangers are inefficient if there is a large air leak around an uncuffed tracheostomy tube (Tilling & Hayes 1987) and do not provide adequate humidification for infants. If the secretions of a patient using a heat and moisture exchanger become tenacious a more effective form of humidification will be required. The humidifier must be changed immediately if it becomes soiled with secretions and at least every 24 hours.

Nebulizers

A nebulizer for humidification may be a jet nebulizer or ultrasonic nebulizer. Nebulizers produce an aerosol mist of droplets (Shelly et al 1988). Some jet nebulizers can have a heater incorporated in the system (Fig. 8.49). This increased temperature raises the relative humidity, is less irritative for patients with hyper-reactive airways and is less likely to increase airflow obstruction than cold humidification. When a jet nebulizer is powered by oxygen the amount of air entrained by the nebulizer will often depend on the oxygen concentration required. If the concentration of oxygen is not important, consideration should be given to the density of mist and flow required by the individual.

The mist particles delivered with a venturi closed (98% setting) appear more dense, but the total flow (approximately 10 l/min) will be insufficient to meet the patient's inspiratory requirement and additional room air will be entrained through the holes in a face mask or mouthpiece, effectively reducing the degree of humidification. A 35% setting on a venturi system will produce a flow of approximately 40 1/min. This would provide a higher degree of humidification as it would meet the inspiratory demand of the patient most of the time.

Many ultrasonic nebulizers do not have a heater but the mist is at ambient temperature and warmer than that produced from a jet nebulizer powered from compressed piped gas. There is often an airflow control valve in addition to a control for the density of the mist. By regulating .these two controls a density of mist can be obtained that the patient can inhale comfortably.

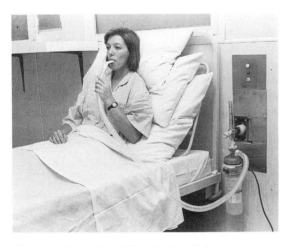

Fig. 8.49 Heated humidification by nebulization (Theramist Medic-Aid Ltd).

Sterile normal saline (0.9%) is an isotonic solution and probably the most acceptable to patients inhaling from a nebulizer. Sterile water can be used if saline is unavailable, but has been shown to cause bronchoconstriction in patients with hyperreactive airways (Schoeffel et al 1981).

Bubble-through humidifiers

A device containing cold water through which the inspired gas is bubbled is not an effective means of humidification. If connected to an oxygen mask with narrow-bore tubing it may alter the oxygen concentration as water condenses in the tubing. A bubble-through humidifier is often connected to nasal cannulae, but there are neither objective nor subjective benefits from this form of humidification (Campbell et al 1988).

Steam inhalations

Inhalation of steam may be useful in patients with postoperative sputum retention if they are encouraged to breathe deeply. Precautions must be taken to avoid spilling the hot water.

Delivery to the patient

Patients with retained secretions postoperatively or those with excess viscous secretions due to. a chronic bronchopulmonary infection may benefit from a period of 10–20 min high humidification before physiotherapy to assist the clearance of secretions. If the concentration of oxygen required by the patient is not critical, a *mouthpiece* with a hole for entrainment of additional air is simple and comfortable to use (Fig. 8.49). Deep breathing interspersed with · tidal volume breathing will encourage peripheral deposition of an aerosol, while avoiding hyperventilation.

If a patient requires an oxygen concentration of 28% or more, a *face mask* can be connected by wide-bore tubing to a nebulizer head and the venturi of the nebulizer should be set to the appropriate concentration.

Patients requiring an inspired oxygen concentration of 24% will probably wear a venturi mask connected to the oxygen by narrow-bore tubing. It is impossible to give high humidification through a narrow-bore tube due to condensation within the tubing. Effective humidification can be obtained by using a *humidity adaptor* which allows the air entrained by the mask to be humidified. It is a cuff fitted over the air entraining holes of the mask and connected by wide-bore humidity tubing to a humidifier powered by an air source. This can be piped compressed air if it is available, or an air cylinder or an electric air compressor capable of continuous use ('continuously rated') (Fig. 8.50). An ultrasonic nebulizer, set at a high flow, can be used and is quieter than a jet nebulizer system. A humidity adaptor can be used to give humidification to ventimasks delivering accurate higher concentrations of oxygen (e.g. 28% or 35%), but is unsatisfactory with a 60% ventimask because the air-entraining holes are too small to entrain the humidity. For humidification with 60–100% oxygen two nebulizing units in parallel may be used (p. 155).

If a patient is breathing spontaneously through a tracheostomy, a *tracheostomy mask* may be attached to a humidifier or nebulizer via wide-bore tubing.

Humidification through a *head box* (Fig. 13.8, p. 292) is often used in the treatment of spontaneously breathing infants. With the narrow airways of an infant the risk of mucus plugging is higher than in adults. Humidity to a head box may be either from a heated water bath humidifier or a heated nebulizer system.

Hazards of humidification

Inhalation of cold mist or water (a hypotonic solution) may cause bronchoconstriction in patients with hyperreactive airways (Schoeffel et al 1981). Heated humidification and normal saline solution are less likely to cause this problem. Peak flow recordings or spirometry should be carried out before and immediately after the first treatment.

Water reservoirs may become infected with *Pseudomonas* and other organisms, many of which multiply rapidly at 45°C. Some control of infection can be obtained by using an operating temperature of 60°C (Oh 1990). Regular disposal, disinfection or sterilization of all humidification equipment is essential to prevent infection.

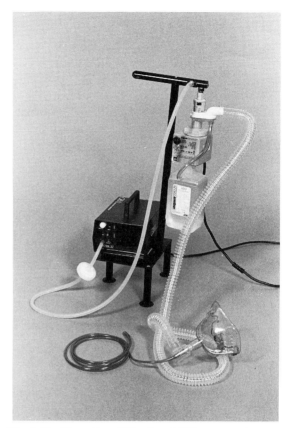

Fig. 8.50 Heated humidification of 24% oxygen using a humidity adaptor (Vickers, Kendall, Medic-Aid).

OXYGEN THERAPY

Oxygen therapy is indicated when tissue oxygenation is impaired. The physiotherapist frequently treats patients requiring added inspired oxygen and may be involved with the setting up of oxygen therapy equipment. Oxygen is a drug and should be prescribed by a medical practitioner and monitored using arterial blood gas analysis or oxygen saturation recordings. When a patient is on continuous oxygen therapy the mask should be removed only briefly for expectoration, eating and drinking, and sometimes during these periods oxygen therapy may be continued using nasal cannulae.

Devices for administering oxygen therapy may be divided into fixed and variable performance devices (Hinds 1987b). A *fixed performance device* will deliver a known inspired oxygen concentration (FiO_2), by providing a sufficiently high flow of premixed gas which will exceed the patient's peak inspiratory flow rate. A venturi system allows a relatively low flow of oxygen to entrain a large volume of air and the mixed gas is conveyed to a large volume mask (Fig. 8.51). For most patients the entrained room air provides sufficient humidification, but occasionally additional high humidification is indicated (p. 153). A bubble-through humidifier attached to the narrow-bore tubing of a ventimask may alter the oxygen concentration as water condenses in the narrow tubing.

On rare occasions when a spontaneously breathing patient requires an oxygen concentration, as near as possible to 100%, two venturi humidification systems set at 98–100% can be run in parallel with a Y-connection leading to a face mask (Fig. 8.52). The two systems are necessary to provide an adequate flow (approximately 30–40 l/min in an adult) to exceed the patient's inspiratory flow. The face mask should have large

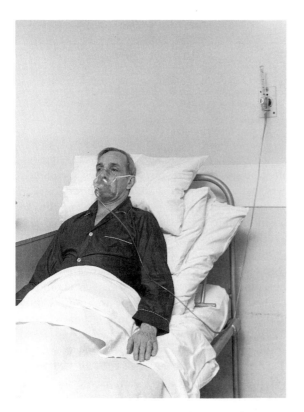

Fig. 8.51 Fixed performance device for oxygen therapy (Venturi mask).

side holes into which are inserted two pieces (approximately 10 cm long) of wide-bore tubing. These will fill with oxygen in the pause between expiration and inspiration and should any air entrainment during inspiration be required it will have an oxygen concentration of 98–100%.

A variable performance device supplies a flow of oxygen which is less than the patient's minute volume. The inspired oxygen concentration (FiO_2) will vary with the rate and volume of breath, and considerable variations between and within subjects have been demonstrated (Bazuaye et al 1992). Commonly used variable performance devices are the simple face mask and nasal cannulae. Nasal cannulae are often preferred as the patient can eat, drink and speak more comfortably and finds it less claustrophobic than a mask. Although high flows of oxygen can be delivered to nasal cannulae, 1–4 l/min (approximately 24–36%) is the range for patient comfort, as higher flows tend to irritate and dry the nasal mucosa. A higher inspired oxygen concentration may be obtained by using a fixed performance device or a combination of face mask and nasal cannulae. This combination has the advantage that the patient will still receive some additional oxygen if the face mask is removed.

Effective humidification cannot be provided by narrow-bore tubing, and if high humidification is required the mask should be attached via wide-bore tubing to a humidifier or nebulizer. The bubble-through humidifier often attached to nasal cannulae does not provide any additional humidification.

When accurate delivery of oxygen is required, especially at low concentrations, a fixed performance device is essential because wide variations in inspired oxygen concentration have been shown to be produced by variable performance devices, even with the recommended flows (Jeffrey & Warren 1992).

Nebulizers for the delivery of drugs in hospital are frequently powered by piped oxygen, but in the patient dependent on his hypoxic drive to breathe, air should be used as the driving gas. Occasionally, in the severely hypoxic patient, who is also hypercapnic and dependent on a controlled 24% oxygen mask, the patient should not be deprived of this added oxygen while

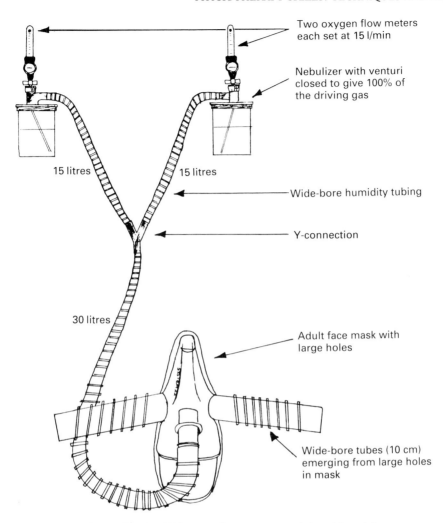

Two oxygen flow meters each set at 15 l/min

Nebulizer with venturi closed to give 100% of the driving gas

15 litres   15 litres

Wide-bore humidity tubing

Y-connection

30 litres

Adult face mask with large holes

Wide-bore tubes (10 cm) emerging from large holes in mask

Fig. 8.52 Equipment for 98–100% oxygen for a spontaneously breathing adult.

using a nebulizer. One to two litres of oxygen can be added through a T-piece into the tubing connecting the air compressor to the nebulizer. The level of oxygen entrained to maintain the baseline oxygen saturation can be monitored using a pulse oximeter.

For most patients an *intermittent positive pressure breathing device* (IPPB) should be driven by compressed oxygen. Starke et al (1979) demonstrated that in hypercapnic patients oxygen can be used as the driving gas (p. 136). In hypoxic patients without hypercapnia, for example in acute asthma, oxygen is required and it is dangerous to use air alone as the driving gas for IPPB.

An *oxygen concentrator* (Fig. 8.53) is a convenient and efficient means of providing long-term oxygen therapy in the home, and the oxygen tubing can be fitted in areas of the home to allow for mobility. An oxygen cylinder is necessary for emergency use. Humidifiers are sometimes fitted to oxygen concentrators but care must be taken as these are a potential source of infection (Pendleton et al 1991).

Small *portable oxygen cylinders* can be used for short trips outside the home. These may be transported on a lightweight trolley (Fig. 8.54) or carried over the shoulder. Portable cylinders can be refilled from a larger oxygen cylinder using a special adaptor, but they cannot be refilled from

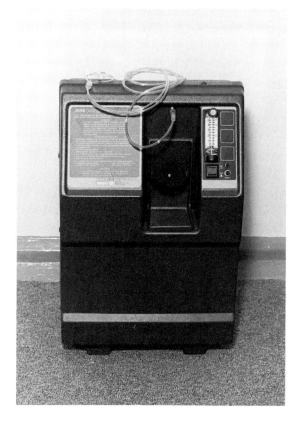

Fig. 8.53   An oxygen concentrator.

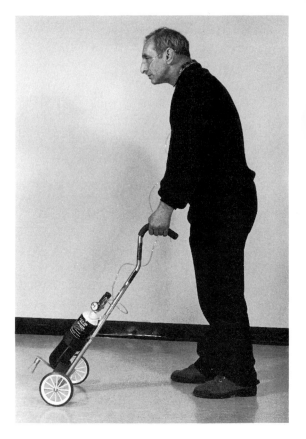

Fig. 8.54   Portable oxygen with variable performance device (nasal cannulae).

an oxygen concentrator. Careful instruction must be given in refilling the portable cylinder, as this can be a frightening and difficult procedure until the patient or his carer are familiar with it.

In an attempt to give patients who are dependent on oxygen greater mobility and the opportunity to participate in activities outside the home, an *inspiratory phased delivery system* or *oxygen by transtracheal catheter*, may be considered (Shneerson 1992). A microcatheter inserted into the trachea will reduce the dead space and decrease the requirement for oxygen. Some patients find this more cosmetically acceptable than nasal cannulae, but there is the increased possibility of infection.

The physiotherapist may be involved in *assessing* patients who may benefit from portable oxygen. Repeated walking tests, for example the 6 minute walking test, with the patient 'blind' to whether he is using oxygen or air during the walk, can be used as a means of assessment in conjunc-

tion with a visual analogue scale of breathlessness. The measurement of oxygen saturation using a pulse oximeter may also be included in the assessment.

Heliox

A mixture of helium (79%) and oxygen (21%) is sometimes used on a temporary basis to relieve respiratory distress in patients with upper airways obstruction, for example a tumour causing partial obstruction of the trachea. Helium is lighter than the nitrogen in air and the mixture passes more easily through the narrowed airway requiring less effort from the patient (Vater et al 1983). A side-effect of heliox is an alteration in the pitch of the voice, due to its effect on the vocal cords. This is only temporary, but should be explained to the patient before use of heliox to avoid unnecessary concern.

MANUAL HYPERINFLATION

The technique of manual hyperinflation may be indicated to mobilize and assist clearance of excess bronchial secretions and to reinflate areas of lung collapse in the intubated patient. It is sometimes known as 'bag squeezing' but differs from the 'bagging' carried out during a resuscitation procedure or when transferring an intubated patient to a mechanical ventilator. The technique was described by Clement and Hübsch (1968) and consists of a series of deep breaths with a quick release of the bag to simulate the effect of a cough.

For an adult, a 2 litre rebreathing bag connected to a flow of 10–15 l/min of oxygen is commonly used. Frequent adjustment to the valve allows the operator to inflate the lungs to an appropriate volume and the elasticity of the rebreathing bag allows her to feel the compliance of the patient's chest.

An alternative to a rebreathing system is a self-inflating bag, such as an Ambu or Laerdal bag, where room air inflates the bag through a valve and additional oxygen is entrained through a connector (Hack et al 1980). The more compliant material of the rebreathing bag allows the physiotherapist to 'feel' the compliance of the lung which will be different for each patient and may alter with treatment. For those inexperienced in adjusting the control valve in a rebreathing circuit a self-inflating bag may be easier to use (Jones et al 1991).

In the spontaneously breathing adult the dependent lung is preferentially ventilated, but it is the uppermost lung that is preferentially ventilated in the patient receiving intermittent positive pressure ventilation (Rehder et al 1972). It is therefore more effective to treat the patient in the side lying position than in the supine position, unless a change of position is contraindicated. If there are signs of collapse only in one lung this side would be positioned uppermost for treatment.

Before treatment an alert patient may require sedation and analgesia to avoid undue discomfort. Entonox is sometimes used instead of oxygen for manual hyperinflation, and if sedative drugs are not indicated Entonox could be considered.

Having positioned the patient and explained the procedure to him, the manual hyperinflation bag is connected to the endotracheal or tracheostomy tube. The bag is squeezed to inflate the lungs with a slow deep inspiration, and after a momentary pause at full inspiration the bag is released quickly to allow a high expiratory flow rate. Compression, vibrations or shaking of the chest wall can augment the expiratory flow and assist clearance of secretions (Fig. 8.55). To achieve maximum effect the compression should be applied at an instant fractionally before the bag is released. If the patient is taking spontaneous breaths it is important to coincide inflation of the bag with the patient's inspiratory effort.

As soon as secretions in the upper airways are audible, or after 6–8 breaths, suction is applied. An alert patient should be encouraged to attempt to cough actively when the catheter is inserted and chest compression or support of a wound is given during the suction procedure.

Following suction the patient can be reconnected to the mechanical ventilator for a rest before the procedure is repeated. Alternatively, the patient may be more comfortable with ventilation continued at tidal breathing using the inflation bag. The number of times the manual hyperinflation and suction sequence is repeated during a treatment session cannot be specified as it must depend on the individual patient's condition. Treatment is similar for the intubated patient who is not requiring mechanical ventilation. He can be encouraged to breathe in during the period of manual hyperinflation and to try one or two huffs before airway suction.

If a high level of positive end expiratory pressure (PEEP) is being used (10 cm or more) it should probably be maintained during manual hyperinflation, although only occasionally would manual hyperinflation be indicated. A level of PEEP can be maintained either by not allowing a rebreathing bag to empty completely or by attaching a PEEP valve to a self-inflating bag (Hack et al 1980).

Assessment should be made of the quantity and colour of the bronchial secretions aspirated and of the breath sounds before and after treatment.

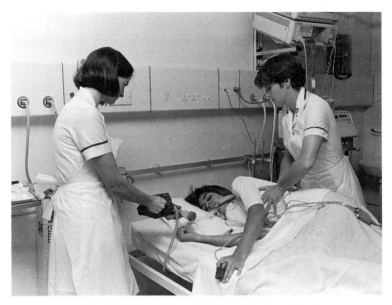

Fig. 8.55   Manual hyperinflation with chest vibrations.

The same principles of manual hyperinflation can be used in treating an intubated infant or child, but the inflation bag must be of appropriate size. A 0.5 litre bag connected to 4–6 l/min of oxygen is used for an infant. Instead of a mechanical control valve on the proximal end of an adult rebreathing bag, the distal end of the infant's bag remains open and the leak is controlled by the physiotherapist's hand. The bag should not be completely emptied during the procedure allowing some positive expiratory pressure to be maintained to avoid airway collapse. It is particularly important in an infant to use a slow inflation to avoid a high peak inspiratory pressure which has the risk of barotrauma.

Instillation of 2–3 ml of normal saline (0.9%) into the trachea before manual hyperinflation may help to loosen tenacious secretions. If there is a persistent area of collapse a more effective way to instil saline is from a syringe via a catheter inserted into the airways and a Coudé tip or a left bronchial catheter should be used for a left lower lobe collapse. The collapsed area should be dependent to allow maximal insufflation of the saline and then the patient should be repositioned with the collapsed area uppermost. The technique of manual hyperinflation is then used.

In an infant with viscid secretions saline can be inserted via a catheter, but it is important to insert only a small known volume. A catheter can be filled with saline and, leaving the syringe attached, it is inserted into the endotracheal tube as far as possible. It is then withdrawn 1 cm to ensure that it is above the carina and then 0.5 ml can be instilled from the syringe.

Manual hyperinflation can produce a fall in cardiac output as the increase in intrathoracic pressure may reduce the venous return to the heart. It is therefore important to watch the monitored recordings of arterial blood pressure, heart rate, oxygen saturation, transcutaneous oxygen and transcutaneous carbon dioxide, depending on which measurements are available.

Manual hyperinflation may be used following assessment if there is an indication for its use, but no pre-existing contraindication. Contraindications include an unstable cardiovascular state, acute pulmonary oedema, severe bronchospasm and surgical emphysema. In infants it would be contraindicated if the lungs are stiff and requiring high inflation pressures and in preterm infants where there is a high risk of pneumothorax. If manual hyperinflation is contraindicated in the intubated patient, appropriate positioning, chest shaking during expiration and suction should be considered.

Weaning from a ventilator

It is usually the consultant doctor who is responsible for the weaning process but the physiotherapist will be involved if respiratory problems develop during this period. In the intubated patient manual hyperinflation may be continued until the patient can cooperate effectively with the active cycle of breathing techniques. Huffing and expectoration of secretions should be encouraged as soon as possible and suction can then be discontinued.

Many cuffed tracheostomy tubes can be converted to speaking tubes, but it is essential to deflate the cuff fully before inserting the speaking cannula.

Following removal of a tracheostomy tube a dressing that will provide an air-tight seal is necessary for effective huffing and coughing. Intermittent positive pressure breathing may be of value in the early stages following extubation to assist in the clearance of secretions.

AIRWAY SUCTION

Airway suction is usually necessary to clear secretions from the intubated patient with an endotracheal tube, tracheostomy, minitracheostomy or the patient with an airway. It is also required in the non-intubated infant and small child unable to clear secretions effectively and occasionally in the non-intubated adult who has retained secretions.

It is well known that airway suction causes damage to the tracheal epithelium (Czarnik et al 1991) and that this can be minimized by the appropriate choice of catheter and technique.

Effective suction and minimal trauma to the mucosa can be achieved using a catheter with a terminal eye and two small cylindrical side holes which prevent adherence of the catheter to the airway walls (Uno Plast 1991).

The diameter of catheter selected for an intubated patient should not exceed half the internal diameter of the endotracheal tube. For adults the most common sizes are 12 and 14 French Gauge (FG) and for children sizes 4, 6 and 8 FG. The catheter should be long enough to exceed the length of an endotracheal tube.

The vacuum pressure should be kept as low as possible, and usually in the range 60–150 mmHg (8.0–20 kPa), but this will vary with the viscosity of the mucus. A built-in finger tip control or Y-connector is recommended to allow a more gradual build up of suction pressure than is possible by the release of a kinked catheter tube.

Before any suction procedure it is important to give an explanation to the patient.

For suction in paediatrics see Chapter 13 (p. 289).

The intubated patient

Preoxygenation by increasing the FiO_2 of the ventilator, or by manual hyperinflation with 100% oxygen may help to avoid a fall in the arterial oxygen tension (Riegel & Forshee 1985, Walsh et al 1989, White et al 1990), but the advantages remain unproven. Suction (Fig. 8.56) should be carried out using a sterile technique and each disposable catheter should be discarded after one insertion. Non-disposable catheters are used occasionally and should be resterilized after a single use.

The catheter is inserted into the endotracheal or tracheostomy tube until it has reached just beyond the end of the tube, when it will probably be on the carina and a cough will be stimulated. The catheter should be withdrawn slightly before the suction pressure is applied. Suction is then maintained while the catheter is gently withdrawn. There is no evidence that intermittent suction is either more effective or less traumatic than continuous suction. A rotating action is unnecessary with the type of catheter described earlier which minimizes adherence to the mucosa.

Aspiration of secretions from the left lung is more difficult, owing to the anatomical position of the left main bronchus. A left bronchial or Coudé tip catheter with a curve at its distal end will facilitate entry to the left main bronchus. After insertion into the trachea the curved tip should point towards the left. Aspiration of secretions from the right lung can usually be carried out effectively using a straight tracheal catheter.

The duration of a single suction procedure should not exceed 15 seconds in order to minimize

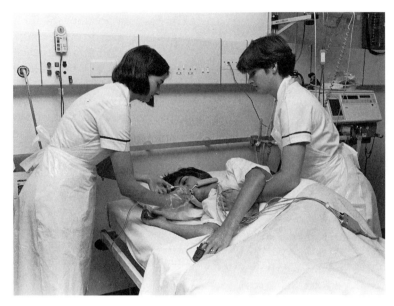

Fig. 8.56   Endotracheal suction (wtih chest support).

the possibility of causing hypoxaemia. In the occasional hypoxic patient, who may be on PEEP, and in whom it would be dangerous to lower the oxygen tension with disconnection for suction, a closed-circuit catheter may be used which permits suction while mechanical ventilation continues (Clark et al 1990). An alternative is an adapted catheter mount through which the catheter can be passed without allowing an air leak.

On occasions there is difficulty passing a catheter down an endotracheal tube. Alteration of the patient's head and neck to a more extended or slightly rotated position may facilitate this procedure. With fenestrated tracheostomy tubes the inner cannula should be reinserted for suction to avoid mucosal trauma if the catheter should inadvertently pass through the fenestration.

Instillation of 2–5 ml normal saline before suction may be indicated in intubated patients when the secretions are viscid. It appears to act as a lubricant and should help to maintain patency of the tube, but probably of more importance than the instillation of saline is systemic hydration and humidification of the inspired gas as the upper airway is bypassed (Ackerman 1985).

The colour and quantity of secretions should be noted during the suction procedure. Following suction the catheter is discarded and the tubing

from the suction apparatus is flushed with sterile water.

A sputum specimen can be obtained by connecting a specimen trap between the suction catheter and the tubing leading from the suction apparatus.

If secretions collect in the oropharynx or nasopharynx, suction will be necessary. A rigid sucker (Yankauer) can be used for the oropharynx and if the patient is capable he may prefer to do this himself. The nasopharynx is cleared using a flexible catheter of similar size to that used for the endotracheal suction.

In the patient who requires monitoring of the cardiovascular system any changes in the cardiovascular state should be noted, for example bradycardia, and the suction procedure should be modified to minimize the effect. Extreme care should be taken if suctioning a patient with a postsurgical anastomosis in the large airways, for example following a pneumonectomy, lung transplantation or replacement of the trachea.

Patients with long-term tracheostomy can often be taught to do their own tracheal suction. Mains electrical suction apparatus is obtainable for domiciliary use and portable battery operated equipment for patients when travelling, and for emergency or community use.

Nasotracheal suction

Nasotracheal suction is a means of stimulating a cough, but is an unpleasant procedure for the patient and should only be performed when absolutely necessary. The indication for suction is the inability to cough effectively and expectorate when secretions are retained. It may be necessary, for example, when an acute exacerbation of chronic bronchitis has led to carbon dioxide narcosis and respiratory failure (p. 226), in neurological disorders, postoperative complications or laryngeal dysfunction. It is contraindicated when there is stridor or severe bronchospasm.

A flexible catheter of suitable size, usually 12 FG in adults, is lubricated with a water soluble jelly and gently passed through the nasal passage so that it curves down into the pharynx. Occasionally a cough may be stimulated when the catheter reaches the pharynx, suction can then be applied, the secretions aspirated and the catheter withdrawn. More often it is necessary to pass the catheter between the vocal cords and into the trachea to stimulate coughing. The catheter is less likely to enter the oesophagus if the patient's neck is extended, and if he is able to cooperate it is often helpful if he can put his tongue out. The catheter should be inserted during the inspiratory phase and if it passes into the trachea will stimulate vigorous coughing.

Oxygen should always be available during the suction procedure and the patient observed for signs of hypoxia. If it has been difficult to insert the catheter and the patient looks cyanosed, instead of withdrawing the catheter from the trachea suction should be stopped and oxygen administered until the patient's colour has improved. Suction can then be restarted.

Adults nursed in the sitting position can be suctioned in that position, but comatose patients should be suctioned in side lying to avoid the possibility of aspiration if vomiting occurs.

Using the technique of nasotracheal suction it is important to be aware of the possibility of causing laryngeal spasm (Sykes et al 1976) or vagal nerve stimulation which may lead to cardiac arrhythmias (Jacob 1990). Provided that suction is carried out carefully and oxygen is always available it is a valuable technique and may avoid the

need for the more invasive treatments of bronchoscopy, endotracheal intubation or minitracheotomy. However, it should not be undertaken until every attempt to achieve effective coughing has failed.

Suction via the nose is contraindicated in patients with head injuries where there is a leak of cerebrospinal fluid into the nasal passages. Oropharyngeal suction through an airway would be an alternative method. An oropharyngeal airway is a plastic tube shaped to fit the curved palate. It is inserted with its tip directed towards the roof of the mouth and is then rotated so that the tip lies over the back of the tongue.

Although retention of secretions may be a problem in patients with respiratory muscle paralysis there is no benefit in using suction in an attempt to stimulate an effective cough. It is the lack of volume of air that prevents clearance of secretions in these patients and it is the combination of gravity-assisted drainage positions, chest compression and intermittent positive pressure breathing or glossopharyngeal breathing (p. 127) which will provide an effective means of clearance.

Minitracheotomy

A minitracheotomy (Fig. 8.57) may be considered when a spontaneously breathing patient is retaining bronchial secretions. It has been used successfully in surgical and medical patients (Preston et al 1986). Nasotracheal suction may have been successful in clearing some secretions but is unpleasant and traumatic for the patient if it needs to be repeated frequently. A minitracheotomy is a means of clearing secretions more easily while avoiding the more invasive techniques of bronchoscopy, endotracheal intubation or tracheostomy (Ryan 1990).

A cannula with an internal diameter of 4 mm is inserted into the trachea through the cricothyroid membrane (Matthews & Hopkinson 1984). The procedure can be carried out under local anaesthesia and the minitracheotomy allows tracheal suction as often as necessary.

With the small tube in position the patient is able to breathe normally through the mouth and nose and the inspired air is humidified as it passes

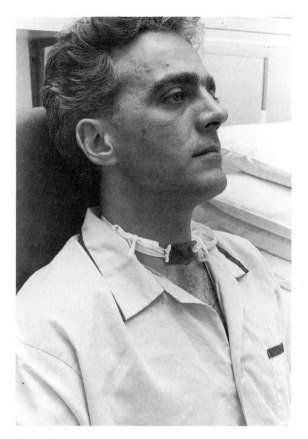

Fig. 8.57 Minitracheotomy.

through the nasal passages. The patient can talk, eat and drink normally and the tube does not prevent him from coughing effectively. Oxygen can be administered by a face mask or nasal cannulae if required.

With a minitracheotomy a size 10 FG suction catheter is the maximum size that can be used. Size 8 FG is usually too narrow to clear secretions effectively. Normal saline solution (1–2 ml) is instilled via the minitracheotomy before suction to assist in maintaining patency of the tube. The catheter is gently inserted either until a cough is stimulated or the carina is reached and suction is applied when starting to withdraw it. There may be copious secretions which will take longer to clear using this small catheter, but the patient is able to breathe with the narrow tracheal tube in situ and the procedure should not be distressing.

As soon as the patient is capable of clearing his secretions effectively without becoming exhausted

the minitracheotomy is removed and the small incision heals quickly.

The size of the minitracheotomy was designed for the adult trachea and is not recommended for children under the age of 12 years (Preston et al 1986).

PHYSIOTHERAPY TECHNIQUES FOR PAIN RELIEF

Entonox

Entonox is premixed nitrous oxide and oxygen, 50% nitrous oxide and 50% oxygen. It is administered by inhalation using a patient demand valve and a mask or mouthpiece (Myles 1970).

The inhalation of Entonox has an analgesic effect which is easily and rapidly induced. The exact mode of action is unknown, but the maximal analgesic effect has been observed 1–2 min (10–15 breaths) after the beginning of the inhalation and more prolonged inhalation does not increase the degree of analgesia. A measurable degree of analgesia does not persist for more than 2–4 min after the end of administration.

Physiotherapy techniques (e.g. thoracic expansion exercises, huffing and coughing) can be facilitated by the inhalation of Entonox when pain which cannot be adequately controlled by other forms of analgesia is a limiting factor.

The time of inhalation varies from approximately 30–120 seconds (5–15 breaths) and, if used in combination with other forms of analgesia, the time of administration of these should be considered. For example, following an intramuscular injection of an analgesic agent the optimum time to obtain a maximal effect from the inhalation of Entonox would be approximately 30 –60 min later and following an intravenous injection approximately 10–15 min later.

Contraindications to the inhalation of Entonox include pre-existing nausea as this can be exacerbated by Entonox, and pneumothorax, lung abscess, emphysematous bullae and gaseous abdominal distension as Entonox may diffuse into these air pockets. It should not be used in patients requiring more than 50% oxygen or patients relying on their hypoxic drive to breathe.

With the intermittent, short-term use of Entonox the most common side-effect is a tendency to feel and appear sleepy, but others which have occasionally been reported include nausea, euphoria (although some may describe this sensation as 'unpleasant'), tingling, numbness, dizziness, spinning and auditory disturbances.

Sitting is probably the best position for the patient if appropriate, especially if the Entonox is being used to encourage thoracic expansion exercises, huffing and coughing. The patient should hold the mask in position and should he become drowsy the mask will fall from his face.

The inhalation of Entonox may be indicated with manual hyperinflation or intermittent positive pressure breathing in some patients in whom other methods of pain control have not been effective.

The two gases tend to stratify when exposed to freezing temperatures. The cylinders should be stored in a horizontal position and it is good practice to invert the cylinder three times before use (British Oxygen Company 1990) to ensure delivery of a consistent mixture of nitrous oxide and oxygen.

Transcutaneous electrical nerve stimulation

Electrical stimulation has been used in the treatment of pain for many years, but it was not until the early 1970s following publication of the gate control theory (Melzack & Wall 1965) that transcutaneous electrical nerve stimulation (TENS), as a form of treatment, was given recognition in clinical practice.

TENS consists of a small battery operated pulse generator and one or two pairs of electrodes. The electrodes are placed transcutaneously and electrical stimuli can be passed into the skin.

There are several methods of applying TENS, which has perhaps contributed to the confusion surrounding this technique. These are acupuncture-like TENS, brief intense TENS and conventional TENS, although it is the latter that is most frequently used.

In conventional TENS, low-intensity, high-frequency stimuli are used to activate the large diameter Aβ fibres. These excite interneurons within the substantia gelatinosa of the spinal cord,

and transmission of pain via the small diameter nociceptive fibres is presynaptically inhibited.

There is also some evidence to suggest that Aβ fibre stimulation may additionally modulate pain via a central descending pathway. Briefly, the mechanism for this is that Aβ fibre stimulation also results in activation of neurons within the periaquaductal grey matter of the brainstem. A group of fibres from this area descend and synapse on enkephalinergic interneurons within the spinal cord. Excitation of these results in the release of enkephalins and subsequent inhibition of small diameter nociceptive activity, but Woolf et al (1978) showed that naloxone did not reverse this effect.

The most commonly encountered situations for the use of TENS in the area of respiratory care are those of rib fractures, and following thoracic surgery where pain inhibits the patient's ability to expand the lung fully and to huff and cough effectively. Conventional TENS has been used in these patients. The intensity and frequency dials on the pulse generator are adjusted to deliver low-intensity, high-frequency stimuli. The pulse width is usually fixed at about 200 microseconds.

The application of the TENS electrodes varies considerably and remains a matter of 'trial and error'. Following rib fractures or thoracotomy incisions, electrodes are usually applied either above or below the fracture site or the incision, respectively, or over the nerve trunk and along its corresponding dermatome. The electrodes, which usually consist of a carbon–silicon compound, are adhered to the skin using adhesive tape and an intervening layer of conductive gel. When the machine is positioned and switched on, the patient should feel a mild, comfortable, tingling sensation.

A number of studies have looked at the effects of TENS following thoracotomy incisions (Stratton & Smith 1980, Ho et al 1987, Stubbing & Jellicoe 1988). Stratton and Smith (1980) measured forced vital capacity (FVC) before and immediately after 10 min of TENS on the first postoperative day following surgery and found a significant increase. Ho et al (1987) demonstrated effective pain relief with TENS in the first 3 days following thoracotomy, as measured by lung function and the greater ability of the patients to generate an effective cough. Stubbing and Jellicoe (1988) could find no difference between postoperative subjects using TENS and a postoperative control group in either peak expiratory flow or opioid requirements, but postoperative nausea and vomiting was reduced in the TENS group. These variations in results may reflect the lack of a standard technique of application.

TENS is a non-invasive form of electrical stimulation. Contraindications include patients with cardiac pacemakers, patients with known heart disease or arrhythmia, and application over the carotid sinus. TENS should not be used over broken skin, or applied over anaesthetized areas. Care should also be taken if it is used in the intensive care unit as TENS may cause interference with monitoring equipment.

Despite conflicting reports, TENS does seem to have a place in the control of pain following thoracic trauma and surgery, intercostal neuritis, post-herpetic neuralgia, pleuritic pain and the pain associated with neoplastic lesions (Frampton 1988, Woolf 1989). However, its greatest use is as a supplementary form of pain control rather than as the only form of pain control.

Acknowledgement

We are grateful to Karen Peebles for this section on TENS from her thesis (1991).

MANUAL THERAPY SKILLS

Alterations in chest wall mechanics result from changes in lung volume (hyperinflation) and shortening in some of the respiratory muscles. These changes can cause joint dysfunction (Vibekk 1991) and chest wall pain (Wyke 1970) in patients with chronic lung disease. Afferent information from joint tissues in the thorax has a reflex effect on the chest wall muscles at spinal and brain stem levels (Wyke 1970) and this can potentially alter respiration.

Manual therapy is a method of treating these neuromuscular and skeletal changes by specific mobilizations, manipulations, postural correction and exercise, and the stretching of muscle, ligamentous and neural tissue (Maitland 1986). The techniques are selected according to the assessment findings. Manual therapy would probably be contraindicated if there is evidence of osteoporosis, metastatic disease on the chest radiograph or the presence of cord signs.

Pilot studies by Vibekk (1991) have shown improvements in lung function, in subjects with cystic fibrosis, using these techniques. Hamberg and Lindahl (1981) have shown improvements in chest wall pain, due to thoracic spine disorders, following manual therapy techniques. These techniques need further validation in subjects with chronic respiratory disease and with postoperative chest wall pain, but clinical evidence suggests that they could be more widely practised.

RESPIRATORY MUSCLE TRAINING

Respiratory muscle training devices have been used to increase strength and endurance in the muscles of either inspiration or expiration (Leith & Bradley 1976, Pardy et al 1981, Pardy et al 1988). Whether this 'training' effects exercise ability, activities of daily living, morbidity or mortality has yet to be determined and once training ceases the effect of conditioning declines (Pardy et al 1990, Smith et al 1992).

The patient breathes through a mouthpiece or a face mask with a resistance applied to either the inspiratory or expiratory limb of a valve. The valve may be 'flow resistive' or 'threshold loading'. With a 'flow resistive' device the patient breathes in and out through an aperture. Alteration in the size of the aperture alters the load on the respiratory muscles, provided the frequency of breathing, tidal volume and inspiratory or expiratory time are kept constant. The load is increased by decreasing the size of the aperture. If the patient breathes more slowly and deeply the pressure exerted on the respiratory muscles will be less than if he breathes more quickly and not as deeply (Pardy et al 1990).

A threshold loading device requires a predetermined pressure to initiate either inspiration or expiration and this is dependent on the magnitude of the threshold load. When inspiration or expiration has been initiated the pressure required to keep the valve open is constant and independent of the flow rate. To provide a maximal training effect, inspiratory or expiratory time and the frequency of breathing should be controlled (Pardy et al 1990). Threshold loading devices will increase the pressure generated by the inspiratory or expiratory muscles and are more reliable as training devices (Flynn et al 1989, Morrison et al 1989).

On assessment the appropriate resistance is selected for an individual patient. By increasing the length of time for treatment, endurance may be improved and by increasing the resistance, muscle strength may be increased.

The studies by Flynn et al (1989) and Morrison et al (1989) were undertaken in patients with chronic airflow limitation. In patients with severe respiratory disease it is possible that they will already have 'trained' their respiratory muscles as a result of the increased load created by the increased work of breathing, and further respiratory muscle training would be of limited value (Pardy et al 1990, Moxham 1991).

In conditions of respiratory muscle weakness the underlying cause of the weakness should be treated, for example myasthenia gravis, malnutrition and electrolyte imbalance (Moxham 1991). Disuse atrophy may result from resting the respiratory muscles during prolonged assisted ventilation. Many factors will contribute to improvement in muscle strength and endurance such as nutrition, the treatment of infection and other underlying disease processes. It is possible that inspiratory muscle training may assist the weaning process in these subjects (Abelson & Brewer 1987, Aldrich et al 1989).

In cervical and high thoracic spinal injuries, progressive resistive exercises are recommended for increasing respiratory muscle strength and endurance (Gross et al 1980, Morgan et al 1986).

The response to treatment can be monitored by measuring maximal inspiratory mouth pressures (P_iMax) or maximal expiratory mouth pressures (P_eMax). Further rigorous clinical trials are necessary to identify the place of respiratory muscle training. Does it significantly improve respiratory muscle strength, endurance and exercise performance, and if so in which patient groups?

CARDIOPULMONARY REHABILITATION

Rehabilitation of the respiratory patient is not isolated to the respiratory system alone. Cardiopulmonary rehabilitation is a more accurate description than pulmonary rehabilitation as the cardiac and respiratory systems are interdependent.

Cardiopulmonary rehabilitation embraces a wide range of activities including education of patients in their condition and correct use of their prescribed drugs, encouragement and support to discontinue smoking, breathing control and positioning to reduce breathlessness (p. 113), clearance of bronchial secretions (p. 121), graduated exercise programmes, nutritional advice and psychological support.

The goals of cardiopulmonary rehabilitation are to maximize independence, productivity and quality of life, and to minimize clinical deterioration as far as possible (Donner & Howard 1992). In patients with light to moderate obstructive airways disease ($FEV_1 \geq 60\%$ predicted) it is the cardiovascular system and/or peripheral muscle function which limit exercise ability. With severe obstruction ($FEV_1 = 40–60\%$ predicted) the pulmonary system limits exercise (Donner & Howard 1992).

A successful rehabilitation programme should reduce breathlessness on exertion and improve exercise tolerance. Lung function may not alter, but changes may be detected in measurements of breathlessness using a rating of perceived exertion scale (p. 326) or questionnaire (p. 59). Exercise tolerance can be measured using the 6 minute walking or shuttle tests (p. 60) and quality of life by a questionnaire (Hyland et al 1992).

Before a cardiopulmonary rehabilitation programme is designed, individual assessment is essential in order to identify the patient's problems and any factors such as cardiac disease which may limit a programme. Follow-up assessments for revision of an exercise programme and remotivation are essential if the improvements gained are to be maintained. Care must be taken not to place too much emphasis on outcome measures when patients with deteriorating lung conditions, for example a musculoskeletal disorder, lung cancer or fibrosing alveolitis, are included in an exercise programme.

Rehabilitation for the very sick patient may begin with the exercise and effort of moving, with assistance, from the bed to the chair (Ch.7,

p. 99). For the patient who has been on long-term bed rest a tilt table (Fig. 8.58) may be useful and the patient can learn to stand and then to walk. Assisted ventilation can be continued as necessary (Fig. 8.59).

Breathlessness is the most disabling symptom in patients with chronic lung disease and leads to decreasing activity. With inactivity the level of fitness deteriorates and a vicious circle of breathlessness and decreasing activity is set up. The benefits of exercise programmes have been documented in patients with cystic fibrosis (Dodd 1991) (p. 411), chronic airflow limitation and asthma (Cockcroft 1988), patients awaiting heart/lung transplantation (p. 350) and in the elderly (Zadai 1991).

A graded stair climbing programme has been shown to increase exercise tolerance in patients with chronic bronchitis and emphysema (McGavin et al 1977). A walking programme can be used if stairs are not available. These programmes (Webber 1981), outlined in Table

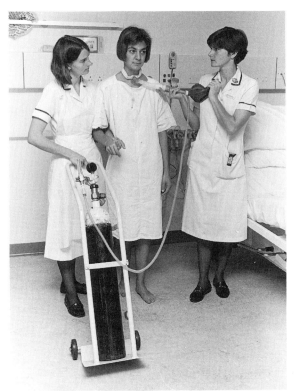

Fig. 8.59   Assisted ventilation while walking.

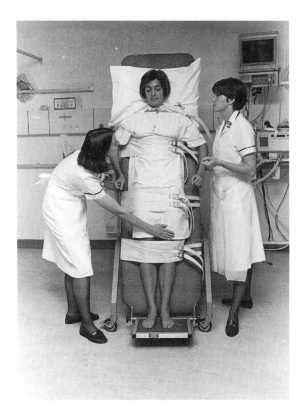

Fig. 8.58   Standing assisted by a tilt table.

8.3, help to overcome the fear of breathlessness and break the vicious circle of inactivity. If walking on the level, the patient is instructed to walk fast enough to make himself moderately breathless, but not so fast that he has to stop. For example in week 1, after 2 min of brisk walking, he should stop for a rest using breathing control before walking briskly for a further 2 min.

Table 8.3   Graduated exercise programme

| Week No. | Stairs | | Walking on level |
	No. of steps	Time (min)	(min)
1	5	2	2 + 2 (4)
2	5	2	3 + 3 (6)
3	5	5	5 + 3 (8)
4	5	5	5 + 5 (10)
5	10	5	5 + 5 (10)
6	10	5	10 + 5 (15)
7	10	10	10 + 5 (15)
8	10	10	10 + 10 (20)

The patient is advised to exercise at least once a day and record in a diary card the number of stairs or the distance achieved. After a programme of 8 weeks some form of daily exercise is encouraged, perhaps a 15 min walk to the shops. One day a week the patient should repeat the training programme and if he is unable to achieve the maximum level he had reached he should be encouraged to do the programme more regularly. If a patient develops a chest infection during the programme he should discontinue the progressive exercise programme for a period of time and then restart at a lower level, gradually building up his exercise tolerance again.

The programme must be adapted to the individual. Some patients will not be able to achieve the suggested target by the eighth week. Booker et al (1985) found that patients with severe emphysema were unable to make any progress with the stair climbing programme. The use of breathing control while walking increasing distances was of greater benefit to these individuals. A training target will be more effective if it has a purpose for the individual, for example to walk 100 metres to a club to meet friends or to walk to the corner shop.

For patients using the progressive exercise programme it is important to explain the difference between exercise training or testing where breathlessness is expected, and walking or stair climbing with breathing control (p. 116) which should be used at all other times to try and avoid breathlessness and allow these normal activities to be more comfortable.

Many aspects of cardiopulmonary rehabilitation can be undertaken as a group activity. Education, exercise and relaxation are important components. An exercise class may take the form of modified aerobic exercises, accompanied by music, where with the encouragement and advice from a physiotherapist and motivation from others in the group, patients who are markedly disabled with breathlessness often improve their physical fitness and morale. Before starting an exercise session, patients should do some warm-up muscle stretching exercises to help to prevent injuries and, at the end of the exercise period, a cool-down phase of more gentle activity.

Studies need to be undertaken to determine the value of classes, but patients and therapists comment on the psychological, motivational and physical benefits of group work.

Cardiopulmonary rehabilitation has many components and the priorities will be different for individual patients, depending on their problems and on the underlying pathology. A small increase in exercise tolerance can lead to a marked improvement in quality of life (Cockcroft 1988).

REFERENCES

Abelson H, Brewer K 1987 Inspiratory muscle training in the mechanically ventilated patient. Physiotherapy Canada 39: 305–307

Ackerman M H 1985 The use of bolus normal saline instillations in artificial airways: is it useful or necessary? Heart & Lung 14: 505–506

Aldrich T K, Karpel J P, Uhrlass R M et al 1989 Weaning from mechanical ventilation: adjunctive use of inspiratory muscle resistive training. Critical Care Medicine 17: 143–147

Althaus P, Leuenberger P H 1988 A new method in positive expiratory pressure, the Flutter. Paper presented at the 5th meeting of the European Society of Respiratory and Cardiovascular Therapy, Villars, Switzerland (unpublished)

Andersen J B 1987 Personal communication

Andersen J B, Olesen K P, Eikard B et al 1980 Periodic continuous positive airway pressure, CPAP, by mask in the treatment of atelectasis. European Journal of Respiratory Diseases 61: 20–25

Ayres S M, Kozam R L, Lukas D S 1963 The effects of intermittent positive pressure breathing on intrathoracic pressure, pulmonary mechanics, and the work of breathing. American Review of Respiratory Disease 87: 370–379

Bazuaye E A, Stone T N, Corris P A, Gibson G J 1992 Variability of inspired oxygen concentration with nasal cannulas. Thorax 47: 609–611

Bendefy I M 1991 Home nebulisers in childhood asthma: survey of hospital supervised use. British Medical Journal 302: 1180–1181

Booker H, Harries D, Rehahn M, Collins J 1985 Progressive exercise training: subjective and objective changes. Physiotherapy Practice 1: 31–36

Bott J, Keilty S E J, Noone L 1992 Intermittent positive pressure breathing—a dying art? Physiotherapy 78: 656–660

British Oxygen Company 1990 Entonox fact sheet. Guildford, Surrey

Burge P S 1986 Getting the best out of bronchodilator therapy. Patient Management July: 155–185

Campbell A H, O'Connell J M, Wilson F 1975 The effect of chest physiotherapy upon the FEV_1 in chronic bronchitis. The Medical Journal of Australia 1: 33–35

Campbell E J, Baker D, Crites-Silver P 1988 Subjective effects of humidification of oxygen for delivery by nasal cannula. Chest 93: 289–293

Chatburn R L 1987 Physiologic and methodologic issues regarding humidity therapy. Journal of Pediatrics 114: 416–420

Chatham K, Marshall C, Campbell I A, Prescott R J 1993 The Flutter VRP1 device in post-thoracotomy patients, Physiotherapy 79: 95–98

Chuter T A M, Weissman C, Starker P M, Gump F E 1989 Effect of incentive spirometry on diaphragmatic function after surgery. Surgery 105: 488–493

Chuter T A M, Weissman C, Mathews D M, Starker P M 1990 Diaphragmatic breathing maneuvers and movement of the diaphragm after cholecystectomy. Chest 97: 1110–1114

Clark A P, Winslow E H, Tyler D O, White K M 1990 Effects of endotracheal suctioning on mixed venous oxygen saturation and heart rate in critically ill adults. Heart & Lung 19: 552–557

Clarke S W 1988 Inhaler therapy. Quarterly Journal of Medicine New Series 67 (253): 355–368

Clarke S W 1990 Physical defences. In: Brewis R A L, Gibson G J, Geddes D M (eds) Respiratory medicine. Baillière Tindall, London, ch 3.1, p 176–185

Clay M M, Pavia D, Newman S P, et al 1983 Assessment of jet nebulizers for lung aerosol therapy. Lancet ii: 592–594

Clement A J, Hübsch S K 1968 Chest physiotherapy by the 'bag squeezing' method. Physiotherapy 54: 355–359

Cockcroft A 1988 Pulmonary rehabilitation. British Journal of Diseases of the Chest 82: 220–225

Cole P 1990 Bronchiectasis. In: Brewis R A L, Gibson G J, Geddes D M (eds) Respiratory medicine. Baillière Tindall, London, ch 18, p 732–733

Conway J H 1992 The effects of humidification for patients with chronic airways disease. Physiotherapy 78: 97–101

Conway J H, Fleming J S, Perring S, Holgate S T 1992 Humidification as an adjunct to chest physiotherapy in aiding tracheo-bronchial clearance in patients with bronchiectasis. Respiratory Medicine 86: 109–114

Currie D C, Munro C, Gaskell D, Cole P J 1986 Practice, problems and compliance with postural drainage: a survey of chronic sputum producers. British Journal of Diseases of the Chest 80: 249–253

Czarnik R E, Stone K S, Everhart C C, Preusser B A 1991 Differential effects of continuous versus intermittent suction on tracheal tissue. Heart & Lung 20: 144–151

Dab I, Alexander F 1979 The mechanism of autogenic drainage studied with flow volume curves. Monographs of Paediatrics 10: 50–53

Dail C W 1951 'Glossopharyngeal breathing' by paralyzed patients. California Medicine 75: 217–218

Dail C W, Affeldt J E, Collier C R 1955 Clinical aspects of glossopharyngeal breathing. Journal of the American Medical Association 158: 445–449

David A 1991 Autogenic drainage—the German approach. In: Pryor J A (ed) Respiratory care. Churchill Livingstone, Edinburgh, p 65–78

Dean E 1985 Effect of body position on pulmonary function. Physical Therapy 65: 613–618

Dodd M E 1991 Exercise in cystic fibrosis adults. In: Pryor J A (ed) Respiratory care. Churchill Livingstone, Edinburgh, p 27–50

Donner C F, Howard P 1992 Pulmonary rehabilitation in chronic obstructive pulmonary disease (COPD) with recommendations for its use. European Respiratory Journal 5: 266–275

Editorial 1988 Nebulisers and paradoxical bronchoconstriction. Lancet ii: 202

Falk M, Andersen J B 1991 Positive expiratory pressure (PEP) mask. In: Pryor J A (ed) Respiratory Care. Churchill Livingstone, Edinburgh, p 51–63

Falk M, Kelstrup M, Andersen J B et al 1984 Improving the ketchup bottle method with positive expiratory pressure, PEP, in cystic fibrosis. European Journal of Respiratory Diseases 65: 423–432

Flower K A 1980 Personal communication

Flower K A, Eden R I, Lomax L et al 1979 New mechanical aid to physiotherapy in cystic fibrosis. British Medical Journal 2: 630–631

Flynn M G, Barter C E, Nosworthy J C et al 1989 Threshold pressure training, breathing pattern, and exercise performance in chronic airflow obstruction. Chest 95: 535–540

Frampton V 1988 Transcutaneous electrical nerve stimulation and chronic pain. In: Wells P E, Frampton V, Bowsher D (eds) Pain: management and control in physiotherapy, ch 10, p 89–112

Freitag L, Bremme J, Schroer M 1989 High frequency oscillation for respiratory physiotherapy. British Journal of Anaesthesia 63: 44S–46S

Gallon A 1991 Evaluation of chest percussion in the treatment of patients with copious sputum production. Respiratory Medicine 85: 45–51

George R J D, Geddes D M 1985 High frequency ventilation. British Journal of Hospital Medicine June: 344–349

George R J D, Howard R S, Geddes D M 1984 Oral high frequency oscillation improves exercise tolerance and recovery from breathlessness. Thorax 39: 717

George R J D, Johnson M A, Pavia D et al 1985a Increase in mucociliary clearance in normal man induced by oral high frequency oscillation. Thorax 40: 433–437

George R J D, Winter R J D, Johnson M A et al 1985b Effect of oral high frequency ventilation by jet or oscillator on minute ventilation in normal subjects. Thorax 40: 749–755

George R J D, Pavia D, Woodman G et al 1986 Oral high frequency oscillation (OHFO) as an adjunct to physiotherapy (PHYSIO) in cystic fibrosis (CF), Thorax 41: 235–236

Gherini S, Peters R M, Virgilio R W 1979 Mechanical work on the lungs and work of breathing with positive end-expiratory pressure and continuous positive airway pressure. Chest 76: 251–256

Girard J P 1989 Therapeutic trials with the VarioRaw S A Flutter VRP1 for bronchial asthma. Department of Immunology and Allergy, Geneva University Cantonal Hospital, Switzerland (unpublished)

Gleeson J G, Price J F 1988 Nebuliser technique. British Journal of Diseases of the Chest 82: 172–174

Goldman J M, Teale C, Muers M F 1992 Simplifying the assessment of patients with chronic airflow limitation for home nebulizer therapy. Respiratory Medicine 86: 33–38

Gormezano J, Branthwaite M A 1972 Pulmonary physiotherapy with assisted ventilation. Anaesthesia 27: 249–257

Green M, Moxham J 1985 The respiratory muscles. Clinical Science 68: 1–10

Gross D, Ladd H W, Riley E J et al 1980 The effect of training on strength and endurance of the diaphragm in quadriplegia. The American Journal of Medicine 68: 27–35

Gunawardena K A, Patel B, Campbell I A et al 1984 Oxygen as a driving gas for nebulisers: safe or dangerous? British Medical Journal 288: 272–274

Hack I, Katz A, Eales C 1980 Airway pressure changes during

'bag squeezing'. South African Journal of Physiotherapy 36: 97–99

Hall J C, Tarala R, Harris J et al 1991 Incentive spirometry versus routine chest physiotherapy for prevention of pulmonary complications after abdominal surgery. Lancet 337: 953–956

Hamberg J, Lindahl O 1981 Angina pectoris symptoms caused by thoracic spine disorders. Clinical examination and treatment. Acta Medica Scandinavica (suppl) 644: 84–86

Higgens J M 1966 The management in cabinet respirators of patients with acute or residual respiratory muscle paralysis. Physiotherapy 52: 425–430

Hinds C J 1987a Intensive care. Baillière Tindall, London, p 26–27

Hinds C J 1987b Intensive care. Baillière Tindall, London, p 205–207

Ho A, Hui P W, Cheung J, Cheung C 1987 Effectiveness of transcutaneous electrical nerve stimulation in relieving pain following thoracotomy. Physiotherapy 73: 33–35

Hodson M E, Penketh A R L, Batten J C 1981 Aerosol carbenicillin and gentamicin treatment of pseudomonas aeruginosa infection in patients with cystic fibrosis. Lancet ii: 1137–1139

Hofmeyr J L, Webber B A, Hodson M E 1986 Evaluation of positive expiratory pressure as an adjunct to chest physiotherapy in the treatment of cystic fibrosis. Thorax 41: 951–954

Howard P, Cayton R M, Brennan S R, Anderson P B 1977 Lignocaine aerosol and persistent cough. British Journal of Diseases of the Chest 71: 19–24

Hyland M E, Bott J, Singh S J et al 1992 A disease specific questionnaire for assessing quality of life in patients suffering from chronic obstructive pulmonary disease. Proceedings of the 2nd international conference on advances in pulmonary rehabilitation and management of chronic respiratory failure, Venice

Jacob W 1990 Physiotherapy in the ICU. In: Oh T E (ed) Intensive care manual, 3rd edn. Butterworths, Sydney, ch 4, p 24

Jeffrey A A, Warren P M 1992 Should we judge a mask by its cover? Thorax 47: 543–546

Jones A Y M, Jones R D, Bacon-Shone J 1991 A comparison of expiratory flow rates in two breathing circuits used for manual inflation of the lungs. Physiotherapy 77: 593–597

Keeley D 1992 Large volume plastic spacers in asthma. British Medical Journal 305: 598–599

Kelleher W H, Parida R K 1957 Glossopharyngeal breathing. British Medical Journal 2: 740–743

Kieselmann R, Bolde A, Hüls G, Lindemann H 1991 A comparison of physiotherapy methods: Flutter VRP1 versus autogenic drainage. Abstracts 17th European Cystic Fibrosis Conference, Copenhagen, Denmark

Langlands J 1967 The dynamics of cough in health and in chronic bronchitis. Thorax 22: 88–96

Leith D E, Bradley M 1976 Ventilatory muscle strength and endurance training. Journal of Applied Physiology 41: 508–516

Lewis R A, Fleming J S 1985 Fractional deposition from a jet nebuliser: how it differs from a metered dose inhaler. British Journal of Diseases of the Chest 79: 361–367

Liardet C 1990 VarioRaw S A, Aubonne, Switzerland. Personal communication

Lindner K H, Lotz P, Ahnefeld F W 1987 Continuous positive airway pressure effect on functional residual capacity, vital capacity and its subdivisions. Chest 92: 66–70

Loddenkemper R 1975 Dose- and time-response of Sch 1000 MDI on total (R_t) and expiratory (R_e) airways resistance in patients with chronic bronchitis and emphysema. Postgraduate Medical Journal 51 (suppl 7): 97

Lyons E, Chatham K, Campbell I A, Prescott R J 1992 Evaluation of the Flutter VRP1 device in young adults with cystic fibrosis. Thorax 47: 237P

McDonnell T, McNicholas W T, FitzGerald M X 1986 Hypoxaemia during chest physiotherapy in patients with cystic fibrosis. Irish Journal of Medical Science 155: 345–348

McGavin C R, Naoe H, McHardy G J R 1976 Does inhalation of salbutamol enable patients with airway obstruction to walk further? Clinical Science and Molecular Medicine 51: 12–13

McGavin C R, Gupta S P, Lloyd E L, McHardy G J R 1977 Physical rehabilitation for the chronic bronchitic: results of a controlled trial of exercises in the home. Thorax 32: 307–311

Macklem P T 1974 Physiology of cough. Transactions of the American Broncho-Esophalogical Association: 150–157

Maitland G D 1986 Vertebral manipulation, 5th edn. Butterworths, London

Martin C J, Ripley H, Reynolds J, Best F 1976 Chest physiotherapy and the distribution of ventilation. Chest 69: 174–178

Matthews H R, Hopkinson R B 1984 Treatment of sputum retention by minitracheotomy. British Journal of Surgery 71: 147–150

Mead J, Turner J M, Macklem P T, Little J B 1967 Significance of the relationship between lung recoil and maximum expiratory flow. Journal of Applied Physiology 22: 95–108

Mead J, Takishima T, Leith D 1970 Stress distribution in lungs: a model of pulmonary elasticity. Journal of Applied Physiology 28: 596–608

Melzack R, Wall P D 1965 Pain mechanisms: a new theory. Science 150: 971–978

Menkes H, Britt J 1980 Rationale for physical therapy. American Review of Respiratory Disease 122 (suppl 2): 127–131

Menkes H A, Traystman R J 1977 Collateral ventilation. American Review of Respiratory Disease 116: 287–309

Mestitz H, Copland J M, McDonald C F 1989 Comparison of outpatient nebulized vs metered dose inhaler turbutaline in chronic airflow obstruction. Chest 96: 1237–1240

Morgan M D L, Silver J R, Williams S J 1986 The respiratory system of the spinal cord patient. In: Bloch R F, Basbaum M (eds) Management of spinal cord injuries. Williams & Wilkins, Baltimore, p 78–115

Morrison N J, Richardson J, Dunn L, Pardy R L 1989 Respiratory muscle performance in normal elderly subjects and patients with COPD. Chest 95: 90–94

Moxham J 1991 Respiratory muscle weakness—its recognition and management. Respiratory Disease in Practice April/May: 12–17

Myles P V 1970 Use of the entonox machine in post-operative chest physiotherapy. Physiotherapy 56: 559–560

Nelson H P 1934 Postural drainage of the lungs. British Medical Journal 2: 251–255

Newman S P, Pellow P G D, Clarke S W 1986 Droplet size distributions of nebulised aerosols for inhalation therapy. Clinical Physics and Physiological Measurement 7: 139–146

Newman S P, Weisz A W B, Talaee N, Clarke S W 1991 Improvement of drug delivery with a breath actuated pressurised aerosol for patients with poor inhaler technique. Thorax 46: 712–716

Oberwaldner B, Evans J C, Zach M S 1986 Forced expirations against a variable resistance: a new chest physiotherapy method in cystic fibrosis. Pediatric Pulmonology 2: 358–367

Oberwaldner B, Theissl B, Rucker A, Zach M S 1991 Chest physiotherapy in hospitalized patients with cystic fibrosis: a study of lung function effects and sputum production. European Respiratory Journal 4: 152–158

O'Driscoll B R, Kay E A, Taylor R J, Bernstein A 1990 Home nebulizers: can optimal therapy be predicted by laboratory studies? Respiratory Medicine 84: 471–477

Oh T E 1990 Humidification. In: Oh T E (ed) Intensive care manual, 3rd edn. Butterworths, Sydney, ch 24, p 169–173

Oikkonen M, Karjalainen K, Kähärä V et al 1991 Comparison of incentive spirometry and intermittent positive pressure breathing after coronary artery bypass graft. Chest 99: 60–65

Pardy R L, Rivington R N, Despas P J, Macklem P T 1981 The effects of inspiratory muscle training on exercise performance in chronic airflow limitation. American Review of Respiratory Disease 123: 426–433

Pardy R L, Reid W D, Belman M J 1988 Respiratory muscle training. Clinics in Chest Medicine 9: 287–296

Pardy R L, Fairbarn M S, Blackie S P 1990 Respiratory muscle training. Problems in Respiratory Care 3: 483–492

Partridge C, Pryor J, Webber B 1989 Characteristics of the forced expiration technique. Physiotherapy 75: 193–194

Pavia D, Thomson M L, Clarke S W 1978 Enhanced clearance of secretions from the human lung after the administration of hypertonic saline aerosol. American Review of Respiratory Disease 117: 199–203

Pavia D, Webber B, Agnew J E et al 1988 The role of intermittent positive pressure breathing (IPPB) in bronchial toilet. European Respiratory Journal 1 (suppl 2): 250S

Peebles K 1991 Methods of pain control following posterolateral thoracotomy incisions. Thesis submitted to the University of London

Pendleton N, Cheesbrough J S, Walshaw M J, Hind C R K 1991 Bacterial colonisation of humidifier attachments on oxygen concentrators prescribed for long term oxygen therapy: a district review. Thorax 46: 257–258

Preston I M, Matthews H R, Ready A R 1986 Minitracheotomy. Physiotherapy 72: 494–497

Pryor J A, Webber B A 1979 An evaluation of the forced expiration technique as an adjunct to postural drainage. Physiotherapy 65: 304–307

Pryor J A, Webber B A 1992 Physiotherapy for cystic fibrosis —which technique? Physiotherapy 78: 105–108

Pryor J A, Webber B A, Hodson M E, Batten J C 1979 Evaluation of the forced expiration technique as an adjunct to postural drainage in treatment of cystic fibrosis. British Medical Journal 2: 417–418

Pryor J A, Parker R A, Webber B A 1981 A comparison of mechanical and manual percussion as adjuncts to postural drainage in the treatment of cystic fibrosis in adolescents and adults. Physiotherapy 67: 140–141

Pryor J A, Wiggins J, Webber B A, Geddes D M 1989 Oral high frequency oscillation (OHFO) as an aid to physiotherapy in chronic bronchitis with airflow limitation. Thorax 44: 350P

Pryor J A, Webber B A, Hodson M E 1990 Effect of chest physiotherapy on oxygen saturation in patients with cystic fibrosis. Thorax 45: 77

Pryor J A, Webber B A, Hodson M E, Warner J O An investigation into the use of the Flutter VRPI as an adjunct to chest physiotherapy in cystic fibrosis (in press)

Ranasinha C, Empey D, Shak S et al 1993 Preliminary report on a phase 2 double-blind placebo controlled study of the pulmonary function and the safety of aerosolised recombinant DNase in adults with stable stage cystic fibrosis. Thorax 48(4): (in press)

Rehder K, Hatch D J, Sessler A D, Fowler W S 1972 The function of each lung of anesthetized and paralyzed man during mechanical ventilation. Anesthesiology 37: 16–26

Reiser J, Warner J O 1986 Inhalation treatment for asthma. Archives of Disease in Childhood 61: 88–94

Ricksten S E, Bengtsson A, Soderberg C et al 1986 Effects of periodic positive airway pressure by mask on postoperative pulmonary function. Chest 89: 774–781

Riegel B, Forshee T 1985 A review and critique of the literature on preoxygenation for endotracheal suctioning. Heart & Lung 14: 507–518

Ruffin R E, Fitzgerald J D, Rebuck A S 1977 A comparison of the bronchodilator activity of Sch 1000 and salbutamol. Journal of Allergy and Clinical Immunology 59: 136–141

Ryan D W 1990 Minitracheotomy. British Medical Journal 300: 958–959

Schoeffel R E, Anderson S D, Altounyan R E C 1981 Bronchial hyperreactivity in response to inhalation of ultrasonically nebulised solutions of distilled water and saline. British Medical Journal 283: 1285–1287

Schöni M H 1989 Autogenic drainage: a modern approach to physiotherapy in cystic fibrosis. Journal of the Royal Society of Medicine 82 (suppl 16): 32–37

Shah P, Dhurjon L, Metcalfe T, Gibson J M 1992 Acute angle closure glaucoma associated with nebulised ipratropium bromide and salbutamol. British Medical Journal 304: 40–41

Sharp J T, Drutz W S, Moisan T et al 1980 Postural relief of dyspnea in severe chronic obstructive pulmonary disease. American Review of Respiratory Disease 122: 201–211

Shelly M P, Lloyd G M, Park G R 1988 A review of the mechanisms and methods of humidification of inspired gases. Intensive Care 14: 1–9

Shneerson J 1992 Transtracheal oxygen delivery. Thorax 47: 57–59

Simonds A K, Parker R A, Branthwaite M A 1989 The effect of intermittent positive-pressure hyperinflation in restrictive chest wall disease. Respiration 55: 136–143

Smaldone G C, Vinciguerra C, Marchese J 1991 Detection of inhaled pentamidine in health care workers. The New England Journal of Medicine 325: 891–892

Smith K, Cook D, Guyatt G H et al 1992 Respiratory muscle training in chronic airflow limitation: a meta-analysis. American Review of Respiratory Disease 145: 533–539

Starke I D, Webber B A, Branthwaite M A 1979 IPPB and hypercapnia in respiratory failure: the effect of different concentrations of inspired oxygen on arterial blood gas tensions. Anaesthesia 34: 283–287

Stock M C, Downs J B, Gauer P K et al 1985 Prevention of postoperative pulmonary complications with CPAP, incentive spirometry, and conservative therapy. Chest 87: 151–157

Stratton S A, Smith M M 1980 Postoperative thoracotomy. Effect of transcutaneous nerve stimulation on forced vital capacity. Physical Therapy 60: 45–47

Stubbing J F, Jellicoe J A 1988 Transcutaneous electrical nerve stimulation after thoracotomy. Anaesthesia 43: 296–298

Sukumalchantra Y, Park S S, Williams M H 1965 The effect of intermittent positive pressure breathing (IPPB) in acute ventilatory failure. American Review of Respiratory Disease 92: 885–893

Sutton P P, Parker R A, Webber B A, et al 1983 Assessment of the forced expiration technique, postural drainage and directed coughing in chest physiotherapy. European Journal of Respiratory Diseases 64: 62–68

Sykes M K, McNicol M W, Campbell E J M 1976 Respiratory failure, 2nd edn. Blackwell Scientific, Oxford, p 153

Thompson B 1978 Asthma and your child, 5th edn. Pegasus Press, Christchurch, New Zealand

Thompson B, Thompson H T 1968 Forced expiration exercises in asthma and their effect on FEV_1. New Zealand Journal of Physiotherapy 3: 19–21

Thoracic Society 1950 The nomenclature of broncho-pulmonary anatomy. Thorax 5: 222–228

Tilling S E, Hayes B 1987 Heat and moisture exchangers in artificial ventilation. British Journal of Anaesthesia 59: 1181–1188

Uno Plast (UK) 1991 Endotracheal suctioning

van der Schans C P, van der Mark Th W, de Vries G et al 1991 Effect of positive expiratory pressure breathing in patients with cystic fibrosis. Thorax 46: 252–256

van Hengstum M, Festen J, Beurskens C et al 1990 No effect of oral high frequency oscillation combined with forced expiration manoeuvres on tracheobronchial clearance in chronic bronchitis. European Respiratory Journal 3: 14–18

Vater M, Hurt P G, Aitkenhead A R 1983 Quantitative effects of respired helium and oxygen mixtures on gas flow using conventional oxygen masks. Anaesthesia 38: 879–882

Vibekk P 1991 Chest mobilization and respiratory function. In: Pryor J A (ed) Respiratory care. Churchill Livingstone, Edinburgh, p 103–119

Walsh J M, Vanderwarf C, Hoscheit D, Fahey P J 1989 Unsuspected hemodynamic alterations during endotracheal suctioning. Chest 95: 162–165

Wanner A 1977 Clinical aspects of mucociliary transport. American Review of Respiratory Disease 116: 73–125

Ward R J, Danziger F, Bonica J J et al 1966 An evaluation of postoperative respiratory maneuvers. Surgery, Gynecology and Obstetrics 123: 51–54

Webber B A 1981 Living to the limit: exercise for the chronic breathless patient. Physiotherapy 67: 128–130

Webber B A 1988 The Brompton Hospital guide to chest physiotherapy, 5th edn. Blackwell Scientific, Oxford, p 43

Webber B A 1990 The active cycle of breathing techniques. Cystic Fibrosis News Aug/Sep: 10–11

Webber B A 1991 The role of the physiotherapist in medical chest problems. Respiratory Disease in Practice Feb/Mar: 12–15

Webber B A, Shenfield G M, Paterson J W 1974 A comparison of three different techniques for giving nebulized albuterol to asthmatic patients. American Review of Respiratory Disease 109: 293–295

Webber B A, Parker R, Hofmeyr J, Hodson M 1985 Evaluation of self-percussion during postural drainage using the forced expiration technique. Physiotherapy Practice 1: 42–45

Webber B A, Hofmeyr J L, Morgan M D L, Hodson M E 1986 Effects of postural drainage, incorporating the forced expiration technique, on pulmonary function in cystic fibrosis. British Journal of Diseases of the Chest 80: 353–359

West J B 1992 Pulmonary pathophysiology, 4th edn. Williams & Wilkins, Baltimore, p 7–13

White K M, Winslow E H, Clark A P, Tyler D O 1990 The physiologic basis for continuous mixed venous oxygen saturation monitoring. Heart & Lung 19: 548–551

Wilson R, Cole P J 1988 The effect of bacterial products on ciliary function. American Review of Respiratory Disease 138: S49–S53

Wolfsdorf J, Swift D L, Avery M E 1969 Mist therapy reconsidered; an evaluation of the respiratory deposition of labelled water aerosols produced by jet and ultrasonic nebulizers. Pediatrics 43: 799–808

Wollmer P, Ursing K, Midgren B, Eriksson L 1985 Inefficiency of chest percussion in the physical therapy of chronic bronchitis. European Journal of Respiratory Diseases 66: 233–239

Woolf C J 1989 Segmental afferent fibre-induced analgesia: transcutaneous electrical nerve stimulation (TENS) and vibration. In: Wall P D, Melzack R (eds) Textbook of pain. Churchill Livingstone, Edinburgh, p 884–896

Woolf C J, Mitchell D, Myers R A, Barrett G D 1978 Failure of naloxone to reverse peripheral transcutaneous electro-analgesia in patients suffering from acute trauma. South African Medical Journal 53: 179–180

Wyke B 1970 The neurological basis of thoracic spinal pain. Rheumatology and Physical Medicine 10: 356–367

Young I, Daviskas E, Keena V A 1989 Effect of low dose nebulised morphine on exercise endurance in patients with chronic lung disease. Thorax 44: 387–390

Zach M S, Oberwaldner B, Forche G, Polgar G 1985 Bronchodilators increase airway instability in cystic fibrosis. American Review of Respiratory Disease 131: 537–543

Zadai C C 1991 Cardiopulmonary ageing and exercise. In: Pryor J A (ed) Respiratory care. Churchill Livingstone, Edinburgh, p 199–226

9. Communication, counselling and health education

Julius Sim

INTRODUCTION

The intent of this chapter is to provide an insight into the part that various features of communication can play in the management of patients with cardiac and respiratory problems. In addition to a general account of the role of communication in the therapeutic relationship, particular attention will be given to two specialist applications of communication, namely counselling and health education. Some of the associated ethical issues will also be touched upon.

In order to examine these aspects of the physiotherapist's work, it is necessary to augment an awareness of the pathophysiological features of cardiorespiratory dysfunction with an understanding of its psychological and social dynamics. Accordingly, it is to these topics that the first part of this chapter is directed.

THE PSYCHOSOCIAL DIMENSION OF CARDIORESPIRATORY DYSFUNCTION

Like all illnesses, those of cardiorespiratory origin have psychosocial as well as physiological dimensions. Thus, at a general level, social factors play a part in the aetiology of many chronic respiratory diseases and, reflecting a general pattern for morbidity and mortality (DHSS 1980), such patients come disproportionately from the lower social classes (Williams 1989, French 1992) and from areas characterized by industrialization. Psychological factors may be similarly implicated, either as aetiological factors in their own right, or as significant cofactors. Once a cardiac or respiratory disease has become established in a particular individual, it impinges on the person's conscious-

ness. The objective biological fact of dysfunction becomes a subjective experience — the disease becomes an illness (Sim 1990a).

Consequently, a problem-oriented or problem-based assessment of the cardiorespiratory patient should encompass psychosocial as well as physical factors. The problems which are identified in the course of the assessment will consist of those to do with the condition as it is subjectively experienced as well as its physical manifestations. Of course, the same clinical feature will very often represent problems of both types, for example breathlessness, and there will be an interaction between the physical and the psychological factors.

Some psychosocial features of cardiorespiratory illness

It will be useful to look briefly at just some of the social and psychological forces that operate in cardiorespiratory illness.

1. *Anxiety* — many of the symptoms experienced by cardiac or respiratory patients are particularly distressing, e.g. breathlessness, palpitations, angina, and bronchospasm. This is not only because of their inherent unpleasantness, but also because their onset is frequently unexpected and unpredictable. The asthmatic patient may be prone to an attack with little warning, and suddenness of onset is perhaps the characteristic most associated with angina. The popular image of conditions such as these tends to exaggerate their more dramatic features; this is likely to have been internalized by the patient and may heighten feelings of anxiety. Stress and anxiety are also

associated with the trajectory of the disease. In cystic fibrosis, for example, there is a combination of a poor prospect of cure and uncertainty as to outcome in the shorter term (Waddell 1982). Aspects of treatment and management can also be anxiety producing. Strange environments such as the intensive care unit can give rise to disorientation, loneliness, fear and helplessness (Hough 1991).

2. *Defence mechanisms* — patients may respond to crises, such as a diagnosis of heart disease or bronchial carcinoma, with a variety of responses. These may include maladaptive psychotic mechanisms such as denial, distortion and projection, or less severe neurotic mechanisms such as displacement, intellectualization and repression (Porritt 1990). In cases of cystic fibrosis, where the family impact of the diagnosis is especially great (Dushenko 1981), these reactions may involve parents as well as patients themselves.

3. *Depression* — reactive depression is relatively common in cases of chronic cardiac and respiratory impairment. Indeed, psychiatric morbidity has been reported in up to 50% of patients with chronic bronchitis (Rutter 1977).

4. *Stigmatization* — symptoms of cardiorespiratory dysfunction may become a source of stigma, owing to their disruptive effect on smooth social interaction (Sim 1990b). An awareness of others' discomfort at their breathlessness may cause patients with advanced emphysema to curtail social contact (Fagerhaugh 1973). A number of clinical features of cystic fibrosis are potentially stigmatizing; for example, coughing, expectoration, and flatus. In addition, diminutive stature, underweight and delayed development of secondary sex characteristics may adversely affect body image (Norman & Hodson 1983). Perceived lack of attractiveness may reduce social confidence and inhibit sexual and emotional relationships, leading to feelings of reduced self-worth. Males with cystic fibrosis are almost always sterile, which may undermine feelings of manhood.

5. *Disruption of family relationships* — although in some cases illness can cause a strengthening of family ties, in other cases it can be a source of stress or conflict. The need to look after a disabled spouse, with the resulting toll on financial, personal and emotional resources, can place strain on the marital relationship. In the case of a child with cystic fibrosis, there may be strong feelings of guilt in the parents, in view of the hereditary nature of the disease, and resentment in the child at the degree of dependency on his or her parents for physiotherapy. Overprotectiveness on the part of the parents may keep the child from normal activities with those of the same age, and lead to a degree of social isolation (Norman & Hodson 1983). Adolescence is a time when family relationships may be especially strained (Dushenko 1981). Clearly, an assessment of the patient which focuses solely on the individual, and neglects his or her family and social context, will necessarily be incomplete.

These, then, are some of the psychosocial features of cardiorespiratory dysfunction. An awareness of these aspects of the individual's illness is crucial to the success of subsequent management and treatment. However, these are processes which have their own important psychosocial dimension, and these too should be understood.

PSYCHOSOCIAL ASPECTS OF CARE AND TREATMENT

There are certain features of the physiotherapist–patient relationship that have an important bearing on issues to do with communication. Above all, it tends to be an unequal relationship, with a differential distribution of power. The physiotherapist has specialized knowledge which the patient usually lacks, thereby creating a competency gap which is reinforced by the fact that, in hospital settings at least, the physiotherapist is on home ground whereas the patient is in an unfamiliar environment.

Coupled with this competency gap in many cases is a status gap. One of the key features of the doctor–patient relationship is the difference in social status that usually exists between the doctor and the patient (Navarro 1978); the same obtains, although to a less marked degree, in the case of the physiotherapist and the patient. When this status gap exists, the professional can use superior social status to enhance his or her status as 'expert' to exert leverage on the client (Friedson

1962). In the process, patients or clients are likely to be inhibited in initiating or discussing their own agenda of topics or concerns (Cartwright & O'Brien 1976), and 'the transmission of information is likely to be halting and imperfect' (Thompson 1984).

There is also a tendency (perhaps more in hospital and acute-care settings than in community health care) for the physiotherapist to act as an 'active initiator', leading the interaction and setting the agenda for treatment, while the patient assumes the role of 'passive responder'. As a result, the physiotherapist will tend to set the agenda for the encounter, and direct the flow and pattern of communication. There may therefore be a neglect of issues which are of concern to the patient, but which the physiotherapist is unaware of or unconcerned with.

Finally, an element of professional distance or detachment characterizes the physiotherapist's role. This is reinforced by such factors as the wearing of uniform, the avoidance of certain kinds of informality, and simple physical distance. There are, however, certain features of the physiotherapist's role which tend to reduce professional distance. Physiotherapists are generally in frequent and prolonged contact with their patients, which may allow a certain degree of informality to develop between them. In addition, they are almost always in a position of close physical proximity, with varying degrees of direct physical contact. The determinants of professional distance can therefore be adjusted when appropriate in order to facilitate the communication process.

Categories of intervention

The physiotherapist's role with respect to the cardiorespiratory patient can be roughly divided into three forms of involvement:

1. *Physical treatment* — this involves the direct use of various physical modalities, such as breathing exercises, postural drainage, chest shaking.
2. *Psychological care* — given that most respiratory conditions have little prospect of ultimate cure, assisting the patient in coming to terms with

the impact of respiratory impairment is an important part of the therapist's role. This may involve some form of counselling.

3. *Education* — by various forms of health education, the physiotherapist can help the patient adapt to the functional constraints imposed by cardiorespiratory impairment, and can encourage preventive strategies which may limit further deterioration.

There is, of course, no real dividing line between these areas of involvement. Physical treatment can have direct psychological benefit, and psychological care can enhance the effectiveness of physical treatment by lessening anxiety and increasing compliance. Similarly, by fostering a sense of purpose, self-confidence and empowerment, health education can provide the patient with psychological support. Above all, these facets of the therapist's role have in common the need for effective communication, and it is to this that we will now turn.

COMMUNICATION

A model of the communication process

Communication is a complex process, involving both verbal and non-verbal elements. Verbal communication can be either oral or written. Non-verbal communication incorporates such factors as facial expression, body language, spatial factors such as the relative position of the participants, and ecological factors relating to the environment in which communication occurs, with its various visual, olfactory and other exteroceptive stimuli. Verbal and non-verbal elements of communication exist in a mutual relationship, such that they can either reinforce or counteract one another.

For a single communication act, there will be an *initiator*, who encodes the intended meaning into a *message* of a certain form (e.g. a sentence with a certain grammatical structure) which is then transferred by means of a *medium* (e.g. the spoken word) to a *recipient*, who decodes the message. This process is subject to slippage at virtually any point — the process of encoding can distort the intended message; the medium can lend changes in emphasis or undertones of meaning (e.g. tone of voice, or its absence in the case of written communication); there can be further distortion as the recipient decodes the message (e.g. words may be taken to have a different meaning or connotation from that intended, or may even be unintelligible); or non-verbal behaviour can be taken as a gloss on the message which may or may not accord with the desired meaning.

Moreover, just as the recipient responds to the message, so the initiator monitors and reacts to the recipient's response in an ongoing feedback process (e.g. signs of non-comprehension are likely to prompt elaboration, whereas apparent understanding will probably encourage the initiator to encode a fresh message). Although it is helpful for the purposes of analysis to look at single communication acts, they are of course not discrete events, like shots in a game of tennis. There is, rather, a constant interplay within as well as between communication acts—the initiator relies on constant feedback from the recipient during the process of encoding, while the recipient similarly relies on various cues from the initiator while decoding. The roles of initiator and recipient are held simultaneously, not sequentially.

For purposes of clarity, the communication process so far has been seen in essentially dyadic terms; needless to say, the intricacy and essential vulnerability of the process increases when more than two participants are involved. The complexity of the communication process suggests:

- that it is likely to take different forms in different contexts and to serve different purposes
- that it requires a considerable degree of skill in the participants if it is to be effective
- that there are a large number of diverse factors which are capable of enhancing or detracting from the process.

It is in the context of these considerations that we now pass on to some more specific aspects of communication.

Purposes of communication

In a therapeutic setting, there are many possible purposes of communication, of which perhaps the foremost are:

- To pass on information
- To gain or extract information
- To establish interpersonal relationships
- To influence another's attitudes, opinions or behaviour
- To express feelings or emotions
- To gain an understanding of others' feelings, emotions, attitudes, etc.
- To create or maintain personal identity.

Any of these purposes can, of course, be held by either physiotherapist or patient, and can exist in virtually any combination. Moreover, they can be held either consciously or subconsciously. They can also be characterized as predominantly either instrumental or expressive. Instrumental communication is that which aims to secure a particular outcome or accomplish a specific task, such as when a physiotherapist asks a patient to take a deep breath, or requests a specific item of factual information. Expressive communication has to do with the communication of emotions or states of mind and does not require (though of course it often obtains) a response from the other participant. Expressive communication is often referred to as 'consummatory', in that 'the goal is achieved by the act of communicating' (Dickson et al 1989, p. 10) Expressive and instrumental aspects of communication often come together in a single communication act. Thus, a physiotherapist may smile at a patient to convey a feeling of caring (expressive goal), or to reassure the patient (instrumental goal), or, of course, for both reasons.

Detractors from effective communication

There are a number of factors which can militate against effective physiotherapist–patient communication.

Inappropriate attitudes. As MacWhannell (1992) argues, a prerequisite for effective communication is a willingness to form a relationship and an accompanying quality of 'openness'. The importance of good communication must be appreciated by both parties.

Inadequate skills. A disproportionate focus

on the acquisition of motor skills and manual techniques during their training may cause physiotherapists to overlook the fact that communication is a skill that can be learnt like any other. Listening skills are just as important as those concerned with the delivery of messages (MacWhannell 1992).

Language-related factors. As part of the competency gap identified earlier, health professionals are in possession of a specialized vocabulary which is likely to be unfamiliar to most patients. The inappropriate use of jargon will hinder effective communication (Porritt 1990), and therapists should learn 'when and how to use professional jargon and translate it into lay terms' (Purtilo 1990, p. 124). Syntax is equally important; complex, lengthy sentences may obscure meaning and confuse the recipient. The term 'register' is defined as 'a variety of the use of language as used by a particular speaker or writer in a particular context' (Darbyshire 1967); the choice of inappropriate register in a therapeutic context will clearly detract from communication.

Emotional factors. Various emotions on the part of one or both participants may obscure or distort intended meanings. Fear, anxiety, defencelessness, embarrassment, hostility and depression are common emotional responses in health care contexts which may prevent good communication, particularly if they are unacknowledged by one or both parties.

Cultural factors. Certain features of verbal and non-verbal communication carry different meanings from culture to culture. As an example, the degree of touch or eye contact acceptable in Latin cultures is greater than in Western Europe (Hyland & Donaldson 1989). Argyle (1988) notes that, during conversation, Arabs will exhibit a far higher degree of mutual gaze than British or American interlocutors, and that black Americans exhibit less eye contact, during both talking and listening, than white Americans. If proper allowance is not made for such cultural variations, communication is likely to be misinterpreted.

Noise. The term 'noise' is applied to any form of extraneous interference to the communication process. It may take the form of: visual, auditory or olfactory distractions; impairment of visual cues between participants; concurrent activity which diverts the attention; physical discomfort; unconducive positioning of participants; etc. It is not hard to imagine how all of these could simultaneously detract from communication in a setting such as an intensive care unit.

Facilitators of communication

To a large extent, factors which facilitate communication are the obverse of those that detract from it. Thus, the appropriate choice of register, judicious selection of vocabulary, absence of 'noise', and the appropriate attitudes will all make for good communication. However, there are also some more specific considerations which will allow positive steps to be taken to improve communication.

Positioning. It is important to consider the appropriate use of physical distance. The anthropologist Edward Hall has defined four basic distances for social interaction (Table 9.1). It is clear that many of the physiotherapist's activities will bring him or her into the intimate distance, with the risk of invading the patient's personal space. At times, such as when implicit permission has not been gained, such intimacy may be a barrier to communication. On other occasions, when more expressive purposes are concerned, such proximity can instil confidence and a sense of caring, and thereby enhance communication; use of public distance in such a case would be clearly inappropriate. Exaggerated physical distance from a patient who is expectorating can easily convey a sense of discomfort or distaste.

Table 9.1 Distances for social interaction, according to Hall (1966)

Intimate distance	
Close phase	In contact
Far phase	6–18 in.
Personal distance	
Close phase	$1\frac{1}{2}$–$2\frac{1}{2}$ ft
Far phase	$2\frac{1}{2}$–4 ft
Social distance	
Close phase	4–7 ft
Far phase	7–12 ft
Public distance	
Close phase	12–25 ft
Far phase	>25 ft

The relative height of participants is also important. MacWhannell (1992) points out that an action such as sitting on the patient's bed facilitates eye contact and promotes a feeling of equality. It also counteracts the feeling of hurriedness that can often seem to characterize therapeutic activities.

Posture and gestures. For the purposes of analysing communication, there are two fundamental types of bodily posture. A closed posture is one which indicates that social interaction is not desired, whereas an open posture signals a willingness to interact (Hyland & Donaldson 1989). Sitting back in a chair with legs closely crossed and arms folded defensively would be a typical closed posture. Gestures, used appropriately, can illustrate meaning and be used as a form of emphasis. Excessive gesturing can constitute a source of 'noise'.

Facial expression and eye contact. Appropriate use of facial expression and eye contact can reinforce communication. Signs of attentiveness on the part of the physiotherapist provide positive feedback and encourage the patient to communicate more openly. Eye contact is often a sign of affinity between individuals, and can therefore be used by the therapist to create empathy. It can also be used to counteract various emotional detractors from communication. Avoiding eye contact can help to eliminate inappropriate levels of arousal, and thus defuse aggression and hostility (Hyland & Donaldson 1989). When engaged in intimate procedures which might cause embarrassment to the patient, minimizing eye contact can help to define the procedure as instrumental rather than expressive, and thus reduce embarrassment. Argyle (1983) notes that excessive eye contact, in the form of 'mutual gaze', can be distracting.

Touch. Judicious use of touch can convey liking and a sense of caring. Porritt (1990, p. 8) notes that the 'laying on of hands has always been synonymous with healing, and these days is an important counter-balance to the technology of health care'. There is, however, a risk that touch may be perceived as inappropriate; Purtilo (1990, p. 145) notes that the health professional, who is accustomed to touching patients, 'probably has so firm a concept of his or her good intentions that the question of inappropriateness or improper familiarity never arises'. Hyland & Donaldson (1989) point out that touching often connotes dependency on the part of the person touched, and that this may not be welcomed. Hargie et al (1987) note that certain groups of individuals, such as elderly people with no close relatives or those who have been widowed (categories which are likely to include many patients with chronic respiratory illness), may rarely experience touch from others, and to this extent are deprived of a certain degree of emotional fulfilment. They point out that health professionals, by the appropriate use of touch, can help to redress this deficiency.

Memory

An important feature of effective communication is the ability of participants to retain information that is imparted. Although it is crucial that communication in the physiotherapist–patient relationship should be a two-way process, specific problems of recall seem to occur most often on the part of the patient. Reflecting this concern, extensive research has been conducted within health care on factors that may either hinder or facilitate memory and thus determine the degree of subsequent compliance (Ley 1988). Table 9.2 summarizes some of the principal steps that can be taken to maximize the information that patients will retain and recall; further discussion of these and other factors can be found in Ley (1988) and Hill (1992). It is important to stress that such techniques, useful though they are, should not be seen as a substitute for the less tangible interpersonal skills and attitudes that help to create the sort of relationship with the patient that is a prerequisite for good communication.

The importance of communication

As Thompson (1984, p. 88) points out, 'dissatisfaction with medical communications remains the most prominent of patient complaints and a major factor in the move to alternative medicine'. Moreover, it is not merely a question of patients' perceptions; ever since Egbert and colleagues' seminal study (Egbert et al 1964), the direct

Table 9.2 Principal factors that can facilitate memory

Utilizing primacy and recency effects	Information given either at the beginning or the end of the encounter tends to be best retained
Limiting the number of items of information given	Too many items can lead to 'overcrowding' of the short-term memory
Emphasizing the key points	This can be done by using repetition or by explicitly highlighting items
Categorization	Information is placed into separate categories, which are explicitly identified to the patient
Simplification	Short words and sentences are generally better, and jargon should be avoided
Being specific	Instructions in particular should be specific rather than general
Providing feedback	This can be either positive or negative
Using written reinforcement	This gives the patient a source of subsequent reference
Making use of 'dual encoding'	The use of both concrete and abstract concepts brings into play both hemispheres of the brain when the information is processed by the listener

therapeutic value of good communication has repeatedly been demonstrated. It is, moreover, important not to take too restricted a view of the role of communication in health care:

First and foremost, all health professionals need to enlarge their repertoire of communication skills. In some circumstances 'controlling' and 'managerial' communication may be required and appropriate, particularly in a crisis, but the other more sensitive communication skills, associated with 'counselling' and 'helping' patients to sort our their own problems and take their own decisions, require quite different training and the development of quite different skills. (Thompson et al 1988)

These authors go on to argue that traditional forms of education and training for health professionals do little to instil these additional skills.

Therefore, good communication on the part of physiotherapists is not only a means of securing patient satisfaction, but is also an essential component of effective care and treatment. The quality of communication is at a particularly high premium in two specialist areas of the cardiorespiratory physiotherapist's work (counselling and health education) to which we will shortly turn. Before doing so, however, it is important to emphasize that communication also has moral significance. Good communication is required not only for the *effectiveness* of the relationship between therapist and patient, but also for the *ethics* of this relationship. In the course of caring for a patient, therapists may come into possession of information which, they may feel, the patient has a right to know (Sim 1986a). For example, a man with unexplained unilateral pneumonia may be found to be suffering from previously undiagnosed bronchial carcinoma, and it may be felt that this should be made known to him. Alternatively, a young woman with cryptogenic fibrosing alveolitis may seem to have unrealistic beliefs as to the prospects of cure. Should she be given a more accurate picture of her future?

Ethical issues also surround consent. Informed consent can be defined as 'the voluntary and revocable agreement of a competent individual to participate in a therapeutic or research procedure, based on an adequate understanding of its nature, purpose, and implications' (Sim 1986b). In some instances, gaining consent to treatment procedures can be accomplished fairly straightforwardly. However, in the case of nasopharyngeal suction, the patient may not be in a state of consciousness that permits explicit consent. Alternatively, the patient may seem to be withholding consent, and a decision must be made whether or not to proceed nonetheless, on the grounds that the patient is expressing a wish that is not fully autonomous, or perhaps on the basis that the therapeutic benefits likely to accrue justify disregarding a lack of consent. Presumably with this latter argument in mind, Hough (1991, p. 93) argues that '[f]orcible suction is unethical, and acceptable only in life-threatening situations'.

COUNSELLING

Henry is a middle-aged man with emphysema who is suffering increasing restriction on his activities due to breathlessness, to the extent that he is unable to participate fully in running the family business. He is experiencing feelings of inadequacy and guilt, and finds that he is losing what he perceives to be his role within the family.

Karla, an 18-year-old woman with cystic fibrosis, recently discovered that another patient of the same age, whom she has got to know very well during the course of several shared in-patient admissions, has died of the disease. The sense of purpose and hopefulness with which Karla previously pursued her treatment now seems to be weakening, and she is becoming increasingly fatalistic about her future.

Gary is a young man with asthma who is subject to acute attacks of moderate severity. He is increasingly unwilling to engage in social activities, anticipating the disruption and alarm that a sudden attack may cause, and fearful of straying from the support of his family, who 'know what to do'.

Each of these vignettes demonstrates the way in which the psychosocial features of respiratory disease may affect the patient. They equally show how the physiotherapist will require skills other than those of direct physical treatment in order to help. The focus here is on the second category of intervention that we identified earlier (psychological care) and in order to accomplish this the physiotherapist may feel the need to assume the role of counsellor in situations such as these. However, it is important first of all to be clear what counselling is, and what it is not. It has been defined thus:

> Counselling is a technique concerned to help people help themselves by the development of a special relationship which leads a client into a greater depth of self-understanding, clarifies the identity of problems and conflicts and mobilises personal coping abilities. (Nichols 1984, p. 142)

Counselling is not just being a passive receptacle for people's anxieties, fears, emotions, problems, etc. Equally, it does not consist in providing specific pieces of advice, guidance or reassurance; indeed, in his classification of helping strategies, Griffiths (1981) explicitly separates counselling from strategies such as 'giving information', 'teaching', and 'giving advice'. Rather, it is a process whereby the patient (or 'client' in counselling parlance) is assisted towards insight and an understanding of his or her own emotional, attitudinal and social situation. Emotions are not suppressed by the counsellor, nor are they permitted to flow in a totally free and unrestrained manner — they are clarified. Instead of providing ready-made strategies, the counsellor helps the

client in setting his or her own goals. The counsellor frequently acts as a catalyst (Nichols 1984).

This all requires specific communication skills, which are as much to do with listening as with talking. Physiotherapists must assess carefully the extent to which they possess such skills. While some sort of counselling role is well within the capabilities of most, if not all, physiotherapists, it is important to recognize the limit of one's expertise, and to refer patients to a more fully trained counsellor, or even to a clinical psychologist, when the case demands.

Essential elements in counselling

Naturally, it is not possible to provide here a practical account of the skills required in counselling. However, it is perhaps worth looking briefly at some of what are generally agreed to be the essential ingredients of effective counselling. It should be remembered that there are many different approaches to counselling, and each approach will tend to attach varying importance to the different factors.

Positive regard. The counsellor should show some degree of detachment. On the one hand, there should be no signs of disapproval, censure or blame. The counsellor should display 'unconditional positive regard' for the client (Burnard 1989), i.e. positive feelings towards the client which do not need to be 'earned', will not be affected by what the client may say or may have done, and which the client should not necessarily feel obliged to reciprocate. Without such openness, acceptance and apparent liking, the client is unlikely to be forthcoming and confide in the counsellor. In the case of Gary, for example, any suggestion by the therapist that his anxieties are inappropriate or exaggerated would be likely to inhibit a counselling relationship. On the other hand, undue sympathy or emotional closeness should be avoided. Explicit emotional identification ('I know just how you feel') may threaten the essential privacy and uniqueness of the client's state of being, and may accordingly be resented.

Non-possessiveness. A young female physiotherapist may be able to identify strongly with a patient such as Karla, and feel that she understands the emotions which she is experiencing. As a result of this powerful sense of empathy, she may experience an intense desire to help. However, the counsellor should not become possessive with regard to the client. Undue sympathy for the client may cause the helper to seek to impose what he or she sees as the optimum solution to the individual's problems, without due regard for what the client would regard as optimum. Dickson et al (1989) see altruism as an essential attribute for the counsellor, and one result of this is that it is all too easy for the counsellor to become paternalistic. Just because the client has permitted access to what are often private and sensitive aspects of his or her life, does not mean that the client has in any way surrendered personal control. The professional has to balance feelings of benevolence and a desire to help against respect for the client's autonomy.

Willingness to yield control. The counsellor should not control the encounter excessively. Indeed, many counsellors adopt a 'non-directive' approach, and try to ensure that the course taken by the consultation is, as far as possible, in the control of the client. At the same time, skilful use of probing questions can facilitate this process, and confrontation techniques may be required if the consultation seems to have reached an impasse, with the client 'going over the same ground without any new insights' (Brearley & Birchley 1986, p. 32). What are termed 'prescriptive interventions' do have a part to play in counselling, but Burnard (1989) warns that they can very easily be overused. Specific practical advice might seem to be useful in the case of someone like Henry. However, it is often only of short-term usefulness, and may encourage dependency. Moreover, if a suggested strategy does not work, the counsellor may be blamed and the relationship may be broken, depriving the counsellor of the opportunity to help further.

Orientation to action. Greater self-understanding on the part of the client is an important aim of counselling, but this is only of value if it in turn leads to a solution (whether partial or total) of the individual's problems. According to Burnard (1989), immediacy is an essential quality in the counselling relationship;

that is, the counsellor should have a concern with the here-and-now, and should discourage the client from undue reminiscing about the past, which may remove the focus from issues of immediate practical concern. Accordingly, many counsellors feel that the client should always leave a consultation with some definite course of action to pursue, however minimal it may appear to be.

Establishing a contract. It is important to clarify mutual expectations. The counsellor should make it understood what sort of help is likely to be forthcoming, so that the client does not bring unrealistic hopes to the relationship (Brearley & Birchley 1986). Similarly, boundaries should be set. The client should understand that, whilst help is freely given, this can only be for a certain period of time, and that the counsellor may not necessarily be available at unarranged times between sessions. As part of an effective working relationship, the client will be expected to confide information relating to often private and intimate aspects of his or her life. The client can only be expected to do so with an assurance of confidentiality on the part of the counsellor (indeed it is unlikely that information will be freely disclosed otherwise). If it is felt that other professionals need to be consulted in order adequately to help the client, the counsellor will need to explain this to the client and obtain consent for information to be revealed to another party. In such a case, the benevolent aim of helping the client does not override the ethical requirement to respect privacy. It should also be remembered that patients may have legal redress in certain cases of breach of confidentiality (Mason & McCall Smith 1987).

Assuming the counselling role

It is fair to say that not all physiotherapists take readily to the role of counsellor. In common with many other practitioners, they may often be 'reluctant to deal with emotional and psychological dimensions of patients' problems' (Dickson et al 1989, p. 126). There may be an unwillingness to explore aspects of patients' lives to do with such areas as intensely felt emotions, their personal fears, and feelings related to their sexuality.

More specifically, the predominant accent within physiotherapy training and education on physical treatment strategies may cause physiotherapists to feel, albeit unconsciously, that they are not performing their proper role if they are apparently 'just talking' to patients. It should be accepted that the process of 'problem-solving' is likely to take a very different form in psychological care from that undertaken in physical treatment. The strategies adopted will often be far less tangible, and may involve, in comparison, little active participation by the physiotherapist. Frequently, the therapist engaged in psychological care will not be providing specific, concrete interventions, but will be involved in a more passive, facilitatory role, involving considerably more response than initiation. Any action to be taken is generally for the client rather than the therapist. Thus, Griffiths describes counselling as 'helping someone to explore a problem, clarify conflicting issues and discover alternative ways of dealing with it, so that they can decide what to do about it; that is, helping people to help themselves' (Griffiths 1981, p. 267).

In a similar way, the sort of dialogue which is likely to be engaged in may often appear to be less purposeful than those to which physiotherapists have become accustomed in the course of physical treatment. Pauses, and even considerable periods of silence, are often not only acceptable but positively beneficial in counselling and other forms of psychological care (Bendix 1982); however, they may initially be a source of unease to therapists who are used to more 'business-like' exchanges with their patients.

Counselling, if it is to be effective, involves a new set of skills for many physiotherapists and, just as important, a new perspective on their professional role. However, appropriate training in counselling skills, and a fuller understanding of the psychosocial dynamics of cardiorespiratory illness, will reveal a wider and more holistic approach to the management of these patients.

HEALTH EDUCATION

Health education and health promotion

The terms 'health education' and 'health promotion' are sometimes used almost interchangeably. However, a valuable distinction can be drawn between them. 'Health promotion' is used to cover a broad spectrum of activities that seek to improve or restore health. The term has been defined by Downie et al (1990, p. 59) as follows:

Health promotion comprises efforts to enhance positive health and prevent ill-health, through the overlapping spheres of health education, prevention, and health protection.

This model of health promotion incorporates three key elements, earlier identified by Tannahill (1985). One of these is *health education*, which we will return to in due course. The notion of *prevention* concerns activities which are designed to reduce the incidence or risk of occurrence of any undesirable health-related state of being— whether this is physical illness, mental illness, physical injury, physical disability, or handicap. Traditionally, prevention has been classified into three types. Gray, for example, speaks of three phases of preventive medicine:

primary preventive medicine, which tries to prevent disease; secondary preventive medicine, which tries to prevent the effects of disease by treatment at an early stage in its course; and the tertiary preventive phase, which tries to prevent the serious consequences of disease by effective treatment. (Gray 1979)

Downie et al (1990) criticize this typology for being unduly centred in the narrow concept of disease, and for identifying prevention with the idea of treatment. They also note the lack of unanimity with which these three phases are used by various commentators. Downie et al (1990) propose, instead, what they call 'four foci of prevention', which give a rather fuller idea of the potentialities of prevention:

- Prevention of the onset or first manifestation of a disease process, or some other first occurrence, through risk reduction
- Prevention of the progression of a disease process or other unwanted state, through early detection when this favourably affects outcome
- Prevention of avoidable complications of an irreversible, manifest disease or some other unwanted state
- Prevention of the recurrence of an illness or other unwanted phenomenon.

The third key element in health promotion is that of *health protection*. This comprises various legal controls, policy initiatives, codes of practice, and other regulatory mechanisms which are designed to improve or restore health.

Health education is therefore just one of the ways in which the goals of health promotion can be pursued. There is, of course, a large degree of interrelation between the three elements; for example, a considerable proportion of health education may concern itself with prevention.

The scope of health education

Downie et al (1990, p. 28) define health education as:

> a communication activity aimed at enhancing positive health and preventing or diminishing ill-health in individuals and groups, through influencing the beliefs, attitudes, and behaviour of those with power and of the community at large.

Thus, health education, like education in other contexts, has three main targets — beliefs (or knowledge), attitudes and behaviour. By seeking to influence one or more of these factors, the health educator hopes to enhance or restore health. Ewles and Simnett (1985) use these factors to construct, respectively, 'knowing', 'feeling' and 'doing' objectives in health education. 'Knowing' objectives are 'concerned with giving information, explaining it, ensuring that the client understands it, and thus increasing the client's knowledge', while objectives about 'feeling' are 'concerned with clarifying, forming or changing the clients (sic) attitudes, beliefs, values or opinions'. Objectives about 'doing' have to do with the client's skills and actions (Ewles & Simnett 1985, p. 21). Under these headings, these authors formulate seven more specific health education goals. Thus, the 'knowing' objectives incorporate what Ewles and Simnett call the 'health consciousness goal' and the 'knowledge goal'; the 'feeling' objectives include the 'self-awareness goal' and the 'attitude change goal'. The 'decision-making goal' comes under the aegis of both 'knowing' and 'feeling' objectives, and the social change goal straddles all three sorts of objectives (Table 9.3).

Table 9.3 Health education objectives and goals, according to Ewles and Simnett (1985)

Goal	Objective		
	Knowing	Feeling	Doing
Health consciousness	✓		
Knowledge	✓		
Self-awareness		✓	
Attitude change		✓	
Decision-making	✓	✓	
Behaviour change			✓
Social change	✓	✓	✓

Ewles and Simnett (1985, p. 23) describe the social change goal as 'the rather complex goal of making "healthy choices easier choices" by changing the physical and/or social environment so that people are encouraged to adopt healthier behaviour'. This illustrates clearly the need for health education not to take a purely individualistic approach, but to concern itself with wider social issues. For example, in the case of children with cystic fibrosis, health education may extend to advising schools of the need for treatment facilities or special diets. In the case of persons with acquired immune deficiency syndrome (AIDS), it may involve attempts to dispel misconceptions and to foster more tolerant attitudes in the wider community. Furthermore, it is not only important that the wider community should be educated about health-related matters; patients themselves need to know about the broader context into which their health (or lack of it) fits.

Draper et al (1980) emphasize this wider remit for health education in their description of three types of health education:

> The first and most common is education about the body and how to look after it . . . The second is about health services — information about available services and the 'sensible' use of health care resources. But the third, about the wider environment within which health choices are made, is relatively neglected. It is concerned with education about national, regional, and local policies, which are too often devised and implemented without taking account of their consequences for health.

They argue that health education that is restricted to the first two types is 'partial to the point of being socially irresponsible'.

At the heart of health education is the notion of empowerment. 'True health education should work to enable people to understand better what they are, what they believe, and what they know' (Seedhouse 1986).

Health education and the physiotherapist

The question now arises as to how, and to what extent, the physiotherapist should incorporate the role of health educator in the management of patients with cardiac and respiratory conditions. There would seem to be a number of factors which suggest that this is a highly appropriate role. First, it must be recognized that, with some exceptions (e.g. acute lobar pneumonia, hyperventilation syndrome), most of these conditions are not amenable to cure. There is, therefore, a need for a programme of long-term management, in addition to any short-term treatment. Second, any physical treatment that is administered is generally only beneficial for these conditions if it is continued between periods of direct contact with the therapist and, in addition, is augmented by self-care strategies on the part of the patient. Effective management of these patients consists therefore as much in what takes place in the patient's personal, domestic and social life as in what occurs in the health care setting. Third, cardiorespiratory disease offers full scope for prevention, under each of the four foci identified by Downie et al (1990), and health education is an important means of implementing preventive health measures. Finally, there are many areas of the individual's life in which changes in behaviour can have a beneficial effect on cardiorespiratory dysfunction, e.g. dietary adjustments, avoidance of possible sources of infection or allergic reaction, the taking of exercise, etc. Here, too, health education has a clear contribution to make.

Accordingly, the physiotherapist involved in the care of patients with cardiorespiratory problems can fulfil the role of health educator in a wide variety of ways, of which just some are:

- by explaining the underlying pathological processes and the significance of these in terms of prevention and treatment

- by advising on means by which general health may be maintained (e.g. adequate nutrition, appropriate balance of rest and activity)
- by teaching treatment modalities which can be carried out independently, such as the active cycle of breathing techniques, and strategies for coping with the physiological demands of the disease, such as breathing control
- by instructing patients in the use of items of equipment, such as air compressors, nebulizers and oxygen concentrators
- by providing information on appropriate health and social services available, including information on patients' statutory rights
- by putting patients in contact with self-help groups and patients' organizations such as those that exist in many countries for patients with cystic fibrosis
- by helping to create attitudes of confidence, self-worth and confidence, thereby empowering patients in their efforts to cope with disability.

In order to achieve such goals, the physiotherapist will need highly developed communication skills, and an awareness of the factors identified previously which may either enhance or detract from the communication process. There are, however, some specific points which should be considered. The first is that health education should not consist of unilateral giving of instruction and advice. It is essential that goals are mutually negotiated, otherwise the patient will not see him- or herself as a partner in the overall process, and will be poorly motivated to carry through recommended courses of action. Second, the therapist must gain a sound insight into the patient's psychological profile and social environment. Patients with a primarily internal locus of control (i.e. those who broadly regard themselves as capable of determining their own destiny) will respond to different forms of goal setting compared with patients who have an external locus of control (i.e. those who see themselves as subject to more fatalistic, external influences). Similarly, ignorance of the patient's social situation may lead the therapist to advocate inappropriate strategies that are incompatible with the individual's lifestyle. In the light of this, talk of 'non-compliant' patients is singularly unhelpful. Locating failures of compliance in the patient is to overlook the fact that compliance is the property of a relationship, not of an individual. If compliance is not achieved, the relevant shortcomings reside in the rapport and understanding that exist (or perhaps do not exist) between therapist and patient. Such rapport and understanding are a shared responsibility.

The third important consideration is that effective health education, like all areas of health work, relies on sound liaison and teamwork. It is important that messages are echoed and reinforced by all those with whom the patient comes into contact. Above all, it should be remembered that team members each have their own agenda, and some sort of compromise must be effected in order that a shared set of priorities can be drawn up. Needless to say, the patient has his or her own agenda, and this should be given full consideration in the process.

This leads us to the final consideration, which concerns a respect for the individual's autonomy. In many instances, the physiotherapist's expertise may allow him or her to identify authoritatively the best means of achieving a certain health-related goal. However, this does not mean that the therapist is in a privileged position to identify this as a valuable goal in the first instance. Such goals only have value in the context of the person's total state of being, and the ultimate authority on what matters to a given individual is, necessarily, that individual. The patient's values and priorities may differ from the therapist's. If health education goals are defined disproportionately by the therapist, with insufficient regard for the desires of the patient, and then imposed unilaterally, the recipient's self-determination is likely to be overridden. The physiotherapist must recognize the dividing line between education and indoctrination (Campbell 1990).

CONCLUSION

This chapter has attempted to highlight the role that communication can play in the management of patients with cardiorespiratory problems. Communication skills are fundamental to the three main categories of intervention — physical treatment, psychological care, and health education — and, like other professional skills, can be learnt and further developed in order to improve the quality of patient care.

REFERENCES

Argyle M 1983 The psychology of interpersonal behaviour, 4th edn. Penguin, Harmondsworth

Argyle M 1988 Bodily communication, 2nd edn. Methuen, London

Bendix T 1982 The anxious patient: the therapeutic dialogue in clinical practice. Churchill Livingstone, Edinburgh

Brearley G, Birchley P 1986 Introducing counselling skills and techniques, with particular application for the paramedical professions. Faber & Faber, London

Burnard P 1989 Counselling skills for health professionals. Chapman & Hall, London

Campbell A V 1990 Education or indoctrination? The issue of autonomy in health education. In: Doxiadis S (ed) Ethics in health education. Wiley, Chichester

Cartwright A, O'Brien M 1976 Social class variations in health care and the nature of general practitioner consultations. In: Stacey M (ed) The sociology of the National Health Service. Sociological review monograph 22. University of Keele, Keele

Darbyshire A E 1967 A description of English. Edward Arnold, London, p 23

DHSS 1980 Inequalities in health: report of a research working group (Black report). HMSO, London

Dickson D A, Hargie O, Morrow N C 1989 Communication skills training for health professionals: an instructor's handbook. Chapman & Hall, London

Downie R S, Fyfe C, Tannahill A 1990 Health promotion: models and values. Oxford University Press, Oxford

Draper P, Griffiths J, Dennis J, Popay J 1980 Three types of health education. British Medical Journal 281: 493–495

Dushenko T W 1981 Cystic fibrosis: a medical overview and critique of the psychological literature. Social Science and Medicine 15E: 43–56

Egbert L D, Battit G E, Welsh C E, Bartlett M K 1964 Reduction of postoperative pain by encouragement and instruction of patients. New England Journal of Medicine 270: 825–827

Ewles L, Simnett I 1985 Promoting health: a practical guide to health education. Wiley, Chichester

Fagerhaugh S Y 1973 Getting around with emphysema. American Journal of Nursing 73: 94–99

French S 1992 Inequalities in health. In: French S (ed) Physiotherapy: a psychosocial approach. Butterworth-Heinemann, Oxford

Friedson E 1962 Dilemmas in the doctor-patient relationship. In: Rose A M (ed) Human behavior and social processes: an interactionist approach. Routledge & Kegan Paul, London

Gray J A M 1979 Man against disease: preventive medicine. Oxford University Press, Oxford, p 32

Griffiths D 1981 Psychology and medicine. British Psychological Society/Macmillan, London

Hall E T 1966 The hidden dimension: man's use of space in public and private. Bodley Head, London

Hargie O, Saunders C, Dickson D 1987 Social skills in interpersonal communication, 2nd edn. Routledge, London

Hill P 1992 Communication in physiotherapy practice (2). In: French S (ed) Physiotherapy: a psychosocial approach. Butterworth-Heinemann, Oxford

Hough A 1991 Physiotherapy in respiratory care: a problem-solving approach. Chapman & Hall, London

Hyland M E, Donaldson M L 1989 Psychological care in nursing practice. Scutari Press, Harrow

Ley P 1988 Communicating with patients: improving communication, satisfaction and compliance. Chapman & Hall, London

MacWhannell D E 1992 Communication in physiotherapy practice (1). In: French S (ed) Physiotherapy: a psychosocial approach. Butterworth-Heinemann, Oxford

Mason J K, McCall Smith R A 1987 Law and medical ethics, 2nd edn. Butterworths, London

Navarro V 1978 Class struggle, the state and medicine: an historical and contemporary analysis of the medical sector in Great Britain. Martin Robertson, Oxford

Nichols K A 1984 Psychological care in physical illness. Croom Helm, London

Norman A P, Hodson M E 1983 Emotional and social aspects of treatment. In: Hodson M E, Norman A P, Batten J C (eds) Cystic fibrosis. Baillière Tindall, London

Porritt L 1990 Interaction strategies: an introduction for health professionals. Churchill Livingstone, Melbourne

Purtilo R B 1990 Health professional and patient interaction, 4th edn. W B Saunders, Philadelphia

Rutter B M 1977 Some psychological concomitants of chronic bronchitis. Psychological Medicine 7: 459–464

Seedhouse D 1986 Health: the foundations for achievement. Wiley, Chichester, p 91

Sim J 1986a Truthfulness in the therapeutic relationship. Physiotherapy Practice 2: 121–127

Sim J 1986b Informed consent: ethical implications for physiotherapy. Physiotherapy 72: 584–587

Sim J 1990a The concept of health. Physiotherapy 76: 423–428

Sim J 1990b Stigma, physical disability and rehabilitation. Physiotherapy Canada 42: 232–238

Tannahill A 1985 What is health promotion? Health Education Journal 44: 167–168

Thompson J 1984 Communicating with patients. In: Fitzpatrick R, Hinton J, Newman S, Scambler G, Thompson J (eds) The experience of illness. Tavistock, London

Thompson I E, Melia K M, Boyd K M 1988 Nursing ethics, 2nd edn. Churchill Livingstone, Edinburgh, p 161

Waddell C 1982 The process of neutralisation and the uncertainties of cystic fibrosis. Sociology of Health and Illness 4: 210–220

Williams S J 1989 Chronic respiratory illness and disability: a critical review of the psychosocial literature. Social Science and Medicine 28: 791–803

10. Research in cardiopulmonary physiotherapy

Cecily J. Partridge

INTRODUCTION

This chapter provides an introduction to the process of applied research for therapists. The underlying principles of each stage are outlined and ways of avoiding pitfalls and solving common problems are discussed.

Research is defined in the *Oxford English Dictionary* as 'a careful search or enquiry after, or for, or into ...' (COED 1976) and it is helpful to consider it as a process which involves a sequence of stages; a brief outline is given in Table 10.1.

Table 10.1 Outline of the stages in the research process

Reading and reviewing the literature
Asking questions and developing ideas
Defining the research question
Statement of objectives for the study, or a hypothesis for testing
Deciding on appropriate research design
Obtaining research grants
Writing the research proposal
Ethical committees
Assessment and measurement of study variables
Organization of fieldwork
Pilot work
Main study
Analysis of data collected
Writing the report and presentation of results

Systematic planning is essential in research. In clinical practice it is common for one treatment approach to be tried and if it does not work it is adapted or changed; in research, the plan has to be thoroughly worked out in advance with great attention to detail at each stage.

READING AND REVIEWING THE LITERATURE

Reading journal articles and review papers is a central part of the work of research: the first task after getting ideas for research is to search the literature to find what is already known about the topic and where the new idea fits in.

Finding a good library is essential. They are to be found in larger hospitals, postgraduate medical centres, universities and colleges. Most librarians enjoy helping readers, so it is worth finding a friendly one.

Manual searches can be time consuming but are the best starting point, as they give a feel for the subject and an idea of the depth and breadth of work. Most libraries can access a number of computerized searches, and it is usual to go back about 5 years in the search if there are many references, or perhaps 10 years if little has been written. Each reference on the computer printout is a potential source of more references. It is best not to order too many articles at one time and librarians often restrict numbers of offprints to around ten. It is essential to set up a system either using cards or a computer so that papers can be easily retrieved.

Reading research articles

The ability to read research papers critically and decide the value of the work reported is a key skill for researchers which can only be acquired through practice. Common problems here are spending too much time on papers later rejected as unreliable, and deciding how much value to place on the work of different authors.

A few questions may help in identifying specific points to be considered:

1. *What was the purpose of the study*? Are the objectives and the research question clearly stated.

2. *What methods were used*? This is a central issue, if the design is not appropriate to answer the question or there is insufficient information about what was done the value of the results is diminished.

3. *If a clinical trial, what outcome measures were used*? Variables selected as outcome measures *must* be directly related to the treatment being evaluated. It is also important not to have too many variables in the study, by collecting too much information the real purpose of the study may be lost.

4. *Were the tools of measurement used appropriate*? Were they sensitive enough to measure expected changes?

5. *Were other factors which might influence results taken into account in the analysis*? For example, in studying vital capacity in postoperative patients, were severity of pain, analgesia and type of operation taken into account?

6. *Was there sufficient information about selection of patients, procedures followed and treatments given*? The ideal is for sufficient information to be given for others to be able to replicate the study.

7. *What did they find*? The results should be clearly presented in either tables or text, but not both. It is well to remember that statistical analysis is meant to clarify information from large data sets, not to mystify the reader. Results should be clearly understandable without detailed knowledge of the statistical tests used.

8. *Are the discussion and conclusion sections clear*? This should clearly connect with the introduction and explain the extent to which the purpose of the study has been fulfilled and how the results compare with others in the same field. For conclusions to be valid they must relate only to the results of the study reported.

Writing a review

There is a feeling of achievement when the wads of computer paper and then the articles start to arrive. The next task is to pull the information together and provide a critical review, this again can be a lengthy task. Good reviews pick out the main issues and then discuss the evidence for and against, drawing from the most important work. This ensures that the researcher has a sound background knowledge of the area before starting the project and can learn from the strengths and weaknesses of previous work.

ASKING QUESTIONS AND DEVELOPING IDEAS

Ideas and problems arising from clinical practice are not too difficult to find as a starting point for a research project, but getting from there to the research question is surprisingly difficult. It is essential to identify a good question and time is well spent in trying to get it right.

If there are problems with developing ideas, Buzan (1989) suggests the use of mind maps. The initial idea is put in the centre of the paper and others can flow outwards and interconnect. Figure 10.1 shows an example of a map on the idea of breathlessness.

Hudson (1966) introduced a concept of convergent and divergent thinking, from work undertaken investigating the patterns of thought in schoolboys. He describes convergent thinking as that used in tasks such as the solution of crossword clues where there is only one solution, and intelligence tests which question logical relations in terms of patterns; in both the assumption is that there is a correct answer and thinking works towards it. Divergent thinking, on the other hand, does not seek a logical and correct answer, rather it is imaginative and creative. In research, both types of thinking are needed: in the early ideas stage, divergence is needed so that a wide area is covered and different avenues explored. In the later stages, when the question and purpose of the study have been decided, convergent thinking is more appropriate to follow the plan set out without any distraction. Creative ideas half way through a project are likely to be disruptive.

DEFINING THE RESEARCH QUESTION

Defining a good research question takes time and a lot of careful thought. It must:

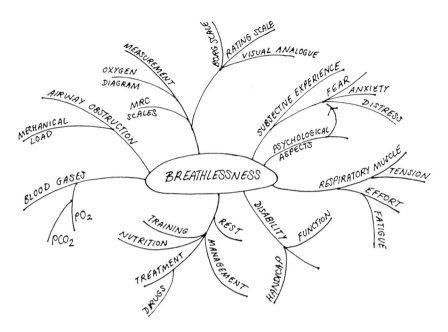

Fig. 10.1   Example of a mind map on the concept of breathlessness.

- Be stated clearly and unambiguously
- Be answerable within the time and resources available
- Have practical implications.

Clear and unambiguous. There is a tendency in physiotherapy to talk about patients 'improving', 'getting better' and 'achieving goals': these are well-understood terms in clinical practice, but in research clearer language is needed as these terms could be interpreted differently.

Answerable within the time and resources available. Many questions may seem both important and interesting, but are not answerable within the time and resources available. Resources include not only finance but also research knowledge and skills.

Has practical implications. Applied research starts with a practical problem and, therefore, the results should have implications which have the possibility of influencing some aspect of practice, education or management. It is also important not to come up with a 'so what?' result, for example a treatment that achieves faster results but requires therapy staff to be trebled.

OBJECTIVES AND HYPOTHESES

Objectives are needed to define the purpose of the study. They should be stated in terms of actions, that is:

- To obtain information about . . . .
- To investigate . . . .
- To find if . . . .

so that work undertaken can be checked against the listed objectives.

If the study is a clinical trial a hypothesis will be tested. Hypotheses are statements about expected relationships and can be stated in two ways. An example of the positive form of a hypothesis is: *Treatment A will reduce breathlessness faster than treatment B*. This expresses an expectation that treatment A is a better treatment for reducing breathlessness than is B. The hypothesis can also be stated in a *null* form: *Treatment A and treatment B are equally effective in reducing breathlessness*.

Although the purpose and work of the study is the same whichever form is used, if treatment A *is* shown to be more efficacious, in the first example the hypothesis will be supported, in the second it will be rejected.

In more descriptive studies, for example investigating patient's opinions about their treatment, the use of stated hypotheses may not be appropriate and, therefore, the list of objectives will lead the work. Practical and specific objectives used as a check list throughout the study help to avoid later problems.

DECIDING ON THE APPROPRIATE RESEARCH DESIGN

The design selected decides the methods to be used to answer the research question and fulfil the study objectives. It provides a plan of action, a blueprint to use during the work of the study, and will decide the format of the procedures to be followed.

Physiotherapists may encounter a number of problems because research methodologies in physiotherapy are not long established or well developed. Applied research into clinical practice can rarely use the methods of the physical sciences, as human subjects are not as amenable to investigation as are cells or microorganisms. Most designs used at present are adapted from other disciplines, for example the clinical trial from medicine, and surveys and single case study design from the social sciences. Designs are not intrinsically good or bad; each has its strengths and weaknesses and the design should be selected on the basis of its appropriateness to answer the research question. For example, if the effects of two methods of treatment are to be compared the design will probably be a clinical trial, whereas if information about patients' attitudes to hospitalization is needed a survey would be the design of choice. Five designs which have been used in physiotherapy are described here in more detail.

Observation and description

Observation and description are key methods of research on their own and are often undertaken as a first stage before later experimental work. Studies may use either method, but each will involve elements of the other; observations must be noted down and described, and observation plays a part in many descriptive studies.

Observational studies

The background knowledge and experience of the observer influences what is observed; for example a specialized respiratory physiotherapist will pick up signs of patient distress or dysfunction that might easily be missed by a therapist not experienced in respiratory care. Therefore, in an investigation using observation as the main method, exactly what has to be observed must be stated very clearly and specifically. For example, if an observation study was undertaken of nursing care on a ward, the behaviour to be observed would be listed and then the frequency of occurrence noted during a specified time period; this might for example be noting the number of times during a 3 hour shift that each nurse checked equipment or spoke to a patient.

Strengths
- Actually observing real-life behaviour provides direct information about the situation
- Provides an excellent starting point for further research
- Encourages accurate monitoring.

Weaknesses
- Observing someone may, of itself, make them change their behaviour
- Time consuming.

Descriptive studies

On their own, descriptive studies provide an essential stage in the development of a professional knowledge base and may be a necessary first stage before starting a study to evaluate treatment effects. Rigorous and systematic planning and clear objectives are needed.

Strengths
- Provides useful insights into a procedure, behaviour or service
- Provides a sound basis for further study.

Weaknesses
- Descriptive studies provide information about *how* things are, but do not *explain* why they are so.

Having said this, many descriptive studies have altered practice by providing facts and figures about service provision in a particular area.

Clinical trials

Clinical trials are based on the classical experimental medical model originally developed to test the effectiveness of new drugs or to compare the effectiveness of two different types of medication. All aspects of the study must be carefully controlled and bias eliminated wherever possible. It is usual to compare two groups of patients receiving different treatments or one group receiving either no treatment or a placebo—called the 'control group'—while the other receives the new treatment under investigation. For physiotherapy, the comparative clinical trial may often be more appropriate, as withholding treatment from the control group can present ethical problems, and placebo physiotherapy treatments are difficult to devise.

Patients in a clinical trial must be selected on the basis of clear criteria both for *inclusion* (who comes into the study) and *exclusion* (who is not allowed to). The patient group for the study must be homogenous, that is all patients must be as similar as possible in all respects so that differences do not bias the results. For example, if patients are all at very different stages of their disease, the severity of the disease may be the most important factor in deciding the outcome of treatment. Other things which must be controlled for include past history, other intercurrent illnesses and age. When a homogenous group has been identified they must be allocated to the different treatment groups by a random procedure to ensure there is no bias in the allocation; for example the researcher might be tempted to allocate people who were likely to do better to the active treatment group. The principle here is that each patient must have an equal chance of being allocated to either treatment group. There are a number of random allocation procedures and the reader is referred to the Further Reading section at the end of this chapter for books which provide more details.

One way of ensuring that patient differences are controlled for is to use each patient as their own control. Measurements are taken on all patients both before and after treatment which helps to control for inter-patient variability, but because of the differences in the before treatment measurements of each patient, group comparisons are more complex.

Strengths
- A rigorous method for providing sound evidence of the effectiveness of different treatments
- If clear results are obtained they have immediate practical implications
- Clinical trials are widely accepted by funding bodies as an acceptable design.

Weaknesses
- Large numbers of subjects are needed
- Double blind conditions are rarely possible in cardiopulmonary physiotherapy, that is a trial where neither patient nor physiotherapist know which patients are receiving which treatment
- Ensuring that patients in control and treatment groups are matched for all important variables is often difficult
- Standardized treatments are often used in clinical trials, yet physiotherapy is rarely standard, each treatment being based on an initial assessment of the individual patient and changing as the patient's condition changes.

Single case study designs

There are a number of variations of this design, the two main ones are multiple phase and multiple baseline. In the multiple phase, known as 'ABAB' or 'reversal' design, the baseline phase A is followed by a treatment phase B, withdrawal of treatment for another baseline A and a final treatment phase B. The withdrawal and reinstatement of treatment enables effects on baseline measurements to be assessed.

In multiple baseline designs treatment is not withdrawn, the baseline is established, and after introduction of the treatments monitoring of key variables continues. If this design is used with a number of subjects and change occurs after the introduction of the treatment in all of them, this suggests the treatment is causing the effect. However, this situation does not establish a causal relationship in the same way as it does in a carefully controlled clinical trial.

Strengths
- Easy to undertake alongside clinical practice
- Design allows for changes to be made and monitored
- Very good in the early stages of investigation.
- Useful for generating hypotheses to be tested in a further study
- Simple descriptive analysis is often all that is required to present results clearly.

Weaknesses
- Often confused with a case report in which the treatment and management of an individual patient with an interesting condition is described but which is not research based
- Not possible to generalize findings to a wider population as conditions for statistical generalization are not present—a small number of patients is unlikely to be representative of most patients with a certain condition
- Baseline measurements need to be established over a period of time before the interventions start, but in many cardiopulmonary conditions the patient's symptoms are not stable for a long enough period of time to establish a stable baseline.

Censuses and surveys

These designs are used to obtain information from populations or samples of populations. Epidemiologists use them to obtain information about disease patterns and public health issues, sociologists investigate social and demographic issues, and they are widely used to explore people's opinions and attitudes.

The term 'population' in research usually refers to the group of interest, for example the study population could be all out-patients with a specific condition who visited hospital X during the previous 12 months. In a different type of study the purpose might be to investigate opinions

of the whole physiotherapy profession; here a subsample is needed, this can be done by choosing for example a 10% or 20% sample selected from the professional register. If equal age representation in the sample is required, a stratified sample can be collected, obtaining a given number from each age band. Information for surveys is usually collected using a questionnaire.

Questionnaires

Many people think designing a questionnaire is a simple, straightforward task, but to obtain clear and useful information a lot of detailed preparation is required.

Questions

Some of the common problems encountered in formulating questions are given by Partridge and Barnitt (1986) and are listed below.

1. Using *complex language*—patients might not be familiar with terms such as 'thoracic expansion' or 'decreased exercise tolerance'.

2. *Embarrassing and personal topics*—different topics are embarrassing for different people; age, finance, medical and sexual matters may all seem too personal, and potentially sensitive topics need extra care.

3. It is easy to *presume knowledge or opinions* when the subject has none. For example, asking 'What is your opinion about community physiotherapy services?' when a patient may have had no experience of them.

4. *Leading questions* introduce bias, for example 'Do you agree that respiratory physiotherapy is important for people with cystic fibrosis?'

5. *Hypothetical questions*—for example 'Do you think your chest problems would be better if you lived in a bungalow?'

6. *Questions involving memory*—the question 'How often have you visited your doctor in the past year?' is unlikely to produce an accurate answer. If the time period is shortened, memory is likely to be more accurate.

7. *The layout of the questionnaire* can cause

problems. It should be clear and user-friendly, and the sequence of questions should have a logical order.

A number of factors will encourage a high response rate, that is the proportion of people who are asked to complete the questionnaire who actually do so. They include convincing would-be respondents that the work is important and that their contribution is valued, explanatory letters addressed wherever possible to individuals by name, and giving a definite return-by date. Avoiding problems raised in points 1–7 above also contributes to ease of completion of the questionnaire.

To avoid problems of analysis of the data, consideration should be given at an early stage as to how the information from the questionnaire is to be presented in the final report and how the data are to be used to fulfil the purpose of the study.

OBTAINING RESEARCH GRANTS

Small projects undertaken alongside clinical practice may not require extra funding, but most research needs some financial support. Each funding body will have different interests, and chances of success can be increased by careful and detailed preparation of the protocol and targeting a funding source that is likely to be interested in the work. Clearly, trusts such as the Cystic Fibrosis Trust have very specific interests, but for others it may be less clear. Written information should be obtained from the funding body about their interests to help target the proposal correctly. First timers need advice from experienced researchers and perusing a successful proposal often helps.

Calnan (1976) listed five points referees ask themselves and these are still relevant:

1. *Is it important?* This would relate to the aims and purpose of the funding body.
2. *Can it be done?* Does the proposal give clear information about the feasibility of the study?
3. *Is the investigator competent to carry out the work?* If the proposer does not have the necessary research track record, it is wise to work with others with appropriate experience and to have their names on the proposal.

4. *Can it be done within the specified time?* Always allow generous estimates, as conditions may change and extra time is often needed.
5. *Are the costs realistic?* Help is usually needed to estimate all costs involved. Common problems are underestimating both the time and costs needed. The list below gives items that often need to be included:

- Salaries of all research staff to be employed with additional costs such as National Insurance and superannuation
- Secretarial help which can be estimated on an hourly or weekly basis
- Equipment which could include measuring devices and computers
- Recurrent expenses such as telephone and postage, stationery, photocopying and computer costs.

WRITING THE RESEARCH PROPOSAL

Clear thinking and time are essential in preparing the proposal or protocol. It provides the plan to follow throughout the project and avoids the problem of 'interesting' additions once the project has started. The proposal must be written in clear English without the use of professional jargon so that it is comprehensible to non-specialists. Headings given by funding bodies usually include the following:

Title

The title needs to be clear and succinct. Time is well spent on getting a good title as it is the first thing anyone sees.

Background

This sets the scene for the whole project and should be a logical and imaginative introduction to the subject with reference to major work in the area, clearly identifying a gap in knowledge that the project will fill. It is usual to spell out the research questions that are being asked and if a clinical trial, the hypothesis to be tested.

Plan of investigation

This section needs to be explicit. It should give sufficient detail to enable the reader to understand what is to be done and demonstrate the researcher's familiarity with the chosen method. If there are going to be particular problems, details of how they are to be overcome are needed.

Items to be mentioned include the overall design, the recruitment of subjects and criteria for their selection, treatments to be given and procedures to be followed. Details of where the study will be undertaken and permissions obtained from other health professionals will also be needed.

ETHICAL COMMITTEES

Research projects often involve ethical issues and most proposals have to be approved by a hospital ethical committee. Problems that arise are often to do with withholding treatment from control group subjects and concern about confidentiality and procedures in the design of the study. Ethical committees meet infrequently and an early application is advisable. Before any patient is recruited into the study they must give *informed consent*. It is the duty of the researcher to provide detailed information about the study to the patient, spelling out exactly what it will entail and the time involved. Without this information the patient cannot give informed consent and this can cause ethical problems.

ASSESSMENT AND MEASUREMENT OF STUDY VARIABLES

Assessment is a clinical skill which is usually highly developed in physiotherapists, and based on their knowledge and experience. Assessment and measurement for research projects is somewhat different and all measurements must be demonstrably objective, that is free from influence or bias. Clinical judgements, though essential in clinical practice, cannot be used as objective measurements in research. If the purpose is to evaluate the outcome of a treatment or procedure,

the value of the results depends critically on the soundness of the measures used and it is essential to differentiate between measurements of objective phenomena such as blood gases or sputum, and subjective phenomena such as opinions, attitudes and sensations. Each is equally valid as data, but in the first instance objective tests can be used, whereas patient reports and rating scales are more appropriate for the second.

There are two main interrelated problem areas in measurement in research; the first relates to selection of measures, the second to their reliability and validity for the study purpose.

Selection of variables to be measured

'Variable' is the term used in experimental investigations for the properties that are being studied and are likely to vary. Common examples are things like sex, height, sputum and blood gases: some variables are mutually exclusive, for example either male *or* female; most others, such as height, occur on a continuum.

Some variables can be measured directly, for example weight or forced vital capacity, but others cannot because they relate to subjective experience such as pain or breathlessness. Many laboratory tests and complex procedures can provide objective results, but sophisticated assessment procedures are not intrinsically better than simple measures, the key issue is their appropriateness for the purpose of the study and medical tests may not be appropriate to assess the outcomes of physiotherapy. The reliability and validity of the scales used are key issues in measurement.

Reliability

'Reliability' refers to three aspects of a test procedure:

- Do different therapists using the test to measure the same variable get similar results?
- Does the same therapist using the test on different occasions on the same person obtain similar scores?
- On retesting after an interval when nothing has changed, are similar scores obtained?

The extent of reliability of a test is calculated by

obtaining the correlation between sets of scores. A score of 1.0 represents perfect agreement and this rarely occurs. Other correlations are all less than one; the nearer to 1.0 the more reliable the measure (for example, 0.9 represents good correlation, 0.4 very little). When measuring the effects of different treatments it is important that the person undertaking the measurements is not involved in the treatments and does not know the group allocation of the patient.

Validity

Validity is a more complex concept and there are a number of ways of considering it. If a scale has *face validity* it means that, on the face of it, it seems correct for its stated purpose. *Construct validity* refers to the central concept being measured. A concept such as breathlessness has to be operationalized so that it can be measured, but the relationship between the measure used and the construct must be clear. For example, walking makes breathlessness worse in patients with chronic airflow limitation and, therefore, walking tests do provide a valid measure of breathlessness as the link between them has been demonstrated. *Criterion validity* is concerned with how the test under consideration compares with others measuring similar concepts. For example, the validity of a new test of pain severity could be examined by comparing scores on the new scale with those of an established test such as a visual analogue scale.

Scales of measurement

Two main types of scale are used in physiotherapy studies: *ratio* scales which are the classic scales of the physical sciences (time, mass and length); and *ordinal* scales which provide a means of rank ordering data, however the numbers cannot be added and multiplied as with ratio scales. Different kinds of statistical tests are used with different scales, parametric tests such as Student's *t*-test with ratio scales and non-parametric tests such as the chi-squared test with ordinal scales. The reader is referred to books listed in the Further Reading section at the end of this chapter which deal with this topic in more depth.

Physiotherapists are often concerned directly with the patient's symptoms, and two problems of measurement that commonly occur are discussed in more depth. Both breathlessness and pain are perceived sensations, i.e. they are subjective experiences that cannot be accessed directly. Holland (1991) comments that the true nature of breathlessness is appreciated only by the person himself.

For both breathlessness and pain, physiological and pathological mechanisms are easier to monitor but do not necessarily reflect the variable of interest, i.e. the patient's breathlessness or the pain.

Breathlessness. Details are given of two different tests used in clinical practice to measure different aspects of breathlessness.

1. *The baseline dyspnoea index* (Mahler et al 1984) uses three categories:

- functional improvement
- magnitude of task
- magnitude of effort.

Five grades are provided for scaling within each category.

2. *The oxygen cost diagram* (McGavin et al 1978) is a visual analogue scale of a 100 mm line with descriptive phrases at points which correspond to oxygen requirements of different activities.

Two different methods are used to operationalize the concept of breathlessness in these examples.

Before using any test the literature must be checked to find whether it is valid for the required purpose and whether there is evidence for its reliability in clinical use with similar patients. It may be necessary to retest for reliability in use with a new study population.

Pain. Many scales used to measure pain assume that it is a unidimensional sensation varying only in intensity, yet the pain experience is clearly multidimensional. Melzack (1975) developed the McGill pain questionnaire which addresses sensory, affective and evaluative aspects: what the pain feels like, how it affects mood and an evaluation of its severity. There are other aspects which are part of the pain experience, for example disruption of sleep, diurnal patterns, and any factors which increase or diminish pain. Present pain is often assessed and this may be appropriate if pain is unremitting. However, if it is intermittent or variable in any way it may be more useful to ask about pain over a specified period, for example 24 hours, or to ask a patient to complete a diary over a week or more.

As with breathlessness, there is not always a direct relationship between severity of injury or disease and reports of pain. Many different factors have been shown to influence perception of pain, including fear, anxiety, previous experiences and individual pain thresholds; cultural factors may also alter the expression of pain.

Tests include visual analogue scales. Huskisson (1974) used a 10 cm line with anchor points of 'no pain' and 'worst pain imaginable'. This provides a rough guide to intensity and is often used to assess present pain in clinical practice, but its weakness lies in the fact that someone could use the top of the scale one day, yet on the next day pain might exceed that of the first occasion. Some patients find it difficult to relate their pain to a 10 cm line. Verbal rating scales can overcome the problem to some extent as they provide an ordinal scale of verbal descriptors appropriate for the particular condition under investigation.

The McGill pain questionnaire (Melzack 1975) provides a comprehensive pain picture, but may be too time consuming for general use in clinical practice.

ORGANIZATION OF FIELDWORK

One of the first tasks of organization is to ensure that everyone who may be involved in the study is contacted and given information about the purpose of the study and how it may affect them; these are likely to be other therapists, nursing staff and doctors, but administrators, ambulance staff and trade union representatives may also need to be included. Permission may also be required from the patient's own doctor. If someone is left out they may hinder the smooth running of the study at a later stage.

Like so many other aspects of research, planning the fieldwork takes much longer than

might have been expected; again meticulous attention to detail avoids problems.

Considering data collection

The actual work of data collection needs to be planned with great care. Forms for collecting data will always be needed and questionnaires are often used on their own or as a part of the data collection. Whatever the type of study, some information will need to be recorded and clear forms will be necessary. A list of the information required should always precede arranging the layout of the forms.

Number of subjects in the study

'How many subjects do I need?' is a very common question asked by researchers, but unfortunately it is only possible to answer in relation to a specific project when the research questions, the design of the study, and measurements to be used have been decided. Consultation with a statistician is necessary about numbers of subjects required in relation to analysis at an early stage.

Availability of subjects

It is a sad fact well recognized by researchers that the minute you start to study a particular condition patients with that condition become scarce. There is always a dilemma between using one's own hospital where everything is familiar or using a number of hospitals. However, although multi-centre studies provide larger numbers of subjects, they also introduce a range of different problems of administration and control. When the number of subjects available over a given period has been carefully worked out, this should be halved as patients are inconsiderate enough to move hospital, acquire other illnesses and even die during the study period. Figures about the availability of subjects must be checked against records, as estimates are notoriously unreliable.

PILOT WORK

This work may be undertaken in stages, with development of methods of measures and trying out of procedures before the pilot study. This is the trial run, everything is done as in the main study with a small sample of subjects. Problems usually arise if this stage is missed. Ironing out wrinkles before the main study ensures a sounder project.

MAIN STUDY

If all preparatory work has been undertaken diligently, this stage should be more straightforward and easier to follow through. However, obstacles may occur and some delays must be expected as research always takes much longer than estimated.

ANALYSIS OF DATA COLLECTED

Good planning of analysis at an early stage should help to avoid problems. A coding frame must be prepared which will detail every piece of information collected and needed for the analysis. In a small study analyses can be undertaken by hand and information displayed in the form of graphs, pie charts, histograms and tables. In a larger study or if complex statistical tests are to be used, using a computer minimizes problems.

It is wise to get a feel for the data by examining raw material before subjecting it to analysis. Analysis should be undertaken to demonstrate the extent to which the purpose of the study has been fulfilled. Statistical tests will provide answers about statistical significance, but clinical judgement will decide whether the results are clinically significant, i.e. will it make a real-life difference—the two are not always the same.

WRITING THE REPORTS AND PRESENTING THE RESULTS

It is very important to write up the completed project and to get it published. Help from experienced authors is useful in the beginning, and it is worth studying the style of a journal before sending in a paper. Expect to have it returned with comments which can be used to improve it before resubmission to the same journal or elsewhere. If the work is to be of value the results must be disseminated as widely as possible so that they may be implemented in practice. It may be a good idea to present papers at conferences of a number of different disciplines, for example medical and nursing conferences as well as physiotherapy meetings.

CONCLUSION

In a chapter of this length it is only possible to provide a brief introduction to some of the pitfalls and problems experienced by clinicians undertaking applied research and to identify underlying principles. Further texts are listed below and they will provide more in depth information on different aspects of research.

REFERENCES

Buzan T 1989 Use your head. BBC Enterprises, London
Calnan J 1976 One way to do research. Heinemann, London
COED 1976 Concise Oxford English dictionary, 6th edn. Oxford University Press, London
Holland L 1991 Breathlessness. In: Pryor JA (ed) Respiratory care. Churchill Livingstone, Edinburgh, ch 1, p 5–26
Hudson L 1966 Contrary imaginations. Penguin, Ho
Huskisson E C 1974 Measurement of pain. Lancet ii: 1127–1131
McGavin C R, Artvinli M, Naoe H et al 1978 Dyspnoea, disability, and distance walked: comparison of estimates of exercise performance in respiratory disease. British Medical Journal 2: 241–243
Mahler D A, Weinberg D H, Wells C K, Feinstein A R 1984 The measurement of dyspnoea contents, interobserver agreement and physiologic correlates of two new clinical indexes. Chest 85: 751–758
Melzack R 1975 The McGill Pain Questionnaire—major properties and scoring methods. Pain 1: 277–299
Partridge C J, Barnitt R E 1986 Research guidelines. A handbook for therapists. Heinemann, London

FURTHER READING

Bryman A 1988 Quantity and quality in social research. Contemporary Social Research 18. Unwin Hyman, London

Calnan J 1984 Coping with research. A complete guide for beginners. Heinemann, London

Holsti O R 1974 Content analysis for the social sciences and humanities. Addison Wesley, Massachusetts

McDowell I, Newell C 1987 Measuring health. A guide to rating scales and questionnaires. Oxford University Press, London

Moses C A, Kalton G 1971 Survey methods in social investigation. Gower, Aldershot

Offenbacher K 1986 Evaluating social change. Williams and Wilkins, Baltimore

Robson C 1974 Experimental design and statistics in psychology. Penguin Education, Harmondsworth

Stacey M 1977 Methods of social research. Pergamon Press, Oxford

Yin R K 1990 Case study research. Design and methods. Sage Publications, London

11. Physiotherapy problems and their management

Jackie Anderson   Susan C. Jenkins

This section identifies the problems and potential problems encountered by physiotherapists in patients with respiratory and cardiac dysfunction. Each problem is introduced and subdivided into categories according to the causative factors. This is followed by a brief discussion of the underlying pathophysiology, interpretation of clinical findings and the medical management of the problem. The role of the physiotherapist in the management of the patient is then discussed.

It is important for the physiotherapist to be aware of problems which may develop in a patient should preventive measures not be undertaken. The problem orientated approach to treatment helps in the identification of existing patient problems, but it is also essential to recognize potential patient problems.

A high risk surgical patient (p. 240) may develop problems of excess bronchial secretions or reduced lung volume but, if preventive treatment is started, for example the active cycle of breathing techniques, during the at risk period, the problems may not develop. Advice given to a patient with asthma can minimize exacerbations of asthma, if the patient understands his condition and knows what steps to take in response to presenting signs and symptoms. In the patient with paralysis or abnormal muscle tone, contractures and joint injury can be prevented by positioning and passive or active assisted movements.

There are conditions for which physiotherapy is not indicated or may be detrimental. Some of these are mentioned, as the physiotherapist should be aware of the pathology and why she cannot offer assistance.

The key to effective physiotherapy management of a patient is accurate assessment which leads to the identification of the patient's problems. If the problem could respond to physiotherapy, treatment should be started. At a certain stage the natural rate of recovery cannot be augmented by the intervention of physiotherapy, and treatment should be discontinued. Patients should be encouraged to take responsibility for their own treatment, and those with chronic physiotherapy problems can usually be taught self-management.

The problems to be discussed are:

- Reduced lung volume
- Breathlessness and decreased exercise tolerance
- Excess bronchial secretions
- Pain.

PROBLEM 1: REDUCED LUNG VOLUME

A reduction in lung volume occurs in a wide variety of conditions and is commonly encountered by the physiotherapist. Sometimes the cause is a disease process affecting the lung parenchyma, but in many situations decreased lung volume arises from processes affecting other structures such as the respiratory muscles or the pleura. The respiratory physiotherapist does not always have a role to play in the management of the problem, for example when the cause of the decrease in lung volume is ascites or pregnancy unassociated with respiratory disease.

A reduction in lung volume may be the result of general anaesthesia and surgery, collapse (atelectasis), abdominal distension, excess fluid and/or air in the pleural space, excess fluid in the extravascular spaces and tissues of the lung, fibrotic lung conditions or abnormalities of the respiratory muscles.

General anaesthesia and surgery

The precise mechanism responsible for the reduced lung volume varies between patients and with different types of surgery. The primary cause may be mucus plugging, progressive regional hypoventilation or intraoperative compression of lung tissue.

The general anaesthetic. An average reduction in fuctional residual capacity (FRC) of 0.5 L or 18% accompanies general anaesthesia. This occurs irrespective of whether the patient is paralysed or breathing spontaneously, and the exact cause is still not known (Rehder & Southorn 1985). Bendixen et al. (1964) proposed that the fall in FRC was due to progressive regional collapse caused by the absence of periodic deep breaths. Respiratory depression is a consequence of general anaesthesia and contributes to the reduction in lung volume (Jones 1987).

Intermittent positive pressure ventilation (IPPV) may accompany or follow surgery. During IPPV the mechanical properties of the lung and chest wall are altered and this leads to changes in the distribution of ventilation (Grimby et al 1975). The FRC is decreased, lung compliance is reduced and gas is preferentially delivered to the more compliant, non-dependent regions of the lung. This produces collapse in dependent portions of the lung. The efficiency of collateral ventilation is substantially reduced at low lung volumes compounding the tendency for hypoventilation of dependent lung regions (Terry et al 1978).

The operation. The site of the operation is the most important factor in determining the extent of lung function abnormalities (Figs 11.1 to 11.3). Incisions to the upper abdomen or thorax significantly alter abdominal and/or chest wall mechanics, and surgery in the vicinity of the diaphragm has been shown to interfere with its contractile properties (Ford et al 1983, Simonneau et al 1983).

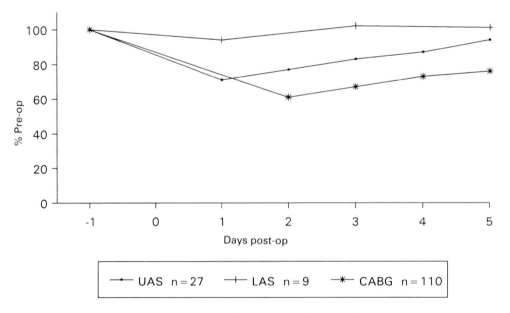

Fig. 11.1 Functional residual capacity (FRC) measured before and after operation. Postoperative values are expressed as a percentage of the preoperative result, taking the preoperative value as 100%. Values are means. UAS, upper abdominal surgery (predominantly cholecystectomy via a right paramedian incision) (Meyers et al 1974). LAS, lower abdominal surgery (Ali et al 1974). CABG, coronary artery bypass graft surgery via median sternotomy (Jenkins et al 1988b). n, Number of patients.

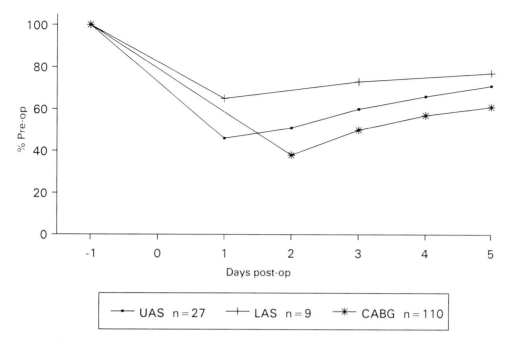

Fig. 11.2 Vital capacity (VC) measured before and after operation. Postoperative values are expressed as a percentage of the preoperative result, taking the preoperative value as 100%. Values are means. UAS, upper abdominal surgery (predominantly cholecystectomy via a right paramedian incision) (Meyers et al 1974). LAS, lower abdominal surgery (Ali et al 1974). CABG, coronary artery bypass graft surgery via median sternotomy (Jenkins et al 1988b). n, Number of patients.

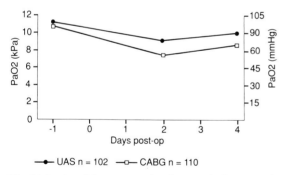

Fig. 11.3 Arterial oxygen tension (mean value) measured before and after operation with the patient breathing room air. UAS, upper abdominal surgery (cholecystectomy) (Morran et al 1983). CABG, coronary artery bypass graft surgery via median sternotomy (Jenkins et al 1988b). n, Number of patients.

The postoperative period. Following surgery several factors may be involved in precipitating and maintaining airway closure (Johnson & Pierson 1986). Mucus transport is impaired and this may lead to retention of secretions, localized airways obstruction and collapse of lung tissue distal to obstructed airways. The rate of the collapse is increased when oxygen is breathed (Dale & Rahn 1952) and the composition of surfactant is adversely affected by high concentrations of inspired oxygen (Johnson & Pierson 1986).

The forces acting to expand the lung may be reduced because of pleural space encroachment by gas or fluid and abdominal distension from any cause will impair diaphragm function.

In the early postoperative period patients are relatively immobile and FRC is reduced by 25–30% in the supine and slumped positions compared with the erect position (Blair & Hickam 1955, Jenkins et al 1988a). This is largely due to changes in the effects of gravity on the abdomen and thorax. In contrast, posture has little effect on closing volume (CV); therefore in positions where FRC is reduced, gas exchange is further compromised by premature airway closure (Leblanc et al 1970, Craig et al 1971). Any factor that causes CV to increase (for example, increased age, cigarette smoking, airways obstruction) or FRC to

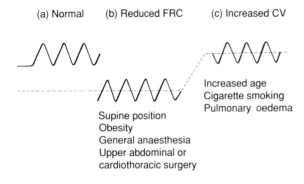

(a) Normal   (b) Reduced FRC   (c) Increased CV

Increased age
Cigarette smoking
Pulmonary oedema

Supine position
Obesity
General anaesthesia
Upper abdominal or
cardiothoracic surgery

In young healthy subjects FRC is greater than CV (a)
If FRC falls (b) or CV rises (c), small airway closure may
occur during normal breathing.

Fig. 11.4   Relationship between closing volume (CV) and
functional residual capacity (FRC). (Adapted from Craig D B,
Anesthesia and Analgesia 1981 60: 46–52 with permission.)

decrease (for example, obesity) enhances the
tendency for airway closure (Fig. 11.4).

The typical breathing pattern of a patient who
has recently undergone surgery to the upper
abdomen or thorax is one of small tidal volume,
increased rate, and absence of periodic deep
breaths (sighs) (Zikria et al 1974). This is the
least painful and most energy efficient pattern.
The tendency to breathe shallowly is
compounded by the treatment of pain with
narcotic analgesics (Egbert & Bendixen 1964).
Tachycardia and mild fever often accompany
collapse. Absence of periodic deep breaths
produces alveolar closure, reduces surfactant
activity and decreases lung compliance (Ferris &
Pollard 1960, Johnson & Pierson 1986).

Postoperative lung function

The arterial oxygen tension (PaO_2) is decreased
and the alveolar–arterial oxygen gradient
(A–aPO_2) increased compared with preoperative
values. The fall in PaO_2 is due to an increase in
the amount of deoxygenated blood reaching the
systemic circulation because of increased ventila-
tion/perfusion ($\dot{V}/\dot{Q}$) mismatching and intrapulmonary shunting. Although compensatory
hypoxic pulmonary vasoconstriction occurs in the
regions of lung collapse, this is insufficient to

prevent the fall in PaO_2. A rise in arterial carbon
dioxide tension ($PaCO_2$) is unusual unless
marked respiratory depression occurs (for
example, following high doses of narcotics). In the
absence of preoperative arterial blood gas results,
a knowledge of the magnitude of the decline in
PaO_2 with age is essential to judge the importance
of hypoxaemia in the postoperative patient.

Average values for PaO_2 range from 11.2 to
13.9 kPa (84–104 mmHg) in individuals aged 25
years and from 9.5 to 12.1 kPa (71–91 mmHg)
for those aged 65 years (Nunn 1987).

The changes in lung function are most severe
within the first 24–72 hours are followed by a
gradual return to preoperative levels. This may
take up to 7 days after upper abdominal surgery
(UAS) and several weeks after cardiac surgery
(Meyers et al 1975, Morran et al 1983, Jenkins et
al 1988b, Locke et al 1990). This is the normal
sequence of events; however, up to 30% of
patients who undergo UAS and around 10% of
patients who have cardiac surgery will develop a
chest infection (these figures assume that preoperative lung function is within the normal range)
(Ali et al 1974, Garibaldi et al 1981, Jenkins et al
1990). In these patients increasing respiratory
distress is accompanied by progressive hypoxia,
tachycardia, pyrexia and a failure of FRC to
increase. The greatest risk of chest infection is in
cigarette smokers, especially if lung function tests
show severe airflow obstruction, and in malnourished patients (Morran et al 1983, Windsor & Hill
1988, Jenkins et al 1990). The elderly, the obese
and those who undergo emergency procedures are
also at greater risk.

Although the changes in lung function are
minimal after operations on the lower abdomen or
the extremities, complications may still occur in
high risk patients.

Management

The postoperative management includes observation of the respiratory and cardiovascular systems
and adequate analgesia. Different types of surgery
require additional specific management, for
example intravenous fluids, inotropic drugs, and
mechanical ventilation. Effective communication
between doctors, nurses, physiotherapists and

other members of the multidisciplinary team is essential if the patient is to receive optimal care.

Physiotherapy problems are most likely to develop in patients in whom the risk of chest infection is greatest. The physiotherapist should identify these patients and, if possible, assess them preoperatively. If the patient is aware of the possibility of postoperative respiratory problems, he is more likely to cooperate with early ambulation which should help to prevent these problems. Preoperative instruction in the active cycle of breathing techniques and wound support may be indicated.

Adequate postoperative analgesia is essential for effective pain control and will further encourage ambulation and cooperation with breathing exercises.

The easiest method of increasing functional residual capacity and preventing lung collapse is appropriate positioning and early ambulation (Jenkins et al 1988a). Most patients can sit out of bed the day after surgery (Fig. 11.5a). If they cannot sit in a chair, they should be encouraged to either sit upright in bed or to adopt a side lying position, but they should not be in a slumped sitting position (Fig. 11.5b). Positioning can also be used to alter ventilation and perfusion. In the adult, both ventilation and perfusion are preferentially distributed to the dependent parts of the lung (West 1992).

To assist in the reinflation of any collapsed areas of lung tissue and to aid the clearance of excess bronchial secretions the patient can be encouraged to use the active cycle of breathing techniques. The thoracic expansion exercises are usually performed with a 3 second 'hold' at the end of inspiration. An inspiratory 'sniff' is sometimes of additional benefit.

Before, during and after the treatment session the physiotherapist must assess and reassess the patient, and evaluate the techniques used. If the problem is resolving the treatment method should be continued, but if there is no change different techniques should be considered.

Intervention by the physiotherapist should be discontinued when the patient is effectively managing his own chest. The physiotherapist must ask herself: Is further intervention necessary if the patient is independently ambulant, huffing

and coughing effectively and on auscultation the breath sounds are improving? If the patient is performing his own breathing exercises effectively, is it necessary to continue chest physiotherapy?

If the patient has reduced breath sounds despite effective breathing techniques, a mechanical adjunct should be considered, for example periodic continuous positive airway pressure (Bourn & Jenkins 1992). As the patient improves, the mechanical adjunct can be withdrawn and the breathing exercises continued for as long as necessary.

The treatment outcome can be monitored by improvements in auscultatory findings and, if available, arterial oxygen saturation or arterial blood gases and the chest radiograph.

Collapse (atelectasis)

An obvious cause of a reduction in lung volumes is collapse or atelectasis of lung tissue. Lobar or whole lung collapse may arise from a variety of causes, for example a bronchus may be blocked by secretions or an inhaled foreign body. Another cause is an enlarged lymph node causing local compression of a bronchus. Several factors predispose to lobar collapse in the postoperative patient. These include mucus plugging, progressive regional hypoventilation and intraoperative compression of lung tissue.

Symptoms resulting from acute lobar collapse depend on the underlying respiratory impairment, the extent of the collapse and the abruptness of onset. A slowly developing segmental or lobar collapse may produce few symptoms if the patient has otherwise normal lungs. If the same degree of collapse was to occur suddenly in a patient with chronic lung disease, severe respiratory distress may develop.

The three important consequences of acute lobar collapse are (Marini 1984):

1. Increased work of breathing — lung compliance is decreased when a sufficiently large region of lung collapses, and consequently the work of breathing is increased.

2. Hypoxaemia — the extent of radiological collapse does not predict the degree of

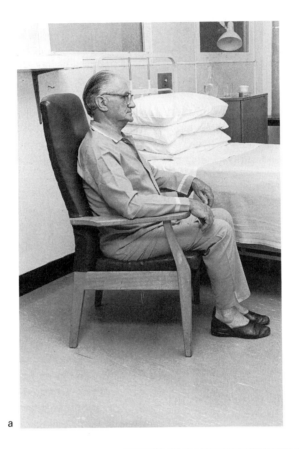

a

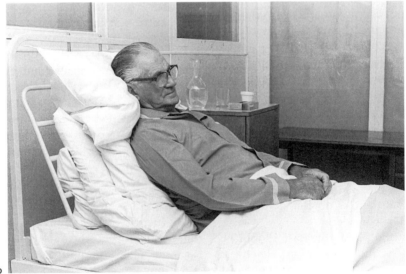

b

Fig. 11.5   Positioning. (a) Sitting upright. (b) slumped position (With permission of the Royal Brompton Hospital.)

hypoxaemia. This is because hypoxic vasocon-striction occurs in the region of collapse and limits the severity of the hypoxaemia (Benumof 1979). The extent to which this happens is variable and is influenced by the rate at which the collapse occurs. Profound desaturation is most likely when collapse occurs suddenly because the full compensatory effect of hypoxic vasoconstriction does not have time to develop (Marini 1984).

3. Predisposition to infection — fever in association with lobar collapse tends to be due to infection developing in stagnant secretions. This is not uncommon in the postoperative patient.

Clinical signs of lobar collapse include absent, diminished or bronchial breath sounds on auscultation, decreased percussion note and characteristic radiological changes (p. 32).

A more diffuse form of collapse is seen in some postoperative patients, for example following cardiac surgery. Radiologically this appears as bilateral basal shadowing.

Management

If the collapse is due to retained secretions, antibiotics and oxygen therapy may be started. If the patient is very hypoxic or breathless continuous positive airway pressure (CPAP) may be indicated (Keilty & Bott 1992). If the problem is caused by obstruction from a tumour, surgery, chemotherapy, radiotherapy or laser treatment may be considered.

If a lobar or whole lung collapse occurs suddenly in a postoperative patient, immediate and effective physiotherapy is indicated. The combination of the active cycle of breathing techniques and a mechanical adjunct, periodic continuous positive airway pressure (PCPAP), is likely to be the most effective and rapid method of reinflating lung tissue. If PCPAP is not available, intermittent positive pressure breathing (IPPB) or incentive spirometry should be considered. Gravity-assisted positions and high humidification may facilitate re-expansion. If mechanical adjuncts are not available, the active cycle of breathing techniques alone in gravity-assisted positions can be used, but the response is likely to be slower.

The physiotherapist's goal should be an immediate response to treatment as demonstrated by increased breath sounds, an improvement in arterial oxygen saturation and chest radiograph, and a pyrexia, if present, should settle.

Some medical chest patients present with a long standing lobar collapse. This should respond to the active cycle of breathing techniques and either PCPAP or IPPB and high humidification, over a period of time.

The diffuse form of postoperative collapse will not respond quickly to treatment, but the active cycle of breathing techniques and ambulation are likely to produce the optimal outcome.

Abdominal distension

Irrespective of the underlying cause, abdominal distension produces a reduction in FRC.

Obesity. This represents a major problem in developed countries. In the UK the prevalence of obesity in adult males and females is 40% and 32% respectively (Garrow 1988). Even in subjects who are only mildly obese the FRC, expiratory reserve volume (ERV) and PaO_2 are reduced and the $A-aPO_2$ is increased compared with normal weight subjects (Fig. 11.6). These changes may be reversed with substantial weight loss (Thomas et al 1989). A large proportion of excess body mass is commonly located around the chest and abdomen and this alters the mechanical properties of the chest wall and diaphragm. The compliance of the respiratory system, particularly that of the chest wall, is decreased and excursion of the diaphragm is restricted (Naimark & Cherniack 1960, Farebrother 1979). Breathing at low lung volumes causes closure of small airways in dependent lung regions. These regions are therefore relatively overperfused and an increase in $\dot{V}/\dot{Q}$ mismatching is responsible for the reduction in PaO_2 (Farebrother 1979). The majority of obese and grossly obese subjects maintain a normal $PaCO_2$.

The decrease in compliance of the respiratory system causes an increase in the work of breathing. Tidal volume is decreased and respiratory frequency is correspondingly increased (Farebrother 1979). Shortness of breath on exertion is a common symptom in many grossly obese subjects (Alexander et al 1962).

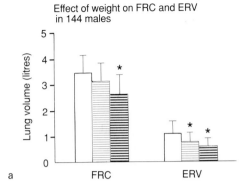

a

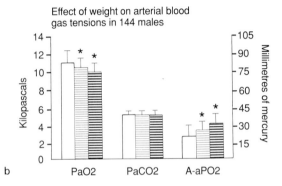

b

Fig. 11.6 **a** Effect of weight on functional residual capacity (FRC) and expiratory reserve volume (ERV) and **b** arterial blood gas tensions in 144 males grouped according to their body mass index (BMI = weight/height^2). Grade 0 obesity = ☐ — mean weight 70.8 kg, $n = 28$; grade I obesity = ▨, mean weight 81.1 kg, $n = 91$; grade II obesity = ■ — mean weight 90.1 kg, $n = 25$. PaO_2, arterial oxygen tension; $PaCO_2$, arterial carbon dioxide tension; A–aPO_2 alveolar–arterial oxygen difference measured with the patient breathing room air. Values are means and standard deviations (SDs). *$p<0.05$ compared with patients of normal weight (Jenkins & Moxham 1991).

Obesity hypoventilation syndrome. A minority (<10%) of severely obese subjects develop the obesity hypoventilation syndrome (OHS). The typical features are alveolar hypoventilation, hypercapnia, hypersomnolence, periodic breathing, cyanosis, polycythaemia and right sided heart failure. These subjects show a reduced ventilatory response to inhaled carbon dioxide.

Reduced lung volumes in conditions analogous to obesity. A reduction in FRC and ERV together with hypoxaemia occur in several conditions in which the causative mechanisms might be considered to be analogous to those occurring in obesity.

These include abdominal swelling due to ascites, peritoneal dialysis and the later stages of pregnancy (Abelmann et al 1954, Gee et al 1967, Norregaard et al 1989).

During the running-in phase of peritoneal dialysis there is a fall in PaO_2, the magnitude of which correlates with the volume of the dialysing fluid. The PaO_2 recovers during the running-out of the fluid (Goggin & Joekes 1971). These changes are thought to be due to the presence of dialysate in the abdomen causing a degree of basal collapse and, therefore, a change in the relationship of FRC and CV. Small pleural effusions occurring during peritoneal dialysis may contribute to the reduction in lung volume.

Management

Management of the underlying condition causing the abdominal distension may comprise dietary advice and an exercise programme for obese patients; diuretics or haemofiltration for patients with ascites. Positioning may improve the $\dot{V}/\dot{Q}$ ratio.

If there is a respiratory problem requiring physiotherapy while a patient is having peritoneal dialysis, treatment will be more effective if given during the running-out phase than when the abdomen is distended during the running-in phase.

Pleural disorders

Lung volumes will be decreased when the pleura is invaded by:

- fluid (effusion)
- pus (empyema thoracis)
- air (pneumothorax).

Pleural effusion

In health, around 600–800 ml of pleural fluid is formed each day. Transport of fluid in and out of the pleural space depends on the balance of hydrostatic and oncotic pressures in the capillary networks of the parietal and visceral pleurae. The oncotic pressures are equal, but the higher hydrostatic pressure in the parietal pleura results in fluid being transferred to the pleural space from which it is reabsorbed by the lower pressure visceral capillary network. Protein in the pleural space is principally removed by lymphatic drainage. The total volume of pleural fluid is less than 20 ml.

When the balance of formation and absorption is affected to favour formation, excess fluid accumulates in the pleural space. When the fluid accumulation is caused by systemic conditions which alter the hydrostatic pressures or oncotic pressures across the pleural membrane, the fluid (a transudate) has a low protein content and is clear or light yellow (straw coloured). Effusions may be bilateral or unilateral. Severe congestive cardiac failure is the most common cause of a bilateral effusion. Small pleural effusions often occur after cardiothoracic or abdominal surgery and during peritoneal dialysis.

Exudates arise as a result of increased capillary permeability. They have a higher protein content (>3 g/dl) and are dark yellow or orange in colour. The fluid is often slightly cloudy and may clot on standing. Effusions due to exudates are usually unilateral.

Pleural fluid is in a dynamic state with between 30% and 75% of the water being turned over each hour. The turn over of protein is much less rapid. Transudates therefore tend to clear quickly if the underlying cause is resolved or in response to diuretics. The higher protein content in pleural exudates means they clear more slowly.

The underlying cause, amount and rate of accumulation of the fluid determine the symptoms of an effusion. Unless accompanied by pleurisy, small pleural effusions are often symptomless, as also may be larger ones if they accumulate slowly. Breathlessness tends to occur when a large effusion accumulates rapidly and/or there is displacement of the mediastinal contents towards the unaffected side (mediastinal shift). The clinical features of mediastinal shift include cough, breathlessness, hoarseness and stridor. The trachea and apex beat are displaced towards the opposite side.

Effusions of at least 500 ml produce the characteristic signs of decreased movement on the affected side, stony dullness to percussion and absent breath sounds over the effusion. Clinical features may include fever and haemoptysis, depending on the nature of the underlying condition. The chest radiograph is diagnostic of the condition but not of the cause.

The accumulated fluid decreases the volume of the underlying lung and the weight of the fluid restricts movement of the diaphragm. A restrictive ventilatory defect occurs and when the effusion is large gas exchange is impaired (Yoo & Ting 1964). Removal of fluid relieves breathlessness, increases the PaO_2 and decreases the A–aPO_2 (Perpina et al 1983). The improvements in gas exchange probably result from improved $\dot{V}/\dot{Q}$ matching arising from expansion of previously compressed lung tissue. Occasionally there is a short lived decrease in PaO_2 following removal of a large amount of fluid. If this occurs the cause is worsening of the overall $\dot{V}/\dot{Q}$ matching in the underlying lung because of an uneven return of ventilation and perfusion towards normal.

Blood may accumulate in the pleural cavity. The most usual cause is a penetrating injury or blunt trauma to the chest. Haemothorax may complicate pneumothorax when rupture of vessels within pleural adhesions occurs.

Empyema thoracis

Three stages occur in the development of an empyema:

- dry pleurisy with pain and pleural rub
- serous exudate (parapneumonic effusion)
- empyema.

Empyema complicating a bacterial pneumonia gives rise to a persistent or recurrent fever, a raised white cell count, general malaise and chest pain over the involved area. Digital clubbing occurs within a few weeks. Diagnosis is made on the appearance of the chest radiograph, clinical signs and by aspiration of fluid. With a large empyema there is decreased or almost absent chest movement on the affected side and unilateral elevation of the diaphragm. If this becomes chronic the fibrous capsule of the encysted empyema contracts and local rib fixation occurs. Gas exchange is impaired as the underlying lung is poorly ventilated and pulmonary function tests show a restrictive defect.

Pneumothorax

Spontaneous pneumothorax occurs predominantly in two situations:

1. In healthy, young males, especially tall individuals. The cause is rupture of a subpleural bleb usually located at the apex.
2. Complicating lung disease, particularly chronic airflow limitation.

Trauma to the chest wall may be complicated by pneumothorax and often there are associated rib fractures.

The signs and symptoms depend on the size of the pneumothorax, the presence of any lung disease and associated injuries to the chest wall. Pleuritic chest pain, usually localized to the affected side, and breathlessness are common. The breathlessness often improves before the pneumothorax has had time to resolve.

A large pneumothorax causes hypoxaemia due to areas of increased $\dot{V}/\dot{Q}$ mismatching in the collapsed lung. The $PaCO_2$ is usually normal or low due to hyperventilation, except when a pneumothorax complicates chronic airflow limitation. In this situation the $PaCO_2$ rises and respiratory failure may be precipitated. Breath sounds are reduced or absent over the affected area and the percussion note is more resonant. Tachycardia occurs in association with moderate or large pneumothoraces. Diagnosis of a pneumothorax is made on the appearance of the chest radiograph.

A tension pneumothorax occurs when the ruptured visceral pleura remains unsealed and a valve forms allowing air into the pleura on inspiration but preventing its escape on expiration. This is a life threatening emergency. Displacement of the mediastinal contents towards the opposite side causes cardiorespiratory distress with hypoxaemia and cyanosis, systemic hypotension and shock.

Management of pleural disorders

The medical management depends on the severity of the signs and symptoms. If the effusion or pneumothorax is small, that is less than 10% of the lung field and the patient symptomless, it would be observed and a repeat chest radiograph taken the next day. If this shows that the pneumothorax or effusion is resolving or remains the same, intervention will probably not be necessary. If the patient develops symptoms or the appearance of the radiograph deteriorates, an intercostal drain would be inserted. This would be placed apically for a pneumothorax and basally for an effusion. A vacuum pressure (suction) may be applied to the drainage bottle to encourage faster evacuation of the air or fluid into the bottle.

Treatment for the underlying cause of the effusion would be started, for example anticoagulants for a pulmonary embolus, diuretics for cardiac failure, or antibiotics for an empyema. With an empyema, drainage via an intercostal tube may be difficult as the fluid (pus) is usually too viscous to move freely through the tube. If the empyema does not resolve, open drainage or surgery may be considered. With surgical decortication, the thick fibrotic pleura is removed and the underlying lung can then re-expand.

Physiotherapy is usually indicated in patients with an intercostal tube. Ambulation should be encouraged, keeping the drainage bottle below the level of entry of the intercostal tube in the patient's chest.

Following chest trauma, for example a stab wound in a young patient, vigorous exercise should be encouraged after insertion of the intercostal tube. Brisk walking up and down stairs, or running, will assist drainage of fluid and re-expansion of the lung (Eales 1991). If suction is applied, mobility exercises may include the use of cycle pedals, steps, marching on the spot, or a static bicycle (Fig. 11.7). Occasionally specific positioning determined by the chest radiograph will assist drainage of air or fluid through the intercostal tube. Huffing and coughing will increase the intrathoracic pressure and assist drainage. Breathing exercises will be indicated in the older patient with underlying pulmonary pathology.

Every patient with an intercostal tube should maintain full range of movement of the ipsilateral shoulder. The exercises may be active, active-assisted, assisted-resisted or auto-assisted. Thoracic mobility and posture exercises particularly trunk rotation, will also be indicated.

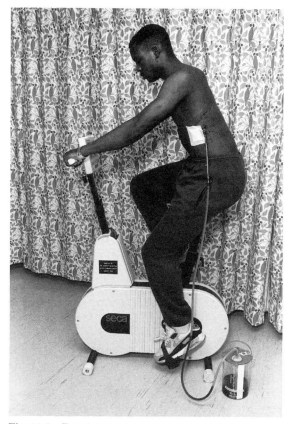

Fig. 11.7 Exercise with intercostal drainage (with permission of the Royal Brompton Hospital).

Evaluation of successful treatment would include increased breath sounds, normal percussion note and improvement on chest radiograph. The patient should have full range of shoulder movement on the affected side and be independently mobile.

Pulmonary oedema

Pulmonary oedema is the accumulation of excess fluid in the extravascular spaces and tissues of the lung. Fluid can accumulate in two major compartments:

- the interstitial compartment, which includes the thin interstitium of the alveoli and the potential spaces around larger airways and blood vessels
- air spaces in the lung.

The continuous movement of water and solutes from the lung capillaries into the interstitium is regulated by the differential permeability of its endothelium to water, small ions and protein as well as changes in the balance between the hydrostatic and osmotic forces across its membrane. Hydrostatic forces tend to move fluid out of the capillary, while osmotic forces tend to keep it in.

The most common cause of pulmonary oedema is an increase in hydrostatic capillary pressure. This may be cardiogenic in origin as in acute myocardial infarction and mitral stenosis, or may arise from non-cardiogenic causes such as absolute hypervolaemia following excessive and rapid transfusion of saline, plasma or blood.

Increased permeability of the alveolar/capillary membrane allows excess fluid to filter into the interstitium and this is the next most common cause of pulmonary oedema. A wide variety of diverse agents may damage the membrane either directly or indirectly, for example following gastric aspiration, inhalation of toxic gases and vapours, in pulmonary oxygen toxicity or in septicaemia. Increased membrane permeability is responsible for pulmonary oedema occurring in adult respiratory distress syndrome (ARDS).

Two other mechanisms by which the formation of pulmonary oedema may be precipitated are:

- decreased plasma protein osmotic pressure (for example due to hypoproteinaemia as in the nephrotic syndrome)
- obstruction of the pulmonary lymphatic drainage system (for example silicosis or immediately following lung transplantation).

In some cases the underlying mechanism is unknown, for example when pulmonary oedema occurs following rapid ascent to high altitude and after injuries to the central nervous system (neurogenic pulmonary oedema).

Irrespective of the underlying aetiology, the sequence of fluid accumulation appears to be similar. When the onset is gradual the four stages described below occur in sequence (Fig. 11.8). In fulminating cases the condition may first appear as the fourth stage (Nunn, 1987).

In the first two stages the interstitial compartment is filled with fluid. At first fluid accumula-

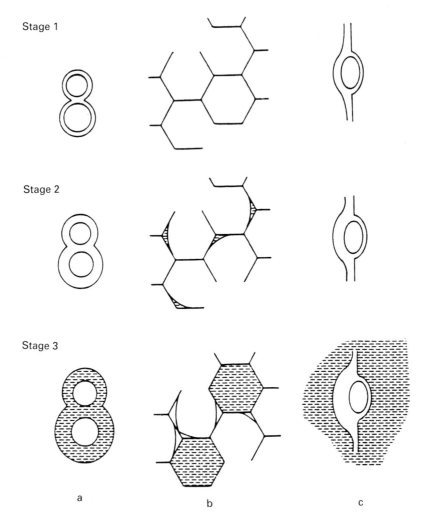

Fig. 11.8   Stages in the development of pulmonary oedema. **1** Cuffs of distended lymphatics. **2** Interstitial oedema and crescentic filling of alveoli. **3** Alveoli filling. (**4** Fluid in airways—not shown.) **a** The development of the cuff of the distended lymphatics around the branches of the bronchi and pulmonary arteries. **b** The appearance of inflated alveoli by light microscopy. **c** The appearance of a pulmonary capillary by electron microscopy. (From Nunn J F 1987 Respiratory failure, 3rd edn, Butterworth-Heinemann, London. With permission.)

tion is restricted to the formation of cuffs of distended lymphatics around the vessels and airways (stage 1). This progresses to filling of the interstitium of the alveolar walls and fluid begins to pass into the alveolar lumen where it first appears as crescents in the angles of adjacent septa (stage 2). In the early stages of pulmonary oedema physical signs may be absent and gas exchange is not grossly abnormal.

In stage 3 alveolar filling occurs. Some alveoli are totally flooded while others only have the crescents of fluid described above or are unaffected. Alveolar flooding tends to occur in the dependent parts of the lung. The flooded alveoli are unable to participate in gas exchange and hence the PaO_2 falls. Finally, the fluid moves into the small and large airways (stage 4) from which it may be expectorated.

Lung function and clinical features in pulmonary oedema

The oedematous lung shows a mixture of a restrictive and an obstructive pattern with the former predominating. The restrictive component arises from the decreased lung compliance due predominantly to vascular congestion, and to a lesser extent interstitial oedema. Dilution of surfactant by oedema fluid contributes to the loss of compliance. The vital capacity (VC) is reduced by interstitial oedema and the reduction is more severe if alveolar oedema is also present. Cardiac enlargement often contributes to the loss of lung volume.

Three factors may contribute to the obstructive component (West 1992):

- peribronchial cuffing around smaller airways causing airway compression
- reflex bronchoconstriction from stimulation of irritant receptors in the bronchial walls
- narrowed airway lumen due to oedema fluid (when severe this may cause wheezing).

Shortness of breath is the characteristic symptom of pulmonary oedema, although with mild oedema breathlessness may occur only on exercise. Typically breathing is rapid and shallow, the increased stimulation to breathing arising from an increased hypoxic ventilatory drive and the stimulation of J receptors in the alveolar walls. In an attempt to reduce the work of breathing the patient breathes shallowly and fast. Orthopnoea is common and paroxysmal nocturnal dyspnoea (PND) may occur (see p. 220).

Initially the cough is dry but progresses to the coughing up of large quantities of white frothy fluid. This may turn pink or bright red in colour due to the presence of erythrocytes which pass into the alveolar lumen.

Interstitial oedema causes fine inspiratory crackles occurring in late inspiration. In the advanced stages audible wheezing may be heard with the unaided ear and the chest sounds 'bubbly'.

The typical changes in blood gas tensions are a decrease in PaO_2, an increase in the A–aPO_2 and, except in the late stages, a normal or low $PaCO_2$. Peribronchial cuffing of small airways increases closing volume (Fig. 11.4) so that the dependent lung regions are only intermittently ventilated and this accounts for the hypoxaemia in interstitial oedema. In alveolar oedema the hypoxaemia chiefly arises from blood flow to units that receive no ventilation, either because they are filled with fluid or because they are supplied by airways obstructed by oedema fluid. The magnitude of the true shunt is decreased by compensatory hypoxic pulmonary vasoconstriction but may approach 50% or more of total blood flow in severe oedema (West 1992). Increased ventilatory drive accounts for the low $PaCO_2$, but in the very advanced stages the $PaCO_2$ rises and respiratory acidosis develops (Avery et al 1970). When pulmonary oedema accompanies acute myocardial infarction, the hypoxia is often aggravated by a low cardiac output which decreases the PaO_2 in the mixed venous blood.

Diagnosis of pulmonary oedema is made on clinical and on radiological signs (p. 42).

Management

The medical management of pulmonary oedema will depend on the underlying cause. Most patients will require diuretics and possibly fluid restriction. If the primary cause is cardiac, inotropic support may be necessary; if the origin is renal, drugs may be used to increase the renal blood flow.

Physiotherapists are often asked to treat patients with pulmonary oedema because they sound 'chesty', but this is not a physiotherapy problem as the cause cannot be affected by physiotherapy. The physiotherapist may be involved in maintaining strength and mobility by exercises in bed or by encouraging ambulation, and may need to treat a superimposed chest infection. Explanation of the role of the physiotherapist with this type of problem, to the medical and nursing staff, is essential and may prevent inappropriate referrals.

Fibrotic lung conditions

These are a diverse group of conditions which tend to be classified together because of common clinical, radiological or pathological features. Irrespective of the underlying aetiology, the pathological changes share considerable similarities. In most of the conditions, alveolitis (accumulation of inflammatory cells in the alveolar septae and air spaces), destruction of the alveolar septae and fibrosis occur. Because many patients develop fibrosis, the term 'fibrotic lung disease' is often used, but alternative classifications include infiltrative disease or interstitial lung disease.

In about 50% of cases the aetiology is unknown, for example sarcoidosis and idiopathic pulmonary fibrosis. In others, the cause may be occupational or environmental inhalants, for example inorganic dusts or chemical fumes.

The characteristic lung function abnormalities seen in these conditions are a low VC, FRC, total lung capacity (TLC), a normal or increased FEV_1/FVC ratio and a reduced transfer factor (TLCO) (p. 48). Except in very mild cases the PaO_2 is usually low, as also is the $PaCO_2$.

Management

The medical management of these patients remains a difficult problem. In some cases the use of steroids is beneficial and occasionally immunosuppressants are helpful. Antibiotics would be used to treat an infection and oxygen therapy and sedation may be considered in the advanced stages of the disease.

Physiotherapists can assist the patient by teaching relaxation positions and breathing control at rest, when climbing stairs and during other forms of exercise. The active cycle of breathing techniques may be taught for use during an infection.

The respiratory muscles

Lung function abnormalities associated with respiratory muscle weakness include a reduction in VC and in the presence of severe diaphragmatic weakness the VC typically falls by more than 30% in the supine position (normal decrease in VC from erect to supine is 5–10%). The fall in supine VC is due to the weight of the abdominal contents in this position pushing up against the diaphragm (Green & Laroche 1990). Since the ability to both maximally inhale and exhale is reduced, TLC is decreased and the RV is normal or raised. The

RV/TLC ratio is therefore higher than normal but in contrast to diseases characterized by airflow limitation the FEV_1/FVC ratio is not reduced (Green & Laroche 1990). When corrected for lung volume the gas transfer is normal or high and a restrictive defect with a high carbon monoxide transfer coefficient (KCO) is very suggestive of respiratory muscle weakness. Measurement of VC is especially useful in the management of progressive disorders such as Guillain–Barré syndrome.

Global respiratory muscle strength can be assessed by measuring maximum inspiratory and expiratory mouth pressures (PiMax and PeMax), but for accurate diagnosis and quantification of diaphragmatic weakness the transdiaphragmatic pressure (Pdi) must be measured (p. 51).

Shortness of breath on exertion is a common sign of respiratory muscle weakness (p. 218). Patients with bilateral diaphragmatic paralysis or severe weakness are markedly orthopnoeic. However, symptoms are usually absent in the adult patient when only one hemidiaphragm is involved.

In severe diaphragmatic weakness paradoxical inward movement of the anterior abdominal wall occurs during inspiration and is most easily observed with the patient supine. Chest radiography and fluoroscopy of the diaphragm during sniffing are useful diagnostic tools in hemidiaphragm weakness. The affected side is raised and moves paradoxically upwards on sniffing. Radiography and fluoroscopy are less useful when the problem is bilateral (Green & Laroche 1990). Severe weakness may lead to alveolar hypoventilation and ventilatory failure (Table 11.1).

Hypercapnia occurring in patients with severe weakness of the respiratory muscles often develops insidiously at night. Muscle tone and respiratory drive are decreased during sleep and the effects are most marked during periods of rapid eye movement (REM) sleep. Tidal volume is decreased by around 25% and breathing is irregular during REM sleep (Nunn 1987). In normal subjects these changes are sufficient to cause a fall in PaO_2 of 1–2 kPa (7.5–15 mmHg) and a modest rise in $PaCO_2$ of 0.4 kPa (3 mmHg) (Stradling et al 1985, Nunn 1987). Transient hypoxaemia during REM sleep is a normal occurrence in healthy older subjects.

Table 11.1 Examples of common causes of respiratory failure

Type I	Hypoxaemic respiratory failure: PaO_2<8.0 kPa (60 mmHg); $PaCO_2$ normal or low
Lungs and airways	Acute asthma Chronic bronchitis and emphysema Pneumonia Pulmonary fibrosis Pulmonary vascular disease Adult respiratory distress syndrome
Type II	Hypercapanic (ventilatory) respiratory failure: PaO_2< 8.0 kPa (60 mmHg); $PaCO_2$>6.6 kPa (50 mmHg)
Lungs and airways	Chronic bronchitis and emphysema★ Severe acute asthma Severe acute pneumonia
Central nervous system	Drugs Trauma
Neuromuscular system	Weak respiratory muscles
Thoracic cage and pleura	Crushed chest Thoracoplasty Kyphoscoliosis

★Most common cause

Nocturnal desaturation in patients with respiratory muscle weakness is mainly due to hypoventilation. An additional mechanism in some patients may be alterations in $\dot{V}/\dot{Q}$ matching arising from the small fall in FRC which occurs during sleep (Hudgel & Devadatta 1984). Early morning headaches and daytime somnolence are suggestive of nocturnal hypoventilation.

With progressive hypoventilation signs of hypercapnic respiratory failure develop. A raised $PaCO_2$ is responsible for the flapping tremor of the outstretched hands (asterixis). The cardiovascular system responds to mild hypoxia with tachycardia and hypertension. Severe hypoxia results in bradycardia and hypotension. Hypoxia is a potent stimulus to pulmonary vasoconstriction, hence pulmonary hypertension may occur (West 1992). Raised levels of CO_2 in the blood greatly increase cerebral blood flow causing headache, raised cerebrospinal fluid pressure and sometimes papilloedema. The net result of a combination of hypoxia and hypercapnia on the central nervous system is restlessness, confusion, slurred speech, tremor, fluctuations of mood and drowsiness.

Management

The medical management will depend on the underlying cause and the severity of the signs and symptoms. For some patients oxygen therapy will be necessary, and possibly some form of ventilatory assistance. The latter may be required only at night (Ellis et al 1987). The use of nasal intermittent positive pressure ventilation (NIPPV) or negative pressure devices is advocated to avoid the complications of intubation and to enable the patient to be managed on the ward or at home (Branthwaite 1991, Elliott & Moxham 1991, Shneerson 1991). If such equipment is not available, or if it fails to restore blood gas tensions to acceptable levels, the patient will require transfer to the intensive care unit for intubation and ventilation.

The active cycle of breathing techniques can be used to assist in the clearance of secretions, and advice be given regarding appropriate positioning to relieve breathlessness and optimize $\dot{V}/\dot{Q}$ matching. Abdominal support with an upwards pressure may make huffing and coughing more effective.

If the patient is unable to perform the active cycle of breathing techniques due to weakness or fatigue, IPPB can be used to increase tidal volume and assist in the mobilization and clearance of secretions. This may be sufficient to prevent intubation and mechanical ventilation.

Efficacy of treatment would be shown by a lowering of the $PaCO_2$, an increase in PaO_2, an increased tidal volume and an improved mental state.

PROBLEM 2: BREATHLESSNESS AND DECREASED EXERCISE TOLERANCE

Breathlessness, both on exertion and at rest, is a frequent presenting complaint in patients seeking medical help. On occasions it may be difficult to distinguish, from subjective findings alone, whether the symptoms are of cardiac or respiratory origin as in both situations the patient may complain of breathlessness on exertion and of acute episodes of breathlessness at rest.

Although it can be appreciated how breathlessness leads to decreased exercise tolerance and poor quality of life (Fig. 11.9), the understanding of the mechanisms responsible for the sensation of breathlessness and dealing with its management pose considerable difficulties.

Breathlessness ('dyspnoea' in the Greek language) is a sensation perceived by an individual. It may be defined as an awareness of increased respiratory effort which is unpleasant and recognized as inappropriate (Brewis 1991). Breathlessness is not tachypnoea (increased rate of breathing), hyperventilation (breathing in excess of metabolic needs) or hyperpnoea (increased breathing). The last three terms all describe ventilation in response to different stimuli. Although hypoxia and hypercapnia may force the patient to breathe more deeply, chemoreceptor signals are not directly subject to conscious appreciation (Holland 1991). The sensation of breathlessness arises from the ventilatory response rather than from the stimulus itself (Nunn 1987).

Different terms used by patients to describe their breathlessness include 'difficulty in breathing', 'chest tightness' and 'difficulty in filling the lungs' and it is likely that the term 'breathlessness' embraces several types of sensation (Howell 1990).

In 1963, Campbell and Howell put forward the length–tension inappropriateness theory to explain the origin of breathlessness, and this continues to be accepted (Burki 1988). This theory proposes that a subject develops the sensation of breathlessness when the output of the respiratory muscles (ventilation) is inappropriate, in the individual's experience, to the central inspiratory motor command.

There is a poor correlation between the severity of breathlessness and the results of pulmonary function tests (McGavin et al 1978; Mahler et al 1984). Some patients with gross abnormalities of lung function may not be severely breathless and may report little difficulty in carrying out activities of daily living. Conversely, in others with only minimal disturbance of lung function, even mild activity is greatly hampered by breathlessness.

Quantification of a sensation such as breathlessness is difficult. The methods most frequently used to assess breathlessness are the oxygen cost diagram, the Borg scale of perceived exertion and visual analogue scales (McGavin et al 1978, Holland 1991). Questionnaires are usually employed to assess functional activity and quality of life in patients with respiratory disease (Guyatt et al 1987, Jones 1991). Exercise tolerance is

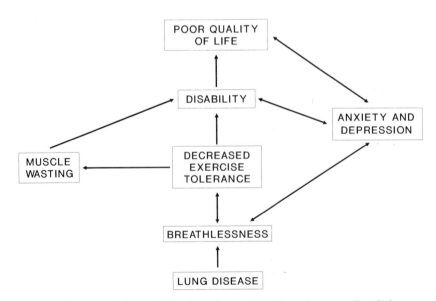

Fig. 11.9 Pathways linking lung disease, disability and poor quality of life.

often measured by recording the distance walked in a given time (usually 6 min) (McGavin et al 1976, Butland et al 1982, Singh et al 1992) or by measuring the maximum distance walked before the patient is stopped by breathlessness (Davidson et al 1988). In patients with heart disease, scales such as the New York Heart Association (NYHA) scale is used to grade the degree of exertion which causes breathlessness (Tunstall Pedoe & Walker 1990). Tests to assess breathlessness and decreased exercise tolerance are described in Chapters 1, 3 and 14.

Bronchospasm

Breathlessness in patients with asthma is due to the difficulty in meeting the increased ventilatory demands produced by an increase in the work of breathing. Airflow limitation and hyperinflation require the patient to generate greater than normal pressures during tidal breathing, but the ability of the inspiratory muscles to achieve the required pressure is compromised by muscle shortening, decreased diaphragmatic curvature, increased velocity of shortening and abnormal rib cage geometry (Moxham 1991).

During an acute attack of bronchospasm the FRC, TLC and RV are increased and all indices of expiratory flow rate are markedly reduced. Except when an attack is very severe, wheezes are heard on auscultation. The chest radiograph may be normal or show signs of hyperinflated lungs. Poorly controlled asthma in childhood may lead to chest deformity. $\dot{V}/\dot{Q}$ mismatch causes hypoxaemia. In the early stages hyperventilation leads to hypocapnia, but as an attack of acute severe asthma progresses, hypercapnia develops. In some patients physical signs are absent between attacks and exercise tolerance is normal. In others, especially older patients, there may be some degree of residual disability. An important sign of asthma, especially in children and young adults, is acute bronchoconstriction following exercise. Wheezing and chest tightness occur 1–2 min after the end of the exercise. If the exercise is prolonged, asthma may develop during the activity. After such an episode there is a refractory period during which, if a second episode of exercise is undertaken, it is much harder to induce the bronchoconstriction.

Certain forms of exercise, for example running, are more likely to provoke exercise-induced asthma (EIA) than others, such as swimming, despite an equivalent amount of energy being expended. Airway cooling is thought to be important in the genesis of EIA, but it remains uncertain whether the mechanism is cooling per se or the development of hypertonicity of the airway lining fluid or cells caused by evaporation of water to saturate the inspired air (Barnes & Holgate 1990).

Management

The medical management will include bronchodilator therapy, probably corticosteroids and possibly prophylactic drugs, for example sodium cromoglycate (Intal).

The physiotherapist should assess the patient's ability to use the prescribed inhalation device. It is essential that the patient uses the device correctly and understands the importance and relevance of each drug.

Patients will often find it helpful to use breathing control at rest in relaxation positions, and during exercise. The active cycle of breathing techniques, with particular emphasis on the periods for relaxation and breathing control, is taught for use when excess secretions are present.

Hyperreactive airways, for example in asthma (Ch. 19), are sensitive to cold temperatures and to hypertonic or hypotonic solutions. If high humidification is indicated this should be warmed and an isotonic solution of normal saline used in the humidifier (Schoeffel et al 1981).

A positive response to treatment can be assessed by improvements in lung function, auscultation and exercise tolerance.

Chronic airflow limitation

Breathlessness develops slowly over several years and initially is present only during exercise. The most likely cause of the breathlessness is overinflation of the lungs and thorax. This causes an increase in the work of breathing by three possible mechanisms (Howell 1990):

1. Hyperinflated lungs are less compliant.
2. The inspiratory muscles are shortened

because of an increase in FRC. This reduces the maximum tension that can be developed.

3. The diaphragm is low and flat. This places the diaphragm at a mechanical disadvantage and, instead of increasing the transverse and antero-posterior diameters of the chest, in severe hyperinflation contraction of the diaphragm may cause the lower lateral rib margins to be pulled in (Hoover's sign).

Typically, the breathing pattern is of a short inspiration and prolonged expiration. Some patients may purse their lips during expiration in an attempt to keep the airways open.

Clinically, it is possible to distinguish two patterns of chronic airflow limitation which represent the ends of a disease spectrum with many intermediate stages. These patterns (type A and type B) are not related to the relative proportions of chronic bronchitis (p. 225) and emphysema (p. 226).

Breathlessness is most severe in the type-A patient (pink puffer) and these patients are usually thin and have signs of marked hyperinflation and muscle wasting. Some patients with α_1-antitrypsin deficiency develop similar signs and symptoms. Hypoxaemia is only mild and the $PaCO_2$ is normal or low.

Examination of the patient with established disease shows signs of hyperinflation:

- high shoulders
- increase in anteroposterior diameter of the chest
- use of accessory muscles
- shortening of the distance between the cricoid cartilage and the suprasternal notch to less than three-fingers breadth
- indrawing of intercostal spaces and supraclavicular fossae on inspiration (this is due to excessive lowering of the intrapleural pressure which is necessary to ventilate the lungs).

The above signs are more evident during exercise as the patient struggles to breathe at lung volumes close to TLC.

Wheezes may be present. The breath sounds may be decreased and the percussion note is hyperresonant, but these signs are unreliable as the disease affects both sides of the chest and the ability to compare the two sides is lost. The chest radiograph shows signs of hyperinflation (see Fig. 2.17).

There is a proportionately greater decrease in FEV_1 than FVC such that the FEV_1/FVC ratio is reduced. The FRC, RV and RV/TLC ratio are increased and in severe emphysema the TLC may be grossly elevated.

The type-B patient (blue bloater) has a poor respiratory drive and may not be especially short of breath, at least not at rest. Cough, sputum and recurrent bronchial infections are more common than in type-A patients. In general, the patients are overweight and may suffer from fatigue and daytime somnolence. Type-B patients are hypoxaemic, have an elevated $PaCO_2$ and may develop dependent oedema, engorged neck veins and cor pulmonale. Hypercapnic respiratory failure may develop during an infective exacerbation. The injudicious use of oxygen therapy in type-B patients is an important cause of increasing $PaCO_2$ as the main ventilatory drive in these patients comes from hypoxaemia. Giving high concentrations of inspired oxygen may abolish the hypoxic ventilatory drive and the ensuing respiratory depression will lead to very high levels of arterial carbon dioxide. The rise in alveolar oxygen level occurring when oxygen enriched air is breathed, releases hypoxic vasoconstriction in poorly ventilated, lung regions and contributes to worsening gas exchange (West 1992).

Hypoxaemia in chronic airflow limitation is principally due to $\dot{V}/\dot{Q}$ mismatch. However, two mechanisms operate to limit the extent of the hypoxaemia from this cause (West 1992): extensive collateral ventilation, which enables air to reach regions supplied by obstructed airways; and localized hypoxic vasoconstriction, which limits the perfusion of poorly or unventilated lung regions (West 1992). Other factors that may contribute to hypoxaemia in chronic airflow limitation are alveolar hypoventilation in patients with respiratory failure and impaired diffusion (West 1992).

Management

Oxygen therapy may be indicated. For type-B

patients the inspired oxygen must be carefully controlled (often 24%) as many of these patients have become accustomed to a high arterial carbon dioxide level and the respiratory stimulus is a low PaO_2. For type-A patients the stimulus to breathe remains an elevated arterial carbon dioxide level and, on occasions, a higher inspired oxygen level may be recommended. High humidification (p. 149) may be indicated.

The medical management would also include bronchodilator drugs, antibiotics for infection, and sometimes a small dose of morphine may provide marked relief of breathlessness. Type-B patients who develop cor pulmonale may need diuretics and may require venesection if the haematocrit is elevated.

The medical team will be involved in the education of the patient with regard to the adverse effects of cigarette smoking, including passive smoking, and adequate nutrition. A domiciliary visit would highlight the problems experienced at home by the breathless patient and his family. Long-term oxygen therapy in selected patients with chronic airflow limitation has been shown to improve survival, exercise tolerance, mental function and quality of life (Nocturnal Oxygen Therapy Trial Group 1980, Medical Research Council Working Party 1981). The expected gradual progression of pulmonary hypertension associated with this condition is slowed down, provided that the oxygen is used at a low flow rate for a minimum of 15 hours per day.

In the acute exacerbation of chronic airflow limitation, where breathlessness is the main problem, the physiotherapist should encourage the pattern of breathing control in well supported and comfortable positions. This will often be combined with the inhalation of nebulized bronchodilator drugs.

Patients with chronic airflow limitation may show signs of reversible airflow obstruction (bronchospasm) which will respond to treatment. Although many of these patients have mainly irreversible airflow obstruction, small increases in FEV_1 and particularly in FVC or VC often give relief of breathlessness and an increase in exercise tolerance. This will usually not be detected using a peak flow meter (p. 148).

The patient can be taught relaxation and breathing control in positions to alleviate breathlessness. Breathing control during walking and stair climbing will help to reduce breathlessness on exertion and increase exercise tolerance. A respiratory walking frame (Fig. 11.10), with or without portable oxygen, may assist ambulation in the very breathless patient.

A progressive exercise programme, for example walking or stair climbing (McGavin et al 1977), can be used to increase exercise tolerance and can be carried out at home, but should be reassessed at intervals.

As a result of treatment, the physiotherapist will hope to see an increase in the distance the patient can walk, for example using the 6 min walking test or by measuring the maximum distance and/or in the activities of daily living.

Excess secretions are frequently another problem in patients with chronic airflow limitation. Following delivery of the bronchodilator

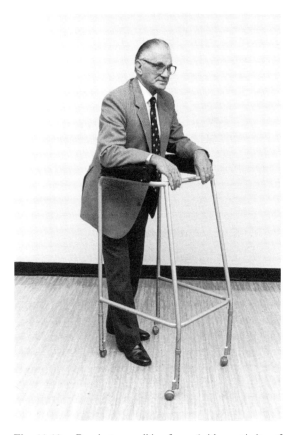

Fig. 11.10 Respiratory walking frame (with permission of the Royal Brompton Hospital).

drugs the active cycle of breathing techniques can form part of the treatment programme.

In the semicomatose and confused patient with excess secretions the problem of retained secretions is of immediate and primary importance, but during the recovery period the problem of breathlessness should be addressed.

Pleural disorders

Pneumothorax. Breathlessness due to pneumothorax is rapid in onset and the severity of the breathlessness relates to the size of the pneumothorax, the presence of any lung disease and of any associated injuries to the thorax. Pleuritic pain is common on the affected side.

Pleural effusion. Breathlessness occurs most often when large effusions accumulate rapidly or there is mediastinal shift. The mechanisms responsible for the breathlessness are probably a decrease in compliance of the affected lung(s) due to volume loss and a decrease in chest wall compliance. Small effusions, unless accompanied by pleurisy, are not usually symptomatic.

Management of pleural disorders

The medical management is discussed on page 208. The physiotherapist can assist the problem of breathlessness by encouraging breathing control in well supported comfortable positions.

Fibrotic lung conditions

Patients with fibrotic lung conditions typically breathe with a small tidal volume and increased rate. This pattern is adopted in an attempt to decrease the work of breathing imposed by the reduction in lung compliance.

One of the earliest symptoms is breathlessness on exertion accompanied by hypoxaemia. This finding may be present even when lung volumes and the chest radiograph are normal. In the majority of patients $\dot{V}/\dot{Q}$ mismatching, and not diffusion impairment, is thought to be the major factor causing exertional hypoxaemia. In a minority, a small contribution to the widened

A–aPO_2 gradient seen during exercise may be accounted for by diffusion impairment (Fulmer 1990). This arises because exercise reduces the time spent by the red blood cell in the pulmonary capillary from around three-quarters of a second to one-third of a second and thus the time available for oxygen diffusion is reduced. As the disease progresses, hypoxaemia at rest develops and this is often extremely severe. The $PaCO_2$ is generally below normal except in the late stages when hypercapnia may occur.

Management

The medical management is discussed on page 212. Physiotherapists can assist the patient by teaching relaxation positions and breathing control at rest, when climbing stairs and during other forms of exercise. The active cycle of breathing techniques can be taught for use during an infective episode characterized by excess secretions.

Weakness of the respiratory muscles

Breathlessness on exertion is common in patients with respiratory muscle weakness. In cases of moderate weakness of the diaphragm, breathlessness in the erect position is usually not a problem. The exception to this is when standing in water up to the chest, for example when entering a swimming pool (Mier et al 1986). Normally, descent of the diaphragm in the erect position is assisted during inspiration by the downward pull of gravity on the abdominal contents. During expiration, patients contract their abdominal muscles, thereby pushing the abdominal contents up into the chest and raising the diaphragm. When standing in deep water the weight of the water prevents adequate abdominal expansion and thus descent of the diaphragm is impeded.

If bilateral paralysis of the diaphragm or severe weakness is present, marked orthopnoea prevents patients lying supine for more than a few minutes. The adult patient with paralysis or weakness of one hemidiaphragm is often asymptomatic unless there are pre-existing problems such as lung disease or obesity.

Management

In addition to the medical management outlined on page 213, nutritional advice and possibly respiratory stimulants may be included. In severe cases of bilateral diaphragmatic paralysis with severe breathlessness, diaphragmatic pacing may be attempted.

Instruction in positioning by the physiotherapist will help to relieve breathlessness and optimize $\dot{V}/\dot{Q}$ matching. Guidelines only can be given for positioning as the optimal position will vary among individuals. In patients with generalized muscle weakness the length–tension status of the diaphragm will improve with the patient lying supine, but with bilateral diaphragmatic paralysis the optimal position may be high side lying with the patient rolled slightly forward. When the diaphragm is paralysed any increase in length and tension would hinder rather than facilitate breathing and a more vertical position which reduces the pressure of the abdominal contents on the diaphragm should reduce breathlessness. In unilateral diaphragmatic paralysis breathlessness is not usually marked, but if there is an underlying pulmonary condition and breathlessness is a problem, positioning in high side lying with the unaffected side dependent may be the most comfortable.

A visual analogue scale of breathlessness could be used to monitor the patient's perceived breathlessness.

Impaired gas exchange

Changes in ventilation arise in response to chemical stimuli such as hypercapnia, hypoxia and changes in acid–base balance. Although these produce changes in ventilation, breathlessness is not necessarily present. An example of this is the hypoxic patient with interstitial oedema in whom breathlessness may be due to the increased work of breathing imposed by the reduction in lung compliance rather than to the hypoxia per se.

The ventilatory response to hypoxia and hypercapnia varies considerably among subjects (West 1990). Hypercapnia is a powerful respiratory stimulant and, under normal conditions, the carbon dioxide tension of the arterial blood is the most important factor in the control of ventilation. This is not the case in some patients with chronic carbon dioxide retention in whom the hypoxic drive to ventilation is very important. When the $PaCO_2$ is normal there is little increase in ventilation until the oxygen tension of the arterial blood has fallen below 8 kPa (60 mmHg) (Weil et al 1970). The ventilatory response to hypoxia is enhanced in the presence of hypercapnia, and is enhanced during exercise, even though the $PaCO_2$ may be normal or low (West 1990).

Changes in acid–base balance affect ventilation. Metabolic acidosis, as may occur in diabetes mellitus due to the accumulation of acid ketone bodies in the circulation, stimulates respiration. In metabolic alkalosis ventilation is depressed and the $PaCO_2$ rises.

Management

Examples of causes of impaired gas exchange include consolidation, lobar collapse, and adult respiratory distress syndrome (ARDS). Oxygen therapy will be necessary to treat hypoxaemia, and antibiotics are likely to be used if there is evidence of bacterial infection. Patients with ARDS will probably require prolonged intubation and mechanical ventilation (p. 276).

Physiotherapy cannot influence the clearance of inflammatory exudate within the alveoli and, therefore, cannot influence the breathlessness of these patients. The physiotherapist should be involved only if there is a physiotherapy problem, for example a superimposed infection with excess bronchial secretions or lobar collapse. It may be the physiotherapist who would be involved with the provision of high humidification with oxygen therapy.

Pulmonary embolism

The majority of pulmonary emboli arise from obstruction to the pulmonary artery or one of its branches by a thrombus formed in the deep veins of the lower limbs. Other sites include the right side of the heart, as in atrial fibrillation, and the pelvis. Non-thrombotic emboli such as fat, air and amniotic fluid are much less common. Emboli involve the lower zones of the lung more frequently than the upper zones. Pulmonary infarction does not always occur because adequate oxygenation to the distal lung may be provided via the bronchial arterial blood supply and the airways. When there is disease of the airways or of the bronchial circulation, pulmonary infarction is more likely.

The clinical features depend on the size of the embolus. Breathlessness of sudden onset is a characteristic finding and is usually followed by pleuritic chest pain and haemoptysis. Hyperventilation is almost always present, and hence the $PaCO_2$ is usually low. The increased drive to breathe is due to hypoxaemia from $\dot{V}/\dot{Q}$ mismatch and the presence of pleuritic pain. The patient is tachycardic and fever develops within a few hours of infarction.

Small emboli may go unrecognized, but if they occur repeatedly the pulmonary capillary bed is reduced in size causing pulmonary hypertension. This leads to marked breathlessness on exercise.

Management

The patient will often have a $\dot{V}/\dot{Q}$ scan to confirm the diagnosis and will probably receive oxygen therapy and anticoagulants. If the patient is unconscious or not fit enough to walk several times a day, active, active-assisted or passive leg exercises should be performed when anticoagulant therapy is established.

Cardiac failure

Fatigue and breathlessness are the principal symptoms of cardiac failure. Cardiac failure is a clinical syndrome consisting of symptoms and signs which develop when the heart is unable to generate an output sufficient to meet the metabolic needs of the body. Either side of the heart may fail independently or, more commonly, left-sided heart failure leads to right-sided failure (Tunstall Pedoe & Walker 1990). The principal causes of heart failure are given in Table 11.2.

In clinical practice cardiac failure is manifested by a decrease in cardiac output or by damming up of blood in the veins behind the right or the left side of the heart. Pulmonary congestion is a

Table 11.2 Principal causes of heart failure

Left-sided failure
(a) Increased load
Systemic hypertension
Mitral and aortic valve disease
Cardiac arrhythmia
High output states — (anaemia, thyrotoxicosis)
Overtransfusion

(b) Myocardial damage
Ischaemic heart disease
Myocarditis
Cardiomyopathy
Cardiac depressant drugs

Right-sided failure
Pulmonary hypertension
Right ventricular infarction
Right-sided involvement in cardiomyopathy and myocarditis
Pulmonary and tricuspid valve disease

cardinal feature of left-sided failure. When the right side fails the characteristic sign is dependent oedema.

Breathlessness. The mechanisms by which breathlessness may arise in cardiac failure are as follows (Sutton 1989):

1. Pulmonary congestion increases the work of breathing because lung compliance is reduced and airways resistance is increased. The reasons for this are discussed on page 211. The patient with pulmonary oedema typically breathes with a small tidal volume and increased frequency in an attempt to reduce the work of breathing. Reflex hyperventilation may be due to hypoxia or from stimulation of the J receptors in the alveolar walls.

2. A reduction in lung volume may occur because of pleural effusion (usually bilateral), ascites or because of cardiomegaly or pulmonary venous congestion. The decrease in lung volume may then be responsible for the increased work of breathing. Less commonly, breathlessness may be due to a severely reduced cardiac output resulting in inadequate perfusion of the respiratory muscles and subsequent fatigue. In some patients, pulmonary disease (for example chronic airflow limitation) may be responsible for causing heart failure, and thus breathlessness may be of cardiac and respiratory origin.

3. Orthopnoea and paroxysmal nocturnal dyspnoea (PND) (acute breathlessness waking

the patient at night) arise in cardiac disease because of a high pulmonary venous pressure. Right atrial filling pressure is increased in the supine position and the increased filling of the right atrium and ventricle is passed on into the lungs. This causes an increase in pulmonary venous congestion and decreases lung compliance. The mechanism responsible for PND is similar to orthopnoea, but because sensory awareness is depressed during sleep severe interstitial and alveolar oedema can accumulate. PND may be confused with nocturnal asthma because it causes patients to wake breathless at night and also because some patients with left-heart failure develop wheeze. In severe left ventricular failure Cheyne–Stokes respiration may occur. This is characterized by a smooth rhythmic waxing and waning of tidal volume interspersed with periods of apnoea, the whole cycle lasting 30–60 seconds.

Fatigue and decreased exercise tolerance. The cause of fatigue in heart failure is not fully understood. When cardiac output is inadequate the demands of the exercising muscle cannot be met by compensatory increases in peripheral blood flow. In chronic heart failure an increase in resistance to blood flow in skeletal muscles has been demonstrated at rest and on exercise (Poole-Wilson 1989).

A fall in lean body mass and hence muscle bulk occurs in long standing peripheral oedema and contributes to the decrease in exercise capacity. Patients with chronic right-heart failure may become cachectic, probably secondary to loss of appetite and to a degree of malabsorption from venous congestion of the gut. When heart failure is due to myocardial damage, as in ischaemic heart disease (IHD), angina may contribute to the decrease in exercise tolerance.

Anxiety and depression frequently accompany heart disease, especially in patients with IHD, and may contribute to the decrease in exercise tolerance and a heightened perception of breathlessness.

Management

Medical management will include diuretics and possibly a potassium supplement. Vasodilators may be used to reduce the afterload and maintain good coronary artery blood flow. Inotropic support may be needed and in severe cases the intra-aortic balloon pump may be required to improve cardiac performance and myocardial perfusion. Oxygen therapy is required and continuous positive airway pressure (CPAP) via a face mask has been shown to benefit some patients with severe cardiogenic pulmonary oedema (Bersten et al 1991). Some patients will be referred for coronary artery bypass graft surgery or valve replacement. Individual exercise programmes, including breathing control where necessary, will help to reduce breathlessness on exertion and increase fitness and confidence.

Fear and anxiety

The psychological state of an individual is important in the perception of breathlessness. High levels of anxiety and depression are common in patients with chronic respiratory disease, and in such patients breathlessness may be disproportionately severe in relation to the degree of lung disease.

Management

The physiotherapist will meet patients in whom breathlessness has no true organic cause and she may be the professional who can advise and increase the patient's confidence by using graduated exercise programmes, relaxation, breathing control and advice regarding sleeping positions. Reassessment of the patient's activities of daily living and sleep patterns will provide evaluation of the efficacy of treatment. Hyperventilation syndrome is discussed in Chapter 18 (p. 377).

PROBLEM 3: EXCESS BRONCHIAL SECRETIONS

In the healthy lung, approximately 100 ml of mucus is produced each day (Moxham & Costello 1990). Mucus is produced from four main sources of which the first two are by far the most important (Clarke 1990):

- the submucosal glands located chiefly in the cartilagenous airways
- the goblet cells lining the trachea, bronchi and bronchioles
- Clara cells (non-ciliated bronchiolar cells) found in the small bronchi, bronchioles and terminal bronchioles
- tissue fluid transudate.

The composition of mucus is 95% water. The remaining 5% is glycoproteins, carbohydrates, lipids, deoxyribonucleic acid (DNA), some cellular debris and foreign particles (Clarke 1990). The glycoprotein content of the mucus is responsible for its distinctive physical characteristics.

Mucus is carried upwards by the integrated action of the cilia, the major mechanism for clearing particles from the airways, and eventually swallowed. In situations where mucus secretion is greatly increased (for example, very dusty environments) clearance of secretions is augmented by cough and expectoration. Absorptive mechanisms operating at the alveolar level are responsible for clearing some of the peripheral secretions. When the volume of mucus reaching the larynx and pharynx has increased to the extent that an individual becomes conscious of its presence on coughing or 'clearing the throat' then the mucus is defined as sputum. The presence of sputum is abnormal.

A number of factors influence the rate of mucociliary clearance. The rate declines with age by as much as 60% and is slowed during sleep. Brisk exercise is thought to enhance clearance (Clarke 1990). Atmospheric pollutants including cigarette smoke disturb clearance. Clearance is slowed in a variety of diseases (p. 224). Inhaled β_2 agonists stimulate clearance, especially when given in high doses (Clarke 1990). Physiological saline has little effect on clearance but hypertonic saline (7.1%) enhances the rate of clearance (Pavia et al 1978). Jet nebulized water administered over 30 min has been shown to significantly increase sputum clearance in bronchiectatic patients (Conway 1992).

Bronchial secretions become a problem only when they are excessive or are difficult to eliminate. Many patients expectorate foul thick sputum postoperatively, but this is not a problem if the patient is conscious, able to huff and cough effectively and ambulant. These factors are of importance in a postoperative assessment.

Inability to clear secretions

An intact cough mechanism is almost essential to life. Much of the value of cough lies in its reflex nature. Reflex coughing is initiated by the stimulation of irritant receptors in the lung and upper airway. Receptors in the proximal respiratory passages (larynx, tracheal bifurcation, and carina) are especially sensitive to mechanical stimuli, whereas those in the terminal bronchioles and alveoli respond to chemical stimuli, for example noxious gases. Receptors in both sites show some adaptation when subjected to continuous stimulation as in the smoker who only coughs after the first cigarette of the day. Afferent impulses from the receptors travel mainly via the vagus nerve to the medulla from where an automatic sequence of events (the cough reflex) is triggered:

1. An inspiratory gasp is followed by sudden closure of the glottis lasting 0.1–0.2 second during which expiratory muscle contraction raises abdominal and intrathoracic pressures to 50–100 mmHg.
2. The glottis then suddenly opens so that the air under pressure is rapidly expelled (the rate of this may exceed 12 L/s in health). During this stage the trachea narrows to one-sixth of its normal diameter (Fig. 11.11) and the rapid flow combined with the narrowing, increases the explosive force of the expelled air. This has the effect of dislodging mucus and foreign particles and bringing them to the pharynx.

Clinical features of sputum retention. Retained secretions predispose to infection, and thus fever and tachycardia are common. The presence of secretions in the lumen of the airways increases airways resistance and the work of breathing. If an airway is completely blocked, collapse of lung distal to the blockage may occur. The trapped gas is gradually absorbed and the rate at which this takes place is greatly increased if a high concentration of oxygen is breathed (Dale & Rahn 1952). Collateral ventilation may delay or

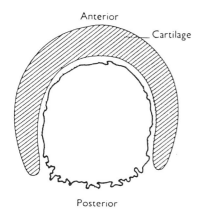

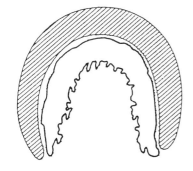

a

b

Fig. 11.11   Cross-section of trachea: **a** during normal breathing; **b** during cough. (With permission of the Royal Brompton Hospital)

prevent the process of absorption collapse by providing an alternative pathway for gas to enter the obstructed region. However, the collateral channels may be obstructed by disease processes. The dependent lung regions are most likely to collapse because gravity will cause secretions to collect there and because the airways and alveoli are relatively poorly expanded.

The presence of secretions and collapse cause hypoxaemia. This arises due to an increase in $\dot{V}/\dot{Q}$ mismatching and intrapulmonary shunting. The severity of the hypoxaemia is somewhat limited by hypoxic vasoconstriction in the poorly ventilated regions. Hypercapnia does not always occur, for example in the conscious postoperative patient $PaCO_2$ is usually low or normal. Conversely, CO_2 retention may be profound when sputum retention occurs in a patient with chronic bronchitis.

General management

Medical treatment would include appropriate antibiotic therapy, bronchodilators if indicated, oxygen therapy in hypoxic patients, analgesia if pain is a problem, and sufficient fluids if the patient is dehydrated. In some centres nasal intermittent positive pressure ventilation (NIPPV) may be used (Bott et al 1992).

The ability of the patient to cooperate in the clearance of excess bronchial secretions influences the physiotherapy techniques which can be used. In the alert and cooperative patient the active cycle of breathing techniques and exercise can be used to maintain airway clearance, but in a number of conditions additional techniques are indicated. In the confused or unconscious patient the use of adjuncts is necessary.

Ineffective cough or failure of the cough reflex

The causes of ineffective cough or failure of the cough reflex and the appropriate treatments are described below.

Depression of the central nervous system. This occurs in coma, general anaesthesia or following drugs such as morphine. Drowsiness due to carbon dioxide retention is a cause of ineffective cough in patients with chronic bronchitis and emphysema who develop respiratory failure. If morphine is the cause of drowsiness, a respiratory stimulant may be used to reverse the effects. If retention of secretions becomes a problem the mechanical effect of intermittent positive pressure breathing (IPPB) will increase tidal volume and allow the physiotherapist to augment the expiratory flow rate by using chest shaking during expiration. This can be vigorous unless contraindicated, for example by an incision or wound. Gravity-assisted positioning may be indicated to help the mobilization of secretions. When secretions have reached the upper airways, nasopharyngeal or nasotracheal suction may be required to clear them. If the secretions are tenacious high humidification should be instigated. If this condition persists a minitracheotomy may be indicated. Positions to improve $\dot{V}/\dot{Q}$ relationships, and passive or active assisted movements to maintain joint range and muscle length may be needed.

Bypassing the upper airway. When the upper airway is bypassed with an endotracheal or tracheostomy tube the normal mechanism by which the inspired air is humidified is bypassed. High humidity should be considered. The self-ventilating patient will maintain airway clearance by use of the active cycle of breathing techniques and endotracheal or tracheal suction. Optimal airway clearance in the patient unable to cooperate or requiring mechanical ventilation will be achieved by manual hyperinflation with chest shaking, unless one or other technique is contraindicated (Ch. 8, p. 157).

Inhibition of cough due to pain. This is a common cause of sputum retention following trauma to the chest wall and after surgery, especially via the upper abdomen and thorax. Postoperative patients are unwilling to take deep breaths and this interferes with the mobilization of secretions by limiting the extent to which air can flow via collateral channels to regions of lung distal to an obstructed airway (Menkes & Britt 1980). The problem is compounded if the patient has a chronic lung disease associated with the excess production of secretions such as cystic fibrosis, chronic bronchitis or bronchiectasis. It is inappropriate for the physiotherapist to attempt treatment if the patient's pain is poorly controlled. When the pain is controlled the patient will be able to cooperate with the active cycle of breathing techniques. Further assistance can be given by pressure applied over or around the painful site. On occasions periodic continuous positive airway pressure (PCPAP) and/or high humidity may be indicated. Ambulation should be encouraged as soon as possible.

Damage to the glossopharyngeal and vagal nerves. These nerves, which carry the afferent impulses from the irritant cough receptors, may be damaged by trauma to the base of the skull. A depressed cough reflex may necessitate the use of the techniques of IPPB with chest shaking and gravity-assisted positions, nasopharyngeal, nasotracheal or minitracheotomy suction, and high humidification.

Paralysed vocal cords. Damage or disease affecting the laryngeal nerve will cause paralysis of the vocal cords. If the active cycle of breathing techniques alone is not effective, the techniques of IPPB with chest shaking and gravity-assisted positions, nasopharyngeal or nasotracheal suction or a minitracheotomy may be indicated.

Laryngectomy. Surgical excision of the larynx may be indicated for treatment of a tumour in this area. In the early postoperative stage high humidification is usually indicated in addition to the active cycle of breathing techniques and tracheal suction. In the long term the upper respiratory tract adapts to reduced humidity, and added humidification is rarely required. Instructing patients to perform their own suction is an important aspect of patient care.

Weakness of the inspiratory or expiratory muscles. This may arise due to either disease processes or trauma, or following muscle relaxants. When the inspiratory muscles are weak the mechanical effects of IPPB are helpful and the increase in tidal volume is often enough to initiate an effective cough. If the expiratory muscles are affected, abdominal support with an upward pressure will make huffing and coughing more effective.

Increasing age. This renders the cough reflex less sensitive. The physiotherapist should be aware of this potential problem with clearance of secretions in the elderly, especially when pain may already be inhibiting the cough.

Impaired clearance and/or excess production of secretions

These may be associated with the following conditions.

Bronchiectasis. Bronchiectasis is defined as 'chronic dilatation of one or more bronchi'. The cause may be congenital or acquired, but the largest single group of patients is that where no cause is found. Congenital factors include cystic fibrosis, immune deficiency syndromes (for example hypogammaglobulinaemia) and primary ciliary dyskinesia. Bronchiectasis may occur following a variety of infective processes in the lung caused by *Klebsiella pneumoniae, Mycobacterium tuberculosis, Pseudomonas aeruginosa* and *Staphylococcus*, or by pertussis. Immunological processes causing inflammation, as in broncho-pulmonary aspergillosis (p. 395), are important causes of bronchiectasis.

The principal sign of bronchiectasis is the production of large amounts of purulent sputum, which is often associated with haemoptysis. The most common infecting organism is *Haemophilus influenzae*.

Physiotherapy for airway clearance in bronchiectasis is discussed in Chapter 20 (p. 400).

Cystic fibrosis. The lungs are morphologically normal at birth and the onset of pulmonary involvement may occur at any time. The basic airway abnormality in cystic fibrosis is a combination of chloride impermeability and excess sodium and water transport from the airway lumen. The ion transport abnormality leads to impaired local defence mechanisms in the respiratory tract which permit bacterial colonization, damage to the bronchial wall and bronchiectasis. The first pathogen is usually *Staphylococcus aureus*, but as the lung disease progresses *Pseudomonas aeruginosa* becomes established. *Haemophilus influenzae* is also a common infective organism.

Impaired mucociliary clearance follows the lung damage. Large volumes of sputum are produced and mild haemoptysis is a common finding in older patients. The early pathological changes consist of hypertrophy of bronchial glands, goblet cell hyperplasia, metaplasia of the bronchiolar epithelium and plugging of the airways with mucopurulent secretions which may cause segmental or lobar collapse. As the disease progresses the chest radiograph shows signs of bronchiectasis and fibrosis.

The physiotherapy for cystic fibrosis is discussed in Chapter 20 (p. 407).

Primary ciliary dyskinesia. Primary ciliary dyskinesia is an inherited condition in which there are a number of underlying defects of the cilia. The cilia beat in an uncoordinated manner and at a much slower rate, sometimes as little as 50% of normal. Mucociliary clearance is severely impaired or absent.

Physiotherapy is discussed in Chapter 20 (p. 403).

Acute bronchitis. In the absence of coexisting lung disease, acute bronchitis is associated initially with a dry irritating cough which after about 2 days progresses to the production of moderate amounts of mucopurulent sputum. Retrosternal discomfort, wheeze and slight fever are common findings. The chest radiograph is normal. The main complication of acute bronchitis is the development of pneumonia.

Following an acute respiratory tract infection, mucociliary clearance may take 2–3 months to return to normal, especially after influenza and mycoplasma infections (Clarke 1990). Bronchial hyperresponsiveness can occur and may last for several weeks. When this happens the patient complains of a dry cough and wheeze which are provoked by exposure to dry air, cold air, fumes or dust.

The physiotherapist may be involved with the administration of bronchodilator drugs. These should be given before using the active cycle of breathing techniques, in an appropriate position which may be sitting, high side lying or side lying, if the patient has difficulty expectorating the secretions.

Chronic bronchitis. Chronic bronchitis is a clinical diagnosis in which there is cough productive of sputum on most days for 3 months of the year for 2 or more years, which is not due to a specific respiratory disease such as bronchiectasis (Moxham & Costello 1990).

Hypertrophy and hyperplasia of the submucosal glands in the large airways occurs and there is an increase in the number and extent of the distribution of the goblet cells. In the absence of infection the sputum in chronic bronchitis is mucoid and the predominant cell is the macrophage.

An acute exacerbation of chronic bronchitis occurs most frequently during the winter and *Streptococcus pneumoniae* and *Haemophilus influenzae* are the most common pathogens.

The patient usually complains of worsening breathlessness. The amount of sputum produced increases and it is often thick and more purulent causing difficulty in expectoration. There is an increase in the number of neutrophils in the sputum seen under the microscope.

In the cooperative patient the active cycle of breathing techniques is used following the inhalation of bronchodilators. The patients are usually dehydrated as they are too breathless to eat or drink. Increasing the fluid intake will reduce the viscosity of the secretions. Controlled oxygen therapy is likely to be necessary and additional humidification can be given, for example using a humidity adaptor attached to a venturi mask (p. 153).

The patient with a high $PaCO_2$ may be confused and unable to cooperate. While positioned in side lying if tolerated, or high side lying, IPPB with a mask or flange mouthpiece can be used to increase tidal volume. The dry driving gas should be humidified by either a prescribed bronchodilator solution or normal saline in the nebulizer of the intermittent positive pressure breathing (IPPB) circuit. Provided adequate ventilation is achieved, it is safe and beneficial to use oxygen as the driving gas (Starke et al 1979). Chest shaking during expiration will assist in the mobilization of secretions by augmenting the expiratory flow rate.

Secretions mobilized to the upper airways may stimulate the cough reflex, but nasopharyngeal or nasotracheal suction may be required if coughing does not occur spontaneously. This regimen should be repeated approximately every 2 hours until the patient becomes more alert, and then the frequency of treatment can be reduced. As soon as the patient becomes cooperative and can huff and cough effectively the regimen of the active cycle of breathing techniques can replace the more passive IPPB treatment.

In between exacerbations, the excess secretions can usually be cleared effectively in the sitting or side lying positions. A graded walking programme can be used to increase exercise tolerance and to further assist in the mobilization of secretions. Patients should be encouraged to take responsibility for their treatment programme for the clearance of bronchial secretions together with a progressive exercise regimen.

Emphysema. Emphysema is defined by its pathology and is characterized by destruction of respiratory tissue, and permanent enlargement of the unit of lung distal to the terminal bronchioles (the acinus) (Moxham & Costello 1990). With emphysema there is a reduction in the maximal expiratory flow rates resulting from loss of elastic recoil. The clearance of secretions during an episode of infection can be assisted by the active cycle of breathing techniques. The pauses for the periods of breathing control should be emphasized and paroxysmal coughing should be discouraged.

Asthma. There is evidence that mucociliary clearance is decreased in asthma even during remission (Bateman et al 1983). Mucus in asthma is often tenacious and contains many eosinophils, epithelial cells and bronchiolar casts (plugs). These plugs are very viscous and may completely occlude the airway lumen.

The modification of the techniques used in airway clearance are discussed in Chapter 19 (p. 392).

Pneumonia/pneumonitis. These terms both mean inflammation of the lung, but in general the former is used for bacterial infections in which intra-alveolar exudate is the predominant lesion. The term 'pneumonitis' is reserved for other kinds of pulmonary inflammation such as those due to chemical or physical injury. Many organisms are responsible for causing infection of lung tissue. The old system for classifying pneumonia by radiological findings or by the causative organism provides little practical help in the management of the condition. A useful system for classification considers the circumstances in which the pneumonia is acquired (for example community or hospital) and the type of patient affected (for example pneumonia in the immunocompromised host) (Moxham & Costello 1990, MacFarlane 1991).

Bacterial infection is the most common cause of consolidation (filling of the alveoli with exudate such that the microscopic appearance of the lung is of solid tissue). The consolidation may be patchy and centred around the terminal bronchioles (bronchopneumonia) or may involve the whole of one or more lobes (lobar pneumonia). The condition is called 'interstitial pneumonitis' when the inflammation is predominantly in the alveolar walls with only secondary changes in the alveoli. For many patients with pneumonia acute pleuritic pain and not secretions is the main problem. However, in some, for example patients who develop pneumonia after surgery, retained secretions are a major problem. These patients become increasingly distressed, tachypnoeic, tachycardic and progressively more hypoxic. Several factors increase the risk of postoperative pneumonia, including cigarette smoking, increased age, obesity, emergency surgery and poor nutrition.

Persistent pneumonia is often a complication of bronchial carcinoma and arises when secretions behind the obstruction become infected. As the majority of patients affected are cigarette smokers, sputum clearance is often a problem.

In patients with pneumonia the medical management may include antibiotics and non-steroidal anti-inflammatory drugs (NSAID) if the pleuritic pain is severe. The physiotherapist is often asked to see these patients, but treatment is appropriate only if there is the physiotherapy problem of excess secretions and then the active cycle of breathing techniques can be used together with adequate analgesia. Physiotherapy cannot affect the inflammatory process occurring in the alveoli and it is therefore illogical to attempt treatment in the absence of excess bronchial secretions.

Lung abscess. This is most commonly caused by aspiration from the oropharynx. Situations predisposing to oropharyngeal aspiration include impaired consciousness from any cause and disease of the nose, mouth, pharynx, larynx or oesophagus. Other causes are bronchial obstruction (for example from a tumour), pneumonia (especially *Staphylococcus aureus* and *Klebsiella*), blood-borne infections and an infected pulmonary infarct. Lung abscesses are common in *Mycobacterium* tuberculosis infections.

The onset, duration of illness and the signs and symptoms depend on the underlying cause. Patients with *Klebsiella* pneumonia are acutely unwell, febrile and produce foul, blood stained sputum. In contrast, the onset is more gradual following oropharyngeal aspiration, the main clinical features being general malaise, weight loss and fever. Chest pain of a pleuritic nature may be present and finger clubbing can occur. The initial radiological signs are of a rounded homogenous opacity, but an air–fluid level appears when drainage via a bronchus has become established. The most common complication of an untreated abscess is empyema.

These patients tend to avoid positions that make them cough. Assessment of the chest radiograph will indicate the position of the abscess and a lateral view is often helpful. It must be remembered that the abscess can distort the bronchial tree and the gravity-assisted position indicated may need modification. The patient should be encouraged to clear secretions using the active cycle of breathing techniques. Foul, black/brown sputum is often expectorated.

Occasionally the contents of the abscess will not move and this may be due to the orifice of the cavity being too narrow to allow the passage of the necrotic tissue, or because a gas-producing organism gives a false air–fluid level in the absence of a communication between the abscess and a bronchus.

Resolution of an abscess would be recognized by absence of pyrexia and clearing on the chest radiograph.

Pulmonary tuberculosis. Post-primary tuberculosis ('TB'), reactivation of a tubercular infection, is the most frequently encountered form of the disease in adults. Cough is the most common non-systemic manifestation and, although it may be non-productive in the early stages, as the lesions become more extensive and involve the airways sputum is produced.

The treatment of tuberculosis will probably consist of a combination of antibiotics, as tuberculosis easily becomes resistant if a single antibiotic is used.

The physiotherapist may assist in the induction of a sputum specimen, but chest physiotherapy is unlikely to be necessary unless there is a concurrent bacterial infection resulting in excess bronchial secretions which can be treated using the active cycle of breathing techniques.

The majority of patients are relatively fit and ambulant, but occasionally a debilitated patient will require a graduated exercise programme, nutritional assessment and advice.

Pulmonary oedema. Except in the early stages, patients with pulmonary oedema have a cough productive of frothy white fluid turning pink or red in colour if erythrocytes are present.

Physiotherapy is not indicated unless there is a superimposed infection when the active cycle of breathing techniques can be used in a comfortable, well supported sitting or high side lying position.

Evaluation of physiotherapy for excess bronchial secretions

Evaluation of the positive effects of treatment can be seen in an increase in arterial oxygen saturation and arterial oxygen tension. In the hypercapnic patient an improvement in mental state and a lessening of the flapping tremor often accompany a lowering of the arterial CO_2 tension. There will be a reduction in tachypnoea and tachycardia, and a settling of pyrexia if present. The volume and purulence of the sputum will decrease and early inspiratory crackles heard on auscultation will clear. Activities of daily living and exercise tolerance should increase.

PROBLEM 4: CHEST PAIN

Chest pain of respiratory origin

In contrast to the presence of cough in a smoker, chest pain is unlikely to be ignored unless it has a familiar and recurrent pattern. Chest pain of respiratory origin may arise in the:

- pleura
- chest wall
- tracheobronchial tree.

Pleural pain. This is a sharp pain which is rhythmic in nature. The pain is related to breathing and is increased on deep inspiration, laughing or coughing. The most likely source is stretching of the inflamed parietal pleura and this explains why the pain is worse during inspiration than expiration.

The parietal pleura is supplied with afferent pain fibres, but the visceral pleura and lung parenchyma contain no pain fibres. When inflammation affects the upper portion of the pleura the pain is localized to the chest. The lower portion of the pleura, including the outer segment of the diaphragmatic pleura, is innervated by the lower six intercostal nerves. As these nerves also supply the abdominal wall, inflammation in this region gives rise to pain in the upper abdomen or loin. When the central portion of the diaphrag-

matic pleura (innervated by the phrenic nerve) is involved the pain radiates to the neck and to the tip of the shoulder.

Important causes of pleuritic pain are pneumonia, cancer (bronchial, pleural, or metastatic), tuberculosis, pulmonary infarction and pneumothorax.

Chest wall pain. All the structures in the thoracic wall, including the skin and subcutaneous tissues, can potentially give rise to pain felt in the chest wall. Most commonly the pain is due to strain, inflammation, malposition of, or injury to the muscles, ligaments, cartilage or bone. Occasionally, the pain may mimic pleurisy, for example following a muscle tear. Usually, however, an area of tenderness can be elicited over the affected site.

Patients with chronic cough and breathlessness frequently complain of chest pain. Asthmatic patients during an exacerbation often describe muscular aches around the lower rib cage.

Tumours involving the ribs or soft tissues usually cause a dull ache which is progressive in nature and unrelated to respiratory or other movements.

Pain from the chest wall occurs following lateral and sternal incisions and chest wall trauma. Intercostal drains may cause localized chest wall pain. Pain may also be a problem in musculoskeletal disorders such as costochronditis (Tietze's syndrome).

Tracheobronchial tree. Sensations arising in the tracheobronchial tree are much less easy to characterize as pain and are generally described as a raw, retrosternal discomfort which is increased on coughing. This occurs in acute inflammation due to infection or from inhalation of irritant fumes.

Management

There are many methods of administering analgesia and the physiotherapist should familiarize herself with the different routes of administration, different drugs and their mechanisms of action, time of onset of action, duration of effect, the effects on other systems and the preference within the hospital or in the community. Some hospitals will have a pain team involved in the care of patients with severe chronic pain, post-operative patients or terminally ill patients.

The routes available for the administration of analgesia (with onset of action) are:

- oral or sublingual (20–30 min)
- intramuscular (20–30 min)
- intravenous (immediate)
- epidural (on going)
- nerve blocks (immediate/on going)
- inhalation (1–2 min)

Cryotherapy can be used at the end of an operation to reduce postoperative pain, particularly following thoracotomy, but some patients complain of numbness for a considerable period of time.

Patient controlled analgesia (PCA) is used in some centres to give intravenous analgesia. The patient presses a button to trigger an infusion pump which releases a predetermined dose of analgesia. The control system is programmed to limit the total amount of drug that can be delivered to the patient and also the time interval between successive doses. Both the dose and the time interval can be changed to the needs of the individual patient.

If the patient has severe pain, potent analgesics such as opiates may be indicated. The level of consciousness of the patient, his blood pressure and, if possible, the arterial CO_2 tension should be considered before this type of analgesia is administered.

If the patient has pain of an inflammatory nature, the use of non-steroidal anti-inflammatory drugs (NSAID) may be beneficial.

The preceding forms of analgesia must be prescribed by a doctor. Other forms of analgesia are available to physiotherapists. These include Entonox (gas mixture of 50% nitrous oxide and 50% oxygen) (p. 162), transcutaneous nerve stimulation (TNS) (p. 163) and acupuncture (Jackson 1991). Entonox is particularly useful following fractured ribs and, in some patients, following surgery to provide additional analgesia if adequate pain control has not been obtained. TNS may be useful in patients with chronic chest disease presenting with fractured ribs, repetitive strains from coughing, thoracotomy pain or pain from a carcinoma. Acupuncture can be used successfully postoperatively by physiotherapists,

and is often combined with relaxation techniques.

If pain is not controlled it can cause or exacerbate respiratory problems such as reduced lung volume or retained secretions. The physiotherapist could evaluate the efficacy of pain control by using a pain measurement scale (Huskisson 1974), the patient's ability to cough and his increased mobility.

Chest pain of non-respiratory origin

There are several possible causes of pain in the chest other than respiratory ones and this sometimes presents difficulty in reaching a diagnosis. The common causes are described below.

Angina pectoris. This is caused by hypoxia of the myocardium. The pain of acute myocardial infarction (MI) is similar to angina but lasts longer (more than 30 min), is usually more severe and is not relieved by glyceryl trinitrate (GTN).

The myocardium becomes hypoxic when the blood supply via the coronary circulation is insufficient to meet the myocardial demands. The supply may be insufficient because there is a restriction to blood flow through the coronary arteries which is either fixed (as in narrowing due to atherosclerosis) or episodic (as in coronary artery spasm). Alternatively, the myocardial demand may be so great that even a normal supply is not adequate (for example in hypertrophy of the myocardium).

Angina is classified as:

1. *Stable* — when the pain is repetitively induced by the same provocative factor, for example when an increase in cardiac work is invoked either because of physical exertion, excitement, emotion or digestion (after a heavy meal).

2. *Unstable* — when myocardial ischaemia occurs spontaneously (for example in coronary artery spasm) or if the pattern of the angina changes from a previously repetitively provoked pattern to one that is unpredictable.

The pain from myocardial ischaemia is usually felt in the centre of the chest but may radiate to the left side of the chest and down the left arm. Other locations of the pain include the upper abdomen, the right side of the chest and the right arm, the shoulders, back, neck, jaws and teeth. Pain presenting in these regions may be part of the radiation or the sole location of the pain. Some patients with myocardial ischaemia do not complain of pain but instead report tightness or discomfort in the chest or, alternatively, complain only of breathlessness.

The physiotherapist should be able to identify this type of pain and should advise the medical staff if she suspects angina. The management of patients following myocardial infarction is discussed in Chapter 14.

Pericarditis. The visceral pericardium is insensitive to pain but inflammation of the parietal pericardium gives rise to a sharp, stabbing pain which may be central or felt on the left side of the chest, the left arm and may radiate to the neck, back and upper abdomen. The duration of the pain depends on the nature of the underlying inflammatory process (for example viral, bacterial, neoplastic, or after myocardial infarction). The development of an effusion tends to decrease the severity of the pain. Sitting upright and leaning forwards tends to decrease the pain, but taking a deep breath increases the pain. Pericardial pain is treated with anti-inflammatory drugs.

Aortic dissection. The pain associated with this is usually even more severe than that with acute myocardial infarction. The pain often presents in the upper back but may also radiate to the neck and face. Surgery may be indicated.

Neural, muscular or skeletal pain. Examples of causative factors are disc degeneration, bony metastases, muscle injuries, inflammation of soft tissues and disorders of the costal cartilages. Treatment depends on the underlying cause.

Herpes zoster (shingles) is the result of reactivation of the varicella zoster virus which has lain dormant in a posterior nerve root ganglion following chickenpox in earlier life. The presence of the virus in the skin causes severe continuous pain, tingling and numbness accompanied by a reddened area with vesicles throughout the dermatome. As the vesicles fade the pain usually subsides, but persistent intractable postherpetic neuralgia may be a complication. This presents as a burning continuous pain responding poorly to analgesics. It may respond to transcutaneous electrical nerve stimulation (Nathan & Wall 1974).

Oesophageal pain. The causes of pain arising from the oesophagus are:

1. *Spasm* — when this occurs the pain may last for up to 1 hour and there may not be an obvious provoking factor. The pain closely resembles that of unstable angina and is often relieved by glyceryl trinitrate.

2. *Oesophageal tear* — this may occur in association with prolonged vomiting and the pain is felt centrally. Surgery may be indicated.

3. *Gastro-oesophageal reflux* — this gives rise to pain felt in the centre of the chest and the epigastrium. The pain is increased when lying down and relieved by sitting upright and by taking antacids. The most common cause is hiatus hernia.

Peptic ulceration and gallbladder disease. Diseases of the stomach, duodenum or biliary system may give rise to pain felt in the chest, although it is more commonly confined to the abdomen. With peptic ulceration the pain is burning in nature, related to meals and relieved by antacids. The postprandial pain occurring with gastric ulceration may resemble angina following heavy meals.

Pain of biliary origin is usually like that associated with colic and felt on the right side of the abdomen, and the front and back of the chest. The pain may be related to the ingestion of certain foods.

REFERENCES

Abelmann W H, Frank N R, Gaensler E A, Cugell D W 1954 Effects of abdominal distension by ascites on lung volumes and ventilation. Archives of Internal Medicine 93: 528–540

Alexander J K, Amad K H, Cole V W 1962 Observations on some clinical features of extreme obesity, with particular reference to cardiorespiratory effects. American Journal of Medicine 32: 512–524

Ali J, Weisel R D, Layug A B et al 1974 Consequences of post-operative alterations in respiratory mechanics. American Journal of Surgery 128: 376–382

Avery W G, Samet P, Sackner M A 1970 The acidosis of

pulmonary oedema. American Journal of Medicine 48: 320–324

Barnes P J, Holgate S T 1990 Pathogenesis and hyperreactivity. In Brewis R A L, Gibson G J, Geddes D M (eds) Respiratory medicine. Baillière Tindall, London, p 558–603

Bateman J R, Pavia D, Sheahan N F et al 1983 Impaired tracheobronchial clearance in patients with mild stable asthma. Thorax 38: 463–467

Bendixen H H, Bullwinkel B, Hedley-Whyte J, Laver M B 1964 Atelectasis and shunting during spontaneous ventilation in anesthetized patients. Anesthesiology 25: 297–301

Benumof J L 1979 Mechanism of decreased blood flow to atelectatic lung. Journal of Applied Physiology 46: 1047–1048

Bersten A D, Holt A W, Vedig A E et al 1991 Treatment of severe cardiogenic pulmonary edema with continuous positive airway pressure delivered by face mask. New England Journal of Medicine 325: 1825–1830

Blair E, Hickam J B 1955 The effect of change in body position on lung volumes and intrapulmonary gas mixing in normal subjects. Journal of Clinical Investigation 34: 383–389

Bott J, Keilty S E J, Brown A 1992 Nasal intermittent positive pressure breathing. Physiotherapy 78: 93–96

Bourn J, Jenkins S 1992 Post-operative respiratory physiotherapy: Indications for treatment. Physiotherapy 78: 80–85

Branthwaite M A 1991 Non-invasive and domiciliary ventilation: positive pressure techniques. Thorax 46: 208–212

Brewis R A L 1991 Lecture notes on respiratory disease, 4th edn. Blackwell Scientific, Oxford

Burki N K 1988 Dyspnoea: mechanisms, evaluation and treatment. American Review of Respiratory Disease 138: 1040–1041

Butland R J A, Pang J, Gross E R et al 1982 Two-, six- and 12-minute walking tests in respiratory disease. British Medical Journal 284: 1607–1608

Clarke S W 1990 Physical defences. In: Brewis R A L, Gibson G J, Geddes D M (eds) Respiratory medicine. Baillière Tindall, London, p 176–189

Conway J H 1992 The effects of humidification for patients with chronic airways disease. Physiotherapy 78: 97–101

Craig D B, Wahba W M, Don H F et al 1971 Closing volume and its relationship to gas exchange in seated and supine positions. Journal of Applied Physiology 31: 717–721

Dale W A, Rahn H 1952 Rate of gas absorption during atelectasis. American Journal of Physiology 170: 606–615

Davidson A C, Leach R, George R J D, Geddes D M 1988 Supplemental oxygen and exercise ability in chronic obstructive airways disease. Thorax 43: 965–971

Eales C 1991 Personal communication

Egbert L D, Bendixen H H 1964 Effect of morphine on breathing pattern. Journal of the American Medical Association 188: 485–488

Elliott M W, Moxham J 1991 Non-invasive ventilation. In: D M Mitchell (ed) Recent advances in respiratory medicine. Churchill Livingstone, Edinburgh, p 23–43

Ellis E R, Bye P T B, Bruderer J W, Sullivan C E 1987 Treatment of respiratory failure during sleep in patients with neuromuscular disease. American Review of Respiratory Disease 135: 148–152

Farebrother M J B 1979 Respiratory function and cardiorespiratory response to exercise in obesity. British Journal of Diseases of the Chest 73: 211–229

Ferris B G, Pollard D S 1960 Effect of deep and quiet breathing on pulmonary compliance in man. Journal of Clinical Investigation 39: 143–149

Ford G T, Whitelaw W A, Rosenal T W et al 1983 Diaphragm function after upper abdominal surgery in humans. American Review of Respiratory Disease 127: 431–436

Fulmer J D 1990 Interstitial lung diseases. In: Stein J M (ed) Internal medicine, 3rd edn. Little Brown and Company, Boston, p 675–683

Garibaldi R A, Britt M R, Coleman M L et al 1981 Risk factors for post-operative pneumonia. The American Journal of Medicine 70: 677–680

Garrow J S 1988 Obesity and related disorders. Churchill Livingstone, Edinburgh

Gee J B L, Packer B S, Millen J E, Robin E D 1967 Pulmonary mechanics during pregnancy. Journal of Clinical Investigation 46: 945–952

Goggin M J, Joekes A M 1971 Gas exchange in renal failure. II. Pulmonary gas exchange during peritoneal dialysis. British Medical Journal 2: 247–248

Green M, Laroche C M 1990 Respiratory muscle weakness. In: Brewis R A L, Gibson G J, Geddes D M (eds) Respiratory medicine. Baillière Tindall, London, p 1373–1387

Grimby G, Hedenstierna G, Lofstrom B 1975 Chest wall mechanics during artificial ventilation. Journal of Applied Physiology 38: 576–580

Guyatt G H, Berman L B, Townsend M et al 1987 A measure of quality of life for clinical trials. Thorax 42: 773–778

Holland L 1991 Breathlessness. In: Pryor J A (ed) International perspectives in respiratory care. Churchill Livingstone, Edinburgh, p 5–26

Howell J B L 1990 Breathlessness In: Brewis R A L, Gibson G J, Geddes D M (eds) Respiratory medicine. Baillière Tindall, London, p 221–228

Hudgel D W, Devadatta P 1984 Decrease in functional residual capacity during sleep in normal humans. Journal of Applied Physiology 57: 1319–1322

Huskisson E C 1974 Measurement of pain. Lancet ii: 1127–1131

Jackson D A 1991 Acupuncture In: Wells P E, Frampton V, Bowsher D (eds) Pain: management and control in physiotherapy. Butterworth-Heinemann, Oxford

Jenkins S C, Moxham J 1991 The effects of mild obesity on lung function. Respiratory Medicine 85: 309–311

Jenkins S C, Soutar S A, Moxham J 1988a The effects of posture on lung volumes in normal subjects and in patients pre- and post-coronary artery surgery. Physiotherapy 74: 492–496

Jenkins S C, Soutar S A, Moxham J 1988b Effect of coronary artery bypass graft surgery on functional residual capacity and blood gas tensions. American Review of Respiratory Disease 137 (2 pt 2): abstr 267

Jenkins S C, Soutar S A, Loukota J M et al 1990 A comparison of breathing exercises, incentive spirometry and mobilisation after coronary artery surgery. Physiotherapy Theory and Practice 6: 117–126

Johnson N T, Pierson D J 1986 The spectrum of pulmonary atelectasis: Pathophysiology, diagnosis and therapy. Respiratory Care 31: 1107–1120

Jones J G 1987 Mechanisms of some pulmonary effects of general anaesthesia. British Journal of Hospital Medicine November: 472–476

Jones P W 1991 Quality of life measurement for patients with diseases of the airways. Thorax 46: 676–682

Keilty S E J, Bott J 1992 Continuous positive airways pressure. Physiotherapy 78: 90–92

Leblanc P, Ruff F, Milic-Emili J 1970 Effects of age and body position on airway closure in man. Journal of Applied Physiology 28: 448–451

Locke T J, Griffiths T L, Mould H, Gibson G J 1990 Rib cage mechanics after median sternotomy. Thorax 45: 465–468

MacFarlane J T 1991 Pneumonia. Medicine International 90, part 3, p 3732–3739

McGavin C R, Gupta S P, McHardy G J R 1976 Twelve-minute walking test for assessing disability in chronic bronchitis. British Medical Journal 1: 822–823

McGavin C R, Gupta S P, Lloyd E L, McHardy G J R 1977 Physical rehabilitation for the chronic bronchitic: results of a controlled trial of exercise in the home. Thorax 32: 307–311

McGavin C R, Artvinli M, Naoe H, McHardy G J R 1978 Dyspnoea, disability, and distance walked: comparison of estimates of exercise performance in respiratory disease. British Medical Journal 2: 241–243

Mahler D A, Weinberg D H, Wells C K, Feinstein A R 1984 The measurement of dyspnea: Contents, interobserver agreement, and physiologic corrleates of two new clinical indexes. Chest 85: 751–758

Marini J J 1984 Postoperative atelectasis: Pathophysiology, clinical importance, and principles of management. Respiratory Care 29: 516–528

Medical Research Council Working Party 1981 Long term domiciliary oxygen therapy in chronic hypoxic cor pulmonale complicating chronic bronchitis and emphysema. Lancet i: 681–686

Menkes H A, Britt J 1980 Rationale for physical therapy. Part 2 American Review of Respiratory Disease 122 (2): 127–131

Meyers J R, Lembeck L, O'Kane H, Baue A E 1975 Changes in functional residual capacity of the lung after operation. Archives of Surgery 110: 576–583

Mier A K, Brophy C, Green M 1986 Out of depth, out of breath. British Medical Journal 292: 1495–1496

Morran C G, Finlay I G, Mathieson M et al 1983 Randomized controlled trial of physiotherapy for post-operative pulmonary complications. British Journal of Anaesthesia 55: 1113–1116

Moxham J 1991 Respiratory muscles. Medicine International 91: 3793–3797

Moxham J, Costello J F 1990 Respiratory disease. In: Souhami R L, Moxham J (eds) Textbook of medicine. Churchill Livingstone, Edinburgh, p 451–542

Nathan P W, Wall P D 1974 Treatment of post-herpetic neuralgia by prolonged electric stimulation. British Medical Journal 3: 645–647

Naimark A, Cherniack R M 1960 Compliance of the respiratory system and its components in health and obesity. Journal of Applied Physiology 15: 377–382

Nocturnal Oxygen Therapy Trial Group 1980 Continuous or nocturnal oxygen therapy in hypoxemic chronic obstructive lung disease: a clinical trial. Annals of Internal Medicine 93: 391–398

Norregaard O, Schultz P, Ostergaard A, Dahl R 1989 Lung function and postural changes during pregnancy. Respiratory Medicine 83: 467–470

Nunn J F 1987 Applied respiratory physiology, 3rd edn. Butterworths, London, p 381–384, 430–439, 450–459

Pavia D, Thomson M L, Clarke S W 1978 Enhanced clearance of secretions from the human lung after the administration of hypertonic saline aerosol. American Review of Respiratory Disease 117: 199–203

Perpina M, Benlloch E, Marco V et al 1983 Effect of thoracentesis on pulmonary gas exchange. Thorax 38: 747–750

Poole-Wilson P A 1989 Chronic heart failure: Causes, pathophysiology, prognosis, clinical manifestations, investigations. In: Julian D G, Camm A J, Fox K M, Hall R J C, Poole-Wilson P A (eds) Diseases of the heart. Baillière Tindall, London, p 48–57

Rehder K, Southorn P A 1985 Influence of anaesthesia on the thorax. In: Roussos C, Macklem P T (eds) The thorax. Marcel Dekker, New York, vol 8, part B, p 923–938

Schoeffel R E, Anderson S D, Altounyon R E C 1981 Bronchial hyperactivity in response to inhalation of ultrasonically nebulised solutions of distilled water and saline. British Medical Journal 283: 1285–1287

Shneerson J M 1991 Non-invasive and domiciliary ventilation: negative pressure techniques. Thorax 46: 131–135

Simonneau G, Vivien A, Sartene R et al 1983 Diaphragm dysfunction induced by upper abdominal surgery. American Review of Respiratory Disease 128: 899–903

Singh S 1992 The use of field walking tests for assessment of functional capacity in patients with chronic airways disease. Physiotherapy 78: 102–104

Starke I D, Webber B A, Branthwaite M A 1979 IPPB and hypercapnia in respiratory failure: the effect of different concentrations of inspired oxygen on arterial blood gas tensions. Anaesthesia 34: 283–287

Stradling J R, Chadwick G A, Frew A F 1985 Changes in ventilation and its components in normal subjects during sleep. Thorax 40: 364–370

Sutton G C 1989 Symptoms of heart disease. In: Julian D G, Camm A J, Fox K M, Hall R J C, Poole-Wilson P A (eds) Diseases of the heart. Baillière Tindall, London, p 89–99

Terry P B, Traystman R J, Newball H H et al 1978 Collateral ventilation in man. New England Journal of Medicine 298: 10–15

Thomas P S, Cowen E R T, Hulands G, Milledge J S 1989 Respiratory function in the morbidly obese before and after weight loss. Thorax 44: 382–386

Tunstall Pedoe D S, Walker J M 1990 Cardiovascular disease. In: Souhami R L, Moxham J (eds) Textbook of medicine. Churchill Livingstone, Edinburgh, p 329–450

Weil J V, Byrne-Quinn E, Sodal I D et al 1970 Hypoxic ventilatory drive in normal man. Journal of Clinical Investigation 49: 1061–1072

West J B 1992 Pulmonary pathophysiology — the essentials, 4th edn. Williams and Wilkins, Baltimore

West J B 1990 Respiratory physiology — the essentials, 4th edn. Williams and Wilkins, Baltimore

Windsor J A, Hill G L 1988 Risk factors for post-operative pneumonia. Annals of Surgery 208: 209–214

Yoo O H, Ting E Y 1964 The effects of pleural effusion on pulmonary function. American Review of Respiratory Disease 89: 55–63

Zikria B A, Spencer J L, Kinney J M, Broell J R 1974 Alterations in ventilatory function and breathing patterns following surgical trauma. Annals of Surgery 179: 1–7

FURTHER READING

Lindsay K W, Bone I, Callander R 1986 Neurology and neurosurgery illustrated. Churchill Livingstone, Edinburgh

Souhami R L, Moxham J (eds) 1990 Textbook of medicine. Churchill Livingstone, Edinburgh

Patient groups with specific needs

12. Surgical patients and patients requiring intensive care

Marion Kieran   Patricia McCoy   Barbara A. Webber
Jennifer A. Pryor

INTRODUCTION

Many advances have been made in surgical procedures but surgery still carries considerable risk to
the patient, both adult and child. Children are
discussed in Chapter 13 (p. 281). The critically ill
surgical patient may require a period of time in an
intensive care unit.

The intensive care unit provides highly specialized care for high risk patients. Examples of
patients requiring admission to an intensive care
unit and possibly intubation and mechanical
ventilation are:

- Trauma
  - head injury
  - chest injuries
  - multiple trauma
- Post-surgery
  - *planned*: major thoracoabdominal surgery,
    major cardiac surgery, major vascular
    surgery, some high risk patients, organ
    transplantation surgery
  - *unplanned*: emergency surgery in high risk
    patients, emergency major surgery,
    complications following planned surgery
- Burns
- Acute lung pathology
  - acute severe asthma
  - adult respiratory distress syndrome
  - fat embolism (following fractures)
- Neuromuscular disorders
  - Guillain–Barré syndrome
  - tetanus
- Drug overdose.

Admission to an intensive care unit is normally
confined to patients who will benefit from assisted

ventilation and/or the specialist care provided
within the unit. The team staffing a unit is usually
under the direction of an intensivist, anaesthetist
or trauma specialist who coordinates the many
specialists who are involved in patient care.

On admission to an intensive care unit the
patient is assessed and his immediate needs are
identified. Illness severity scoring systems such as
the Acute Physiology and Chronic Health
Evaluation II (APACHE II) (Knaus et al 1985)
are used to quantify the severity of illness, to
determine the success of different forms of treatment and to predict mortality. The APACHE II
system takes account of the patient's chronological age, the reason for admission, any pre-existing
organ system insufficiency and the worst score
taken from 12 physiological variables during the
initial 24 hours: temperature, mean arterial
pressure, heart rate, respiratory rate,
alveolar–arterial oxygen gradient, arterial pH,
serum sodium, potassium and creatinine, haematocrit leucocyte count and the Glasgow coma score
(Frisby 1990). The APACHE III prognostic
system has been developed to further improve the
prediction of hospited mortality risk in critically ill
adults (Knaus et al 1991).

The physiotherapist must consider the general
condition of the patient and must remember the
possible feelings and fears that he may have in his
unnatural surroundings. Asbury (1985) under-
took a survey of patients' memories of their
experiences in intensive care units and showed
that greater attention should be given to some
aspects of care. Areas of concern were the
inability to speak, little information about their
treatment and loss of perception of time. An
intensive care unit is extremely busy and often

noisy and, as far as possible, attempts should be made to distinguish between day and night, and at night to give the patient the opportunity to sleep. Sleep is essential to maintain physical and psychological functions (Hamilton-Farrell & Hanson 1990). Normal feeding will probably not be possible, but it is essential to provide adequate nutrition to meet the needs of all tissues and vital organs.

Physiotherapy should be timed to coincide with the administration of analgesia and sedation, and turning of the patient. It is essential to remember the total needs of the patient and to explain before starting treatment, even to the unconscious or ventilated patient, the procedures that are going to be carried out. Constant reassurance, especially before taking a patient off a ventilator and before and during suction, should also be given. Staff should take care to avoid general conversation during treatment. Communication systems for use by the conscious patient should be available and a constant reminder of the time helps to orientate the patient.

SURGICAL PATIENTS

Types of anaesthesia

The administration of anaesthesia is not without risk, and in the preoperative assessment the anaesthetist will take note of the patient's general health and particularly any cardiac, respiratory or renal problems. Any adverse reaction such as unexplained jaundice or prolonged apnoea following a previous anaesthetic will influence the choice of anaesthesia.

General anaesthesia

General anaesthesia is administered, by inhalation or intravenously, to achieve a reversible loss of awareness and temporary blocking of response to stimulation such as movement of skeletal muscle and the autonomic effects such as tachycardia and hypertension (Forrest et al 1991). Inhalation anaesthesia is the most common, but its disadvantages are that it irritates bronchial mucosa, increases bronchial secretion, inhibits ciliary movement and reduces lung compliance.

Local anaesthesia

Local anaesthesia involves the use of a local anaesthetic to block the transmission of impulses along sensory nerve fibres by altering the permeability of the nerve membrane. It is widely used for minor surgical procedures and has the advantage of reducing postoperative risk of pulmonary complications. Local anaesthesia also has considerable value in controlling postoperative pain (Forrest et al 1991).

Spinal and epidural anaesthesia

Spinal and epidural anaesthesia involves the injection of local anaesthetic agents, such as lignocaine or bupivacaine, into the subarachnoid or epidural spaces. For spinal anaesthesia the agent is injected through a lumbar puncture needle inserted between L3 and L4. Leakage of cerebral spinal fluid may occur and this can cause headache. The patient should lie flat in bed for at least 12 hours after the spinal anaesthesia.

Epidural anaesthesia is administered by a needle inserted into the epidural space. A fine catheter can be inserted through the needle before it is withdrawn and this permits the continuous infusion of local anaesthesia to control postoperative pain. This mode of anaesthesia is often used during surgical procedures to the pelvis and legs.

Regional anaesthesia

Regional anaesthesia is induced by injecting a dilute solution of local anaesthetic into a vein while the limb is kept ischaemic by a tourniquet. This method is often used to reduce closed fractures and for other simple surgical procedures on the extremities. The anaesthetic effect lasts for 30–60 min.

Incisional sites

There are common incisional sites (Fig. 12.1) but surgeons will have individual variations.

Sutures

There are two main types of suture: non-absorbable and absorbable. Non-absorbable

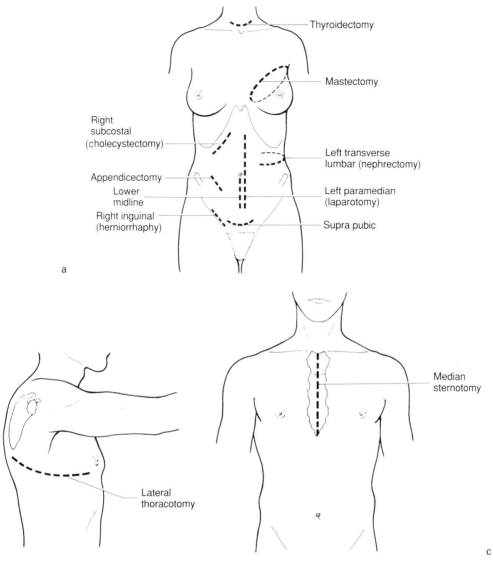

Fig. 12.1   a Common surgical incisions — anterior view. **b** Lateral thoracotomy. The incision passes approximately 5 cm below the angle of the scapula and lies below the breast tissue. It passes through latissimus dorsi and serratus anterior and the rib cage is opened through the sixth intercostal space. The excision may be extended anteriorly, i.e. anterolateral thoracotomy or posteriorly, i.e. posterolateral thoracotomy. **c** Median sternotomy. This is an anterior midline incision through the presternal aponeurosis and the upper rectal sheath with longitudinal division of the sternum. It extends from the substernal notch to approximately 4 cm below the xiphisternum. Closure of the median sternotomy requires five or six steel wire sutures to achieve firm apposition of the sternal bone, together with normal suturing of the soft tissue layers.

sutures are braided natural fibres (e.g. silk), synthetic monofilaments, nylon, prolene, or braided synthetics (e.g. mersiline, ethibond, braided nylon). Absorbable sutures such as catgut, Dexon, Vicryl are rarely used for skin closure.

The recommended times for suture removal (Forrest et al 1991) are:

- Face and neck 4 days
- Scalp 7 days
- Abdomen and chest 7–10 days
- Limbs 7 days
- Feet 10–14 days

Good cosmetic results are obtained by removing sutures in half of the above times and replacing them with adhesive strips, e.g. Steristrip, Clearol.

High risk factors in surgical patients

Preoperative assessment is essential to identify any factors which may lead to complications after surgery.

Pre-existing respiratory disorder

Patients with chronic chest disease are at risk of developing postoperative respiratory complications. These include patients with bronchiectasis and cystic fibrosis who have excess bronchial secretions and patients who have compromised lung function, either obstructive or restrictive, for example patients with chronic bronchitis, emphysema, asthma, pulmonary fibrosis or chest deformity.

Smoking

Chronic cigarette smoking causes damage to the ciliated epithelium and increases the risk of postoperative alveolar collapse (Rigg 1981). Garibaldi et al (1981) found that the risk of developing postoperative pneumonia in patients with chronic obstructive pulmonary disease was doubled by smoking. Patients should be encouraged to cease smoking when the decision is made to operate, and the longer the interval between cessation of smoking and operation the lower the risk of postoperative complications (Forrest et al 1991).

Obesity

The obese patient has a higher incidence of pulmonary complications following surgery than normal subjects. Obesity, particularly when combined with immobility in the supine position, predisposes the patient to inadequate lung expansion with resultant small airway closure and retention of secretions (p. 205).

Patient age

Musculoskeletal changes in the rib cage with ageing decrease the potential expansion of the lungs (Ham & Marcy 1983). Muscle fibres decrease in strength and the decrease in the number of muscle motor units influences the functional patterns by decreasing coordination and speed of muscle contraction (Lewis & Bottomley 1990). The incidence of osteoporosis of the ribcage and vertebrae increases and calcification of the costal cartilages occurs. With age the lungs become less elastic and the alveolar capillary membrane thickens and air ducts increase in size. Response to hypercapnia is reduced (Peterson et al 1981). These changes combine to reduce the respiratory reserve capacity with advancing age.

Cardiovascular disease

Atherosclerosis and ischaemic heart disease are common in the older patient. It is advisable for all patients over the age of 55 years to have a preoperative electrocardiogram (ECG). Patients with clinical signs of cardiac failure are carefully assessed and the operation is delayed until it has been corrected by digitalization and diuretics (Forrest et al 1991). Cardiac arrhythmias occurring preoperatively may be due to myocardial ischaemia, although ventricular extrasystoles can be a feature of sudden withdrawal of nicotine in a patient who is a heavy smoker (Forrest et al 1991).

Haemophilia

Operations in patients with haemophilia are potentially dangerous. The level of antihaemophilic globulin (factor VIII) must be kept between 30 and 40% of normal, by transfusions of fresh blood or plasma or concentrates of human antihaemophilic globulin.

Care must be taken in patients with bleeding disorders so that bleeding is not precipitated, particularly if suctioning is required.

Nutritional status

Poor nutritional status has been shown to cause an increased incidence of pneumonia in the postoperative patient. Protein and vitamin deficiencies impair the synthesis of collagen and delay the healing of wounds. Dehiscence of wounds and disruption of anastomoses are more common in the malnourished patient (Forrest et al 1991). The impaired production of antibodies reduces the patient's resistance to infection. The patient's nutritional state should be improved before surgery if possible, otherwise full nutritional support must be given postoperatively. This is achieved by the use of oral dietary supplements. If oral feeding is not possible, as in patients with gastric or oesophageal obstruction, enteral feeding via a nasogastric tube or by gastrostomy is necessary. If oral and enteral feeding is inadequate or impossible, intravenous (parenteral) feeding is indicated. Malnutrition causes an increase in muscle fatigue and alters the pattern of muscle contraction and relaxation (Lopes et al 1982).

Alcohol abuse

Alcoholics are susceptible to malnourishment and it is advisable that their nutritional state be improved before surgery by an adequate calorie intake and multivitamins. Liver function tests are carried out and, if abnormal, the prothrombin time is assessed; if it is prolonged vitamin K is given.

Patients with a history of alcohol abuse require larger doses of anaesthesia. Withdrawal symptoms can cause problems postoperatively and include disorientation, hallucinations, tremor, sleep disturbance and autonomic disturbances. Sedation is important and is achieved by the administration of diazepam (Valium) and chlormethiazole (Heminevrin) (Forrest et al 1991). Phosphate depletion associated with hypoventilation and muscle weakness may be a cause of pulmonary complications in alcoholic subjects who are given intravenous dextrose and gastric antacids which contain magnesium and aluminium (Newman et al 1977).

Mental changes

Elderly patients often become disorientated in a strange environment, especially at night, but it must always be remembered that it may indicate hypoxia. Mental changes occur in septicaemia (toxic psychoses) and may be the first sign of septicaemic shock (Forrest et al 1991). Surgery that causes mutilation or alters body image, e.g. mastectomy, can cause depression. Anxiety causes diaphragmatic splinting and increases the surgical risk and extends the hospitalization period.

Diabetes

Diabetic patients are normally admitted 1–2 days prior to surgery to ensure that there is adequate control. General anaesthesia may induce ketosis which can be further affected by starvation (preoperative fasting) and the trauma of surgery.

Factors which may complicate the postoperative period

Incisional site

Upper abdominal surgery causes reflex inhibition of the diaphragm and increases the risk of respiratory complications (Simonneau et al 1983). Following upper abdominal surgery, patients have more pulmonary problems than those following lower abdominal surgery (Dureuil et al 1987). The reduced tidal excursion of the lung close to the diaphragm leads to subsegmental lung collapse, infection and retention of secretions in the basal lung areas (Ford & Guenter 1984). Vertical incisions impede mobility because movement produces increased strain on the wound compared with the strain exerted on transverse incisions (Garcia-Valdecasas et al 1988).

Postoperative pain

Regular assessment of pain is essential for effective pain control (Gould et al 1992). Pain is an important factor in reducing lung volume and inhibiting the clearance of bronchial secretions (p. 201). It may cause defensive spasm of the trunk muscles and inhibit breathing.

The control of pain by effective narcotic drug therapy results in improved ventilation and gas exchange. Patient controlled analgesia (PCA) allows small self-administered doses of an analgesic, to be delivered as required, to maintain adequate and constant pain control. Some studies indicate a reduction in the amount of drug required when the technique is compared with intramuscular injections (Lange et al 1988) and an increase in ambulation and cooperation, associated with a decrease in hospital stay (White 1988). Other studies report that intermittent intramuscular injections given on a regular basis and continuous intravenous infusions may be as effective as PCA (Kleiman et al 1988, Gould et al 1992).

Reduction in functional residual capacity

Patient position affects functional residual capacity. It is greatest in the upright sitting position and is probably greater in side lying than either slumped sitting or supine lying (Jenkins et al 1988). Positional change for the postsurgical patient and early ambulation are important (Jenkins et al 1989).

Indwelling tubes and drains

Drains are used in the drainage of air and fluid and in contaminated wounds. The presence of drains, tubes and drips increase patient anxiety and discomfort. A nasogastric tube frequently interferes with coughing and expectoration. Care must be taken to prevent kinking or dislodgement of drainage tubes, and particularly when the patient's position is changed.

Deep venous thrombosis and pulmonary embolus

A deep venous thrombosis (DVT) is a clot which forms in a deep vein and if the veins of the pelvis or lower limb are involved there is a serious risk of pulmonary embolus (PE). This may be fatal.

Important risk factors which predispose a patient to the development of DVT are previous history of DVT or PE, advanced age, malignant disease, varicose veins, venous stasis, obesity, oral contraceptives and hypercoagulability of the blood. For reasons not fully understood, smokers have a lower risk of postoperative DVT than do non-smokers (Forrest et al 1991). Operations which carry a high risk of developing DVT are hip reconstruction, spinal operations, major abdom-

inal or pelvic operations and operations associated with malignancy, sepsis and trauma. The diagnosis of DVT is difficult and it is frequently asymptomatic, especially in the first few days. The principal symptoms are tenderness, swelling and increased warmth of the calf and a positive Homans' sign (pain in the calf on dorsiflexion of the foot). Differential diagnosis includes lymphoedema, dependent oedema, tumour obstruction cellulitis, muscle strain and arterial occlusion. If DVT is suspected, many non-invasive tests are available, including directional Doppler ultrasound, but the most accurate test is phlebography when a non-irritant contrast medium is injected into the vein on the dorsum of each foot or the femoral veins. This will show up the extent of the thrombosis. A lung scan will determine whether the clot is embolizing. Treatment of acute DVT is aimed at relieving the acute symptoms, protecting against pulmonary embolism and facilitating resolution.

A commonly used treatment regimen is the application of graduated elastic stockings combined with intravenous administration of a bolus of heparin followed by a constant infusion to increase the partial prothrombin time to 2–3 times above normal. After a few days, oral anticoagulation (warfarin) is started and is continued for several months. Heparin is discontinued.

If phlebography indicates the presence of thrombus in the femoral or iliac veins, embolism can be averted by inserting a filter into the inferior vena cava percutaneously via the femoral or jugular vein, alternatively fibrinolysis may be used.

Pulmonary embolism may occur if a venous thrombus becomes dislodged. Sudden onset of severe breathlessness is the most common sign and it may be followed by pleuritic or central chest pain, cyanosis, haemoptysis and collapse. Pulmonary angiography may be used to confirm the diagnosis. Heparin is administered for 7–10 days and warfarin is started a few days before heparin is stopped and continued for 3–6 months. Occasionally, embolectomy is carried out using cardiopulmonary bypass. The incidence of fatal pulmonary embolism postoperatively varies between 0.1% and 0.8% and is relatively uncommon in ambulant patients (Dalen et al 1986).

Prophylactic treatment with low dose heparin is often used for high risk patients. Some centres apply thromboembolic deterrent stockings routinely after major surgery to try and prevent the occurrence of DVT.

Renal function

Retention of urine can impair diaphragmatic excursion. Hypotension must be avoided postoperatively because of its detrimental affect on renal function. Protracted periods of poor kidney perfusion after surgery will result in acute renal failure. It can be caused by sepsis and hypovolaemia. Adequate fluid replacement is important to maintain a urine output of at least 30–40 ml/hour. Elderly patients are particularly susceptible to impaired renal function and to the development of acute tubular necrosis.

Stress

The development of superficial ulcers in the duodenum or stomach can occur as a result of surgery, severe illness or injury. Ulceration of the stomach or duodenum after neurosurgical illness or surgery (Cushing's ulcer) and duodenal ulceration in patients who have suffered severe burns (Curling's ulcer) are specific forms of stress ulcer. Patients are stressed by illness and this can be a serious contributor to delayed patient recovery (Swann 1989). Gastric secretion is suppressed by the use of such drugs as Zantac to prevent and heal stress lesions.

Physiotherapy for the surgical patient

Patients at risk from postoperative complications should be identified and when possible seen preoperatively by a physiotherapist. Assessment (p. 3) and reassessment until physiotherapy is no longer indicated are the keys to effective management.

Preoperative assessment. This will identify any pre-existing problems and potential problems. Pre-existing problems, for example excess bronchial secretions and reversible airflow obstruction, should be treated. The effects of the anaesthetic and surgical procedures are outlined in order that the patient has an understanding of the importance of postoperative breathing exercises and early ambulation.

Instruction in breathing techniques, including breathing control, thoracic expansion exercises with a hold at full inspiration, and the forced expiration technique (the active cycle of breathing techniques, p. 116), and instruction in wound support should be given. The patient should be reassured that the effort required for huffing or coughing will not harm the stitches, drainage tubes or operation site, and that analgesia will be given for pain control.

Postoperative assessment. Problems likely to be identified include:

- pain
- difficulty in clearing bronchial secretions
- reduced mobility.

A treatment plan is formulated for the individual patient's problems. Pain should always be controlled by appropriate analgesia.

Positioning can be used to counter the postoperative reduction in functional residual capacity, and as soon as possible patients should be encouraged to sit upright and out of bed in a chair, rather than in a slumped position. Positioning can also be used to improve ventilation and perfusion.

Early ambulation will minimize postoperative complications (Bourn & Jenkins 1992). For many patients this will be either on the day of surgery or on the first postoperative day.

Sometimes a mechanical adjunct, for example periodic continuous positive airway pressure or intermittent positive pressure breathing, can be used to increase lung volume and to assist in the clearance of excess bronchial secretions.

GENERAL SURGERY

Cholecystectomy

Patients with an acute attack of cholecystitis frequently require urgent cholecystectomy, but operations are usually delayed for up to 72 hours or 6 weeks after an attack of acute cholecystitis

(Forrest et al 1991). The surgical treatment of gallstones involves removal of the gallbladder and its stones and may be the open procedure, but in recent years the technique of laparoscopic cholecystectomy (which is less invasive) has been developed.

Open cholecystectomy

For open cholecystectomy the gallbladder is approached through a right subcostal paramedian or midline incision. Following the surgical procedure a T-tube is inserted in the incision and left in situ for approximately 48 hours to permit drainage of bile or blood into a drainage bag. A nasogastric tube, which may interfere with coughing, is passed and connected to a drainage bag. Many surgeons do not permit patients to drink while a nasogastric tube is in situ, but others allow the drinking of small measured amounts at regulated intervals. The main abdominal postoperative complications are the slow recovery of intestinal motor function (peristalsis), leakage at the operation site, occult bleeding or abscess formation. The presence of bowel sounds and the free passage of flatus indicate return of peristaltic activity.

Pulmonary complications can result from the diaphragmatic dysfunction associated with upper abdominal surgery (Simonneau et al 1983). It is suggested that the reduced tidal excursion leads to retention of secretions and subsegmental collapse of the right lower lobe.

Physiotherapy key points
• The nasogastric tube should be aspirated before chest physiotherapy.
• Effective breathing exercises will minimize subsegmental lung collapse, the right lower lobe being more susceptible.
• Many of these patients tend to be overweight. This causes reduced lung compliance and decreased lung volumes, and can predispose to postoperative pneumonia (Garibaldi et al 1981).

Laparoscopic cholecystectomy

Sauerbruch & Paumgartner (1991) estimate that 80% of all patients undergoing elective cholecys-

tectomy are suitable for the laparoscopic technique which involves the use of a laparoscope and insertion of instruments through trocars. This minimal access approach avoids the traditional incision and its inherent problems. Wolfe et al (1991) claim that the advantages of this technique are less pain, early ambulation, reduced hospital stay, a faster return to work and a better cosmetic result. It minimizes the risk of respiratory complications and problems associated with immobilization, and physiotherapy may not be necessary. The main problem associated with the technique is injury to the bile duct and intestine which is not always immediately apparent following surgery. It is likely that the use of laparoscopic surgery will increase as it reduces costs and allows return to work and normal activity in 1 or 2 weeks.

In abdominal laparoscopic surgery, carbon dioxide is used to distend the abdominal wall, i.e. pneumoperitoneum, thus permitting the intestinal contents to drop away from the point of insertion of the trocar. Many patients complain of shoulder or chest pain following this procedure. This is due to irritation of the diaphragm by the insufflation of carbon dioxide (Dunnihoo 1990).

Laparoscopic techniques are also commonly used for appendicectomy, repair of duodenal ulcer and tubal ligation sterilization. Thoracic surgeons employ laparoscopes for pleurectomy and bullectomy.

Colostomy

This is an artificial opening in the large bowel which diverts the faeces to the exterior where they are collected in a disposable adhesive bag. The procedure is usually carried out because of obstruction or disease of the large intestine caused by carcinoma, Crohn's disease, diverticular disease or ulcerative colitis. A colostomy can be temporary or permanent. A temporary colostomy is often placed in the transverse colon and the permanent one is usually placed as distally as possible.

Ileostomy is similar to colostomy but the opening is on the right side of the lower abdominal cavity and involves more extensive resection of the colon than a colostomy. The most common reasons for ileostomy are ulcerative colitis or Crohn's disease.

Following resection of the rectum or lower sigmoid rectum a urinary catheter is usually inserted for 4–5 days. Patients who have a permanent colostomy may have problems adjusting to it. Most hospitals have specially trained nurses who educate and counsel patients in the management of their colostomy. All members of the team responsible for the care of the patient after a colostomy should help to allay the patient's fears and provide support and reassurance.

Many of the complications associated with colostomy are similar to those which follow cholecystectomy, for example a nasogastric tube and slow recovery of intestinal motor function. Pulmonary complications are less likely with lower abdominal wall surgery than with upper abdominal wall surgery because there is less reflex inhibition of the diaphragm (Dureuil et al 1987).

Gastrectomy

The incision is usually left paramedian or midline. A partial gastrectomy is a common treatment for gastric ulceration which fails to respond to medical treatment. Carcinoma of the stomach usually requires a total gastrectomy. Duodenal ulceration is usually treated by pyloroplasty or gastroenterostomy together with vagotomy. When there is duodenal and gastric ulceration the surgeon may perform a partial gastrectomy and vagotomy. The aim of vagotomy is to reduce acid and pepsin secretion.

A nasogastric tube is passed before surgery to ensure that the stomach remains empty and to prevent postoperative gastric distension. It is normally removed by the second postoperative day. The incision site will determine the degree to which lung expansion is restricted.

Physiotherapy key points
- Many of the patients requiring a gastrectomy are debilitated and fatigue easily. Treatments may have to be of short duration and given frequently.
- Effective breathing exercises will minimize subsegmental lung collapse, the left lower lobe being more susceptible.

Hernias

A hernia or rupture is a swelling caused by the protrusion of part of an organ or other tissue through an abnormal opening. It can affect any viscera, i.e. intestine, and can take its name from the organ involved, e.g. small bowel hernia, or from the aperture through which it has occurred, e.g. hiatus hernia (p. 262).

Abdominal hernias

Hernias occur at natural openings in the abdominal wall where structures enter and leave the abdominal cavity, e.g. inguinal and femoral canals and the umbilicus. Other hernias may protrude through an area of abdominal weakness which may be due to weakness of the abdominal muscles or linea alba.

An *inguinal hernia* can be direct or oblique (indirect) and consists of a protrusion of a peritoneal sac containing omentum or bowel. The oblique hernia is commonly congenital and passes through the length of the inguinal canal. The direct hernia projects through a weakness in the posterior wall of the canal medial to the internal ring and is often precipitated by increased intraabdominal pressure from coughing in patients with chronic airflow limitation, obesity, chronic constipation or strain on lifting.

For the direct hernia a herniorrhaphy is performed which involves reducing the herniation and repairing the weakness in the posterior wall. In young children with oblique hernia, simple excision of the sac, i.e. herniotomy, is all that is required, but in older patients where the posterior wall of the canal is stretched and weakened repair of the weakness is required, i.e. herniorraphy.

The repair of inguinal hernia is often carried out as a day case, thus avoiding overnight hospitalization.

A *femoral hernia* projects through the femoral canal and pushes the extra-peritoneal fat and peritoneum through the femoral ring and down the femoral canal. It normally contains omentum, small bowel or both. It is more common in women and may be precipitated by stretching of the pelvic ligaments and widening of the femoral ring during pregnancy. A femoral hernia is particularly susceptible to strangulation and surgery is necessary.

A *strangulated hernia* occurs if the vessels supplying the loop of bowel contained in the hernia are compressed by the neck of the sac (common in inguinal hernia) or constriction of the femoral ring (common in femoral hernia). If a portion of the bowel has become gangrenous through devitalization, it is resected and the remainder is returned to the abdomen, the sac is excised and the hernia is repaired.

An *umbilical hernia* is more common in children but it can occur in older obese patients with weak abdominal muscles, particularly women who have had multiple pregnancies. The sac which protrudes through the linea alba may contain omentum and loops of large and/or small bowel. These can become constricted and strangulation of bowel is common. Surgery is necessary.

An *incisional hernia* occurs where the peritoneum and abdominal contents protrude through a weakened area in an abdominal scar from a previous operation, particularly if the wound had been infected. Midline vertical incisions are most often affected especially those below the umbilicus. Postoperative abdominal distension may be a precipitating factor. Surgery is necessary to repair the hernia.

Physiotherapy key points

• Patients with chronic airflow limitation in whom coughing may have been the precipitating factor in the development of an inguinal hernia will have an increased risk of developing pulmonary complications.

• Patients should be instructed in correct lifting techniques, particularly when the history indicates that lifting may have been a precipitating factor in causing the hernia. Heavy lifting should be avoided for 3 months and any lifting at all for at least 6 weeks.

Mastectomy

Mastectomy involves removal of part or the whole of one breast because of a malignant or benign growth. Breast cancer is the most common cancer affecting females in Western countries. Early diagnosis is essential for optimal treatment.

Benign growths can sometimes be removed without removing the whole breast and may cause minimal disfigurement. Malignant tumours require more extensive surgery and the extent of surgery is dependent on the stage of the disease. A *simple mastectomy* removes the breast and, if necessary, may include the removal of the axillary lymph nodes. A *radical mastectomy* removes the breast, lymph nodes and pectoral muscles. Radical mastectomy is performed less often now as the success rate is no greater than the less radical procedures (Forrest et al 1991). Radiotherapy and/or chemotherapy is frequently given after surgery.

Cancer of the breast may cause psychological stress. Many of the problems are related to the mutilation caused by mastectomy, but fear of the disease and uncertainty about the future play an equally important part. Good counselling is vital. The surgeon and specialist nurses should keep the patient informed about the nature of the disease, its treatment and the best type of prosthetic support. All members of the care team, including the physiotherapist, should be aware of the likely emotional distress of these patients and be supportive. Various forms of breast reconstruction are available. In its most simple form a prosthesis (i.e. silicone gel) is inserted under the pectoral muscles. If tissue loss is extensive it may be necessary to bring up a musculocutaneous flap of latissimus dorsi to form new skin covering for the prosthesis.

Physiotherapy key points

• The chest wall will be painful following surgery and the patient will be reluctant to breathe deeply or cough. Adequate analgesia is essential.

• The danger of developing a stiff shoulder postoperatively is possible, particularly if surgery has been extensive. Some surgeons prefer the arm not to be abducted for 1–2 days after surgery. Exercises should include shoulder shrugging, static deltoid contractions, hand and elbow exercises. Shoulder abduction and elevation is started as soon as the surgeon allows.

• Lymphoedema of the arm is a possible

complication of breast cancer particularly following radical surgery and radiotherapy. Intermittent compression with an inflatable plastic arm cuff and a supportive elastic stocking over the arm, are given together with full range active shoulder exercises.

Fractured femur in the elderly

Fracture of the neck of femur occurs mainly in elderly women whose bones are osteoporotic. The trauma can result from a fall or even as a result of a stumble, when the patient catches the foot, twists the hip and the rotational force breaks the neck of femur. There is marked displacement in most cases, though in others some of the fragments are impacted and the patient can walk but it is painful.

A patient's ability to withstand long periods of immobilization depends on their physiological age rather than their chronological age. The older the patient the greater the risks of prolonged immobilization. The elderly patient is particularly at risk of pneumonia, thromboembolism and decubitus ulceration.

Displaced fractures will not unite without internal fixation and as impacted fractures can become displaced surgery is necessary. Operative treatment permits accurate reduction, secure fixation and early mobilization. If the fracture cannot be correctly reduced it is necessary to perform a hemiarthroplasty or a total hip replacement. There is a high incidence of avascular necrosis in fractured neck of femur, particularly if the fracture has been displaced and total hip replacement is required.

Intertrochanteric fractures are also common in the elderly, particularly in women who have osteoporosis. Such fractures are almost always the result of a fall. Unlike the intracapsular neck fractures, the extracapsular trochanteric fractures unite well and seldom cause avascular necrosis. These fractures are almost always treated by internal fixation with the use of an angled plate and screws which permits early mobilization with partial weight bearing on the second or third postoperative day.

Following the surgical treatment of fractures of the proximal end of the femur in the elderly, patients sit out in a chair on the first postoperative day and begin walking with a frame or crutches on the second postoperative day.

Femoral shaft fractures though more common in the young adult do occur in the elderly patient. The 'closed' treatment entails reduction and prolonged skeletal traction.

It is important to relieve pressure over an area of skin which lies close to the bone, to prevent tissue necrosis. This can cause decubitus ulcer formation which can lead to damage of muscle, bone and skin, and cause infection. There is also an increased risk of deep vein thromboses in these patients.

Physiotherapy key points
- As most of these patients are elderly there is an increased risk of developing pulmonary complications and the active cycle of breathing techniques can be used to minimize these.
- With the high risk of circulatory complications, leg exercises are important until frequent ambulation is possible.
- A home visit will highlight adaptations and the support required to assist the patient to return to their usual life-style.

GYNAECOLOGICAL SURGERY

Hysterectomy

Total hysterectomy involves removal of the uterus and one or both fallopian tubes (salpingectomy). One or both ovaries (oophorectomy) may also be removed if indicated. An extended operation, i.e. Wertheim's hysterectomy, includes removal of the uterus, fallopian tubes, ovaries and a lymphadenectomy. Hysterectomy is carried out through an abdominal or vaginal route. The abdominal incision is usually a lower midline or transverse suprapubic, i.e. 'bikini' incision, although it is sometimes necessary to use a vertical median or paramedian incision.

Hysterectomy is used for the management of benign disease such as dysfunctional uterine bleeding when the use of hormone replacement therapy (HRT) has failed or for the removal of a large uterine cyst or ovarian endometriomal cysts. It is also the treatment of choice for endometrial carcinoma and carcinoma of the cervix.

Repair procedures

Repair procedures are corrective surgical procedures for uterine prolapse. Prolapse is a type of
herniation which occurs if there is failure of the
supporting structures of the muscular vagina and
transverse cervical ligaments. Prolapse is most
common at the menopause when muscular
atrophy occurs, although it can occur in
premenopausal women. Consequently, operative
repair procedures are more common in patients
over the age of 45 years.

Vaginal prolapse may damage the anterior wall
of the vagina with resultant herniation of the
bladder (cystocele). Damage to the posterior wall
can cause herniation of the rectum (rectocele).

Uterovaginal prolapse is a more extensive
prolapse of the vagina and it is equally associated
with the development of cystocele and rectocele.

Colporrhaphy is the repair procedure of the
vagina. Anterior colporrhaphy includes repair for
cystocele and posterior includes repair for rectocele. *Manchester repair* combines colporrhaphy
with amputation of the cervix and shortening of
the transverse ligaments.

Physiotherapy key points

• There is an increased incidence of deep
venous thrombosis in pelvic surgery and particular attention should be given to early ambulation, and leg exercises if the patient is not able to
walk several times a day.

• Pelvic tilting is performed slowly to prevent
protective muscle spasm in abdominal and back
muscles which can cause increased pain. Gentle
abdominal exercises help to restore abdominal
muscle tone. Both exercises are normally started
following the removal of the drains.

• Pelvic floor exercises are given to restore
muscle tone (Laycock 1987). Following hysterectomy and some repair operations, catheterization
is commonly required for up to 48 hours to drain
the bladder and allow resting of the repaired
tissue. Many surgeons prefer pelvic floor exercises
to be delayed until the catheter is removed.

• A list of graduated exercises to strengthen the
back and abdominal muscles should include
crook lying with knee rolling, proceeding eventually to crook lying with a sit up. Pulling and
pushing heavy objects should be avoided for 2–3
months and the lifting or carrying of anything
other than light objects should be avoided for at
least 6 weeks.

• Correct lifting techniques should be demonstrated with particular emphasis on holding the
object close to the body, feet apart, back straight
and using the legs to lift. The surgeon will advise
the patient on return to work and the period can
vary from 6 to 12 weeks depending on the nature
of the patient's occupation. Normally, after 12
weeks the patient is free to return to her usual
lifestyle, although it is important to take care
while performing heavy household tasks and
sports activities for at least 1 year after surgery.

SURGERY FOR THE LUNGS, CHEST WALL AND PLEURA

Many thoracic surgical procedures and traumatic
conditions require intercostal drainage. This
allows continuous drainage of air or fluid through
a tube. Two types of drainage are used: open and
closed.

Open drainage

A small tube is inserted into a pocket of fluid, e.g.
pus as in empyema, which drains into a plastic
drainage bag. This allows the patient to be
ambulant.

Closed drainage

This is used to drain air and/or fluid from the
pleural cavity. This type of drainage using a water
seal (Fig. 12.2) is necessary following thoracic
surgery to maintain the pleural cavity as a potential space. The one-way mechanism prevents air
or fluid from entering the pleural space.

An unobstructed chest tube of adequate
diameter, with eyelets in the patient end of the
tube, is placed inside the pleural cavity and passes
down to a tight fitting connector on the container
neck. This is connected to a rigid tube inside the
container which is below the water level, i.e.
underwater seal. This system allows fluid and
gas/air to leave the chest and at the same time
prevents fluid or gas/air movement into the
pleural cavity. The water seal container must be

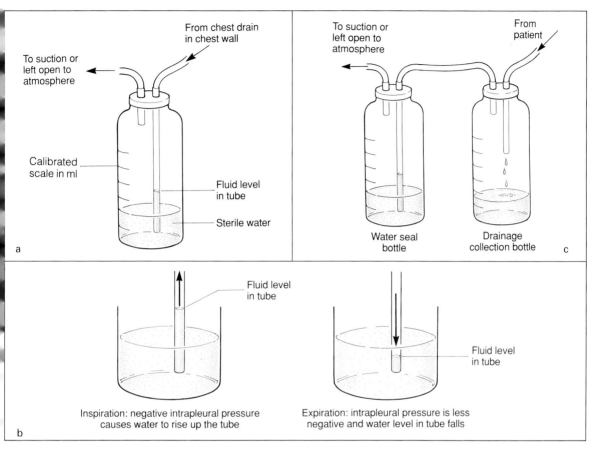

Fig. 12.2 Chest drainage. **a** Underwater seal drain. **b** Oscillation of fluid level with drainage bottle open to the atmosphere. **c** Two-compartment drainage system.

vented to prevent a build up of pressure within it and must be positioned below the level of the chest.

Water seal drainage systems can have one, two or three compartments. With the simplest form (Fig. 12.2a) one bottle serves as a collection container and a water seal. In a two-compartment system (Fig. 12.2c) fluid flows into one container from a chest tube (basal tube) and air flows, usually from a second tube (apical tube), through to the second container. Both containers have underwater seals. This system permits accurate observation of the volume and type of drainage. Another method consists of both tubes (apical and basal) being connected to a Y-piece and connected to a single water seal bottle.

Venting of the container to atmosphere, allows fluid to drain by gravity. Air flow is governed by the relationship of intrapleural pressure to atmospheric pressure. When the pressure in the pleural cavity is below atmospheric pressure (during inspiration), the water level will rise slightly in the water seal and when the pressure is above atmospheric pressure (during expiration), air will flow into the drainage container (Fig. 12.2b). Pressures below atmospheric pressures can be achieved in the water seal container by connecting the venting tube to a suction apparatus. This improves air evacuation from the pleural space by creating a pressure that is less on the non-patient side of the water seal. The suction action decreases the threshold at which the water seal acts as a one-way valve.

Fluctuations in the level of the water column (i.e. the rigid tube inside the underwater container) reflect the changes in pleural pressure.

In a system that is not connected to suction a lack of fluctuation with the breathing pattern may be an indication that the tube is obstructed either by a clot or kinking of the tube, or expanded lung tissue may have blocked the eyelets.

Milking (stripping) of the tubing using rollers is used to re-establish tube patency. The tube is compressed by the rollers and in their release a pulse of suction is created which clears the blockage. This procedure is indicated when the tube appears to be obstructed by clotting blood. If the tube is impinging on lung tissue, the suture holding it to the chest wall is released and the tube is withdrawn a few centimetres to establish patency and the tube is resutured to the chest wall.

Clamping of chest tubing is performed when there is the need to identify an air leak, to replace the drainage containers, if the drain has been inserted following a pneumonectomy, or during chemical pleurodesis. It is also indicated if the tubes become detached from the container in which case they must be quickly reconnected and unclamped. Patients with pleural leaks are at risk of developing a tension pneumothorax when the tubing is clamped and this should be done only for very short periods of time.

Patients can be ambulant with indwelling chest tubes (if they are not connected to a suction pump), if the bottle/containers are hand held below the level of entry of the chest tubes to the pleural cavity. Alternatively, the containers can be placed on a low level trolley to facilitate ambulation (Fig. 12.3).

Failure of closed chest drainage to maintain the normal negative pressure (-5 to -20 cmH$_2$O) in the pleural cavity will lead to collapse of the underlying lung. The positive pressure in one hemithorax will push the mediastinum to the opposite (i.e. unaffected) lung causing further impairment of respiratory function. Consequently, inadequate pleural drainage following surgery can lead to problems in both lungs.

If only blood is expected to drain, a drainage tube placed just above the diaphragm is sufficient. If air leakage is anticipated, a second tube is inserted through a separate incision and placed so that its tip lies high in the pleural cavity (Fig. 12.4). When two drains are inserted, to avoid

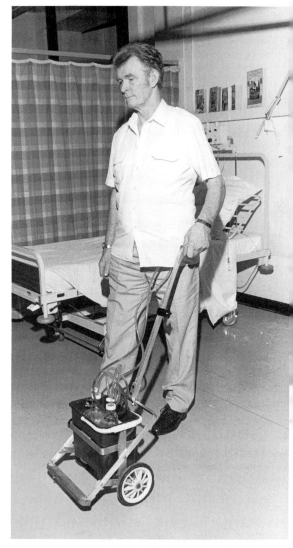

Fig. 12.3   Ambulation with trolley for drainage bottles. (Reproduced with permission of the Royal Brompton Hospital.)

confusion, they are frequently labelled A for the apical tube to drain air, normally placed anteriorly to another tube, and B for the basal tube, normally placed towards the back to drain blood and other fluids.

Usually when suction is applied, low negative pressures of -5 to -10 mmHg will promote fluid drainage, while higher pressures of -30 mmHg are frequently necessary to drain air leaks.

Chest drainage usually ceases after a few days and the drains are removed with the precaution of

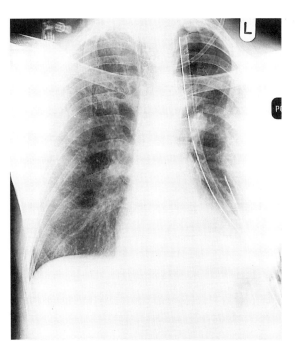

Fig. 12.4 Chest radiograph showing apical and basal chest drains.

pre- and post-removal chest radiographs to ensure that the lung remains expanded. Drainage may have to be continued for a longer period, especially in the emphysematous patient, until all air leakage has ceased.

Important observations

Air leakage. If bubbles continue after the lung has re-expanded there is an air leak arising from a hole in the tubing. Alternatively, if the patient is asked to take a deep breath and cough, and bubbles appear, there is a continuing air leak.

Oscillation of water in the drainage container. When suction is used the water level remains constant, but if there is no suction the water level rises on inspiration and falls on expiration. When the lung is fully expanded oscillation ceases in the drainage container. If oscillation ceases at an inappropriate early stage it is likely to indicate tube blockage or kinking. A chest radiograph will indicate the degree of lung expansion.

Failure of chest drainage.
- The drain is not correctly located in the pleural cavity or it is incorrectly connected to the underwater drainage container

- The fluid and/or air is accumulating at a rate greater than that at which it can be removed and suction must be increased
- The underlying lung is incapable of expansion because of retained bronchial secretions
- Lung expansion may be prevented by pus or solid fibrous slough which accompanies an empyema.

Removal of drains

1. If the chest drain was inserted to drain fluid, it is removed when fluid drainage is 10–20 ml/hour or less.

2. Tubes draining pus are removed slowly, for example about 5 cm every week, depending on the extent of the empyema. The tube is shortened externally and allowed to drain into a bag if drainage has to be prolonged. Removal of the tube for empyema is only begun when there is evidence that the underlying lung is fully expanded.

3. Air drainage tubes are removed when the lung is fully re-expanded and there is no evidence of an air leak. In young patients with a spontaneous pneumothorax the drain usually stops bubbling in approximately 24 hours. Many older patients have severe underlying lung disease such as emphysema and the diseased lung is slower to re-expand and the tube may be required for some weeks. When the leak does stop a clamp may be put on the drain for a period of 12–24 hours and a repeat chest radiograph is used to confirm that the underlying lung has remained expanded before the drain is removed. If the lung does not remain inflated, the tube is unclamped and a further period of drainage is required.

Portable closed chest drainage devices

These, for example the Heimlich valve, can be used for a persistent small air leak to encourage ambulation. The disadvantage is that they do not allow for monitoring of the air leak and a water seal drain should probably be used at night.

Lung surgery

Resection of the lung or a part of the lung may be performed for excision of a malignant or benign tumour, sequestrated lobe or localized bronchiectasis. A bullectomy may be performed for bullous lung disease which severely restricts lung function. Types of lung resection include lobectomy, sleeve resection, segmental or wedge resection and pneumonectomy.

A double lumen endotracheal tube is used to maintain gas exchange during lung resection. This allows continued ventilation of the unaffected lung while the affected lung is collapsed during surgery.

Most lung operations are performed through a posterolateral or anterolateral thoracotomy incision (Fig. 12.1b). A *posterolateral* incision follows the vertebral border of the scapula and the line of a rib (usually the sixth rib) so that it lies below the angle of the scapula and below the tissues of the breast. The muscles incised are trapezius, latissimus dorsi, rhomboids, serratus anterior, intercostals and erector spinae. The ribs are usually retracted, but a rib may be removed or 2–4 cm of a rib may be resected to facilitate easy access to the thorax to prevent the risk of rib fracture.

An *anterolateral* incision starts close to the midline in front, continues along the line of a rib, below the breast to the posterior axillary line and cuts through pectoralis major and minor, serratus anterior and the internal and external intercostal muscles.

A *median sternotomy* (Fig. 12.1c) involves dividing the sternum longitudinally in the midline and no muscles are cut other than the aponeuroses of pectoralis major.

Lung cancer

The term 'lung cancer' covers a number of specific malignancies. There are four major cell types:

- squamous (epidermoid) cell (45–55% of the total)
- adenocarcinoma (20%)
- small cell (oat cell) (20%)
- poorly differentiated large cell (15%) (Forrest et al 1991).

The cause of lung cancer is unclear. However, three major risk factors are known to play a major part in the development of the disease:

- cigarette smoking
- industrial risks such as exposure to asbestos, uranium, radioactive isotopes, arsenic or chromates
- air pollution such as sulphur dioxide.

There is a higher incidence of lung cancer in men than in women, although the incidence in women is increasing. It is the most common cause of death from cancer in both sexes and occurs most commonly in the age range 50–60 years (Forrest et al 1991).

In the investigation of a lung lesion it is important to establish whether the lesion is malignant. If it is malignant, the cell type and whether there is intrathoracic or extrathoracic spread must be determined.

The American Joint Committee (1977) has designed a staging classification for lung cancer which is based on a TNM system:

T relates to the characteristics of the tumour
N relates to the regional hilar and mediastinal nodal metastases
M relates to the distant haematogenous metastases.

A T_1 lesion is a solitary nodule of less than 3 cm in its greatest diameter, surrounded by normal lung and without bronchoscopic evidence of invasion proximal to a lobar bronchus.

A T_2 lesion is greater than 3 cm in diameter or a tumour of any size which with its associated lung collapse or obstructive pneumonitis, extends to the hilar region. On bronchoscopy the lesion must be further than 2 cm from the carina and there must not be any evidence of intrathoracic spread.

A T_3 lesion is one of any size with intrathoracic spread (i.e. chest wall, pleura, diaphragm, pericardium, ribs or the mediastinum and its contents).

A chest radiograph and fibreoptic bronchoscopy are needed to define the T characteristics of a lesion.

An N_0 lesion does not extend to hilar or mediastinal nodes.

An N_1 lesion has extended to lymph nodes in the ipsilateral hilar region.

An N_2 lesion has spread to mediastinal nodes.

A combination of chest radiograph, mid-chest

tomography, computerized tomography scan, gallium imaging of the lung and mediastinoscopy are required to define the N characteristics of a lesion.

To define the M characteristics of a lesion it is necessary to assess the history, physical examination and full blood chemistry, including liver function tests. Unless an abnormality is identified following this assessment it is not usually necessary to carry out liver, brain or bone scans.

An M_0 lesion has no distant metastases.

An M_1 lesion has distant haematogenous metastases in the liver, brain, bone or adrenal gland or has lymph node extension to scalene or cervical lymph nodes.

Clinical staging classifications define the tumour size, location and the presence or absence of metastases and facilitate the decision as to which patients should be referred for surgery. The aim of the TNM staging system is to identify those patients who, following resection, will have improved survival compared with the natural history of the disease (Tisi 1985).

Non-surgical treatment of lung cancer. If surgery is not indicated, other treatments include chemotherapy, radiotherapy, endoscopic laser treatment, and for a centrally situated lesion obstructing the large airways the insertion of an expandable stent may be considered together with endobronchial radiotherapy or endoscopic laser treatment (George et al 1990).

Physiotherapy key points
- When the obstruction of the airway is relieved following treatment it is important for the physiotherapist to assist the clearance of secretions which have been trapped behind the obstruction.
- Positioning and the use of breathing control may give some relief of breathlessness to these patients.

Recurrent laryngeal nerve involvement. Hoarseness as a symptom in lung cancer frequently indicates involvement of the recurrent laryngeal nerve. When one recurrent laryngeal nerve is paralysed the vocal fold of the same side remains motionless while the opposite one crosses the median plane to accommodate itself to the affected one. Speech is possible but the voice is altered and weakened. Vocal cord palsy is more common on the left because the intrathoracic course of the left recurrent laryngeal nerve allows it to become involved in bronchial neoplasms, tuberculosis, etc.

Physiotherapy key points
- Palsy of the vocal cord causes a weak or hoarse voice and difficulty in coughing and expectoration because the inability to approximate the vocal cords makes it impossible to build up the necessary intrathoracic pressure needed for an expulsive cough. Huffing and breathing control should be encouraged.

Lobectomy

Lobectomy rather than pneumonectomy is preferable to conserve pulmonary function if the lesion can be completely excised. Lobectomy is the excision of an entire lobe. The lobar vessels are ligated and divided. The bronchus is divided and closed. If the lobectomy is for lung cancer the hilar lymph nodes are dissected and removed.

Two chest drains are inserted to evacuate air, blood and serous fluid. If there is a significant air leak the underwater seal is connected to suction (15–30 cmH$_2$O). Small air leaks usually close after a few days. The remaining lung expands to fill the space and the hemidiaphragm on the side of the resection is usually slightly elevated.

If a tumour has spread into the right main bronchus, a lobectomy by sleeve resection may be performed (Fig. 12.5). This allows maximum preservation of lung tissue as the surgical alternative would be a pneumonectomy. Resection of the affected portion is followed by an end to end anastomosis of the main bronchus with the lower lobe bronchus.

Physiotherapy key points
- The active cycle of breathing techniques in the sitting position, either in bed or in a chair, may be sufficient to maintain effective airway clearance. In some patients who present with reduced breath sounds and subsegmental lung collapse on chest radiograph, positioning, e.g. side lying, may be indicated, or the adjuncts of periodic continuous positive airway pressure or

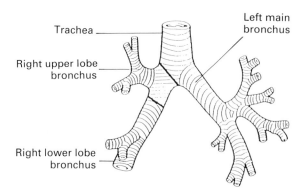

Fig. 12.5   Lobectomy by sleeve resection. (Reproduced with permission of the Royal Brompton Hospital.)

intermittent positive pressure breathing. The airway pressures should be kept low to minimize any possible increase in air leak.

Breathing exercises should be started on the day of surgery. An indication of effective airway clearance following lobectomy is the ability to expectorate blood stained sputum. Occasionally, endotracheal suctioning or the insertion of a minitracheotomy is necessary to clear accumulated secretions.

It is likely that about three treatments will be indicated on the first postoperative day and the patient should be encouraged to continue his own exercises between these sessions.

• Care must be taken to avoid compressing or pulling on the chest drains. The physiotherapist can support the patient when he is huffing and coughing by placing one hand posteriorly below a lateral thoracotomy incision and by giving counterpressure anteriorly. The patient should also be taught how to support his own chest when huffing and coughing (Fig. 12.6).

• The patient should be encouraged to move himself around in bed and this can be assisted by a strap attached to the foot of the bed. Early ambulation, usually starting on the first postoperative day, will minimize pulmonary and circulatory complications.

When the patient is walking with chest drains in situ, care must be taken to keep the drainage container below the level at which the tube enters the chest wall. A low-level trolley is useful (Fig. 12.3). If suction is being applied either the patient should walk 'on the spot' remaining attached to the

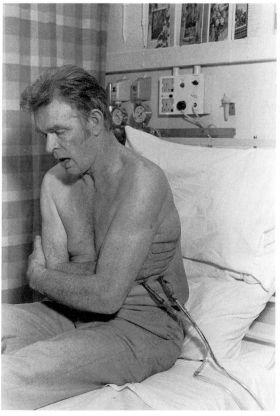

Fig. 12.6   Wound support following thoracotomy. (Reproduced with permission of the Royal Brompton Hospital.)

suction, or he may be allowed to be disconnected from the suction for a short period for ambulation.

As soon as possible exercise is progressed to include stair climbing from about the third postoperative day. If an air leak should persist exercise using a bicycle ergometer may assist lung expansion (Fig. 11.7, p. 209).

• Limitation in shoulder joint movement should be recorded preoperatively. Arm and shoulder girdle movements should be encouraged from the day of surgery. Resisted movements using proprioceptive neuromuscular facilitation techniques are helpful in gaining full range of movement with minimal pain.

• If reversible airflow obstruction is present, inhaled bronchodilators will probably be indicated.

• If secretions are tenacious the patient may be dehydrated and intake of fluids should be encouraged. High humidity may be indicated but steam inhalations may be sufficient.

- Postoperatively there is a tendency to side flex the trunk towards the side of the incision and to lower the shoulder on the operated side. Posture and trunk mobility exercises to correct this tendency and to prevent any permanent defect should be encouraged.
- Persistent chest wall pain may respond to thoracic mobilizations (p. 164) or transcutaneous electrical nerve stimulation (p. 163).
- Advice should be given on management at home. Exercise should be continued until the huff is dry sounding and non-productive and posture, mobility and exercise tolerance are normal for the patient.

Segmentectomy and wedge resection

Segmentectomy is the excision of a bronchopulmonary segment of a lobe performed for localized disease. Wedge resection is the excision of a wedge-shaped section without reference to the anatomical divisions of the lung. This technique is used in open lung biopsy and to resect small non-malignant tumours or cysts (e.g. hamartoma, small hydatid cyst). Occasionally it may be indicated in a patient with a small malignant tumour and poor lung function (Foss 1989).

Physiotherapy key points
- Following a segmental resection there may be a larger air leak and more pleural exudate than after a lobectomy.
- Following a wedge resection a moderate amount of sputum may be expectorated but there is usually a minimal air leak and drainage of fluid.
- Open lung biopsy, although a minor surgical procedure, may be performed on patients with compromised lung function and who may have postoperative respiratory problems requiring physiotherapy.

Pneumonectomy

Pneumonectomy is the removal of an entire lung, often with excision of the mediastinal lymph nodes. Resection of part of the thoracic wall is sometimes included. An exercise tolerance test should be a part of the preoperative assessment if some of the lung to be excised is functional.

Following pneumonectomy, the chest is closed leaving the pleural cavity filled with air, some of which is aspirated to restore normal negative pleural pressures. The cavity fills with fluid and if the air is not reabsorbed quickly enough to keep the mediastinum in the midline, either air or fluid must be aspirated. Many surgeons insert a chest tube in the pneumonectomy side at the time of the operation and leave it in situ for 24 hours to maintain the mediastinum in the correct position. The tube is clamped except for 1–2 minutes every hour. This allows any increased pressure in the hemithorax to be released and the correct mediastinal position maintained. Alterations in the position of the mediastinum can be detected by deviation of the trachea and by the chest radiograph.

During the few weeks following surgery organization and fibrosis take place within the hemithorax. Crowding of the ribs, elevation of the hemidiaphragm and movement of the mediastinum towards the operated side all reduce the size of the hemithorax.

Physiotherapy key points
- The key points postoperatively are similar to those for patients undergoing lobectomy (p. 253), but there will either be no drainage tube or a clamped tube for about 24 hours.
- Deviation of the trachea especially within the first 24–36 hours may cause mechanical difficulty with coughing. Huffing rather than coughing should be encouraged to minimise the intrathoracic pressures generated and the effort involved.
- Occasionally, nasopharyngeal suction to clear bronchial secretions is indicated. When inserting the catheter care must be taken, especially following a right pneumonectomy, to avoid contact with the suture line. A nasopharyngeal airway may facilitate the insertion of a suction catheter. Occasionally a minitracheotomy may be indicated.
- Although breathing exercises will be emphasizing expansion of the remaining lung, after a few days it is important to include bilateral thoracic expansion exercises to encourage mobility and to prevent deformity of the chest wall.

• Most surgeons allow the patient to lie on whichever side is more comfortable.

• Breathing control with stair climbing will probably increase exercise ability.

Bullous emphysema

Various surgical procedures have been developed to relieve the compression of functional lung tissue by large emphysematous bullae. Ligation or plication of the bullae, or resection of lung tissue can be performed via a thoracotomy and sometimes there is marked improvement in lung function (Venn et al 1988) and exercise tolerance.

A less invasive surgical technique is based on Monaldi's procedure in which a tube is inserted into the bullous cavity for several days (Venn et al 1988). The bulla collapses and the space is filled by the previously compressed lung tissue.

Physiotherapy key points

• Patients undergoing these procedures usually have severe underlying lung disease and are at risk of developing postoperative pulmonary complications.

• Re-education in breathing control at rest, while walking and stair climbing should improve exercise tolerance.

Complications following lung surgery

Phrenic nerve palsy. If a tumour involves the phrenic nerve it may be necessary to resect it. This will result in paralysis of the diaphragm on the affected side which reduces the effectiveness of huffing and coughing. Intermittent positive pressure breathing may assist in the clearance of secretions.

Bronchopleural fistula. A bronchopleural fistula is a communication between a bronchus and the pleural cavity. This is occasionally seen following pneumonectomy and more rarely following other lung resections. It tends to arise 5–10 days after surgery and is usually associated with infection and disruption of the bronchial stump. Clinical features include a cough producing a bloody/brownish fluid, tachycardia and spiking temperature.

Medical management includes aspiration of infected fluid, or the insertion of a drainage tube and instillation of antibiotics. Resuturing of the bronchial stump may be necessary if healing does not occur. The patient should always turn with the affected side at a lower level than the unaffected side.

Cardiac arrhythmias. Supraventricular arrhythmias can occur in patients following pulmonary resection, particularly pneumonectomy and older patients are more susceptible. Medical treatment is by digitalization.

Surgical emphysema. If there is a communication between the lungs and the pleura and air pressure builds up in the pleural space, air may track into the tissue layers producing surgical or subcutaneous emphysema. This presents as a crackling sensation when the area is palpated. From the site of a drainage tube or suture line it may spread into adjacent tissues causing swelling of the chest wall and neck. In severe cases this may extend to the face and eyelids. Surgical emphysema usually subsides with correct chest drain management. Huffing to clear secretions is more appropriate than coughing as the intrathoracic pressure is less with huffing because the glottis remains open.

Pleural effusion. Following lung surgery most of the postoperative pleural fluid will be removed through chest drainage. Occasionally fluid reaccumulates after removal of the drainage tube and aspiration may be necessary.

Chest wall surgery

Thoracoplasty

Thoracoplasty involves the resection of ribs to collapse the underlying lung. It was used as a means of treatment for tuberculosis to produce permanent collapse of diseased lung to allow healing to take place. It is now rarely used because tuberculosis can be treated effectively by drugs. Occasionally it is used in the treatment of chronically infected cavities where conservative treatment has failed, for example chronic empyema.

If extensive rib resection is required the operation may be carried out in two stages to reduce the risk of respiratory failure. If the first rib is not removed, the neck remains more stable because the scalene muscles retain their insertion. A firm pad should be applied if there is paradoxical movement of the chest wall.

Physiotherapy key points

• The key points postoperatively are similar to those for patients undergoing lobectomy (p. 253).

• Posture correction and re-education is of particular importance because of the risk of deformity following thoracoplasty. If the first rib has been removed, the distal attachments of the scalene muscles are removed. This results in the muscles of the opposite non-operated side pulling the head and neck over to the non-affected side. The shoulder is raised on the affected side and rotated medially because the rhomboids have been cut. The trunk leans towards the affected side to balance the head displacement and the spine is pulled into a long curve which is concave to the non-operated side. Consequently, posture correction is essential and should be started from the first postoperative day. A mirror is useful for postural correction exercises.

• Shoulder girdle and arm movements should include depression of the shoulder girdle on the side of the thoracoplasty, retraction of the scapulae, bilateral full range arm movements and neck lateral lean towards the side of the operation.

• The corrected posture can often be maintained when standing still but many patients require further practice to maintain this when walking. Posture correction exercises should be continued for about two months.

Pectus carinatum and pectus excavatum

Disturbance of the growth pattern of the sternum and adjacent costal cartilages may lead to deformity of the rib cage (Forrest et al 1991). While the anatomical arrangement of the underlying intrathoracic structures may be unaffected the cosmetic effect may cause considerable distress to the patient. The sternum may be bowed anteriorly (pectus carinatum) or it may be depressed (pectus excavatum).

Lung function and cardiac function are rarely impaired and if surgery is indicated it is usually for cosmetic reasons. Surgical correction involves resection of the costal cartilages and repositioning of the sternum which may be supported by a metal bar placed behind the sternum.

Physiotherapy key points

• In adolescent patients the use of an incentive spirometer may assist thoracic expansion.

• Excess bronchial secretions are rarely a problem as there is usually no underlying chest disease.

Chest wall tumours

Chest wall tumours which are usually metastases or extensions of visceral tumours are not normally removed surgically unless pain is a major problem. The removal of the tumour and adjacent tissue will cause a defect in the chest wall which may lead to respiratory failure. If a large segment is resected a rigid plate is normally inserted to prevent the occurrence of a flail chest.

Pleural surgery

Pleural surgery is usually performed to improve the function of the underlying lung. Surgical procedures include intercostal drainage for pneumothorax, pleurectomy, pleurodesis and excision of an empyema.

Intercostal drainage for spontaneous pneumothorax

Spontaneous pneumothorax can result from one of two mechanisms:

1. A visceral pleural 'tear' caused by rupture of a subpleural bleb or by a parenchymal process that erodes the visceral pleura, e.g. necrotizing pneumonia.

2. Partial bronchial obstruction which may behave as a 'check valve' leading to progressive hyperinflation of distal air spaces. Eventually air travels along the bronchovascular spaces into the hilum of the lung and then directly into the mediastinum with a resulting pneumomediastinum. If the process continues, air will escape in one of two directions. It may pass through the fascial planes in the neck causing surgical emphysema or pass through the visceral pleura in one or both pleural spaces causing a pneumothorax.

Spontaneous pneumothorax occurs in otherwise healthy individuals following a rupture of subpleural apical blebs. The peak incidence is in the age range 20–30 years and there is a 4:1 male predominance. It tends to occur in tall thin individuals and there is an increased incidence in cigarette smokers. In most cases symptoms develop during sedentary activity, although it can be associated with strenuous activity or with a forceful cough or sneeze. Spontaneous pneumothorax is relatively common in patients with emphysema, particularly those with the bullous type. Symptoms depend on the size of the pneumothorax and include sudden onset of chest pain, breathlessness and decreased breath sounds on the involved side. Patients with a 'check valve' mechanism often complain of substernal pressure and discomfort which may be misinterpreted as cardiac in origin. Diagnosis is made by a chest radiograph taken on expiration.

Management depends on the absence or presence of complications such as haemothorax (which is evidenced by blunting of the costophrenic angle and which requires the presence of more than 200 ml of fluid) or underlying lung disease.

Spontaneous pneumothorax without complications and no underlying lung disease is treated by the insertion of a chest tube to an underwater seal for 1–3 days which normally results in prompt re-expansion.

A pneumothorax with complications, e.g. haemothorax, requires a thoracotomy to explore and repair the bleeding site. Failure to re-expand the collapsed lung with the tube drainage is also an indication for thoracotomy. If visceral leaks persist for more than 7–10 days they will not seal without surgical intervention.

Recurrence of a pneumothorax in otherwise healthy patients occurs in approximately 30%, and after a second episode the incidence of a third pneumothorax is 70% (Forrest et al 1991). After the second recurrence pleurodesis or pleurectomy is recommended.

Pleurectomy

Pleurectomy involves the removal of the portion of the parietal pleural layer from an area of the chest wall leaving a raw surface to which the visceral layer will adhere. Identifiable blebs and bullae are oversewn.

Pleurodesis

A pleurodesis is the obliteration of the pleural space by an inflammatory process. This may be produced by rubbing the pleural surfaces with an abrasive material or by insufflating a chemical irritant, e.g. iodized talc or kaolin. This procedure is usually reserved for patients who are not surgical candidates because the effect of these irritants may compromise a subsequent surgical approach.

Decortication

Decortication of the lung involves stripping off the layers of pleura that have become thickened due to chronic inflammation from pleurisy which restricts chest wall movement and lung expansion. If an empyema is not successfully treated by drainage, the whole pleura is stripped to remove the chronic pus-filled area and the surrounding fibrous tissue.

Physiotherapy key points
- The key points postoperatively are similar to those for patients undergoing lobectomy (p. 253).
- Following decortication of the lung there may be a marked increase in movement of the chest wall and breathing exercises will assist rapid expansion of the lung.

CARDIAC SURGERY

Heart disease may be either congenital or acquired and surgery has an important part to play in the management of many of these conditions either to improve cardiac function thereby relieving symptoms or to alter the natural history of the disease (Forrest et al 1991).

Surgical procedures requiring cardiopulmonary bypass include coronary artery bypass grafting, valvotomy, valve replacement and repair, atrial or ventricular septal defect closure (p. 310), excision of ventricular or aortic aneurysm, correction of

Fallot's tetralogy, removal of cardiac myxoma and heart transplantation.

Cardiac surgical procedures where cardiopulmonary bypass is not used include ligation of persistent ductus arteriosus, excision of coarctation of the aorta, Blalock–Taussig shunt for Fallot's tetralogy when symptomatic in early life (p. 310), and pericardiectomy.

Cardiopulmonary bypass permits the removal of the systemic venous blood from the body via a cannula in the right atrium. The machine oxygenates the blood and returns it to the arterial system via a cannula in the ascending aorta. Myocardial protection is effected by cooling and arresting the heart (cardioplegia) with the infusion of cold (4–10°C) isotonic crystalloid solution with a high potassium content. Consequently, the surgeon can operate on a 'still' heart (Forrest et al 1991).

Vertical sternotomy is the most usual approach for heart surgery with the insertion of pericardial and mediastinal chest drains. A lateral thoracotomy incision is often used in non-bypass procedures and drains are inserted in the pleural cavity.

Coronary artery bypass grafting

Both medical and surgical approaches are used in the treatment of angina or myocardial infarction without angina. Following a 10-year survival study, Proudfit et al (1990) concluded that surgery had a higher survival rate. Bypass grafting is used to revascularize the myocardium, thereby improving its function.

Either the patient's saphenous vein or his internal mammary artery may be used as a conduit between the aorta and the coronary artery distal to the occlusion. The patency of the internal mammary artery graft is higher than that for the saphenous vein, but for multiple grafts there is often insufficient material (Grondin 1984, Angelini & Bryan 1992). The internal mammary artery is usually used to bypass the occluded left anterior descending coronary artery (Angelini & Newby 1989).

Coronary artery bypass grafting is effective in reducing angina, but functional impairment frequently continues following surgery (Allen 1990).

Percutaneous transluminal coronary angioplasty

When there is a localized proximal and incomplete block in a coronary artery, angioplasty may be considered. A small balloon is inserted via a peripheral artery under radiological control. When the balloon is positioned across the stenosis it is inflated and reduction in the stenosis can be obtained. Long-term studies comparing angioplasty with bypass grafting are in progress.

Valvular heart disease

Defects in heart valves may be congenital or due to rheumatic fever, connective tissue disorders (Marfan's syndrome), ischaemic heart disease, or infection (e.g. infective endocarditis). The defects range from minor distortion to severe stenosis, often with calcification, regurgitation or a combination of both. Valvular stenosis and incompetence lead to breathlessness and cyanosis, but with aortic valve stenosis symptoms may be absent.

The surgical procedures include valvotomy, annuloplasty, valvuloplasty and valve replacement using a homograft, xenograft or mechanical valve. Surgery has been shown to give symptomatic relief and improve longevity (Forrest et al 1991).

Coarctation of the aorta

Resection of coarctation of the aorta is undertaken to avoid the complications and risks of hypertension. The aorta is clamped above and below the coarctation and the narrowed segment of the aorta is resected. Usually the ends are anastomosed, but occasionally a dacron graft may be inserted.

Medical management

Following heart surgery the patient may be in a recovery room for a few hours, or an intensive-care unit for 12–24 hours before returning to the postoperative ward when cardiovascularly stable.

Until stable, continuous monitoring of pulse rate, blood pressure, and right atrial pressure or central venous pressure are necessary. In some units left atrial and pulmonary arterial wedge pressure measurements are available. Inotropic and chronotropic drugs are given to support cardiac output as necessary.

Some patients will require mechanical ventilation for a few hours, but occasionally longer periods of assisted ventilation are necessary if the patient's cardiovascular state remains unstable or hypoxaemia persists. Pinilla et al (1990) describe the use of nasal continuous positive airway pressure in patients with persistent hypoxaemia.

Complications of cardiac surgery

Respiratory

1. *Pulmonary infection.*
2. *Collapse or consolidation of part or whole of a lung.* Lower lobe collapse particularly in the left lower lobe is common in patients following coronary artery bypass graft surgery. This is due to compression of the lower lobe during surgery and/or damage to the phrenic nerve or cold injury from cardioplegia (Efthimiou et al 1991).
3. *Reduction in lung volumes* postoperatively have been studied in patients following coronary artery surgery. The restrictive ventilatory defect is thought in part to be due to alterations in rib cage mechanics (Locke et al 1990).
4. *Pulmonary oedema* is usually due to excessive fluid replacement to correct hypovolaemia, or to right ventricular failure.
5. *Pneumothorax/haemothorax* is always a risk following opening of the chest.

Cardiovascular

1. *Low cardiac output* is manifested by poor urinary output (less than 0.5 ml/kg body weight per hour), a fall in skin temperature, low arterial blood pressure (diastolic pressure of less than 70 mmHg) and developing metabolic acidosis. The causes of low cardiac output may be cardiogenic (failure of the heart as a pump) or hypovolaemic (inadequate filling of the heart due to an inadequate volume of circulating blood). Measurement of central venous pressure (CVP) will distinguish between cardiogenic and hypovolaemic low cardiac output. If the CVP is less than 5 mmHg hypovolaemia is probably present, and if it is 20 mmHg or more it is likely to be cardiogenic (Smith 1984).

2. *Cardiac arrhythmias* may develop, causing a reduction in ventricular performance and cardiac output. The optimal rhythm is sinus with a rate of 79–100 beats/min in the adult. A tachycardia is defined as a rhythm of over 100 beats/min. This is common after heart surgery but a sudden onset with the pulse rising to 160–180 beats/min indicates supraventricular arrhythmias, for example atrial fibrillation or atrial flutter. Possible causes are hypoxia, hypovolaemia, cardiac tamponade, pain and anxiety (Smith 1984). Bradycardia of below 70 beats/min may occur following cardiac surgery. If this gives rise to ventricular extrasystoles the heart rate needs to be increased by the use of atrial pacing or chronotropic drugs. Sinus bradycardia can also result from carbon dioxide retention.

Irritability of the myocardium may cause ventricular fibrillation and this is probably due to a fall in serum potassium. Unless corrected promptly cardiac arrest may occur. In patients with a very low cardiac output which has not responded to treatment, the intraaortic balloon pump may be used to improve cardiac performance and myocardial perfusion (p. 88).

3. *Cardiac tamponade* is due to haemorrhage into the pericardial cavity causing pressure on the heart and preventing it from filling during diastole. If untreated it can lead to cardiac arrest. It is suspected if there is excessive bleeding or erratic drainage from the chest drains. Tachycardia, hypotension and high atrial pressure usually develop quickly. These symptoms together with heavy blood loss distinguish tamponade from heart failure. If tamponade is suspected the chest wall is immediately reopened to remove clots and control bleeding (Forrest et al 1991).

4. *Deep venous thrombosis* is not common because anticoagulants are both used in cardiac surgery during cardiopulmonary bypass and to prevent thromboembolism from prosthetic valves.

Renal failure

Acute renal failure results from impaired renal perfusion. If the mean blood pressure drops below 70 mmHg, renal artery constriction occurs and urinary output falls, i.e. below 0.5 ml/kg body weight per hour. Inotropic drugs can cause vasoconstriction. The average adult should excrete at least 30–40 ml urine per hour. Treatment to improve cardiac output should be initiated. If renal failure is more than transient peritoneal dialysis, haemodialysis (Forrest et al 1991) or haemofiltration is necessary.

Wound

1. *Infection*
2. *Poor healing and failure of the sternum to unite* following sternotomy can be felt or heard as a 'click' of the sternum when the patient breathes deeply. Sometimes if it does not stabilize rewiring of the sternum is necessary.

Cerebral injury

Cerebral injury can range from minor disturbances of concentration and mood to severe cerebral lesions, i.e. failure to regain consciousness, and/or hemiplegia. The minor disturbances are probably due to inadequate cerebral perfusion during cardiopulmonary bypass. Hemiplegia may be due to air embolism, arterial thromboembolism or cerebrovascular accident occurring during the altered perfusion of cardiopulmonary bypass (Forrest et al 1991).

Physiotherapy key points

• Most cardiac surgical patients will be seen preoperatively by a physiotherapist. The guidelines for pre- and post operative physiotherapy are similar to those discussed for the surgical patient (p. 243). If appropriate, it may be helpful to take the patient to the intensive care unit and to introduce him to the staff who will be caring for him. It is also helpful to teach the techniques of moving about in bed and moving from bed to chair to standing.

• Table 12.1 lists the observations which will assist the physiotherapist in her assessment of the patient.

• For patients who are intubated and mechanically ventilated for a short period of time, physiotherapy will probably not be indicated. If complications develop and mechanical ventilation is continued, physiotherapy may assist the clearance of excess bronchial secretions and help to re-expand areas of lung collapse when the patient is cardiovascularly stable. The technique of manual

Table 12.1   Postoperative observations following cardiac surgery

Respiration: spontaneous or mechanical
Level of consciousness
Colour
Arterial blood gases(SaO_2)
Pulse and temperature
Blood pressure/central venous pressure
Urinary output
ECG
Pacemaker/intra-aortic balloon pump
Drugs including analgesia
Incisions and drains
Chest radiograph
Bronchial secretions
Auscultation

hyperinflation may be indicated (p. 157), positioning for optimal ventilation and perfusion (Dean 1985) should be considered together with passive, active assisted or active limb movements.

• The head down position increases venous return to the heart and increases atrial pressure. It is usually unsuitable and rarely indicated for patients following cardiac surgery.

• Following resection of coarctation of the aorta the patient may experience periods of hypertension, although the reason for this is unknown. Positions which would increase hypertension, e.g. head down position, should be avoided. If the side lying position is indicated the blood pressure should be monitored during treatment.

• Adequate relief of pain will facilitate physiotherapy.

• Breathing exercises and early ambulation are indicated (Bourn & Jenkins 1992).

• If breath sounds are reduced or bronchial, positioning to improve ventilation and perfusion matching may be indicated, for example positioning in right side lying for a left lower lobe collapse.

• Periodic continuous positive airway pressure may be effective if lung collapse persists in a spontaneously breathing cooperative patient, and intermittent positive pressure breathing in a patient unable to cooperate with the active cycle of breathing techniques.

• Support of the wound by the physiotherapist or the patient himself, or the use of a pillow held over the wound, or a 'cough-lok' or towel, may assist huffing and coughing. This is especially important if there is delayed healing of the sternum and a sternal click has developed following a vertical sternotomy incision.

• Posture, trunk and shoulder girdle exercises should be encouraged. For patients following a lateral thoracotomy the objective should be full range of movements before discharge (p. 254).

• Stair climbing is introduced when the patient is cardiovascularly stable when walking on the level. Some centres monitor exercise using pulse rate, but it is of unknown validity.

• If chest wall pain of musculoskeletal origin persists, manual therapy techniques (p. 164) or transcutaneous electrical nerve stimulation (p. 163) may help to relieve this.

• Before discharge the patient is given advice regarding activities of daily living. It is generally recommended that during the first week at home visitors should be kept to a minimum, and a short walk should be taken each day, provided the weather is not cold or windy. The length and pace of the daily walk should be steadily increased until by 6 weeks the patient is walking 3–4 miles. If the patient lives in hilly terrain the distance and pace may need to be modified, or if it is possible the patient should be driven to an area of flatter ground.

A rest, not necessarily in bed, for 1–2 hours during the day is generally recommended for the first 6 weeks following surgery. Patients are normally advised not to drive during the first 6 weeks to allow complete healing of the sternum. Normal sexual activity is quite safe and may be resumed as soon as the patient feels able. Lifting of heavy weights and any type of heavy work should be avoided for 3 months.

Most patients are allowed to return to work at about 3 months following surgery, but some patients whose work involves heavy lifting may be advised to seek alternative employment.

In the longer term, encouragement should be given to include some form of isotonic exercise in the daily routine; swimming, walking and cycling are all suitable.

Some centres provide cardiac rehabilitation classes for patients following coronary artery vein graft surgery and after myocardial infarction (p. 319). These include exercise programmes, as well as comprehensive advice on modifying risk factors. There will be variations in rehabilitation between individuals in different centres and following other cardiac surgical procedures.

SURGERY FOR THE DIAPHRAGM AND OESOPHAGUS

Diaphragm

Traumatic diaphragmatic tears or ruptures can result from direct penetrating injury or from a blunt non-penetrating injury to the abdomen or chest. Over 90% of traumatic injuries to the diaphragm occur on the left side because of the protection given by the liver on the right side. Herniation of abdominal contents can lead to respiratory distress and severe substernal pain. The most common clinical signs are frequently related to associated injuries such as ruptured spleen, perforation of abdominal viscera or fractured ribs. Strangulation of herniated intestine may occur acutely or some years after the injury. Laceration of the diaphragm is repaired with multiple thick sutures through a thoracotomy and/or an abdominal incision.

Hiatus hernia

In this condition there is herniation of part of the stomach through the oesophageal opening in the diaphragm. Symptoms vary depending on the type of hernia. In the sliding type varying lengths of the stomach lie in the chest causing the symptoms of reflux, i.e. heartburn, retrosternal pain and vomiting. The rolling type, where part of the fundus of the stomach lies anterior to the oesophagus, is less common and gives rise to abdominal discomfort, nausea and a feeling of being overfull after a meal.

Conservative management with antacids, weight reduction, elevation of the bed head and small meals at night, often control the condition. If this is not successful or if the hernia is large with the associated risk of strangulation, surgery may be undertaken.

The incision may be abdominal or thoracic and

the most common operation is a Nissen fundoplication. The fundus of the stomach is mobilized and 'wrapped around' the lower oesophagus to enclose the oesophagogastric junction and lower oesophagus. The enclosed segment is compressed as the pressure rises within the stomach and reflux is prevented (Forrest et al 1991).

Oesophagectomy

Cancer of the oesophagus can be treated surgically, by irradiation, or by a combination of the two depending on the size and location of the tumour. Prognosis and resectability are determined by tumour size. Of tumours which are longer than 5 cm, 90% have node involvement. The operative mortality following resection is 10–20% and the overall survival rate 1 year after the diagnosis of oesophageal cancer is 20%. The 5-year survival rate is less than 5% (Forrest et al 1991).

The operative procedure may involve a laparotomy, thoracotomy and neck incision (posterior to sternomastoid). The tumour combined with a portion of the oesophagus above the lesion and a portion of the stomach below it are removed. Some surgeons prefer to carry out a total oesophagectomy. Following resection of the tumour a tube of stomach is brought up to the neck and anastomosed to the oesophageal stump, or alternatively anastomosed to the pharynx (total resection).

Following the thoracotomy a chest drain and underwater seal are usually in situ for about 24 h. There is a risk of leakage at the anastomosis and the possibility of pleural effusion. Following a long period of difficulty with swallowing, the patient is usually poorly nourished and very weak.

Physiotherapy key points

- The key points postoperatively are similar to those for patients undergoing lobectomy (p. 253).
- Following oesophageal surgery the head down position is usually avoided as gastric reflux could affect healing of the anastomosis.
- Patients with a nasogastric tube in situ will probably find huffing and coughing difficult and secretions may be viscid owing to restricted fluids.

High humidification may assist the clearance of secretions.

- If nasopharyngeal suction is indicated, extreme care must be taken to avoid disturbing the anastomosis and minitracheotomy may be preferable.
- Neck extension should be discouraged to avoid unnecessary tension on the anastomosis.

HEAD AND NECK SURGERY

Laryngectomy

Carcinoma of the larynx is a common malignant tumour in Westernized countries (Serra et al 1986). Surgery involves removal of the larynx and occasionally the hyoid bone. If the tumour has invaded the glands of the neck and other structures, more extensive surgery will be necessary to preserve life (Forrest et al 1991). Laryngectomy results in loss of speech and a permanent tracheostomy.

Physiotherapy key points

- Preoperatively it is important that the patient understands that the normal cough will be lost and that suction will be used to clear secretions via a tracheostomy tube. It is usually helpful for the patient to meet others who have had similar surgery to help allay fears and provide encouragement.
- Postoperatively it must be remembered that although the patient cannot speak, he can still hear and can respond using other systems of communication.
- In the early postoperative period humidification via a tracheostomy mask will compensate for the loss of humidification by the upper airways.
- Secretions should be cleared using a sterile suction technique. This should be carried out when necessary, but not at routine intervals. Before discharge the patient and his family/carer should be familiar with the suction technique and confident that they can manage at home.
- With speech therapy the use of an oesophageal voice or speech aid should be possible.
- The psychological effects of loss of voice and alteration of body image must be considered.

• In many parts of the world there are support clubs for patients who have had a laryngectomy and patients, friends and interested professionals can find these of value.

Head and neck procedures. These are many and varied, and many of the patients will have pre-existing lung disease. If a tumour has invaded tissues of the neck, a more radical surgical resection is required probably involving skin grafting. Postoperatively a tracheostomy tube is likely to have been inserted, but care must be taken with both oral and tracheal suction to avoid damage to any suture lines. Posture exercises must be included but these may be delayed until the graft has taken, and strain on the brachial plexus must be avoided.

VASCULAR SURGERY

Aortic aneurysms

An aneurysm is a localized abnormal dilatation of an artery. It is commonly acquired, but may be congenital (Forrest et al 1991). Atheromatous disease may manifest itself in the development of aortic aneurysms as atheromatous plaques weaken the wall of the aorta. These aneurysms occur most commonly in the abdominal aorta but can also affect the thoracic aorta. An aneurysm may be quite large before symptoms appear.

The thoracic aorta is fixed to other structures at its origin and a sudden deceleration motion may tear the aorta at these points. The common tear is above the aortic valve and death is usually instantaneous. Following a tear at the site of insertion of the ligamentum arteriosum the blood may be contained within an aneurysm (traumatic aneurysm) (Leatham et al 1991).

A dissecting aortic aneurysm occurs when there is haemorrhage into the wall of the aorta causing the media to separate from the intima and the adventitia. Branches of the aorta may be occluded.

Indications for surgery are aneurysms greater than 5 cm in diameter, tender aneurysms, severe chest pain, back pain or abdominal pain suggestive of recent enlargement of the aneurysm (Mannick & Whittemore 1989). Patients who present with signs of a ruptured abdominal aortic aneurysm constitute a medical emergency and require immediate surgery to try to prevent life-threatening haemorrhage into the peritoneum.

Surgery for an enlarged or enlarging thoracic aneurysm consists of excision of the aneurysm and replacement by dacron graft. This is usually via a lateral thoracotomy incision.

For an abdominal aortic aneurysm, a midline incision is made extending from the pubis to the xiphoid process of the sternum (Mannick & Whittemore 1989). The aorta is clamped above the aneurysm and clamps are also placed on the common iliac arteries. Some surgeons prefer to clamp the external and internal iliac arteries instead as the common iliac vessels are often calcific or aneurysmal (Campbell 1991). The aorta is opened longitudinally and all thrombi and atherosclerotic material are carefully removed. A tube graft of woven dacron is sutured into the aorta. If the iliac arteries are involved in the aneurysm a trouser graft may be used.

Following elective surgery for abdominal aneurysms postoperative mortality is around 5% (Campbell 1991) and most commonly attributable to cardiac causes. Many of these patients have coexisting ischaemic heart disease, have a high risk of developing cardiac problems during and after surgery, and are usually nursed in the intensive care unit for the first postoperative night.

Physiotherapy key points
• Many of the patients with an abdominal aortic aneurysm are over 70 years of age, have a history of respiratory disease and are at risk of developing postoperative complications.

• Effective analgesia will facilitate positioning, effective breathing exercises and mobilization. As soon as the patient is cardiovascularly stable a more upright sitting position should be encouraged to increase functional residual capacity. Following surgery for an abdominal aortic aneurysm sitting should be limited to an angle of 45° from the supine position, for at least the first 48 hours to prevent occlusion of the graft.

• Breathing exercises alone may be effective in preventing subsegmental lung collapse but sometimes adjuncts such as periodic continuous positive airway pressure, intermittent positive pressure breathing or humidification may be indicated. If there is reversible airflow obstruction, bronchodilators should be given.

• Ambulation should be encouraged after about 48 hours.

• Correct lifting techniques should be taught before discharge and heavy lifting should be discouraged for at least 6 weeks.

• Following surgery for a thoracic aortic aneurysm via a lateral thoracotomy or median sternotomy, shoulder girdle and arm exercises should be included.

Ischaemia of the lower limbs

The formation of atheromatous plaques in the vessels of the lower limbs causes narrowing of the lumen, with subsequent stenosis, occlusion or embolisms (Tunstall Pedoe & Walker 1990). The first sign is usually cramp in the calf muscles on walking, which disappears on rest. As the disease progresses shorter distances produce cramp which may also be present in the thighs and buttocks.

The development of collateral vessels may improve the symptoms, but as the disease process develops pain may be present even at rest indicating that tissue perfusion is inadequate. At this stage there is danger that the patient will develop gangrene and arterial assessment is carried out to ascertain if the patient is likely to benefit from thrombolysis, angioplasty or vascular reconstruction.

If these treatments fail or if the patient is unsuitable for them, amputation is the likely outcome. There has been an increase in arterial reconstruction and angioplasty, but the total number of amputations is also increasing due to the increasing elderly population and the prevalence of obliterative arterial disease (Ruckley 1991).

Physiotherapy key points

• Following reconstructive surgery assessment will identify any cardiorespiratory problems and ambulation should be encouraged as soon as possible.

• When the decision for lower limb amputation has been made a rehabilitation programme

including an appropriate prosthesis should be planned (Engstrom & Van de Ven 1985).

CHEST INJURIES

Chest injuries may result from either penetrating wounds or blunt chest trauma.

Blunt chest injuries

Blunt injury to the chest can result in the fracture of one or more ribs. Multiple fractures of ribs do not necessarily produce an unstable chest wall and resultant 'flail chest' unless each rib is broken in two or more places.

Rib fractures

Rib fractures may be associated with underlying arterial or visceral damage. They usually heal well and poor union is uncommon. The main complication of a simple rib fracture is the intense pain which it causes. This pain restricts the depth of breathing, huffing and coughing and impairs normal tracheobronchial clearance. There is a risk of subsegmental lung collapse and pneumonia. Adequate pain relief is essential and this may be achieved by intercostal nerve block or by direct injection of local anaesthetic to the fracture site.

Pneumothorax

Pneumothorax can result if the sharp end of the fractured rib penetrates the parietal and visceral pleura and punctures the underlying lung. It is treated by the insertion of an intercostal drain connected to an underwater seal and may be placed on suction (p. 249).

When a positive pressure develops within the pleural space the mediastinum is displaced to the opposite side compressing the opposite lung and a tension pneumothorax is produced. This is a life threatening condition and requires urgent insertion of an intercostal drain.

Haemothorax

Haemothorax may occur following rib fractures. A simple or tension pneumothorax may also be present (haemopneumothorax) and treatment is the same as for pneumothorax. Normally there is a large blood loss into the drainage bottle as the accumulated blood is drained. The drainage rapidly decreases as the underlying lung re-expands to the chest wall and the lacerations are compressed. If the bleeding persists above 500 ml/h for 3 or more consecutive hours, a thoracotomy is indicated to remove clotted blood within the hemithorax.

Flail chest

Flail chest occurs when the rigidity of the chest wall is destroyed by fractures of the ribs or costal cartilages. When a segment of the chest wall moves in on inspiration and out on expiration breathing is paradoxical. This leads to marked respiratory problems in ventilating the underlying lung. The degree of respiratory embarrassment depends on the age and fitness of the patient.

The flail segment must be stabilized. Intubation and mechanical ventilation may be necessary to achieve adequate ventilation if the segment is large. Most small flail segments stabilize after a few days though large segments may require about 3 weeks to allow the fractures to heal sufficiently and restore the rigidity of the chest wall.

Surgical emphysema

Surgical emphysema is detected by the characteristic feeling of air in the tissues. It is most commonly present in the immediate area of the fracture and indicates that the underlying lung is damaged. Careful observation and a chest radiograph are required to exclude a pneumothorax. Surgical emphysema can spread extensively from the fracture site to the abdominal area and to the face and eyelids. While distressing to the patient it is not in itself dangerous. Extensive emphysema results from a high pressure of gas in the tissues and a pneumothorax is usually present.

Rupture of the trachea or major bronchus

This can occur as the result of a deceleration injury. Airway trauma is suspected if there is air in the mediastinum on chest radiograph, surgical emphysema of the neck and a persistent and uncontrollable air leak preventing full lung expansion.

Vascular injury

Vascular injury in the mediastinum involves damage to the aorta and its major branches, especially the right ventricle which lies immediately posterior to the sternum. Contusion of the myocardium can follow a blunt chest injury and should be suspected if there is a weak pulse and widening of the mediastinum on the chest radiograph.

Cardiac tamponade

Cardiac tamponade is suspected if there is profound shock and low cardiac output. This is manifested by hypotension, tachycardia, elevated jugular venous pressure, poor urinary output and low temperature due to impaired skin perfusion. Treatment requires an emergency thoracotomy to permit aspiration of the blood from the pericardium. If tamponade is excluded, myocardial support is provided by the administration of inotropic drugs such as dopamine.

Penetrating chest injuries

Penetrating chest injuries can cause damage to any intrathoracic organ and to the abdomen, spinal column or neck. These injuries are not usually associated with extensive soft tissue injury in civilian life but are extensive in trauma caused by military or bombing actions. Failure to diagnose the full extent of the injury is possible, particularly if the only sign is a small puncture site on the chest wall.

Lung and bronchial tree damage

This is apparent if there is a tension haemopneumothorax with gross deviation of the trachea to the opposite side. If the lung fails to expand following the insertion of a chest drain and suction, or bleeding fails to stop, a thoracotomy is performed to permit removal of clots in the pleura and suturing of lacerations to the lung parenchyma.

Damage to the heart and major vessels

This is likely if the penetrating injury is at the front of the chest. Emergency thoracotomy is necessary. Most penetrating wounds to the heart and great vessels can be repaired without the need for cardiopulmonary bypass.

Oesophageal tear

An oesophageal tear can cause mediastinitis, but often leads to a hydrothorax on the side of injury. Aspiration of the fluid will permit diagnosis together with radiological contrast studies.

Damage to the diaphragm and abdominal viscera

This is likely if the injury is in the lower thoracic area and will require surgery.

Physiotherapy key points
- Assessment of the patient will identify individual problems.
- Effective pain control will facilitate breathing exercises and ambulation.
- If there are areas of subsegmental lung collapse periodic continuous positive airway pressure may be considered, but if a pneumothorax is present a patent intercostal tube must be in situ.
- High humidification may help to mobilize tenacious secretions and old blood.

MULTIPLE TRAUMA

Multiple trauma can result from road traffic accidents, domestic, industrial or bomb explosions and fireworks explosions. Road traffic accidents remain a major cause of severe multiple injury and death. Road traffic accidents cause as much severe multiple trauma as all industrial, domestic, criminal and sporting accidents combined.

There are many components to the forces that injure the body in violent accidents, blunt and penetrating injuries being the most common. Blunt injuries are the most typical result of road traffic accidents and penetrating injuries are most frequently associated with explosions and interpersonal violence.

Blunt injuries normally occur as a result of shearing, crushing or torsion forces on the body, and hollow and solid viscera are equally susceptible to such injury. For example, the car driver who is in a 'head on' collision and who is not adequately restrained by a seat belt can receive a direct blow to the chest from the steering wheel, shearing injuries to the small bowel due to compression of the abdomen by the seat belt and injury to the cervical spine as the head is flung backwards and then forwards (Forrest et al 1991). Myocardial contusion, liver injury and posterior dislocations of the hip joints are also likely to occur.

Damage from stabbing injuries is confined to the path of the weapon used, but bomb and similar blast injuries combine the effects of flying debris and shrapnel with the pressure wave radiating from the explosion. Such injuries frequently cause damage to the lungs and ears and if the victim is in close proximity to the explosion, the risk of extensive damage such as the loss of limbs is increased. The assessment of blast injuries necessitates careful examination of entry and exit wounds. The absence of an exit wound indicates that the debris/missile is still in the body. Exit wounds vary according to the velocity of the missile with high velocity missiles causing larger exit wounds than the low velocity type.

The priorities in the management of patients with extensive trauma are to detect and correct life threatening disorders and respiration and circulation will take precedence:

1. Airway patency must be established.
2. Ventilation must be maintained. This may include the relief of a tension pneumothorax or the closing of open chest wounds and the instigation of closed chest drainage. If ventilation is inadequate the patient must be intubated and ventilated mechanically if required.
3. The control of haemorrhage and the maintenance of the circulation by intravenous fluid replacement is essential.

Following stabilization of the patient, a detailed clinical examination is carried out to assess the extent of injury. Treatment is directed towards conditions which are a threat to life or function. This may include the relief of cardiac tamponade which is suspected in any patient with thoracic trauma who exhibits a low arterial blood pressure, raised venous pressure and diminished heart sounds.

Two-thirds of road traffic accident victims suffer head injury. The Glasgow Coma Scale is used to assess the level of consciousness and the size and reaction of the pupils of the eyes will indicate the presence or absence of cerebral pressure, together with an assessment of movement, muscle tone and reflex function. Skull radiographs, computerized tomography scanning and intracranial pressure monitoring are used to ascertain the extent and progression of the injury.

Spinal injury (p. 357) is a high risk in multiple trauma and great care should be taken at the scene of injury to support the spine, for example a cervical collar and specific lifting techniques to avoid causing further damage. Follow-up spinal radiographs and computerized tomography scanning are used to determine the degree of trauma.

Suspected abdominal injury usually requires laparotomy for exploration and repair of visceral or vascular damage. Fractures are reduced, debrided and immobilized and soft tissue injuries are debrided and repaired. Peripheral nerve injuries are often caused by penetrating trauma though they can occur in association with fractures and dislocations. Neuropraxia and axonotmesis are managed conservatively with careful splinting and passive movements to preserve joint mobility and prevent contractures. Sequential electrical testing of nerve conduction and muscle activity are used to monitor the return of function. The prognosis is usually good with recovery within 6 weeks. Neurotmesis (i.e. nerve division) requires surgical repair with end-to-end suture of the nerve sheath. Nerve suture has variable results as fibrous tissue formation hinders growth of the axons and regrowth is approximately 1 mm/day.

Physiotherapy key points
- The problems of the patient following multiple trauma will vary considerably with the type, extent and severity of the injury. Assessment and reassessment is crucial to effective treatment.
- Many factors must be considered before positioning a patient and include abnormal muscle tone, spinal cord injury, cardiovascular instability and high risk pressure areas.
- The maintenance of a patent airway is imperative. If the patient cannot effectively mobilize and clear excess bronchial secretions using the active cycle of breathing techniques, suction (p. 159) will be indicated. If the patient is unconscious an oropharyngeal airway may be required. Tidal volume in the unconscious spontaneously breathing patient may be increased by the use of neurophysiological facilitation techniques (Bethune 1991).
- Correct positioning of the patient can assist ventilation (pp. 56 and 102) and prevent limb contractures. Passive, active assisted and active movements should be encouraged where possible to maintain neuromuscular and musculoskeletal function until the patient is ambulant.
- If the cardiovascular state is stable in the mechanically ventilated patient, and an intercostal tube if present is patent, manual hyperinflation may be indicated to assist in the clearance of secretions. Manual support of the chest wall should be given throughout the procedure if necessary.
- The rehabilitation of these patients should be a continuous process from the time of injury until the maximal functional level has been achieved. This will involve all members of the multidisciplinary team.

HEAD INJURIES

Head injuries are a major medical and social problem in developed countries and are the main cause of mortality and morbidity in young people from 15 to 24 years (Thompson 1990). More than half of the deaths from head injury have resulted from motor vehicle accidents.

A blow to the front or the back of the head causes displacement of the brain within the skull relative to the brain stem. This results in tearing and shearing frequently leading to loss of consciousness and sometimes death. With severe brain damage tearing of the small vessels in the brain stem causes ischaemia and interruption of nervous pathways. Increased intracranial pressure leads to cerebral compression and may result from brain swelling, intracranial bleeding or a combination of these. Compound fractures of the skull can allow cerebrospinal fluid to pass through the ear or nose which become potential sites for infection (Forrest et al 1991).

Vigorous intensive care management has been shown to improve the outcome of patients with severe head injuries, without increasing the number of severely disabled survivors (Moss et al 1983).

An initial rapid, but thorough, assessment of the head injured patient is essential to identify primary injuries and to minimize complications from secondary insults, for example hypoxia, hypercapnia and hypotension. Intubation and mechanical ventilation may be indicated. Assessment of the level of consciousness is important in the initial assessment of the patient and to monitor his progress. The Glasgow Coma Scale (p. 9) is a useful international standard.

Intracranial pressure (ICP) monitoring (p. 72) (normal range 0–10 mmHg) identifies changes in ICP. The head down position impairs venous return from the head (70% of blood volume intracranially is in the venous section of the vascular bed) and will result in an increased ICP. The bed head raised 30° and the head maintained in the midline is the best position to prevent kinking of major arteries in the neck, to aid venous drainage and reduce ICP (Jennett & Teasdale 1981, Hay 1992).

ICP can also be controlled by hyperventilation to lower the arterial carbon dioxide level ($PaCO_2$). A raised $PaCO_2$ causes vasodilatation and an increase in ICP, while lowering the $PaCO_2$ causes vasoconstriction of the cerebral arterioles and decreases the ICP.

Adequate nutrition is important as energy requirements are high in the severely head injured patient.

Physiotherapy key points
• There is great potential for recovery in young patients due to the plasticity of the nervous system.
• Before treatment adequate analgesia and sedation should be given to control pain and avoid agitation as these factors can increase ICP. Cerebral perfusion pressure (CPP) (mean arterial blood pressure minus ICP, normal >70 mmHg) is

a more clinically relevant means of monitoring the cerebral effects of chest physiotherapy than a simple ICP measurement. The normal CPP is greater than 70 mmHg, but if ICP is high, CPP will be compromised and cerebral perfusion may be inadequate.
• The intubated and mechanically ventilated head injured patient will probably present with changes on his chest radiograph owing to aspiration, pre-existing chest disease or trauma, and chest physiotherapy will be indicated. Many of these patients are kept dehydrated and secretions will be tenacious. Instillation of normal saline before manual hyperinflation should assist the clearance of secretions. Manual hyperinflation may increase intrathoracic pressure and a restriction of venous return will raise the ICP, but treatment can produce hyperventilation which will lower the $PaCO_2$ and the increase in ICP may not be significant. The removal of secretions and re-expansion of collapsed lung will also lower the $PaCO_2$.
• Chest vibrations and shaking will be contraindicated if chest or spinal injuries are present.
• Suction tends to increase $PaCO_2$ as ventilation is not being maintained, and will cause cerebral vasodilation and an increase in ICP. It should be carried out sparingly and with care. If there is a leak of cerebrospinal fluid through the nose, nasopharyngeal suction is contraindicated owing to the possibility of infection (Garradd & Bullock 1986).
• Occasionally the head down position may be indicated for the clearance of bronchial secretions. Although an increase in ICP may be considered to be a contraindication, if it is accompanied by a rise in mean arterial blood pressure the cerebral perfusion pressure will be maintained (Imle et al 1988).
• Swallowing involves a complex interplay of the cortical, medullary and peripheral sensory and motor tracts, nuclei and receptors. Neurological damage may lead to incompetence of the swallowing reflex and these patients will probably aspirate. Pneumonia may be the first indication (Logemann 1983). A cuffed endotracheal or tracheostomy tube may be necessary to protect the airways. Before the endotracheal or

tracheostomy tube is removed, swallowing should be known to be safe. To test the swallow, the cuff is let down to see if the patient can cope with his saliva. If he appears to be coping, after about 24 hours, the patient may be given a small amount of coloured fluid to drink. This is followed by suction via the tube to detect any fluid which may have entered the lungs (Hay 1992). Proprioceptive techniques may be helpful to improve swallowing (Guymer 1986).

• If the patient remains unconscious but is being weaned from the ventilator, or breathing spontaneously, techniques to facilitate respiration will probably be beneficial (Bethune 1991).

• Humidification for the spontaneously breathing patient may help to mobilize tenacious secretions and suction may be necessary to elicit the cough reflex.

• Rehabilitation of the head injured patient may extend from weeks to months. The relatives play a very important part in the management and also need support and encouragement from the multidisciplinary team. Rehabilitation of the patient will include treatment for a range of physical and emotional problems (Lister 1983, Snyder Smith 1985).

Acknowledgement

We are grateful to Elizabeth Hay, Superintendent Physiotherapist, Addenbrooke's Hospital, Cambridge, for her help with this section on head injuries.

NEUROMUSCULAR DISORDERS

Myasthenia gravis

Myasthenia gravis is a disease characterized by fatiguable weakness in striated muscle which may be local or generalized and is due to a defect of transmission at the neuromuscular junction (Scadding 1990). The first signs are muscle weakness often limited to the external ocular muscles but in time all muscles including those of respiration may become affected. The condition is twice as common in women as in men with the peak incidence in the third decade (Oh 1990).

Anticholinesterase drugs are given to improve muscle power. Thymectomy is most beneficial if undertaken early in the course of the disease and may result in a longer period of remission particularly in younger patients (Scadding 1990). Anticholinesterase therapy is stabilized before surgery. After surgery the patient may have to be intubated and intermittent positive pressure ventilation may be required owing to respiratory muscle weakness.

Physiotherapy key points

• Patients with myasthenia gravis are at risk of developing chest infections. The active cycle of breathing techniques can be taught to assist in the removal of excess bronchial secretions. The exercises should be done soon after the administration of the anticholinesterase drugs in order that the muscles will be maximally functional.

• Respiratory muscle weakness increases the risk of postoperative complications. Following thymectomy the patient may be intubated and mechanically ventilated. The techniques of manual hyperinflation, chest shaking and suction should assist in the removal of secretions, and both during the weaning process and when extubated, intermittent positive pressure breathing will assist secretion clearance by increasing lung volume. Chest compression during expiration will augment the expiratory flow and further assist chest clearance.

• The anticholinesterase drugs frequently lead to excess secretions.

• Care must be taken to avoid tiring the patient. Treatments may need to be short and frequent.

Guillain–Barré syndrome

Guillain–Barré syndrome is an acute generalized polyneuropathy which affects people of all ages. It is thought to be due to an autoimmune response of the peripheral nervous system (Bannister 1985). It is a demyelinating neuropathy which may follow infective illness or may develop without apparent antecedent infection (Walton 1989). The neurological deficit reaches its peak within 1 month of onset. A total of 70% of patients recover within 1 year, 10% die and 20% have residual disability (Ferner et al 1987).

The first symptom is usually paraesthesia of the hands and feet followed by joint pain and motor weakness which progresses to flaccid paralysis. The development of muscle paralysis may be sudden and reach its peak within 24 hours, but it is more usual to worsen gradually over a period of 10–14 days (Scadding 1990). As well as paraesthesia there will be other sensory disturbances such as loss of touch, vibration and position sense and muscle tenderness. Cranial nerves may be involved, and in 40–45% of cases facial palsy is the most common manifestation (Scadding 1990). In some cases the autonomic nervous system is involved and this may cause postural hypotension and/or paroxysmal hypertension, and more rarely urinary and faecal incontinence.

Corticosteroids and other anti-inflammatory drugs have been used but there is no evidence that they affect the course of the disease. Plasma exchange has been found to be beneficial reducing both the median time for ventilation and death rate. Patients treated by plasma exchange also walked earlier than a control group (Tharakan et al 1989).

Once the diagnosis has been confirmed the patient should be observed closely and regular measurements of vital capacity should be taken. As the condition deteriorates the frequency of vital capacity measurements should be increased and if it drops to 1 litre mechanical ventilation is indicated.

The patient should be told that the muscle weakness may progress to complete paralysis and then reach a plateau before recovery begins. It should be emphasized that complete recovery is expected. Most patients make a complete recovery, while some will have a degree of residual weakness, usually mild (Scadding 1990). It should be explained that if swallowing and coughing become impaired it will be necessary to insert an endotracheal tube and if respiration becomes compromised, mechanical ventilation will be applied until respiration recovers. Tracheostomy will be necessary if it is anticipated that ventilation will be required for more than a few days. A speech therapist should be asked to advise on a communication system for the patient while on the ventilator and a communication board is generally used. It is important that all staff are familiar with the communication system used.

Physiotherapy key points

- If the patient is mechanically ventilated manual hyperinflation, chest shaking and suction should be used as indicated to maintain a clear chest.
- During the period of weaning from the ventilator and following extubation, intermittent positive pressure breathing combined with chest shaking should assist the clearance of bronchial secretions. This will be progressed to the active cycle of breathing techniques as voluntary muscle activity returns, but care must be taken to avoid tiring the patient.
- As muscle weakness progresses passive movements and soft tissue stretching are essential to maintain joint range and tissue extensibility. Entonox is sometimes used to counteract the discomfort of these procedures (Clark 1985). Resting splints for joints, particularly the ankles, may be necessary to prevent contractures. Positioning of the limbs is important and all members of the care team should be aware of the optimum position for each joint.
- As the patient recovers physiotherapy is directed towards increasing muscle strength and endurance and improvement of function. Karni et al (1984) provide a useful summary of the main problems relevant to the physiotherapist (Table 12.2).

Tetanus

Tetanus is a condition characterized by general muscle rigidity and convulsions. It is caused by spores which enter the body, usually through an open wound and travel along the peripheral nerves to the brain. Its incidence, which varies throughout the world, is very low in developed countries where most of the population has been immunized. The prognosis is related to the age of the patient, incubation period, the severity of the attack and its progress (occurrence of spasms and complications) (Oh 1990).

The degree of muscle rigidity varies from minor spasms which can be controlled by diazepam, to severe rigidity which may affect the whole muscu-

Table 12.2   Summary of the main problems in Guillain–Barré syndrome

Phase	Measures taken by physiotherapist
Deterioration phase	
1. Poor respiratory function	Chest care, postural drainage, suction
2. Joint and soft tissue pains	Passive and accessory movements, careful positioning, desensitization, e.g. rubbing, vibration, heat, ice
3. Progressing weakness	Assisted and passive movement Positioning
4. Autonomic dysfunction	Awareness of postural hypotension, and cardiac arrhythmias
5. Fear	Time, reassurance, explanation of what to expect
Plateau phase	
1. Pressure areas	Prevention by regular position changes and passive movements
2. Neuropraxias	Awareness. Positioning and explanation to nursing staff
3. Sensory loss	Encouraging patient to observe limbs when moved and to concentrate on movements being performed. Joint approximation
4. Low morale	Reassurance, encouragement and the introduction of ex-patients who have recovered
5. Disorientation	Constant input of time, place, outside news, etc. Continuity
Recovery phase	
1. Weakness	Strengthening exercises and functional activities
2. Joint and soft tissue pains	Ice, heat, vibration, ultrasound. Gentle stretches and mobilizing exercises
3. Tendency to tire	Short sessions with frequent rests
4. Lack of postural sensation	Joint approximation, weight-bearing activities, sensory input, balance re-education and compensatory use of eyes
5. Autonomic dysfunction	Readjustment of blood pressure to upright position with a tilt table
6. Tremor	Reassurance that this will improve as muscle strength returns
7. Emotional lability	Reassurance, understanding and encouragement by gentle but firm approach
8. Incomplete recovery	Provision of aids, e.g. calipers, home treatment programme and periodic reassessment

* Reproduced with permission from Karni et al 1984 *Physiotherapy* 70(8): 288–292.

lature of the body, including the respiratory muscles. External stimuli may cause reflex spasms which in turn affect respiration and most patients will need to be paralysed to prevent this.

Mechanical ventilation is necessary in severe cases and a tracheostomy may be performed. Muscle spasm is controlled by drugs and patients will probably be nursed in a quiet room. Recovery usually takes 3–6 weeks. During the acute phase there is danger of the patient developing pneumonia and cardiovascular problems.

Physiotherapy key points
• If the patient is paralysed, intubated and mechanically ventilated manual hyperinflation, chest shaking and suction should be used as

indicated to maintain a clear chest. Autonomic dysfunction may lead to excessive bronchial secretions and fluctuations in blood pressure.

• Adequate sedation and relaxants must be given to cover physiotherapy treatment.

• While the patient is paralysed joint range and tissue extensibility should be maintained by passive movements.

Poliomyelitis

The disease is caused by one of three related polio viruses. It is spread by droplet or the faecal–oral route, although infection normally occurs via the nasopharynx. The widespread use of oral vaccines has made it less common in developed countries, although it remains a major problem in developing countries (Macleod et al 1987).

The virus can attack the grey matter of the spinal cord, brainstem and cortex, but it has a specific tendency to damage anterior horn cells, particularly those of the lumbar segments (Macleod et al 1987).

The incubation period is 7–14 days, followed by 2 days of a 'flu-like' illness. Initially there is a mild fever and headache which improve within a few days. Many cases do not progress beyond this stage while in others they may, after having felt well for approximately 1 week, again develop headache and fever with associated neck stiffness (Scadding 1990). This is known as the 'pre-paralytic stage'.

The disease varies from a febrile illness with paralysis to severe paralysis, including the respiratory muscles. It is the respiratory paralysis that may cause death.

Of those who reach the pre-paralytic stage, over half continue to the paralytic stage and develop muscle pain and weakness. Paralysis is more severe if there has been strenuous exercise during the incubation period. Sensation is unaffected. Some anterior horn cells are destroyed by the virus, while others, although damaged by oedema, survive and the muscles supplied by them may regain power. Respiratory failure may occur if the diaphragm, intercostal and abdominal muscles are involved. In the bulbar form there is involvement of the pharyngeal and laryngeal muscles.

Patients with bulbar involvement alone will be intubated with a cuffed endotracheal tube. Nasopharyngeal and oropharyngeal suction will be required to clear secretions which will have accumulated above the cuff. A combination of respiratory and bulbar involvement will necessitate intubation and mechanical ventilation. Patients with respiratory muscle paralysis alone may be intubated and mechanically ventilated with intermittent positive pressure ventilation, but negative pressure ventilation using for example a 'tank' ventilator ('iron lung') may be the less invasive treatment.

In all forms of poliomyelitis bed rest is essential in the early stages of the acute phase. Analgesia may be needed for severe myalgia. Gradual recovery can take place over a period of several months, but any muscle which fails to show signs of recovery after 4 weeks is unlikely to gain return of useful function. Recovery may continue for approximately 2 years and any residual weakness after this is probably permanent. Orthopaedic intervention may be appropriate for the treatment of residual paralysis, for example a tendon transfer may be considered for isolated muscle weakness, or flail joints may require arthrodesis.

Physiotherapy key points

• For intubated patients on intermittent positive pressure ventilation manual hyperinflation, chest shaking and suction should be used as indicated to maintain a clear chest.

• The patient in a 'tank' ventilator should be treated in the head down tipped position, in prone where possible or supine. Chest compression in time with the expiratory phase of the ventilator can be used to augment the cough and clear bronchial secretions (Higgens 1966).

• For patients in a 'tank' ventilator with total respiratory paralysis, positive pressure breathing by mouthpiece will be necessary during physiotherapy limb exercise sessions and nursing procedures.

• Passive movements and soft tissue stretching are essential to maintain joint range and tissue extensibility for all patients during the paralytic phase. Positioning of the limbs is important and all members of the care team should be aware of the optimum position for each joint. Resting splints may be applied to prevent contractures.

- Hydrotherapy will probably be useful during the recovery phase. In the recovery phase in patients who are likely to have residual respiratory muscle paralysis, glossopharyngeal breathing should be taught (p. 127).

- Long-term rehabilitation will be required for many of these patients and multidisciplinary team involvement is essential for an optimal outcome.

DRUG OVERDOSE

Drugs may be ingested or inhaled either accidentally or deliberately. On initial assessment of the patient it may be possible to identify the agent, but this will not be easy if several have been taken. Treatment is directed at supportive measures to prevent complications (Routledge & Holmes 1990).

The priority of treatment is the maintenance of an adequate airway and a cuffed endotracheal tube may be necessary to protect the lungs if the patient has no cough reflex. If the cough reflex is present an oropharyngeal tube should be sufficient. Oxygen therapy may be indicated.

The spontaneously breathing patient is usually nursed in the semiprone position to prevent aspiration. In some patients assisted ventilation may be necessary. Medical measures to prevent further drug absorption, for example gastric emptying, may be used.

Physiotherapy key points

- If the spontaneously breathing, semi-comatosed patient has excess bronchial secretions and radiological changes indicating aspiration or lung collapse, physiotherapy will be indicated. Vigorous chest shaking during expiration, with the patient in the semiprone or prone position, may stimulate coughing. Nasopharyngeal or nasotracheal suction may be necessary and if the patient's tidal volume is inadequate intermittent positive pressure breathing may be helpful.

- If the patient is intubated and mechanically ventilated the techniques of manual hyperinflation, chest shaking and suction may be indicated.

- If neurological impairment is present techniques should be used to encourage a return to normal function.

INHALATION BURNS

Respiratory complications occur in 15–25% of patients who suffer significant burns and account for the majority of burn associated mortalities (Bordow & Landers 1985).

Smoke inhalation is indicated by the presence of soot around the mouth and nostrils. The thermal, chemical and hypoxic effects of smoke inhalation cause respiratory and systemic damage.

Heat injury

This results from inhaling hot gases and other products of combustion. Thermal injury, in many cases, is restricted to the pharynx and upper airway. Laryngeal oedema develops following direct thermal injury caused by inhalation of flame, hot gases or steam. Inhalation of hot gases can cause burns down to the terminal bronchioles though only steam can carry sufficient heat into the lungs to cause thermal damage to the alveoli. This is an unusual injury with a poor prognosis.

Chemical injury

This is caused by toxic elements in smoke and can result in oedema of the mucosa, bronchospasm, paralysis of the cilia and loss of surfactant. Materials commonly found in the home produce smoke containing high concentrations of hydrochloric acid, phosgene and cyanide. Polyvinyl chloride (PVC) is widely used in the manufacture of upholstery, floor and wall coverings, clothing, etc., and when it burns it produces a dense smoke which releases 40% of its volume as hydrochloric acid. It also produces phosgene. Polyurethane foam contains corrosive agents and cyanide (Bordow & Landers 1985). The most common cause of pulmonary damage is smoke inhalation and corrosive burning of the lungs is most often due to hydrochloric acid and phosgene. The inhalation of incomplete products of combustion (carbon particles) can lead to pneumonia.

Hypoxia

This may be due to pulmonary damage from thermal injury, inhalation of noxious gases, e.g. carbon monoxide, pulmonary oedema and/or adult respiratory distress syndrome and the restrictive effect caused by circumferential trunk burns.

Carbon monoxide which is produced by the combustion of carbon in a limited air supply combines with haemoglobin preventing the uptake of oxygen and results in tissue hypoxia. Carbon monoxide has a particularly high affinity for haemoglobin (210–250 times greater than oxygen). Small amounts of inspired carbon monoxide have a profound effect on the oxygen carrying capacity of haemoglobin reducing oxygen unloading in the tissues. The oxyhaemoglobin curve shifts to the left (Murray 1976).

The patient may have upper and lower airway obstruction and carbon monoxide poisoning and may present with cyanosis, breathlessness, hoarseness, stridor, wheezing and cough (Bordow & Landers 1985). Carbon monoxide symptoms vary with the level of carboxyhaemoglobin. Carbon monoxide produces toxicity at blood levels over 15% carboxyhaemoglobin. At lower levels (10–30%) headache and nausea are present, and at higher levels (30–40%) dizziness, visual disturbance and ataxia occur (Bordow & Landers 1985).

Medical management

Maintenance of an adequate airway is an immediate priority. If there is no upper airway damage leading to obstruction, the patient is treated with humidified oxygen (Moylan 1980). If there are burns or scalds to the face, airway support is almost always necessary. Endotracheal intubation is instituted if there is any risk to airway patency, e.g. stridor. If upper airway oedema has progressed to the extent that complete obstruction is imminent or there are severe facial burns, a tracheostomy must be performed. Continuous positive airway pressure may suffice to maintain arterial blood gases but intermittent positive pressure ventilation is necessary if arterial blood gases show evidence of respiratory failure (PaO_2<8 kPa, $PaCO_2$>8 kPa). A minitracheotomy may be inserted if a patient has an underlying chest condition and difficulty in clearing secretions. It would not be appropriate if there are burns in the area of the neck due to the high risk of infection spreading to the site of the burns. Bronchodilatation may be needed to relieve bronchospasm.

Intravenous fluid replacement is necessary in the adult if the burns are 15–20% of body surface area or greater. Calculation of the body surface area with second or third-degree burns is made (in the adult) by the 'rule of nines' (Muir et al 1987). Each arm carries 9% of body skin, the front and back of the trunk carry 18% each, the head 9%, legs 18% each and perineum 1%. Adequate fluid replacement is necessary to avoid the onset of shock and to maintain the urine output. Care is taken to avoid fluid overload which could lead to pulmonary oedema particularly in the presence of renal insufficiency. Acute tubular necrosis is a potential complication of extensive burns especially in the elderly (Muir et al 1987).

Nutritional support. This is vital, as a weight loss in excess of 10% of the preburn weight is associated with an increase in complications. Feeding is usually by the oral or nasogastric route but if there is an ileus or gastric dilation calories are administered parenterally. Large doses of insulin may need to be given to control insulin resistant hyperglycaemia which is a feature of the metabolic response to thermal injury. Acute ulceration and multiple gastric erosions which can follow major burns can be avoided by early feeding.

Analgesia. Analgesia in the form of intravenous opiates is used to relieve severe pain. Entonox (50% nitrous oxide, 50% oxygen) inhalation (p. 162) may be used for painful procedures such as positional change and changing of dressings.

Restrictive pulmonary dysfunction. This occurs secondary to circumferential trunk burns and is treated by escharotomy which involves slits being made in the restrictive tissue.

Adult respiratory distress syndrome (ARDS). This syndrome does not always occur, but if it does it tends to occur after a 24–48 hours symptom free period (Bordow & Landers 1985). The cause is not fully understood, although many factors are believed to contribute to it such as inhaled chemical toxins, fluid overload associated with the fluid replacement regimen, heat damage to surfactant, disseminated intravascular coagulation which is suspected if the patient shows signs of spontaneous bleeding and the formulation of multiple small emboli (Muir et al 1987).

Patients who have been burned in explosions, in enclosed spaces or by flames are most at risk of developing ARDS. The patient develops severe breathlessness, tachypnoea, bilateral crepitations and progressive hypoxaemia. Mechanical ventilation is frequently necessary, and surfactant by aerosol may be given.

Pneumonia. This is a common late complication of burn trauma, usually occurring 3–14 days following the injury. The most common infecting organisms are *Pseudomonas* and *Staphyloccus aureus* which can spread from the burn sites. All personnel coming into contact with the burned patient must take the appropriate sterile precautions to minimize the risk of contamination.

Physiotherapy key points

- Adequate pain control should be continuously maintained but analgesia may need to be increased for physiotherapy treatment.
- Following airway damage bronchial secretions are usually thick and tenacious. Humidification will probably be indicated. Intermittent positive pressure breathing or periodic continuous positive airway pressure may be necessary in addition to the active cycle of breathing techniques to assist in the clearance of the secretions which often contain carbonaceous material (sooty plugs).
- If bronchospasm is present, nebulized bronchodilators may be indicated.
- The sitting position is recommended for patients with head and neck burns in an attempt to reduce the oedema (Forrest et al 1991).
- Careful positioning of the patient is important to avoid pressure or tension on the burned areas or skin grafts.
- For a conscious patient full range of motion of all joints affected by the burns are encouraged to prevent contractures and maintain function. Active movements, rather than active assisted, are used where possible as contact by the physiotherapist predisposes the patient to cross infection and can cause an increase in pain. If the patient is unconscious gentle passive movements should be carried out (Leveridge 1991).
- If the patient is intubated and mechanically ventilated manual hyperinflation may be indicated if excess secretions are present, but chest vibrations and shaking will be contraindicated if there are burns over the chest wall.
- Suction should be carried out only in the intubated patient and care should be taken to avoid trauma to the damaged lung tissue. The instillation of normal saline may facilitate the clearance of excess secretions.

ADULT RESPIRATORY DISTRESS SYNDROME

Adult respiratory distress syndrome (ARDS) is characterized by increased pulmonary vascular permeability, decreased lung compliance, progressive hypoxaemia and pulmonary infiltrates on the chest radiograph. It was first described by Ashbaugh et al in 1967. The understanding of the mechanisms of ARDS has increased and intensive care technology has improved, but ARDS is not yet fully understood and mortality remains high (Hunter et al 1989).

The syndrome is initiated in response to a wide variety of conditions. These include the inhalation of noxious gases, shock, sepsis, multiple trauma, aspiration, lung contusion, acute viral pneumonias. The precipitating cause leads to diffuse pulmonary capillary damage which results in an increase in capillary leak across the epithelial/endothelial barrier. There is an increased movement of plasma and red blood cells into the interstitial spaces and alveoli, and the alveoli become filled with proteinaceous and haemorrhagic fluid debris. Eventually a proliferation of fibroblasts leads to interstitial fibrosis.

The clinical features include breathlessness, tachypnoea, cyanosis, fine crackles over the lung fields, increasing hypoxaemia, and bilateral diffuse shadowing on the chest radiograph which may lead to a complete 'white-out'.

If multisystem failure and sepsis develop the prognosis is extremely poor. The medical management is centred around the maintenance of ventilation and many mechanical ventilatory techniques have been tried. Fluid management, cardiac support and nutrition should also be considered as ARDS is a systemic disturbance (Hunter et al 1989, Evans et al 1990, Keogh et al 1990).

High levels of positive end expiratory pressure (PEEP) are often used in an attempt to improve oxygenation. High peak and mean airway pressures may lead to haemodynamic compromise and barotrauma and either minimal effective pressures should be used, or alternative approaches in ventilatory support should be considered (Keogh et al 1990).

Physiotherapy key points

• Accurate assessment of patients with ARDS is imperative as physiotherapy is not indicated unless there is lung collapse and/or excess bronchial secretions which cannot be cleared adequately by suction alone.

• If severe hypoxia is present and there are few secretions, manual hyperinflation is contraindicated as there is no problem which will respond to physiotherapy.

• If excess bronchial secretions or lung collapse are present, manual hyperinflation may be indicated. It is important to avoid high peak airway pressures and a slow controlled hyperinflation should be used. If ventilated with a high level of PEEP this should be maintained during manual hyperinflation (p. 157) and a closed circuit catheter should be used for suction (p. 160).

REFERENCES

Allen J K 1990 Physical and psychosocial outcomes after coronary bypass graft surgery. Heart & Lung 19: 49–54
American Joint Committee 1977 Manual for staging of cancer. American Joint Committee for Cancer, Chicago
Angelini G D, Bryan A J 1992 Saphenous vein grafts: current problems and future prospects. British Journal of Hospital Medicine 47: 726–727
Angelini G D, Newby A C 1989 The future of saphenous vein as a coronary artery bypass conduit. European Heart Journal 10: 273–280
Ashbaugh D G, Bigelow D B, Petty T L, Levine B E 1967 Acute respiratory distress in adults. Lancet ii: 319–323
Asbury A J 1985 Patients' memories and reactions to intensive care. Care of the Critically Ill 1: 12–13
Bannister R 1985 Brain's clinical neurology, 6th edn. Oxford University Press, Oxford, p 421
Bethune D D 1991 Neurophysiological facilitation of respiration. In: Pryor J A (ed) Respiratory care. Churchill Livingstone, Edinburgh, p 121–145
Bordow R A, Landers C F 1985 Pulmonary injury. In: Bordow R A, Moser K M (eds) Manual of clinical problems in pulmonary medicine, 2nd edn. Little Brown, Boston
Bourn J, Jenkins S 1992 Post-operative respiratory physiotherapy. Indications for treatment. Physiotherapy 78: 80–85
Campbell B 1991 How can we prevent complications from elective aortic surgery? In: Barros D'Sa A A B (ed) Vascular surgery current questions. Butterworth-Heinemann, Oxford, ch 7
Clark K J 1985 Coping with Guillain–Barré syndrome. Intensive Care Nursing 1: 13–18
Dalen J E, Paraskos J A, Ockene I S et al 1986 Venous thromboembolism scope of the problem. Chest 89 (suppl): 370S–373S
Dean E 1985 Effect of body positioning on pulmonary function. Physical Therapy 65: 613–618
Dunnihoo D R 1990 Fundamentals of gynecology and obstetrics. Lippincott, Philadelphia, p 246
Dureuil B, Cantineau J P, Desmonts J M 1987 Effects of upper and lower abdominal surgery on diaphragmatic function. British Journal of Anaesthesia 59: 1230–1235
Efthimiou J, Butler J, Benson M K, Westaby S 1991 Bilateral diaphragm paralysis after cardiac surgery with topical hypothermia. Thorax 46: 351–354
Engstrom B, Van de Ven C 1985 Physiotherapy for amputees: the Roehampton approach. Churchill Livingstone, Edinburgh
Evans T W, Turner J S, Hunter D N et al 1990 Adult respiratory distress syndrome. British Medical Journal 301: 1087–1089
Ferner R, Barnett M, Hughes R A C 1987 Management of Guillain–Barré syndrome. British Journal of Hospital Medicine December: 525–530
Ford G T, Guenter C A 1984 Toward prevention of post operative pulmonary complications. American Review of Respiratory Disease 130: 4–5
Forrest A M, Carter D C, Macleod I B 1991 Principles and practice of surgery. Churchill Livingstone, Edinburgh
Foss M A 1989 Thoracic surgery. Austen Cornish, London
Frisby J R 1990 Predicting outcome of critical illness. In: Oh T E (ed) Intensive care manual, 3rd edn. Butterworths, Sydney, ch 2, p 7–12
Garcia-Valdecasas J C, Almenara R, Cabrer C et al 1988 Subcostal incision versus midline laparotomy in gallstone surgery. British Journal of Surgery 75: 473–475
Garibaldi R A, Britt H R, Coleman M L et al 1981 Risk factors for post operative pneumonia. American Journal of Medicine 70: 677–680
Garradd J, Bullock M 1986 The effect of respiratory therapy on intracranial pressure in ventilated neurosurgical patients. Australian Journal of Physiotherapy 32: 107–111
George P J M, Irving J D, Mantell B S, Rudd R M 1990 Covered expandable metal stent for recurrent tracheal obstruction. Lancet 335: 582–584
Gould T H, Crosby D L, Harmer M et al 1992 Policy for controlling pain after surgery: effect of sequential changes in management. British Medical Journal 305: 1187–1193
Grondin C M 1984 Later results of coronary artery grafting. Is there a flag on the field? Journal of Thoracic Cardiovascular Surgery 87: 161–166
Guymer A J 1986 Handling the patient with speech and swallowing problems. Physiotherapy 72: 276–280
Ham R J, Marcy C L 1983 Normal aging: A review of systems/maintenance of health. In: Ham R J, Holtzman J M, Marcy M L, Smith M R Primary care geriatrics. John Wright, PSG, Boston

Hamilton-Farrell M R, Hanson G C 1990 General care of the ventilated patient in the intensive care unit. Thorax 45: 962–969

Hay E 1992 Personal communication

Higgens J M 1966 The management in cabinet respirators of patients with acute or residual respiratory muscle paralysis. Physiotherapy 52: 425–430

Hunter D N, Keogh B F, Morgan C J, Evans T W 1989 The management of adult respiratory distress syndrome: I. British Journal of Hospital Medicine 42: 468–471

Imle P C, Mars M P, Eppinghouse C E et al 1988 Effect of chest physiotherapy (CPT) positioning on intracranial (ICP) and cerebral perfusion pressure (CPP). Critical Care Medicine 16: 382

Jenkins S C, Soutar S A, Moxham J 1988 The effects of posture on lung volumes in normal subjects and in patients pre- and post-coronary artery surgery. Physiotherapy 74: 492–496

Jenkins S C, Soutar S A, Loukota J M et al 1989 Physiotherapy after coronary artery surgery: are breathing exercises necessary? Thorax 44: 634–639

Jennett B, Teasdale G 1981 Management of head injuries. F A Davis, Philadelphia

Karni Y, Archdeacon L, Mills K R, Wiles C M 1984 Clinical assessment and physiotherapy in Guillain–Barré syndrome. Physiotherapy 70: 288–292

Keogh B F, Hunter D N, Morgan C J, Evans T W 1990 The management of adult respiratory distress syndrome: 2. British Journal of Hospital Medicine 43: 26–34

Kleiman R L, Lipman A G, Hare B D, MacDonald S D 1988 A comparison of morphine administered by patient-controlled analgesia and regularly scheduled intramuscular injection in severe, postoperative pain. Journal of Pain and Symptom Management 3: 15–22

Knaus W A, Draper E A, Wagner D P, Zimmerman J E 1985 APACHE II: a severity of disease classification system. Critical Care Medicine 13: 818–829

Knaus W A, Wagner D P, Draper E A et al 1991 The APACHE III prognostic system. Chest 100: 1619–1636

Lange M P, Dahn M S, Jacobs L A 1988 Patient-controlled analgesia versus intermittent analgesia dosing. Heart & Lung 17: 495–498

Laycock J 1987 Graded exercises for the pelvic floor muscles in the treatment of urinary incontinence. Physiotherapy 73: 371–373

Leatham A, Bull C, Braimbridge M V 1991 Lecture notes on cardiology, 3rd edn. Blackwell Scientific, Oxford, ch 12

Leveridge A (ed) 1991 Therapy for the burn patient. Chapman & Hall, London

Lewis C B, Bottomley J M 1990 Musculoskeletal changes with age: clinical implications. In: Lewis C B (ed) Aging: the health care challenge, 2nd edn. F A Davis, Philadelphia

Lister M J (ed) 1983 Head injuries. Physical Therapy 63 (12) 1943–2029

Locke T J, Griffiths T L, Mould H, Gibson G J 1990 Rib cage mechanics after median sternotomy. Thorax 45: 465–468

Logemann J A 1983 Evaluation and treatment of swallowing disorders. College-Hill, San Diego

Lopes J, Russell D M, Whitwell J, Jeejeebhoy K N 1982 Skeletal muscle function in malnutrition. American Journal of Clinical Nutrition 36: 602–610

Macleod J, Edwards C, Bouchier I (eds) 1987 Davidson's principles and practice of medicine, 15th edn. Churchill Livingstone, Edinburgh, ch 15, p 644

Mannick J A, Whittemore A D 1989 In: Greenhalgh R M

(ed) Vascular surgical techniques and atlas. W B Saunders, London

Moss E, Gibson J S, McDowall D G, Gibson R M 1983 Intensive management of severe head injuries. Anaesthesia 38: 214–225

Moylan J A 1980 Smoke inhalation and burn injury. Surgical Clinics of North America 60: 1533–1540

Muir I F K, Barclay T L, Settle J A D 1987 Burns and their treatment, 3rd edn. Butterworths, London

Murray J S 1976 The normal lung: the basis of diagnosis and treatment of pulmonary disease. W B Saunders, Philadelphia

Newman J H, Neff T A, Liporin P 1977 Acute respiratory failure associated with hypophosphetemia. New England Journal of Medicine 296: 1101–1103

Oh T E 1990 Tetanus. In: Oh T E (ed) Intensive care manual, 3rd edn. Butterworths, Sydney, ch 45, p 305–309

Peterson D D, Pack A I, Silage D A, Fishman A P 1981 Effects of aging on ventilatory and occlusion pressure responses to hypoxia and hypercapnia. American Review of Respiratory Disease 124: 387–391

Pinilla J C, Oleniuk F H, Tan L et al 1990 Use of a nasal continuous positive airway pressure mask in the treatment of postoperative atelectasis in aortocoronary bypass surgery. Critical Care Medicine 18: 836–840

Proudfit W L, Kramer J R, Goormastick M, Loop F D 1990 Ten-year survival of patients with mild angina or myocardial infarction without angina: a comparison of medical and surgical treatment. American Heart Journal 119: 942–948

Rigg J R A 1981 Pulmonary atelectasis after anaesthesia: pathophysiology and management. Canadian Anaesthetists' Society Journal 28: 305–313

Routledge P A, Holmes J 1990 Drug overdose, poisoning and drug addiction. In: Souhami R L, Moxham J (eds) Textbook of medicine. Churchill Livingstone, Edinburgh, ch 4, p 45–59

Ruckley C V 1991 Lower limb amputation—time for critical appraisal. In: Barros D'Sa A A B (ed) Vascular surgery current questions. Butterworth-Heinemann, Oxford, ch 16

Sauerbruch T, Paumgartner G 1991 Gallbladder stones: management. Lancet 338: 1121–1124

Scadding J W 1990 Neurological disease. In: Souhami R L, Moxham J (eds) Textbook of medicine. Churchill Livingstone, Edinburgh, ch 23

Serra A M, Bailey C M, Jackson P 1986 Ear, nose and throat nursing. Blackwell Scientific, Oxford

Simonneau G, Vivien A, Sartene R et al 1983 Diaphragm dysfunction induced by upper abdominal surgery. Role of postoperative pain. American Review of Respiratory Disease 128: 899–903

Skowpronski G A 1990 Myaesthenia gravis. In: Oh T E (ed) Intensive care manual, 3rd edn. Butterworths, Sydney, ch 44, p 302–304

Smith G H 1984 Complications of cardiopulmonary surgery. Baillière Tindall, London, ch 6

Snyder Smith S 1985 Traumatic head injuries In: Umphred D A (ed) Neurological rehabilitation. C V Mosby, St Louis, ch 10, p 249–287

Swann P 1989 Stress management for pain control. Physiotherapy 75: 295–298

Tharakan J, Ferner R E, Hughes R A C et al 1989 Plasma exchange in Guillain-Barré syndrome. Journal of the Royal Society of Medicine 82: 458–460

Thompson W R 1990 Severe head injuries. In: Oh T E (ed) Intensive care manual, 3rd edn. Butterworths, Sydney, ch 67, p 427–433

Tisi G M 1985 Neoplastic diseases. In: Bordow R A, Moser K M (eds) Manual of clinical problems in pulmonary medicine, 2nd edn. Little Brown, Boston, ch 11, p 411

Tunstall Pedoe D S, Walker J M 1990 Cardiovascular disease. In: Souhami R L, Moxham J (eds) Textbook of medicine. Churchill Livingstone, Edinburgh, ch 13

Venn G E, Williams P R, Goldstraw P 1988 Intracavity drainage for bullous, emphysematous lung disease: experience with the Brompton technique. Thorax 43: 998–1002

Walton J N 1989 Essentials of neurology, 6th edn. Churchill Livingstone, Edinburgh

White P F 1988 Use of patient controlled analgesia for management of acute pain. Journal of the American Medical Association 259: 243–247

Wolfe B M, Gardiner B, Frey C F 1991 Laparoscopic cholecystectomy. A remarkable development. Journal of the American Medical Association 265: 1573–1574

FURTHER READING

Chartered Society of Physiotherapy 1992 Standards of physiotherapy practice for the management of patients with amputations. Chartered Society of Physiotherapy, London, WC1R 4ED

Edels Y (ed) 1988 Laryngectomy: diagnosis and rehabilitation, Croom Helm Routledge, London

Jennett B, Teasdale G 1981 Management of head injuries. F A Davis, Philadelphia

Muir I F K, Barclay T L, Settle J A D 1987 Burns and their treatment, 3rd edn. Butterworth-Heinemann, Oxford

13. Paediatrics

Annette Parker

INTRODUCTION

Respiratory care in children can be very different from that in adults. There are anatomical and physiological differences which mean that other criteria need to be used for assessment and treatment. The age of the child affects his ability to understand and cooperate with treatment. Fear of the unknown is even more obvious in children than in adults.

At all times children should be handled with care and respect. They should be given information and explanation about their treatment appropriate to their age and understanding.

It is always easier and more pleasant when a child is compliant with treatment. Cooperation can be obtained by persuasion, or by distraction, for example by games, television, cassette tapes, or reading books suited to the child's age and interest. Rewards can also be given for good behaviour or bravery, for example balloons or stickers. Children should never be forced into having treatment. If treatment is deemed essential the child must be treated, despite protest, giving reasons for doing so.

It is important to include parents, relatives, and carers as part of the care team. Parents should always have a full explanation of why treatment is required and how it is to be carried out. Parents are able to refuse physiotherapy treatment for their child but this rarely occurs in practice. Parents of sick children, particularly mothers who have recently delivered an ill baby, are extremely vulnerable to stress and should at all times be handled with tact and understanding. Parental stress may be manifested in different ways, for example hysteria, apparent lack of concern, or anger. Some parents are so distressed they are unable to stay with or visit their sick child and may need special help to express their feelings of fear and panic.

Parents benefit from the physiotherapists' support when they are required to carry out physiotherapy treatment themselves at home. Fathers are often more wary of participating in treatments and may need extra encouragement.

When children and parents are intensively involved in treatment sessions, siblings may often feel left out. It is therefore important to include them in some way, perhaps even in helping with treatment.

A child's awareness of the implications of illness and treatment develops as he grows older. Explanations which are suitable for younger children will need to be expanded as the child grows older and begins to understand how his body works. Teenagers, particularly, have a more sophisticated understanding and may be beginning to think about the future and the impact of illness on school and social life, as well as body image. It is important for them to develop responsibility for their treatment, although they may often object to being told what to do or to being treated like a child.

The physiotherapist treating any child with acute or chronic respiratory problems must be aware of the psychological problems affecting the child and parents and adapt his approach accordingly.

DEVELOPMENT OF THE LUNG

The development of the lung can be divided into four stages (Inselman & Mellins 1981):

- embryonic period (weeks 3–5)
- pseudoglandular period (weeks 6–16)
- canalicular period (weeks 17–24)
- alveolar sac period (weeks 24–40).

Embryonic period (weeks 3–5)

The lung bud starts as an endodermal outgrowth of fetal foregut. The single tube thus formed soon branches into two, forming the major bronchi. By cell division, the process of growth continues until, at the end of this period, the major lung branches are formed.

Pseudoglandular period (weeks 6–16)

During this period the airways grow by dichotomous branching so that by week 16 all generations of the airway from trachea to terminal bronchioles (i.e. the pre-acinus) are formed.

Also during this period the pulmonary circulation develops, cartilage and lymphatic formation occur, and cilia appear (week 10 onwards).

Canalicular period (weeks 17–24)

The respiratory bronchioles, alveolar ducts and alveoli (i.e. the acinus) start to develop during this time, simultaneously with the lung capillaries. The air–blood barrier first appears at week 19 and towards the end of this period surfactant synthesis begins.

Terminal sac period (weeks 24–40)

Development of the pulmonary circulation continues and the respiratory bronchioles subdivide to form air spaces. The air spaces are lined by two different types of cell (types-I and II pneumocytes). Type-I pneumocytes are involved in gas exchange and cover about 90–95% of the surface area. Type-II cells make up the remaining 5–10% and produce surfactant. Surfactant is the phospholipid substance which stabilizes surface tension in the alveolus and prevents alveolar collapse on expiration. Small quantities of surfactant are present at weeks 23–24 of gestation and the amount present gradually increases until there is a surge at about week 30. Birth itself and the

onset of respiration stimulates and matures surfactant production (Dinwiddie 1990).

Towards the end of the terminal sac period, the air spaces have developed into primitive multilocular alveoli. After birth, alveoli increase in size and number. The average number of alveoli in the newborn is 150 million. By the age of 3–4 years, the adult number of 300–400 million alveoli has been reached, but alveolar growth continues until about 8 years of age.

ANATOMICAL AND PHYSIOLOGICAL DIFFERENCES BETWEEN CHILDREN AND ADULTS

There are several anatomical and physiological differences between children and adults that put children at an increased risk of respiratory problems.

Anatomical differences

1. The higher position of the larynx in infants allows them to feed and breathe simultaneously up to approximately 3 to 4 months of age. It has been thought that this effectively makes them 'obligatory nose breathers' so that any nasal blockage by mucus or tubes leads to apnoea (Purcell 1976), although this is now in doubt (Rodenstein et al 1987).

2. The lymphatic tissue (adenoids and tonsils) may be enlarged in the infant. The tongue is also relatively large. These factors may contribute to upper airway obstruction.

3. The smaller diameter airways of infants, particularly those born preterm, offer very high resistance to airflow.

4. Bronchial wall structure is different in infants. Cartilage is less firm and there are proportionately more mucous glands. Both these factors predispose to airway obstruction and collapse.

5. There are fewer alveoli in young children and, therefore, less surface area for gaseous exchange (Reid 1984).

6. The collateral ventilation channels between alveoli, respiratory bronchioles, and terminal bronchioles are poorly developed until 2–3 years of age, predisposing towards lung collapse.

7. Because infants' ribs are horizontally positioned (Fig. 13.1), there is no 'bucket handle' movement of respiration. This position, combined with weak intercostal muscles, means that the diaphragm is the main muscle of respiration. The 'bucket handle' movement does not occur until children walk and spend more time in the upright position, so that gravity pulls the anterior ribs downwards.

8. The horizontal angle of insertion of the diaphragm combined with the compliant cartilaginous rib cage of the infant means less efficient ventilation and distortion of chest wall shape on inspiration (Muller & Bryan 1979).

9. The heart and other organs are relatively large in infants and, therefore, there is relatively less space for lung tissue.

Physiological differences

1. The lungs of infants are less compliant than those of older children and adults, particularly in preterm infants where there will probably be a lack of surfactant.

2. Neonates, especially those born preterm, have irregular breathing patterns which may lead to apnoea. Although short spells of apnoea are considered normal, longer periods and those which require stimulation to restart breathing will need investigation.

3. The compliant rib cage with its lack of bucket handle movement does not allow the infant to increase lung volume so that, when in respiratory difficulties, the infant must increase respiratory rate, rather than depth, to maintain minute volume.

4. Neonates may sleep for up to 20 hours a day and 80% of this time may be in rapid eye movement (REM) sleep. This percentage compares with 20% REM sleep in adults. During REM sleep there is a decrease in postural tone causing a drop in functional residual capacity, thereby increasing the work of breathing (Muller & Bryan 1979).

5. The diaphragm has only approximately 25% fatigue resistant type I muscle fibres in the neonate. The adult has 50%. Preterm infants may have as little as 10% and, therefore, have an increased susceptibility to diaphragm fatigue.

6. Hypoxia in infants causes bradycardia (less than 100 beats/min), rather than tachycardia as in adults.

7. Infants and children preferentially ventilate uppermost lung regions, rather than dependent lung regions as in the adult (Davies et al 1985). This difference may persist up to 10 years of age.

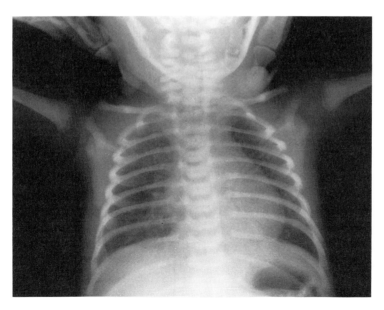

Fig. 13.1 Normal chest radiograph.

In children with unilateral lung disease, the good lung should be positioned uppermost to maximize gas exchange.

8. In the small infant the closing volume exceeds the functional residual capacity so that airway closure occurs following full expiration.

9. Children have a higher resting metabolic rate with greater demand for oxygen. Any further demands placed on them can, therefore, cause hypoxia more rapidly than in adults.

RESPIRATORY ASSESSMENT OF THE INFANT AND CHILD

Careful assessment is essential to identify a problem requiring physiotherapy intervention. Many aspects of assessment will be the same as in adults, but specific differences are listed below.

Medical notes

Information can be extracted from the medical notes relating to present condition and past medical history, etc. When assessing a neonate, the following points are relevant:

1. History of pregnancy, labour, and delivery.
2. The Apgar score, which relates to heart rate, respiratory effort, muscle tone, reflex irritability, and colour, and gives an indication of the degree of asphyxiation suffered by the infant at birth.
3. Gestational age and weight.

Discussion with the relevant carers

Discussion with medical staff, nursing staff, and the parent/guardian is essential to obtain correct information about recent changes. Questions may include:

1. How stable has the child's condition been over the last few hours?
2. How well is handling tolerated? Does the infant become rapidly hypoxic or bradycardic? How long does he take to recover from the handling episode?
3. Is the infant being fed? If so, is it via the oral, nasogastric, or intravenous route? When was the last enteral feed?

4. Is the infant properly rested from the last handling episode?

Nursing charts

From the nursing charts it is important to note:

1. Temperature. If the child is pyrexial, this may indicate a possible respiratory infection. In preterm infants, a temperature of less than 36.5°C indicates that non-essential handling should be delayed until the infant's temperature has risen. The core-to-peripheral temperature gradient should also be noted, particularly in patients following cardiac surgery.
2. Trend of heart rate. A child who is tachycardic may be septic or in shock. If the child is ventilated, inadequate sedation must be excluded. In preterm infants both self-limiting bradycardias and bradycardias requiring stimulation may be due to many causes, but one to be considered is retention of secretions.
3. Apnoeic spells in the infant may indicate respiratory distress, sepsis, or presence of secretions in the upper or lower respiratory tract.
4. The trend of arterial gases and their relationship to oxygen saturation and transcutaneous oxygen and carbon dioxide should be noted together with the type of ventilation and amount of inspired oxygen.
5. Other relevant observations should be made as in adults, e.g. blood pressure, intracranial pressure, urine output, etc.
6. Drug therapy including analgesia, bronchodilators, sedation, etc. Infants may or may not require paralysis in order to be ventilated.

Results of investigations and observations

Results of investigations, e.g. chest radiograph, lung function tests, and bacteriology results, should be referred to as appropriate. Other relevant observations, as in adults, include the presence of intravenous infusions, drains, arterial lines, pacing wires, etc.

Examination

Examination of the older child is similar to that of

the adult. Points which are specific to infants and younger children in the assessment of respiratory distress include:

Observations

1. *Recession*—recession occurs due to the high negative pressure generated on inspiration pulling on the very soft, compliant chest wall and may be sternal, subcostal, or intercostal. Mild recession may be normal, but if the sternum and ribs are severely pulled in, this movement is a sign that the infant is making increased respiratory effort.

2. *Nasal flaring*—this dilatation of the nostrils by the dilatores naris muscles is a sign of respiratory distress in the infant. It may be a primitive response attempting to decrease airway resistance.

3. *Tachypnoea*—respiratory rates greater than or equal to 60 breaths/min indicate respiratory distress in infants. The normal respiratory rate is 35–40 breaths/min in a full-term neonate. The normal respiratory rate for preterm infants varies according to gestational age. The more preterm the infant, the higher the normal respiratory rate.

4. *Grunting*—this noise is made by the infant when breathing out against a partially closed glottis. It is an attempt to increase functional residual capacity and thereby improve ventilation.

5. *Stridor*—this harsh sound is made when there is partial obstruction of the upper trachea and/or larynx. Obstruction may be due to collapse of the floppy tracheal wall, inflammation, or an inhaled foreign body.

6. *Neck extension*—the infant and young child with respiratory distress will often slightly extend the neck in order to lessen airway resistance. Over-extension of the neck in an infant, however, collapses the trachea.

7. *Head bobbing*—when infants are attempting to use the sternocleidomastoid and the scalene muscles as accessory muscles of respiration, head bobbing is seen because the neck extensors of infants are not strong enough to stabilize the head and prevent this movement.

8. *Reluctance to feed*—infants with respiratory distress are often reluctant to feed, needing to take frequent pauses from sucking when very tachypnoeic.

9. *Cyanosis*—is an unreliable sign of respiratory distress in infants and young children as it depends on the relative amount and type of haemoglobin in the blood and the adequacy of the peripheral circulation. For the first 3–4 weeks of life, the newborn infant has an increased amount of fetal haemoglobin in the blood which has a higher affinity for oxygen than adult haemoglobin. This fetal haemoglobin shifts the oxygen saturation curve to the left in an infant.

10. *Pallor*—is commonly seen in infants with respiratory distress and may be a sign of hypoxaemia or other problems including anaemia.

11. *Barrel shaped thoracic cage*—is a result of hyperinflation and air trapping within the lung. This air trapping may occur acutely in the infant with small airway disease such as bronchiolitis, but also may be a sign of chronic obstructive lung disease as seen in asthma.

Auscultation. Auscultation of the infant and young child is difficult due to the easy transmission of sounds. In the preterm infant who is ventilated, referred sounds from the ventilator, including water in the expiratory tubing, make assessment extremely difficult. It is often impossible to hear any breath sounds at all in the preterm infant who is breathing spontaneously.

In the older child, secretions in the nose or throat may lead to referred crackles in both lung fields.

Wheezing in the younger child or infant may be due to bronchospasm, but could also be due to retained secretions partially occluding smaller airways.

Other relevant observations. The behaviour and manner of a child can give important clues about his respiratory state. A child who is sitting up and playing happily is not usually distressed, whereas one who is agitated or irritable may be showing signs of hypoxia. The child in severe respiratory distress may be withdrawn and lie completely still as if saving all his energy for respiration.

It is important to note muscle tone and appearance in the infant or child with respiratory distress. A hypotonic child will have increased difficulty with breathing, coughing and expectorating. Children with hypertonia will also have difficulty with clearing secretions.

Abdominal distension can be a cause of respiratory distress in infants or can worsen an existing respiratory problem because the diaphragm, the main respiratory muscle in infants, is less able to work effectively.

PHYSIOTHERAPY TECHNIQUES IN INFANTS AND CHILDREN

Most physiotherapy techniques used in adults can be applied in children and the same contraindications apply. Differences when using techniques in younger children and infants are as follows:

General points

1. The possible deleterious effects of chest physiotherapy and suction mean that treatment should only be given when indicated and never as a 'routine'.
2. Whenever possible, children and infants should be treated prior to feeds or at least 1 hour following feeds to avoid aspiration of stomach contents.

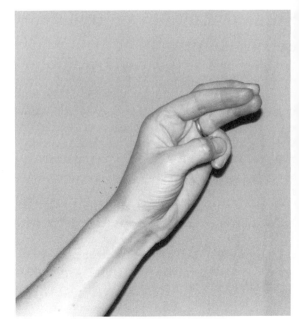

Fig. 13.2   Position of fingers for 'Tenting'.

Chest percussion

Chest percussion includes chest clapping using the hand or chest percussion using, e.g. a face mask. Children up to the age of about 1 year tolerate chest percussion very well—infants will often fall asleep while being treated! Clapping should be one-handed in small children and infants. For preterm infants the first 3 or 4 fingers of one hand may be used, slightly elevating the middle finger (tenting) (Fig. 13.2). Chest percussion can be applied using a cup-shaped object such as a face mask (Fig. 13.3). This mask has a soft plastic cuff and so can be used over bare skin. The face mask has been shown to be a well tolerated means of percussion (Tudehope & Bagley 1980) but is probably not effective in infants bigger than 5 kg. When using the hand for clapping, the chest should always be covered with clothing or a towel.

Vibrations and shaking

These techniques are not generally as well tolerated as percussion in infants and small children. They can be applied using fingertips or the whole hand, depending on the size of the child.

The chest wall is very compliant in infants and young children, so vibrations can be very effective in removing secretions when the respiratory rate is normal or near normal (30–40 breaths/min). If infants are breathing very rapidly, e.g. more than 60 breaths/min, the expiratory phase is so short that vibrations will not be effective.

Precautions for chest percussion and vibratory techniques

1. Children with dietary deficiencies, liver disease, or those who have been born preterm may develop rickets. Skeletal changes in rickets include general osteoporosis and softening of long bones and deformities of the thorax and pelvis. Depending on the circumstances, percussion and vibrations may be contraindicated. This decision should be discussed with the paediatrician.
2. Vibrations during expiration should not be continued beyond functional residual capacity as closing volume exceeds functional residual capacity.
3. Very preterm infants have extremely thin skin which is easily bruised and damaged, thereby predisposing to infection. Chest percussion and vibrations may not be appropriate in these infants.

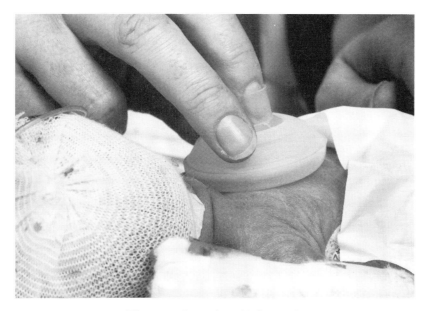

Fig. 13.3 Percussion with face mask.

Gravity-assisted positioning (postural drainage)

Gravity-assisted positions can be used for children in the same way as adults. The upper lobes, particularly the right side, are often more affected by respiratory problems in younger children so gravity-assisted positions for these areas are important, particularly the posterior segments.

Precautions with positioning

1. As children preferentially ventilate the uppermost lung in the side lying position, great care must be taken in putting the affected area uppermost for physiotherapy treatment. This position may cause rapid deterioration in the acutely ill child's condition.

2. Any child with raised intracranial pressure should not be tipped head down.

3. Infants and children with abdominal distension do not tolerate the head down position, because the diaphragm, which is the main inspiratory muscle, cannot work effectively.

4. Newborn infants are better oxygenated when tilted slightly head up (Thoresen et al 1988) and show a drop in PaO_2 if placed flat or tilted head down unless they are fully mechanically ventilated.

5. Preterm infants who are very unstable should not have their position changed for treatment. Those at risk of periventricular haemorrhage should not be tipped head down.

Manual hyperinflation

The same indications and contraindications apply for children as for adults when considering manual hyperinflation as a physiotherapy technique.

500 ml bags are used for infants and 1 litre bags are used for children. Bags may have valves or be open-ended for outlet of excess pressure, controlled by the operator's fingers (Fig. 13.4). Self-inflating bags may be used in some units. Flow rate of gas into the bag depends on the size of the child: 2 l/min for small infants increasing to 8 l/min for children. Oxygen is usually used for manual hyperinflation, but if the child is ventilated on room air the procedure should be carried out using air, unless the child requires preoxygenation. A manometer should ·be placed in the circuit when treating children less than 2 years old so that the amount of pressure being generated can be observed. As a general guideline, the inspiratory pressure should be increased by no more than 20% of the inspiratory pressure on the ventilator. In order to prevent airway collapse, some positive end expiratory pressure (PEEP) should be maintained in the bag.

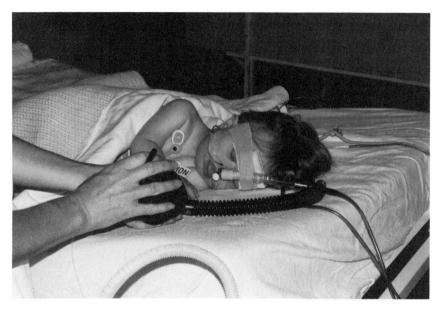

Fig. 13.4 Manual hyperinflation in small child.

Manual hyperinflation should only be carried out in children by staff experienced in its use.

Precautions of manual hyperinflation in children

1. The lack of alveolar and bronchiolar connecting channels in infants and young children means that air will not diffuse from inflated to collapsed alveoli. Manual hyperinflation is therefore likely to overinflate areas already inflated but leave other areas collapsed. This effect also increases the risk of pneumothorax. Particular care should be taken in conditions causing hyper-inflation, e.g. asthma and bronchiolitis.

2. Preterm infants have very delicate lung tissue which is easily damaged by high inflation pressures. Manual hyperinflation should not be used as a physiotherapy technique in these patients.

Breathing exercises

Laughing and crying are very effective means of lung expansion in infants. It is possible to encourage children to deep breathe from about 2 years of age by using bubbles, paper windmills, etc., although whether these 'deep breaths' are effective is debatable. Incentive spirometers are useful pre- and postoperatively or when teaching

inhaler technique. Huffing or 'huffing games' can also be introduced at this age.

Older children can be taught the active cycle of breathing techniques. Since children use the diaphragm as the main inspiratory muscle, they find breathing control very easy. Encouraging them to 'fill up their tummy with air, like a balloon' works well, provided they are reminded not to use their abdominal muscles.

Coughing

Children from about 18 months of age can often mimic coughing if asked to do so, but it is often very difficult to persuade an acutely ill child to cough and expectorate.

Positioning or movement may cause mobilization of secretions which may stimulate a cough reflex. Secretions produced will be swallowed as the ability to expectorate does not often develop before 3–4 years of age.

In children of less than 18 months of age, tracheal compression can be used to stimulate a cough. Gentle pressure with a sideways motion is briefly applied with a finger to the trachea below the thyroid cartilage. This causes apposition of the tracheal walls, which are soft and pliant in this age group, stimulating the cough reflex. This technique must be used with care as the infant may become bradycardic.

If there is no effective cough and there are copious secretions, suction will have to be used.

Suction

Oxygen should be available for use as necessary, and particular points to note for infants and young children are as follows:

1. Preoxygenation is usually important to reduce hypoxia, but care should be taken in preterm infants to avoid hyperoxia. The inspired oxygen should therefore only be increased by about 10% in these infants. Hyperoxia, even for a short time, may lead to retinopathy of prematurity, a condition which can cause permanent blindness (Gandy & Roberton 1987). In infants with increased pulmonary blood flow preoxygenation should be omitted to avoid further dilatation of the pulmonary vasculature.

2. Infants are at particular risk of infection, so great care must be taken with handwashing and wearing gloves, etc.

3. The vacuum pressure should not be excessive but will need to be strong enough to draw secretions up very narrow bore catheters. Recommended values are 10–20 kPa (75–150 mmHg).

4. Most commonly used catheters are 6 and 8 French gauge (FG). Size 5 FG and below are usually ineffective in removing thick secretions. Size 10 FG and above should be reserved for use with older children.

5. Diluents and mucolytics, e.g. saline, acetylcysteine, may be used to loosen thick secretions, as appropriate. The following is a guideline only and indicates the amount to be instilled prior to each passing of a suction catheter:

- Preterm infants   0.5 ml
- Full-term infants   0.5–1.0 ml
- Infants   1–3 ml
- Young children   3–5 ml

In some instances, e.g. blockage of a bronchus by a mucus plug, mini-bronchial lavage may be carried out, instilling up to 10 ml at once. Great care should be taken with this technique.

Diluents may be instilled prior to physiotherapy techniques or, in the acutely ill infant, may need to be instilled directly before passing the suction catheter. Instillation may be directly down the endotracheal tube or via a primed suction catheter (Downs 1989).

6. There is a risk of pneumothorax due to perforation of a segmental bronchus by a suction catheter in intubated preterm infants with severe chronic lung disease (Vaughan et al 1978). To avoid this event, suction catheters should not pass further than the carina in infants. A measured catheter can be attached to the incubator so that staff can gauge how far to pass the catheter.

7. The non-intubated child requiring nasopharyngeal suction should be wrapped in a blanket or held firmly by an assistant to avoid unnecessary struggling. The child should be positioned in side lying to avoid aspiration of gastric contents (Fig. 13.5). Constant reassurance should be given throughout the procedure.

8. Particular care should be taken with nasopharyngeal suction of neonates as reflex bradycardia and apnoea can occur (Cordero & Hon 1971).

9. Nasopharyngeal suction should be avoided if the child has stridor or has recently been extubated as it may precipitate laryngospasm.

Passive movements

Passive movements and two-joint muscle stretches should be given regularly to older children in intensive care, although they are at less risk of developing joint stiffness than adults. Care should be taken when handling children and infants who are hypotonic in order to avoid soft tissue damage. Preterm infants are hypotonic and require minimal handling, so passive movements are not usually indicated.

EQUIPMENT USED IN NEONATAL AND PAEDIATRIC INTENSIVE CARE

Physiotherapists working in an intensive care unit should be familiar with equipment used on that unit (Fig. 13.6). They should be able to respond when a problem is indicated by the equipment

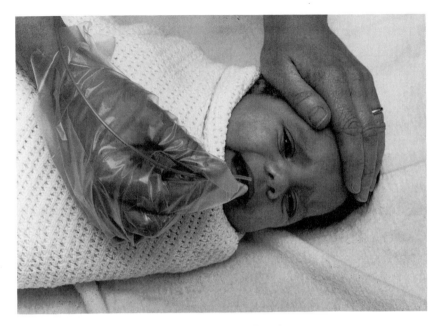

Fig. 13.5   Nasopharyngeal suction.

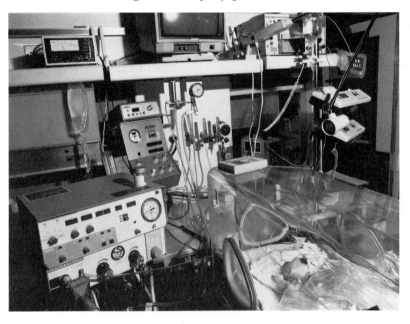

Fig. 13.6   Equipment used in a neonatal intensive care unit.

and be able to ascertain whether the problem is with the patient or the machine.

Mechanical ventilators

These may be specifically designed paediatric ventilators or adult ventilators adapted for paediatric use.

Volume-cycled ventilators are mostly used in older children. The ventilator delivers a set volume of gas to the patient before cycling to expiration. Pressure-cycled and time-cycled ventilators are used in young children and neonates. The pressure-cycled ventilator delivers gas to a preset pressure, the volume of gas delivered being dependent on lung compliance. Time-cycled ventilators deliver a preset pressure for a selected length of time. There is a continuous flow of gas so that the infant is able to breathe spontaneously between ventilator breaths.

Endotracheal tubes

Tubes may be nasal or oral (Fig. 13.7) and are uncuffed for children less than about 8 years old. The lack of cuff reduces the risk of tracheal stenosis but increases the risk of tube displacement and the possibility of aspiration of gastric contents around the tube.

Nasal prong (nasopharyngeal tube)

A nasal prong is a means of delivering continuous positive airway pressure. It is a soft, narrow bore, uncuffed tube which passes through the nose into the pharynx.

Incubators and radiant warmers

Infants may have difficulty maintaining their temperature, especially if they were born preterm. They are therefore nursed in incubators or under radiant warmers.

Incubators are enclosed units of transparent material with portholes in the sides for access. They can be warmed, and humidified air or oxygen can be delivered to the infant inside. The temperature inside an incubator is maintained in the thermoneutral range. This range is the environmental temperature at which oxygen consumption is minimal in the presence of a normal body temperature. It will vary according to the patient's gestation and weight.

A radiant warmer is an open-topped unit with a radiant heating device above it. It allows free access to the infant, but there is more convective heat loss and insensible fluid loss than with an incubator.

Headbox

This is a clear plastic box which is placed over an infant's head to deliver humidifed air or oxygen (Fig. 13.8).

Humidifiers

Humidification is essential for infants and children as narrow bore endotracheal tubes and small airways can easily be blocked by thick secretions. Infants should have heated humidification from humidifiers which can be used with or without ventilators. The temperature of the inspired gas from these humidifiers should be 37–37.5°C at the patient end of the circuit.

Phototherapy unit

These units consist of white or blue lamps which emit light of wavelength 400–500 nm. Light of these wavelengths oxidizes unconjugated bilirubin into harmless derivative and so is very important in the treatment of jaundice in neonates. Infants receiving phototherapy have to be nursed naked, which can cause problems of temperature control. There is also increased insensible fluid loss and a theoretical risk of eye damage, so eye shields should be worn.

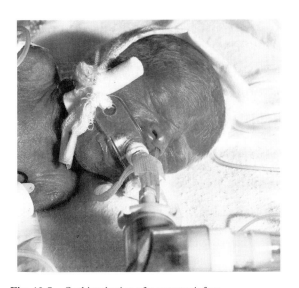

Fig. 13.7 Oral intubation of a preterm infant.

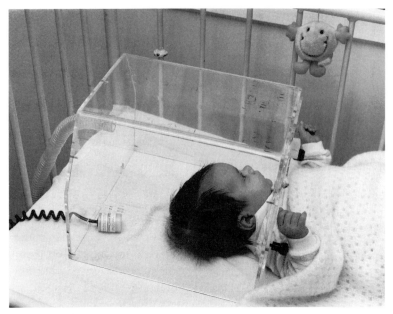

Fig. 13.8   Humidified oxygen delivered via a head box.

Electrocardiogram (ECG), respiratory and blood pressure monitors

These are similar to the monitors used on adults, although normal values vary according to age, (see Table 13.1).

Transcutaneous oxygen monitors

These monitors provide a non-invasive means of measuring the partial pressure of oxygen (PaO_2) in arterialized capillaries through the skin. Transcutaneous oxygen (TcO_2) monitors have electrodes which are heated and placed on an area of thin skin, e.g. the abdomen. The heating produces a superficial erythema so that the PaO_2 in the dilated capillaries can be assessed by the

machine and displayed on a visual monitor. Normal values are 8–12 kPa (60–90 mmHg). Electrodes need to be moved to a different position every 4–6 hours in order to prevent burning.

Transcutaneous carbon dioxide monitors

Transcutaneous carbon dioxide ($TcCO_2$) monitors work on the same principle as TcO_2 monitors and are a useful indication of respiratory status in older infants.

PHYSIOTHERAPY IN THE NEONATAL INTENSIVE CARE UNIT

Physiotherapists who may be called upon to treat infants in a neonatal intensive care unit (NICU) should be fully aware of the problems these infants may have. Reasons for admission to a NICU include:

- Preterm delivery
- Low birth weight
- Perinatal problems
- Congenital abnormalities.

Table 13.1   Normal values of heart rate, respiratory rate and blood pressure according to age

Age group	Heart rate (beats/min)	Respiratory rate (breaths/min)	Blood pressure (mmHg)
Preterm infants	120–140	40–60	70/40
Full-term infants	100–140	30–40	80/40
1–4 years	80–120	25–30	100/65
Adolescents	60–80	15–20	115/60

Preterm delivery

Preterm is defined as less than 37 completed weeks of gestation (full term is 38–42 weeks). In reality those preterm infants who may require admission to a NICU are likely to be less than 32 weeks of gestation and weigh less than 2500 g. Some infants are born after only 23 weeks of pregnancy and may weigh as little as 450 g.

Causes of preterm birth may be antepartum haemorrhage, cervical incompetence, multiple pregnancies, or infection. There is also an association with deprived socio-economic circumstances, and in some cases the cause of preterm delivery is unknown.

Low birth weight

Infants who are born preterm will have a low birth weight, but more mature infants may be of low birth weight due to intra-uterine growth retardation. Causes include placental dysfunction, smoking, and intra-uterine infection, e.g. rubella.

Perinatal problems

Problems occurring at or around the time of birth, e.g. birth asphyxia or meconium aspiration, may lead to an infant being admitted to the NICU.

Congenital abnormalities

Congenital abnormalities include congenital heart disease and diaphragmatic hernia.

General problems of infants in the NICU

Parent–infant bonding

It is accepted modern practice for the newborn to remain with the mother and father, if present, after delivery. Infants who have been resuscitated and transferred to a NICU shortly after birth will not have had the chance for physical contact with their parents.

Bonding is further hindered by the barrier of incubators and other equipment surrounding the infant. Parents should be encouraged to give comfort to their infant by stroking, etc., and to cuddle him when his condition is stable enough to do so.

When parents are confident, they can be involved in their infant's care, e.g. nappy changing.

Handling

Handling of severely ill infants will cause their condition to deteriorate. For this reason, these infants should be left alone as much as possible. Physiotherapy and suction should only be carried out when there are definite indications, e.g. retention of secretions or lung collapse due to mucus plugging. Careful assessment is essential prior to intervention.

Problems of preterm and low birth weight infants

Respiratory distress

The main cause of respiratory distress in preterm infants is respiratory distress syndrome (RDS). The primary cause of this syndrome is lack of surfactant in the immature lung. The more preterm the infant, the higher the incidence of RDS. RDS is seen in 10% of infants of 36 weeks gestation, but in 80% of infants at 28 weeks gestation (Gandy & Roberton 1987).

RDS develops within 4 hours of delivery with sternal and costal recession, grunting, and tachypnoea. The chest radiograph shows a 'ground glass' appearance due to lung collapse (Fig. 13.9). Many preterm infants, however, are 'electively' intubated and ventilated at birth and thus never develop these classical signs.

Treatment includes giving added oxygen to avoid hypoxia, as hypoxia hinders surfactant production. These infants should be handled as little as possible. Mildly affected infants may only require humidified oxygen via a head box, but more severely affected infants will require ventilatory support of some kind such as positive pressure ventilation or continuous positive airway pressure.

The natural history of the syndrome is that surfactant will start to be produced in the lung 36–48 hours after birth, regardless of gestational age. The more mature infant will start to recover at this time. Very preterm infants who have other

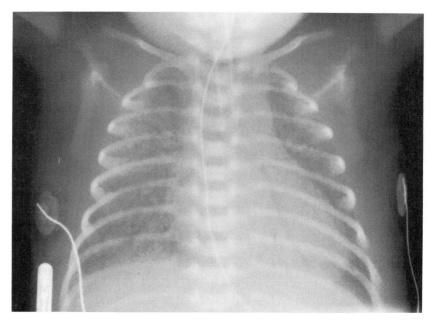

Fig. 13.9 Chest radiograph of respiratory distress syndrome.

problems compounding their respiratory distress or infants who have developed complications of treatment may require ventilatory support for much longer.

During the last decade there have been many trials investigating the use of surfactant therapy to try to prevent or ameliorate RDS (Morley 1991). Natural or artificial surfactant in fluid form is introduced into the endotracheal tube prophylactically or after signs of RDS have appeared. Although these trials have shown a reduction in mortality in very preterm infants given surfactant therapy, it is still unclear which is the best type of surfactant to use and how and when it should be given. Further trials are in progress.

As lung collapse in RDS is primarily caused by lack of surfactant, physiotherapy is not required for this condition. Secretions may become a problem after the infant has been intubated for more than 48 hours due to irritation of the tracheal mucosa by the endotracheal tube. These secretions may be cleared easily by suction alone. Physiotherapy should be given only when suction is not adequately clearing secretions.

Respiratory distress in the preterm infant can also be caused by pneumonia. Organisms causing pneumonia may be bacterial, viral, or fungal and may be acquired before, during or after birth. The most serious bacterial cause is group B *Streptococcus*. The presenting features of this pneumonia are similar to RDS with an indistinguishable chest radiograph. Group B streptococcal pneumonia can be rapidly fatal unless antibiotic therapy is started early. For this reason all infants presenting with respiratory distress are given antibiotics.

Periventricular haemorrhage and periventricular leucomalacia

Periventricular haemorrhage (PVH) is a major cause of mortality and morbidity in very preterm and low birth weight infants. The incidence is inversely proportional to birth weight occurring in about 43% of infants weighing less than 1000 g, 19% of infants weighing between 1000 and 1500 g, and 6% of infants weighing between 1500 and 2000 g (Gandy & Roberton 1987). It may occur spontaneously, but particularly occurs in infants who have had episodes of hypoxia, hypotension, or apnoea. It occurs most frequently and severely in the smallest and least mature infants.

The haemorrhages arise from the fragile capillaries in the floor of the lateral ventricles. Fluctuations of cerebral blood flow are caused by marked changes in blood pressure, arterial oxygen, and carbon dioxide. These fluctuations cause the capillaries to burst and bleed into and around the ventricles.

There are four grades of severity (Gandy and Roberton 1987):

- Grade I—Bleeding into the floor of the ventricle
- Grade II—Bleeding into the ventricle (intraventricular haemorrhage (IVH))
- Grade III—IVH with dilatation of the ventricle
- Grade IV—IVH and bleeding into the cerebral cortex causing areas of ischaemia.

Grades I and II may be asymptomatic and chances of recovery are good. Grades III and IV are likely to cause residual problems such as hydrocephalus or neurological deficit. Severe grade IV haemorrhage may result in the death of the infant.

Prevention of PVH is directed towards minimal handling of 'at risk' infants and avoidance of hypoxic and hypotensive episodes.

Periventricular leucomalacia (PVL) may occur on its own or associated with PVH. Ischaemia of cerebral tissue adjacent to the ventricles causes formation of cystic lesions. There is an association with neurological problems particularly diplegia.

Regular cerebral ultrasound scanning shows the presence of PVH and PVL and their progression.

Temperature control

Preterm and low birth weight infants have difficulty in maintaining their body temperature because they have a large surface area relative to their body mass. They also have a smaller proportion of brown fat in comparison with full-term infants and easily lose heat through the skin by evaporation and radiation.

As hypothermia can cause acidosis, hypoglycaemia, increased oxygen consumption, and decreased surfactant production, it is essential to maintain body temperature. Infants should therefore be kept in a thermoneutral environment.

To maintain a thermoneutral environment, infants are nursed in incubators or under radiant warmers. Heat shields are used to reduce radiant

heat loss and the ambient room temperature is kept high at 27–28°C. Draughts should be avoided and incubator doors should not be left open as the infant's temperature can drop dramatically. If the infant's temperature is less than 36.5°C physiotherapy should not be given unless essential.

Infection

The preterm infant is particularly vulnerable to infection. The skin is very thin and easily damaged. Cellular and humoral resistance to infection are also reduced.

The most important means of preventing and reducing cross infection is by scrupulous hand washing by all staff and visitors. Regular use of a disinfectant solution is also necessary. Visitors should be kept to a minimum, for example parents, siblings, and grandparents. Anyone who has an infectious disease should not enter the unit.

Antibiotic therapy is frequently used to try and prevent infections becoming life threatening.

Jaundice

Physiological jaundice is common in the normal full-term infant due to the breakdown of fetal haemoglobin causing a raised level of unconjugated bilirubin in the blood. Physiological jaundice starts to appear 2 days after birth and has usually disappeared by days 7–10 of life.

If the level of unconjugated bilirubin is high it may diffuse into the basal ganglia and lead to a condition called 'kernicterus'. Kernicterus is characterized by athetoid cerebral palsy, deafness, and mental retardation.

Preterm infants are particularly prone to developing jaundice and run an increased risk of subsequent kernicterus. To avoid this risk, daily serum bilirubin levels are taken by heel prick from jaundiced infants and treatment consists of phototherapy, or in severe cases exchange transfusion. In this procedure, blood is withdrawn from the infant in small amounts (5 or 10 ml) and replaced by donor blood until twice the infant's blood volume has been exchanged.

Nutrition

Adequate calorie intake and weight gain are important in preterm and low birth weight infants to avoid hypoglycaemia, persistent jaundice, and delayed recovery from RDS.

Feeding should be started as soon as possible, either enterally, in those who can tolerate it, or intravenously.

Preterm infants have poor sucking, gag, and cough reflexes so will be fed nasogastrically until these reflexes develop. Continuous infusion of milk is often given rather than bolus feeds as bolus feeds can increase respiratory distress due to abdominal distension. Pooling of milk in the stomach can also lead to regurgitation and aspiration. Orogastric tubes may be used rather than nasogastric ones in order to avoid blockage of the nostril in spontaneously breathing infants with respiratory distress.

Pulmonary haemorrhage

In this condition, fresh blood pours out of the lungs and the infant collapses. It is relatively uncommon but may occur after surfactant therapy.

Physiotherapy is contraindicated, although regular suctioning may be required to keep the airway clear. When fresh blood is no longer being aspirated, physiotherapy techniques may be required to aid removal of residual old blood. Prognosis is often poor.

Perinatal problems

Birth asphyxia

This occurs in about 10% of births. Infants who have been severely asphyxiated may require admission to the NICU. Careful monitoring will be required as these infants may develop cardiac failure, neurological damage, or renal failure. Some may have fits and will need to have anticonvulsant therapy. As these infants are often very irritable, handling should be kept to a minimum.

Meconium aspiration

This usually occurs in full-term infants who become hypoxic due to a prolonged and difficult labour. Hypoxia causes the infant to pass meconium into the amniotic fluid and to make gasping movements so that meconium may be drawn into the pharynx.

If the mother's liquor is meconium stained, a paediatrician should suction the infant's airway as soon as the head is delivered to prevent aspiration when the first breath is taken. Once delivered, the infant may require intubation for further suction. The irritant properties of meconium can cause a chemical pneumonitis and predispose to bacterial infection, especially *Escherichia coli*. A severely affected infant may require assisted ventilation, although ventilation is difficult because of the risk of pneumothorax due to gas trapping.

Physiotherapy is very important when meconium aspiration has occurred in order to remove the extremely thick and tenacious green secretions. Treatment consists of gravity-assisted positioning, as tolerated, with chest percussion and should be carried out as soon as possible after aspiration has occurred, preferably within 1 hour. Physiotherapy is often well tolerated in these cases as removal of meconium plugs allows the infant to be better ventilated.

Congenital abnormalities

Congenital heart disease

This is discussed on page 309.

Diaphragmatic hernia

In this condition loops of bowel herniate through the diaphragm into the thoracic cavity, most commonly on the left side. The incidence is approximately 1 in 3000 births (Dinwiddie 1990). The abnormality may be diagnosed antenatally by ultrasound, or postnatally when the infant presents with respiratory distress (usually soon after birth). A chest radiograph will show abdominal viscera in the thoracic cavity. Unless the herniation has occurred late in pregnancy, which is very unusual, there will be associated pulmonary hypoplasia on the affected side as the abdominal viscera occupy the space normally available for the growing lung. The contralateral lung is also smaller than expected because of compression due to mediastinal shift during pregnancy (Reid 1984).

The infant with diaphragmatic hernia is often very unwell, particularly as the bowel in the chest distends with air and further compresses the lungs, and requires immediate gastric decompression with simultaneous intubation and ventilation. Surgery is not carried out until the infant's condition is fully stabilized. Surgical correction is via a laparotomy. The abdominal viscera are carefully returned to the abdominal cavity and the defect in the diaphragm is closed.

Postoperatively, the infant may require ventilation for some time, depending on the amount of pulmonary hypoplasia. Prognosis is often poor as the mortality for this condition is about 60%. Physiotherapy may be indicated postoperatively if retention of secretions is a problem. Manual hyperinflation is contraindicated because the lungs are hypoplastic and high pressures should be avoided.

Oesophageal atresia with tracheo-oesophageal fistula

This condition may present in several ways, most commonly with the upper end of the oesophagus finishing in a blind pouch, with a fistula between the trachea and the lower section of the oesophagus. The incidence is approximately 1 in 3500 births (Byrne 1991).

The infant presents shortly after birth with respiratory distress due to the inability to swallow saliva which overflows and is aspirated into the trachea. The first feed will cause choking and coughing.

Surgical correction is usually attempted as soon as possible. Preoperatively the airway should be kept clear by continuous suction of the upper pouch, and the infant should be nursed head up to prevent reflux of gastric contents through the fistula.

In most cases surgical treatment consists of primary anastomosis of the oesophagus and closure of the tracheo-oesophageal fistula. Some anastomoses may be performed under tension so that the infant has to be electively ventilated and paralysed with the neck kept in flexion postoperatively. In a few cases, where the gap between the two ends of the oesophagus is too large, primary anastomosis is not possible, and a feeding gastrostomy with cervical oesophagostomy are performed. Oesophageal replacement by colonic, jejunal, or gastric interposition will be carried out at a later date.

Physiotherapy. Preoperatively some patients may require physiotherapy if there are increased secretions or lung collapse due to reflux of gastric contents. Treatment must be carried out in the head up position. Postoperatively the patient will be nursed in the head up position for the first few days. Physiotherapy may be indicated but the head down position should not be used because of the risk of reflux. Care must be taken not to extend the neck, especially in those patients whose anastomosis has been performed under tension. In the non-intubated patient, pharyngeal suction must be used cautiously to avoid passing the catheter into the oesophagus and damaging the anastomosis.

Gastroschisis and exompholus (ompholocele)

These conditions are due to a defect in the abdominal wall and occur in approximately 1 in 6000 births (Byrne 1991). The small and large intestines and sometimes the liver are outside the abdominal cavity (gastroschisis) or enclosed in a sac of amniotic membrane and peritoneum (exompholus). The defect is usually diagnosed antenatally by ultrasound.

Immediately after birth, the abdominal contents are covered and the infant is wrapped in a polythene sheet from axillae to feet to prevent heat and fluid loss until he can be taken for surgery.

Postoperatively the infant usually requires ventilation as the tightly packed, rigid abdomen causes respiratory embarrassment and compromises venous return. These infants often need to be sedated, paralysed, and ventilated for weeks. Primary closure may not be possible, and various means may be employed to stretch the abdominal wall carefully to allow the abdominal contents to be returned. During this time it may not be possible to turn the infant.

Physiotherapy. These infants are particularly at risk from retention of secretions and lobar collapse due to the distended abdomen and lack of position changes. If treatment is required, techniques which increase intrathoracic pressure and consequently increase intra-abdominal pressure, such as vibrations, should be used cautiously, and manual hyperinflation is contraindicated.

Meconium ileus

In this condition, thickened meconium causes blockage of the colon and ileum. The infant presents in the first day of life with abdominal distension, vomiting and failure to pass meconium. The obstruction can sometimes be relieved conservatively by enemas, but laparotomy is often required with formation of a temporary colostomy.

Most patients who present with this condition have cystic fibrosis which will later be confirmed with a sweat test. Of cystic fibrosis patients, 12% present in this way.

Physiotherapy. As a large proportion of these patients have cystic fibrosis, retention of secretions can be a major problem, so physiotherapy intervention is very important. Physiotherapy should be continued even after initial postoperative problems have been resolved, unless the patient has been shown not to have cystic fibrosis.

Congenital anomalies of the lung

Congenital conditions of the lung such as lobar emphysema, lung cysts, and adenomata are very rare. They may be diagnosed by ultrasound antenatally, or by the chest radiograph postnatally. Treatment is usually surgical resection (lobectomy) sometimes as an emergency if there is severe mediastinal shift.

Acquired lobar emphysema and lung cysts are more common as complications of respiratory distress syndrome and its treatment. Most of these cases will resolve with medical therapy and only a few will require resection.

Physiotherapy may be indicated postoperatively if there is sputum retention, but manual hyperinflation is contraindicated if cysts are present.

Pulmonary hypoplasia

This condition occurs in approximately 1 in 1000 births (Dinwiddie 1990) and is associated with oligohydramnios (reduction of amniotic fluid) during pregnancy, secondary to fetal renal problems or due to prolonged rupture of membranes. The prognosis for pulmonary hypoplasia is variable, depending on the severity and underlying cause. The prognosis is worse in those with renal problems.

VENTILATION OF THE NEWBORN

Ventilation is often started from birth in infants of birth weight less than 1000 g but otherwise the indications are (McMahon & Kovar 1990):

1. Deteriorating blood gases indicating respiratory failure, i.e. PaO_2 less than 8 kPa (60 mmHg) with an FiO_2 of 60% and/or $PaCO_2$ greater than 8 kPa (60 mmHg).

2. Recurrent or major apnoea.

3. Major surgery pre- and/or postoperatively, e.g. cardiac lesions, diaphragmatic hernia.

Conventional positive pressure ventilation

Mature infants of birth weight greater than 2500 g can be ventilated at rates of 30–40 breaths/min with time-cycled, pressure-limited, constant-flow ventilators. Preterm, low birth weight infants have been shown to be better oxygenated with fast rate ventilation (60–150 breaths/min) using the same ventilators (Greenough et al 1987). These higher rates mimic the spontaneous respiratory rates of very preterm infants, who may breathe in synchrony with the ventilator, enhancing oxygenation (Greenough et al 1987). Those infants who do not synchronize with the ventilator require paralysis to prevent the development of pneumothorax (Greenough et al 1984).

Ventilator settings are adjusted to maintain the PaO_2 between 7.0 and 9.5 kPa (50–70 mmHg) and the $PaCO_2$ between 4.5–7.0 kPa (35–50 mmHg), although the $PaCO_2$ may be allowed to go higher in infants with chronic lung disease who are being weaned from the ventilator. At all times the PaO_2 levels must be monitored to reduce the risk of retinopathy of prematurity.

Infants may be weaned from ventilation by first reducing the inspiratory pressures and FiO_2 and then the respiratory rate through intermittent mandatory ventilation (IMV) and continuous positive airway pressure (CPAP). More mature infants may be extubated and then require only humidified oxygen via a head box, but low birth weight infants often require CPAP via a naso-pharyngeal airway (nasal prong).

Patient-triggered ventilation

Triggered ventilation has been shown to be useful as an aid to weaning from conventional ventila-tion and in some mature infants during the acute stage of RDS (Greenough & Pool 1988). It is not as useful in the very preterm low birth weight infant whose respiratory efforts are often inade-quate and inconsistent. Modified neonatal venti-lators that respond quickly to small changes in airflow are needed in these infants.

Negative extrathoracic pressure ventilation

Negative extrathoracic pressure ventilation (NEPV) was first used in the treatment of children with respiratory failure due to poliomyelitis. It has now been adapted for use in the management of respiratory failure due to a variety of causes (Samuels & Southall 1989).

The equipment consists of a transparent perspex box in which the infant's body is placed with the head remaining outside. An airtight seal around the neck is essential. There are portholes for access for nursing care and physiotherapy. A negative pressure is applied to the box so that the pressure inside becomes subatmospheric and assists with ventilation. The indications for the use of NEPV are:

- Respiratory failure due to myopathy or other neuromuscular disorder
- Congenital central hypoventilation (Ondine's curse)
- Bilateral phrenic nerve damage
- Weaning from positive pressure ventilation (e.g. in RDS or following cardiac surgery)

- Prevention of further lung damage due to positive pressure ventilation in infants with severe chronic lung disease.

The use of NEPV is at present not widespread.

Extracorporeal membrane oxygenation

Extracorporeal membrane oxygenation (ECMO) is used in the management of infants with severe reversible respiratory failure who are not responding to other forms of ventilatory support. Infants are considered for ECMO if they have a predicted mortality of greater than 80%, are not suffering from serious congenital abnormalities, serious persistent neurological damage, and do not have a high risk of spontaneous bleeding or periventricular haemorrhage. The risk of haemor-rhage makes most preterm infants weighing less than 2000 g ineligible.

Blood is taken from the jugular vein, passed through a membrane oxygenator and returned via the umbilical or femoral vein or via the carotid artery. Positive pressure ventilation is continued, but on minimal settings to prevent lung damage.

ECMO has many complications and in all but a few patients there is still controversy over whether it is more effective than appropriate aggressive conventional therapy.

High frequency jet ventilation and high frequency oscillation (HFO)

High frequency jet ventilation (HFJV) delivers compressed gas through a small bore cannula at rates of between 180–600 per minute. High frequency oscillation (HFO) uses a pump oscil-lator or airflow interrupter to deliver pulses of gas at a rate of 180–3000 per minute (3–50 Hz). The tidal volumes of gas used at these high frequencies are less than the dead space, and gas exchange is thought to occur by diffusion and convection (Sumner 1990).

These techniques have been used in patients with RDS, pulmonary interstitial emphysema, and pulmonary hypoplasia due to diaphragmatic hernia. Boros et al (1986) reported complications of tracheal erosions and necrosis with HFJV.

Further study is necessary to determine which groups of patients will benefit from these types of ventilation.

Complications of ventilatory support

Pneumothorax

Pneumothoraces are a complication of positive pressure ventilation occurring mainly in preterm infants with immature lungs or in association with congenital bullae. A predisposing factor is the hyperinflation of alveoli occurring in conditions such as meconium aspiration and RDS.

Causative factors are high peak inspiratory pressures, positive end expiratory pressure, long inflation times, and active expiration by the infant against the ventilator's inspiration (Greenough et al 1983).

A tension pneumothorax will cause a sudden deterioration in the infant's condition, and should be drained as soon as possible with a chest drain and suction.

Small pneumothoraces may not require drainage but the infant will need close monitoring.

Pulmonary interstitial emphysema

Pulmonary interstitial emphysema (PIE) occurs when gas leaks out of an alveolus, tracks along the cardiovascular bundle and remains trapped forming interstitial gas pockets. PIE is most common in preterm infants; the incidence is inversely proportional to gestational age.

Treatment is fast rate, low pressure ventilation with a longer expiratory than inspiratory time to prevent an increase in air trapping. In severe cases, where ventilation is becoming difficult, needle scarification of the lung surface may be helpful. Unresolved PIE may require surgical resection in severe cases.

Subglottic stenosis

Subglottic stenosis occurs in some infants following prolonged intubation and leads to upper airway obstruction. Stridor is often present and may respond to adrenaline via a nebulizer, but severely affected infants may require tracheostomy until the airway has increased sufficiently in size to allow adequate ventilation. This growth may take years. In order to prevent subglottic stenosis, uncuffed tubes are used and a small air leak should always be present during ventilation.

Retinopathy of prematurity

In this condition the delicate capillaries in the retina proliferate leading to haemorrhage, fibrosis and scarring of the retina. In the most severe form, this may result in permanent visual impairment. The cause is unknown but periods of hyperoxia (exact length of time unknown) with a PaO_2 of above 12 kPa are thought to be a major predisposing factor (Gandy & Roberton 1987).

Continuous oxygen monitoring using a transcutaneous oxygen electrode and oxygen saturation monitor is essential to attempt to prevent this condition.

The damaged retina is treated with cryotherapy.

Bronchopulmonary dysplasia or chronic lung disease

About 15% of infants who require ventilation after birth go on to develop bronchopulmonary dysplasia (BPD). BPD is defined as a requirement for ventilatory support at 1 month of age with typical radiographic changes. Many infants do not fit this original definition and the term 'chronic lung disease' is now more commonly used.

The most common cause of chronic lung disease (CLD) is acute RDS requiring oxygen and ventilatory support. High peak pressures in positive pressure ventilation cause barotrauma, and high inspired oxygen concentrations cause an acute inflammatory response leading to local tissue damage. Other precipitating factors are fluid overload, persistent ductus arteriosus and PIE.

The infant with CLD shows an increased oxygen requirement and carbon dioxide retention and has decreased lung compliance with increased airway resistance. The infant is tachypnoeic with persistent sternal and costal recession. The condition may be progressive, requiring more ventilatory support and eventually leading to respiratory and cardiac failure.

Radiographic appearances can vary but include alternating areas of collapse and hyperinflation, widespread fibrosis, and scarring of the lung with compensatory emphysema.

Treatment consists of appropriate respiratory support which may be IMV, CPAP, HFO, NEPV or added oxygen via a head box or nasal cannulae. Good nutrition is essential and the infant may require fluid restriction and diuretics. Some infants respond to bronchodilators and steroids. Antibiotics may be required as these infants are prone to recurrent chest infections.

The prognosis is variable. Mortality may be as high as 30% in severe cases. Those who survive are often small and underweight, have recurrent upper and lower respiratory tract infections, wheezing and gastric reflux. These abnormalities are particularly common in the first 2 years of life (Sauve & Singhal 1985). Some children may require oxygen for several years and are therefore managed at home if the family is able to cope with home oxygen therapy.

The long-term prognosis for those who survive the first 2 years is good.

Physiotherapy. As infants with CLD are particularly prone to chest infections, physiotherapy may be indicated if excess secretions are a problem. These infants often have severe wheeze and airway collapse and physiotherapy techniques may not be appropriate. Careful assessment is important before any intervention. If wheezing is not too severe, careful treatment may be possible following bronchodilator therapy, providing the infant has a good response (O'Callaghan et al 1986, 1989). Modified gravity- assisted positions with chest percussion may be useful, and suction may be required. Infants having oxygen through nasal cannulae often have a problem with thick, dry nasal secretions. It is not possible to humidify oxygen effectively when using nasal cannulae as the water condenses in the small bore tubing and cuts off the oxygen supply. Humidifiers which bubble oxygen through cold water counteract the absolute dryness of the oxygen to some extent but are not effective in loosening thick secretions. If necessary, the infant should have nasal cannulae while awake during the day to allow social interaction, but should have humidified oxygen via a head box for long periods of sleep. Normal saline via a nebulizer or saline nose drops can also be used but have a limited effect.

Ventilation in children

Children may require ventilation for respiratory failure which may be primary or secondary to other problems, for example cerebral oedema due to head injury. Children may also be electively ventilated following major surgery.

Methods of ventilation and weaning are similar to those in infants, although ventilator rates greater than 60 breaths/min are not usually required.

Indications and risks for the various types of ventilation, for example intermittent positive pressure ventilation IPPV, high frequency positive pressure ventilation HFPPV, ECMO, are the same. The complications of pulmonary interstitial emphysema, chronic lung disease, and retinopathy of prematurity are only seen in the newborn.

RESPIRATORY DISEASE IN CHILDHOOD

Respiratory disease in childhood is very common, comprising about half of all illnesses in children less than 5 years of age and about a third of illness in primary school children (Price 1986). Most of the illnesses are mild, but about 5% are more serious, involving the lower respiratory tract. The highest morbidity and mortality from lower respiratory tract disease occurs in the first year of life.

Respiratory disease is more common in children from a poor socio-economic background, with a family history of respiratory disease, from an urban rather than country environment, with a pre-school age sibling, or with a mother who smokes.

Respiratory disease is more severe in infants with congenital heart or lung abnormalities, immunodeficiency, cystic fibrosis, or chronic lung disease (bronchopulmonary dysplasia).

Asthma

Asthma affects 10–20% of infants and children with a wide range of severity.

Pathology

The main problem is bronchial hyperreactivity, i.e. the bronchial smooth muscle overreacts to normal everyday stimuli. This reaction leads to hypertrophy of smooth muscle in the bronchial wall. There is also an inflammatory response in the mucosa and submucosa, mucus gland hyperplasia and mucus plugging. These changes can lead to chronic and severe airway obstruction and gas trapping (hyperinflation).

Cause

Hereditary and allergic factors play an important part in childhood asthma. A child is more likely to develop asthma if parents or close relatives are asthmatic or atopic (allergic) (Konig & Godfrey 1973). There is an important link between atopy and bronchial hyperreactivity. About 90% of children with asthma also have other atopic features such as eczema, food allergy, hayfever or urticaria. Exposure to specific allergens such as house dust mite, pollen and animal dander can precipitate bronchial hyperreactivity leading to bronchospasm and wheeze. Other factors such as exercise, emotional upset, or upper respiratory tract infections can also have this effect.

Management

Children with mild infrequent asthma need intermittent bronchodilator treatment. The younger child may show more benefit from an anticholinergic agent (Henry et al 1984). Those who have more frequent attacks require additional regular prophylactic treatment with sodium cromoglycate (Intal), theophylline or inhaled steroids. All drugs should preferably be given by inhalation, although children under the age of 2 years may use oral preparations. In order that inhaled drug therapy can be effective, it is essential that the correct mode of delivery is chosen according to the age of the child.

Children under 2 years may use a nebulizer in addition to oral bronchodilator therapy. A metered dose inhaler (MDI) with a spacer device (for example Nebuhaler or Volumatic and face mask) can be used to deliver bronchodilators to infants. Some centres omit the spacer device and use a polystyrene coffee cup for the face mask. The infant is placed in the supine position and the mask is held gently over the nose and mouth with the spacer held vertically. The drug can then drift down through the open valve to be inhaled. As infants can exhibit paradoxical bronchoconstriction following inhaled bronchodilators, the first dose should be given in controlled circumstances, for example in a hospital or clinic (O'Callaghan et al 1986, 1989).

From the age of 2–5 years, the spacer device can be used conventionally with the MDI (Fig. 13.10). Five tidal volume breaths are needed to inhale each dose of the drug (Gleeson & Price 1988). The click of the valve opening will be heard with each breath.

From about 5 years of age, children's inspiratory flow rates will be fast enough to use powdered preparations in devices which are easy to use, such as a rotahaler, diskhaler or turbohaler.

The MDI without a spacer should not be used until the child is able to coordinate activation of the aerosol with inhalation. Children will not usually have this skill before the age of 8 years.

All patients using inhaled steroids should be instructed to rinse the mouth after inhalation to avoid candidiasis (thrush).

Any of the above inhaler devices will be less

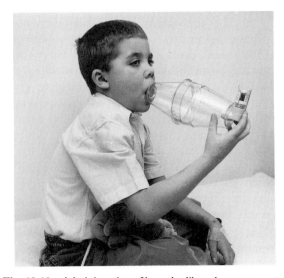

Fig. 13.10   Administration of bronchodilator by spacer device.

effective during an acute attack when inhalation may be difficult. A nebulizer will then be required for drug delivery, preferably with a mouthpiece (when the child is able to use one) to avoid drug deposition on the face.

Children with an acute severe attack may require admission to hospital. Signs of respiratory distress may be apparent, but wheezing may or may not be marked. When there is severe airway obstruction with hyperinflation, airflow is reduced so a wheeze may not be heard.

Initial treatment consists of nebulized bronchodilators. If a good response is not obtained intravenous theophylline will be started. Intravenous steroids and β_2 agonist drugs will be required if initial therapy does not have the necessary effect. Humidified oxygen should be given as required to maintain oxygen saturation at 90–95%.

A few severely affected children who do not respond to these drug regimens may require ventilation.

Physiotherapy management

A crucial part of the management of asthma is education of the child and parents about the condition and its treatment. It is important that the physiotherapist is part of the team involved in that education. Physiotherapists are often involved in teaching children how to take their medication, although in some clinics this role is taken by a specialist asthma nurse.

Physiotherapists can also advise on exercise which is important in the asthmatic child to maintain general fitness. Where exercise-induced asthma (EIA) is a problem, bronchodilators should be taken before beginning exercise. Swimming is the activity least likely to cause EIA and running is the one most likely to cause EIA (Dinwiddie 1990).

Some physiotherapists organize swimming and exercise classes specially designed for asthmatic children. These classes include instruction in drug therapy, progressive exercises to increase exercise tolerance, posture awareness, and breathing control to help cope with breathlessness during an acute attack. Peak flow is monitored regularly to judge effectiveness of treatment.

Apart from physical improvement, classes are also important psychologically, particularly for those with more severe asthma. These children are often afraid to exercise and lack confidence.

Older children who do not have access to such classes should have the opportunity to consult a physiotherapist, if necessary, for education in breathing control and posture awareness.

The child with an acute attack may be severely ill. When bronchospasm is severe, tipping the child head down and encouraging coughing should not be attempted. Even in the ventilated patient it will not be possible to mobilize secretions until bronchodilation has occurred. Younger children will not be able to cooperate with breathing control at this stage, but the physiotherapist may be able to advise on optimum positioning to reduce breathlessness.

When treatment is appropriate it should be given at least 15 min following inhaled bronchodilators and should proceed cautiously. If bronchospasm worsens treatment should be discontinued.

Not all patients will require physiotherapy following an acute attack. Often effective bronchodilation will allow the younger child to cough and clear secretions spontaneously.

Children with persistent areas of lung collapse following an acute attack will respond well to appropriate gravity-assisted positioning and chest clapping with the active cycle of breathing techniques. Parents may need to continue physiotherapy at home if excess mucus production is a chronic problem.

Bronchiolitis

Bronchiolitis is the most common severe lower respiratory tract disease affecting about 1% of infants less than 1 year of age. The peak incidence occurs at 2–4 months of age. It tends to occur in epidemics between October and March. The cause is viral with respiratory syncytial virus (RSV) being the main agent in more than 70% of cases. Other causes include parainfluenza, influenza and adenoviruses.

Pathology

Bronchiolar inflammation occurs with necrosis

and destruction of cilia and epithelial cells leading to obstruction of the small airways. Ventilation and perfusion mismatch causes hypoxia and hypercapnia.

Clinical features

The initial presenting symptoms are coryzal, that is like the common cold. The infant develops a dry irritating cough and has difficulty in feeding. As the disease progresses, the infant becomes tachypnoeic and wheezy with signs of respiratory distress. The chest radiograph shows hyper-inflation and patchy areas of collapse or pneumonic consolidation. Widespread inspiratory crepitations and expiratory wheezes can be heard on auscultation.

Management

Management of this condition is mainly supportive. The infant is nursed in an upright position to assist respiration and is given humidified oxygen via a head box as required. A bronchiolitis chair may be used. Infants with severe respiratory distress will need blood gas monitoring and may require ventilatory support.

Most infants will have difficulty with feeding due to respiratory distress. Milder cases may tolerate small, frequent nasogastric feeds, although the nasogastric tube causes obstruction of one nostril. With enteral feeds the possibility of vomiting leading to aspiration remains. More severely affected infants will require intravenous nutrition.

Antibiotics are not required as the cause of the illness is viral. If the infant is ventilated, there is an increased risk of secondary bacterial infection and many centres would use intravenous antibiotics for the ventilated patient.

Bronchodilators may be used in cases with severe wheeze, but effective response is variable and unreliable.

Ribavirin is an antiviral agent which has been shown to be effective in reducing severity and duration of the disease (Barry et al 1986). It is given in nebulized form for 18 hours per day for 3–5 days, and the drug is expensive. The complicated mode of delivery and cost of this drug means that its clinical use is limited to those infants with pre-existing cardiac or pulmonary problems, immunodeficiency or severe respiratory failure.

Physiotherapy management

Physiotherapy is not indicated in the acute stage of bronchiolitis when the infant has signs of respiratory distress. A study comparing chest physiotherapy and no chest physiotherapy in infants with bronchiolitis showed no benefit in chest physiotherapy given routinely (Webb et al 1985).

The ventilated infant with bronchiolitis needs careful assessment with physiotherapy techniques only being applied when sputum retention is a problem.

Pertussis

Pertussis, commonly called 'whooping cough', is caused by the organism *Bordetella pertussis*. It occurs in epidemics every 3–4 years and is largely preventable by immunization. Following adverse publicity about side effects in the 1970s the uptake of immunization was greatly reduced, leading to an increased incidence of the disease.

Pertussis is particularly dangerous in infants less than 6 months of age and in children with other pulmonary problems, for example asthma and chronic lung disease.

Clinical features

The disease starts with coryza lasting 7–10 days during which the child is most infectious. The cough then becomes paroxysmal and can be provoked by crying, feeding or any other disturbance. It is particularly bad at night. The spasms of coughing may cause hypoxia and apnoea, especially in infants, and may lead to further problems such as convulsions, intracranial bleeding, and encephalopathy.

At the end of the coughing spasm, the inspiratory whoop may occur, followed by vomiting. Some very thick, tenacious sputum may be expectorated. This phase of paroxysmal coughing may last for 6–8 weeks and is exhausting for the child and parents. The Chinese call pertussis the 'hundred day cough'.

Bronchopneumonia is the most common complication, particularly in infants and may be due to the disease itself or due to secondary bacterial infection with *Staphylococcus*, *Haemophilus*, or *Pneumococcus*. The chest radiograph in severe cases shows hyperinflation and patchy areas of collapse and consolidation.

Management

Most children with pertussis will be managed at home. Infants and children with pneumonia may need admission to hospital. Treatment is supportive. Minimal handling in a quiet environment is essential for the infant with pertussis in order to reduce disturbance which may precipitate coughing. Nutritional and fluid support should be given throughout the stage of paroxysmal coughing. Antibiotics do not effect the course of the disease, but erythromycin may reduce infectivity and may also be given prophylactically to close contacts.

A small number of cases, particularly infants who have had frequent apnoeic attacks or hypoxic convulsions, will need intensive care and artificial ventilation.

Physiotherapy management

Any physiotherapy manoeuvre during the acute phase will stimulate the paroxysmal cough. Treatment is therefore contraindicated in infants during this stage and is of little use in older children.

If the child or infant requires ventilation, physiotherapy is very important to remove the extremely tenacious secretions which easily block large and small airways and endotracheal tubes. The paroxysmal cough is not a problem when the child is paralysed in order to be ventilated.

When the stage of paroxysmal coughing is over, there may be persistent lobar collapse. This lung pathology responds to physiotherapy with appropriate gravity-assisted positions, and chest clapping with the active cycle of breathing techniques. Parents can be taught how to treat the child at home.

Pneumonia

The most common cause of pneumonia in the neonate is *Staphylococcus*, in the infant RSV or *Mycoplasma*, and in the child *Mycoplasma*, *Streptococcus*, or *Haemophilus influenzae*. Staphylococcal pneumonia is usually an indication of underlying lung disease, for example cystic fibrosis. Children can become severely ill with pneumonia.

Clinical features

Presenting signs are pyrexia, dry cough, tachypnoea and sometimes recession of the ribs and sternum. The chest radiograph shows areas of consolidation. Chest signs are often minimal compared with the degree of illness. Children with underlying pulmonary disease are particularly at risk from pneumonia.

Management

Treatment is supportive with adequate fluid intake and humidified oxygen, if required. In younger children it is impossible to distinguish between viral and bacterial pneumonia and broad spectrum antibiotics are usually given.

Physiotherapy management

In many cases of pneumonia there is consolidation of lung tissue with no excess secretions. Physiotherapy is therefore not indicated. Where sputum retention is a problem, appropriate gravity-assisted positions with clapping, and in the older child breathing techniques, can be used. Copious amounts of sputum may be cleared in one treatment following which the pyrexia may settle and the child will feel better. Reassessment of the child is often necessary as retention of secretions may become a problem as the pneumonia resolves.

Acute laryngotracheobronchitis (croup)

Croup is a common problem occurring between the ages of 6 months and 4 years. The illness is usually caused by viruses which produce acute inflammation and oedema of the airway.

Clinical features

The presenting symptoms are coryzal and later the symptoms include a harsh barking cough and hoarse voice. There may be fever. Stridor, initially inspiratory only, is much worse at night and may become inspiratory and expiratory. Signs of respiratory obstruction are seen and the severely affected child may develop respiratory failure. The acute stage of respiratory obstruction may only last 1–2 days, but the stridor and cough may continue for 7–10 days. Some children have recurrent bouts of croup.

Management

Mild cases can be managed at home. Extra humidity is often given, for example steam from a kettle, but there is no objective evidence of benefit from this treatment.

More severely affected infants will be admitted to hospital and given humidified oxygen if hypoxic or distressed. Treatment is supportive, but with minimal handling as any disturbance which upsets the child will increase the laryngeal obstruction. Nebulized adrenaline may be given with careful observation. Antibiotics are not usually required unless there is some specific evidence of bacterial cause, for example purulent secretions.

About 3% of children with croup who are admitted to hospital may require intubation to maintain the airway. Some of these, particularly infants, may also require some form of respiratory support, e.g. IPPV or CPAP.

Physiotherapy management

There is no place for physiotherapy in the non-intubated child with croup. Treatment may be required when the child is intubated if sputum cannot be cleared by suction alone.

Acute epiglottitis

Epiglottitis is an uncommon but very dangerous condition occurring between the ages of 1 and 7 years. The cause is usually *Haemophilus influenzae*.

Clinical features

The onset is sudden. A severe sore throat develops with a high temperature. The child is systemically unwell and stridor and dysphagia develop rapidly. The child is unable to swallow saliva, and dribbles. The neck is held extended in an attempt to open the airway. Respiratory difficulty develops with hypoxia and hypercarbia. Acute and possibly fatal obstruction of the airway may develop at any time.

Management

The child with suspected epiglottitis must not be disturbed in any way. No attempt must be made to look down the throat as this may precipitate obstruction. Usual management is intubation with a nasotracheal tube, or tracheostomy if intubation is not possible. Ventilatory support may need to be given if the nasotracheal tube   is very small. Intravenous antibiotics will be given.

The child may only require intubation for 3–4 days following which there is usually complete recovery. Recurrence is rare.

Physiotherapy management

Physiotherapy techniques may be required in the intubated child if secretions cannot be removed by suction alone.

Inhaled foreign body

Aspiration of a foreign body into the respiratory tract can occur at all ages, but is most common between the ages of 1 and 3 years. All types of foodstuffs may be aspirated, for example peanuts, pieces of fruit and vegetables, as well as small plastic or metal toys.

Objects are most commonly aspirated into the right main bronchus. The left main bronchus and trachea are the next most common, and smaller objects may be inhaled into right middle and lower lobe bronchi or occasionally into the left lower lobe bronchus.

When aspiration has been witnessed by parents or carers, the child should be taken immediately to hospital. On examination there may be wheeze and some signs of respiratory distress. Breath sounds may be reduced over the affected lung. The chest radiograph taken on expiration may show gas trapping in the area distal to the blockage.

In some cases the aspiration is not witnessed and the acute changes just described may be assumed to be the onset of a respiratory infection. Further changes then occur. The bronchial wall becomes oedematous, especially if the inhaled object is vegetable matter. Peanuts are particularly irritative (Mitchell 1973). Total obstruction of the bronchus gradually occurs and secondary pneumonic changes develop in the area distal to the blockage. After a few days the child becomes unwell with a persistent cough. An inhaled foreign body should be suspected in a child with a pneumonia which does not respond to conventional treatment.

Management

All children who have aspirated a foreign body into the airway should have an urgent bronchoscopy for removal of the foreign body. If symptoms persist a repeat bronchoscopy may be necessary to ensure complete removal. Occasionally it may be impossible to remove the object by bronchoscopy and thoracotomy and bronchotomy may be required.

Physiotherapy management

Physiotherapy is not indicated to attempt to remove the object before bronchoscopy. Usually physiotherapy is ineffective as the object is firmly wedged in the bronchus. More importantly, if the object is dislodged by physiotherapy manoeuvres it may travel up the bronchial tree and obstruct the trachea leading to respiratory arrest.

Following bronchoscopy gravity-assisted positioning and chest clapping may be necessary to clear excess secretions particularly if the object has been aspirated for some time and secondary bacterial infection has occurred.

Primary ciliary dyskinesia

Primary ciliary dyskinesia is a rare, inherited (autosomal recessive) condition in which cilial motility is severely reduced due to structural defects within the cilia.

Reduced cilial motility can lead to recurrent sinusitis and bronchiectasis due to decreased clearance of secretions. Males are usually infertile because of reduced cilial motility of the sperm tails. A classical triad of sinusitis, bronchiectasis, and infertility is known as 'Kartagener's syndrome', but only about 50% of patients with ciliary dyskinesia present with this picture. Cilia can be examined for motility using nasal epithelial brushings.

Infants with this condition may present in the neonatal period with pneumonia, but many children present later with chronic upper and lower respiratory tract infection.

This condition is not curable, so treatment is directed towards preventing infection and chronic lung damage. Children will require daily physiotherapy (p. 402) similar to children with cystic fibrosis. Appropriate antibiotics will be required during periods of infection.

Cystic fibrosis

Cystic fibrosis is the most common inherited condition in caucasians, occurring in about 1 in 2500 births. The major clinical and diagnostic features result from the abnormalities affecting the exocrine glands. The most important areas affected being the respiratory and digestive tracts.

Children may present at birth with meconium ileus (see p. 298) or may present later with recurrent chest infections and/or failure to thrive.

Physiotherapy is essential from the time of diagnosis to try and prevent progressive lung damage due to excessive mucus production and recurrent chest infections.

Cystic fibrosis is fully described on pages 404–416.

SURGERY IN INFANTS AND CHILDREN

The effects of surgery, anaesthesia and immobility are the same in infants and children as in adults. Due to the anatomical and physiological differences, however, the potential for respiratory complications is greater.

Infants and children undergoing major surgery should, therefore, be regularly assessed by a physiotherapist.

Preoperatively

In some hospitals preoperative visits and handbooks are available to take some of the fear out of being in hospital. Except in emergency situations, children and their parents should be seen by a physiotherapist preoperatively. Explanation of postoperative procedures should be given at a level appropriate to the child's understanding. Overloading the child with information which he does not understand only increases preoperative stress and anxiety. It is important that parents are fully aware of the need for postoperative physiotherapy intervention. Parents can play an important role in encouraging postoperative mobility.

Assessment by the physiotherapist should include respiratory function and motor development. Older children who are able to understand and cooperate may be taught the active cycle of breathing techniques. Incentive spirometry can be very useful in children especially those specifically designed for their use, for example the 'Coach' incentive spirometer which has a spaceship which moves upwards on inspiration (Fig. 13.11).

When a child has pre-existing pulmonary disease, for example cystic fibrosis, he may need to be admitted some time before surgery to clear his chest as effectively as possible. Some children may require physiotherapy and suction in the anaesthetic room following intubation and before entering the operating theatre. Suction is often required before extubation in these patients.

Postoperatively

Children and infants should be regularly reviewed and intervention given as required. Effective pain relief is essential for children postoperatively prior to any intervention. It may be difficult to assess the severity of pain, as crying may be due to other causes, for example hunger. Lack of crying does not necessarily indicate lack

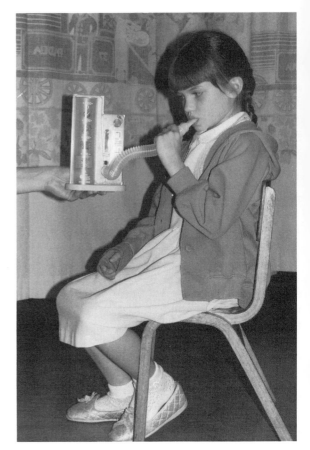

Fig. 13.11   Use of the 'Coach' incentive spirometer.

of pain as children in pain are often totally withdrawn and immobile. Infants in pain may be tachycardic and tachypnoeic. Many children who have a fear of needles will deny pain in order to avoid injections.

Continuous opioid infusion, for example pethidine, is now used regularly in some hospitals following major surgery. It is an effective and continuous means of pain relief and fear of pain is not such a problem. This method of pain control means that the patient requires close monitoring due to the risk of respiratory depression. The amount of drug delivered per hour to the child is gradually reduced as the pain lessens following surgery.

Treatment is directed towards regular position change; the 'slumped posture' position should be avoided at all times. When in bed, children should be comfortably positioned in alternate side lying or sitting upright. As soon as the condition allows, children should be sat out of bed, preferably on the first postoperative day. Walking should be started as soon as possible and drips, drains and catheters can all be carried to allow early ambulation. Attention to posture is important, particularly following thoracotomy when shoulder exercises to the affected side are also essential.

Infants should have regular position changes and should be taken out of bed for a cuddle with parents as soon as the condition allows.

If sputum retention is a problem postoperatively, other techniques such as chest clapping may be required, but there should always be effective pain relief.

A child often prefers not to have his wound supported or to support his wound himself. He may like to press a pillow or favourite soft toy to the area.

At all times firm but sympathetic and gentle handling is important to avoid undue distress.

CONGENITAL HEART DISEASE AND CARDIAC SURGERY IN INFANTS AND CHILDREN

Congenital heart disease is the most common congenital anomaly affecting approximately 8 per 1000 live births (Elliott 1987). The normal anatomy of the heart is shown in Figure 13.12.

Many cardiac anomalies can be diagnosed in utero by ultrasound scanning. Planned delivery of affected infants can then occur in a centre where paediatric cardiac facilities are available, thus optimizing chances of survival. Where defects have not been diagnosed antenatally, infants will present with a variety of clinical signs and symptoms.

Congenital anomalies can be divided into three groups:

1. *Excessive pulmonary blood flow* presents clinically with heart failure, tachypnoea, and poor feeding. It can occur in association with defects such as ventricular septal defect (VSD), atrial septal defect (ASD) or persistent ductus arteriosus (PDA).

2. *Inadequate pulmonary blood flow* is most common in abnormalities affecting the right side of the heart, e.g. tetralogy of Fallot, tricuspid atresia, and transposition of the great arteries.

3. *Increased pressure* due to obstruction, e.g. in conditions such as coarctation of the aorta, pulmonary and aortic stenosis.

Surgery for these conditions may be divided into closed surgery (not requiring bypass) or open surgery (requiring bypass).

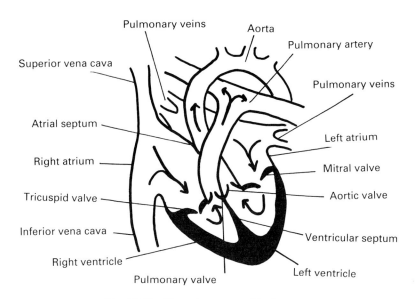

Fig. 13.12 Normal anatomy of the heart.

Preoperatively, echocardiography can be very useful in more accurately assessing defects. If clinical signs and echocardiography do not correlate cardiac catheterization should be performed. This can confirm the haemodynamics by measuring pressures and oxygen saturation in the cardiac chambers.

Excessive pulmonary blood flow

Persistent ductus arteriosus

The ductus arteriosus connects the left pulmonary artery to the descending thoracic aorta in utero. It should contract, close and fibrose into the ligamentum arteriosum by a few days after birth. Occasionally it persists, particularly in preterm infants, and blood will flow from the aorta into the pulmonary system. This flow eventually overloads the left side of the heart, increases the risk of endocarditis and, if long term, can cause pulmonary vascular disease.

Surgery. The persistent duct is ligated via a left thoracotomy incision.

Ventricular septal defect

Ventricular septal defect (VSD) is one of the most common forms of congenital heart disease, but more than 60% of defects will close spontaneously. Large defects will require surgery.

Patients with small defects may be asymptomatic, but large defects may cause breathlessness on exertion and right sided heart failure with systemic venous congestion.

Surgery. Surgical intervention may be palliative in infancy with full correction taking place after 3–4 years of age. If the defect is severe or multiple, full correction may take place earlier. The palliative operation for this defect is pulmonary artery banding via a left thoracotomy or median sternotomy. The pulmonary artery is identified and its lumen restricted by a Teflon band. The tightness of the band is judged by measuring the pressure in the artery beyond the band and by measuring the systemic oxygen saturation. The band is removed later when the defect is repaired.

Corrective surgery is carried out via a median sternotomy. Smaller defects are repaired by direct suture, larger defects by a patch of pericardium or synthetic material.

Atrial septal defect

Atrial septal defects (ASD) may be formed by the ostium primum or ostium secundum failing to close. These ostia allow the passage of blood between the atria in utero.

Ostium secundum defects occur in the region of the foramen ovale and are the most common and simplest to correct. Ideally they should be closed before school age. Lesions may be asymptomatic or give mild breathlessness on exertion.

Surgery. Surgery is corrective with closure by direct suture or patch via a median sternotomy or right thoracotomy incision.

Atrioventricular septal defects

The atrioventricular septum is at the junction of the atrial and ventricular septa. Defects may be partial (i.e. ostium primum ASD) or complete (i.e. atrioventricular canal). Many patients present with significant heart failure because of a large left to right shunt. There is a strong association between these defects and Down's syndrome.

Surgery. Partial defects behave like an ASD unless there is associated abnormality of the mitral valve. These defects always require a patch for repair and there is a significant risk of later mitral regurgitation, and patients need to be reviewed for the rest of their lives.

Complete defects pose difficult surgical problems. Complete repair is usually advocated at whatever age the child presents. The defect may be closed with two patches closing the ASD and VSD separately or as a one patch technique.

Late mitral regurgitation is a significant problem and may be the ultimate cause of death.

Inadequate pulmonary blood flow

Tetralogy of Fallot

Tetralogy of Fallot (Fig. 13.13) is characterized by:

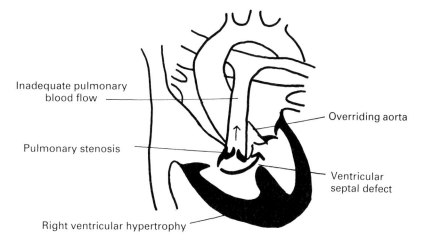

Fig. 13.13   Tetralogy of Fallot.

- VSD
- pulmonary stenosis
- overriding aorta
- hypertrophy of the right ventricle.

These abnormalities result in right to left shunt due to right ventricular outflow tract obstruction (RVOTO) and high right ventricular pressure.

The affected child is small for his age, cyanosed with clubbed fingers and toes, is breathless on exertion and has a tendency to squat.

Surgery. Surgery may be palliative in infancy with total correction before school age. Palliative surgery for this condition is usually a Blalock–Taussig shunt and may be modified by using a piece of 5 mm polytetrafluorethylene (PTFE) tube placed between the subclavian artery and pulmonary artery on the side opposite the ductus arteriosus. The size of the subclavian artery prevents the shunt from giving too much pulmonary blood flow.

Corrective surgery aims to patch the VSD also correcting the overriding aorta, resect the hypertrophied infundibular muscle, and treat pulmonary valvular stenosis either with valvotomy or a patch. Partial reconstruction of the valve may be necessary.

Tricuspid atresia

In this anomaly (Fig. 13.14) the tricuspid valve is deficient or absent and the right ventricle is frequently malformed. Pulmonary blood flow occurs through ASD, VSD, or persistent ductus arteriosis (PDA).

Surgery. The corrective surgery for tricuspid atresia is the Fontan operation. This operation involves either connecting the right atrium with the rudimentary right ventricular chamber or, more commonly, directly connecting the right atrium to the pulmonary artery, excluding the right ventricle. The contraction of the left ventricle alone then provides the impetus for blood flow into the lungs. Any form of left ventricular dysfunction or distortion of the pulmonary arteries is a serious adverse factor.

The Fontan procedure can also be used for other cardiac anomalies such as a single ventricle heart. In this defect a single chamber, from which both arterial trunks arise, receives blood from both atria.

Transposition of the great arteries

Where there is transposition of the great arteries (TGA) (Fig. 13.15), the aorta arises from the right ventricle and the pulmonary artery from the left ventricle. Infants present within the first few days of life and are unable to survive without an ASD, VSD, or PDA. Initial treatment is prostaglandin to keep the ductus arteriosus open and an urgent balloon atrial septostomy to rupture the atrial wall. The septostomy is carried out under echocardiographic control.

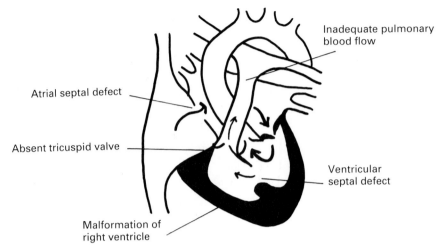

Atrial septal defect

Absent tricuspid valve

Malformation of
right ventricle

Inadequate pulmonary
blood flow

Ventricular
septal defect

Fig. 13.14   Tricuspid atresia.

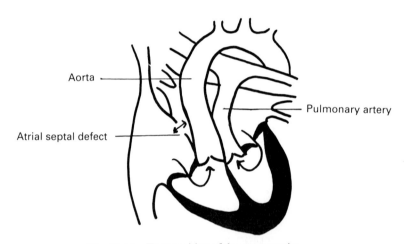

Aorta

Atrial septal defect

Pulmonary artery

Fig. 13.15   Transposition of the great arteries.

Surgery. There are two methods of correction for this condition:

1. Arterial switch procedure in which the aorta and pulmonary artery are reversed, transplanting the coronary arteries into the new aorta.
2. Intra-atrial redirection of blood in which venous return is redirected via an intra-atrial tunnel fashioned from pericardium (Mustard's operation) or from a portion of atrial wall (Senning's operation).

If the TGA is associated with a large VSD, initial treatment will include pulmonary artery banding to protect the pulmonary vascular system from excessive flow. Subsequent corrective surgery of choice is the arterial switch procedure with patching of the VSD.

Other anomalies occurring in association with TGA will require more complicated surgery.

Congenital conditions associated with increased pressure

Coarctation of the aorta

This condition is a constriction of the aorta most commonly located just distal to the origin of the left subclavian artery. There is hypertension proximal to the coarctation which increases with exercise. The hypertension may be associated with headaches, dizziness, tinnitus, and epistaxis due to increased blood pressure in the head.

There is hypotension distal to the coarctation leading to reduced femoral pulses, cold feet, and possible claudication in the lower limbs because of decreased blood flow. Collateral vessels develop to maintain the flow to the lower half of the body.

Some infants present in the neonatal period with severe heart failure so urgent surgery is required.

Surgery. Early surgery gives a greater chance of prevention of late complications such as hypertension and stroke. Two principal surgical techniques are used, both via a left thoracotomy.

1. *Subclavian flap repair* — the constricted portion of the aorta is dissected longitudinally. A portion of the subclavian artery is turned down as a flap and attached to the dissected margins. The PDA is ligated.

2. *Resection and end-to-end anastomosis* — the coarctation is resected and incisions are made along the underside of the aortic arch and lateral aspect of the descending aorta to give an inlay flap to increase the size of the anastomosis.

Pulmonary stenosis

In right ventricular outflow tract obstruction (RVOTO) there is a defect in fusion of the valve commissure, which often occurs in association with infundibular stenosis. The pulmonary circulation is decreased and the work of the right ventricle increased often resulting in right ventricular hypertrophy. Symptoms are breathlessness on exertion and fatigue. Infants may be hypoxic and develop cardiac failure.

Surgery. Pulmonary stenosis may be treated by balloon angioplasty, pulmonary valvectomy or valvotomy (dilatation of the valve via the right ventricle). The patient may require replacement of the pulmonary valve at a later stage.

Aortic stenosis

Left ventricular outflow tract obstruction (LVOTO) may occur at three levels: valvular,

subvalvular, or supravalvular. Although valvular stenosis often does not cause problems until the age of 40–50 years, the narrowed valve orifices in sub- and supra valvular defects cause left ventricular hypertrophy.

Surgery. Valvotomy via the ascending aorta is required for valvular stenosis. Subvalvular stenosis may be corrected by myomectomy via an aortic or ventricular incision. Supravalvular stenosis is relieved by suturing an elliptical gusset of synthetic material into a vertical incision through the constricted portion of the aorta.

Physiotherapy for cardiac surgery

Preoperatively

Whenever possible, patients should be assessed by the physiotherapist to identify respiratory or motor problems and potential problems, and to meet the parents. Some infants who have excessive pulmonary blood flow have increased secretions and are at risk of developing chest infections. Physiotherapy in the form of modified gravity-assisted positioning, clapping and sometimes suction, may be required to clear the chest. Preoxygenation should not be given to these patients to avoid further pulmonary vasodilatation. Preoperative instructions will depend on the age of the child.

Postoperatively

Following open heart surgery patients will require ventilation for varying lengths of time. Children who have had simple procedures, for example repair of an uncomplicated atrial septal defect, may have an uneventful postoperative recovery and require little physiotherapy input. These children should be sat out of bed and taken for short walks as soon as their condition allows. While in bed, appropriate positioning to maximize ventilation and perfusion matching may be all that is required.

Following more complicated procedures, for example Sennings repair of transposition of the great arteries, patients are more likely to develop postoperative complications such as pulmonary oedema which may significantly delay recovery.

Some patients, particularly those who had pulmonary hypertension preoperatively, may be at risk of pulmonary hypertensive crises. These crises are massive, paroxysmal rises in pulmonary artery pressure which exceed systemic arterial pressure and are associated with a low cardiac output and a drop in left atrial pressure. They are precipitated by falling PaO_2 and rising $PaCO_2$, and increased ratio of pulmonary artery pressure to systemic artery pressure and an increased core–peripheral temperature gradient (Kendall 1991).

Physiotherapy treatment should never be given as a routine. Careful assessment is required before physiotherapy intervention. The physiotherapist must understand the effects of surgery on the cardiovascular system, the relevance of monitoring and the effects of the cardiac support drugs.

Treatment techniques for the ventilated child may include manual hyperinflation, positioning, chest clapping, vibrations and suction with or without the instillation of saline. They should be used with care as outlined previously. The modalities used will depend on the indications for treatment.

In some cases physiotherapy may be indicated but patients may be very unstable and treatment should not be attempted during periods of low cardiac output or pulmonary hypertensive crises, unless essential.

Patients should be carefully preoxygenated, and during treatment it is important to evaluate continually the effects of intervention. Oxygen saturation should be maintained to avoid pulmonary hypertensive crises and the other complications of hypoxaemia.

Children who have a low peripheral temperature, measured by a temperature probe on the toe, should remain covered during treatment whenever possible.

In small infants the heart may be very oedematous following surgery so that sternal closure has a tamponade effect. In these cases the sternum will be left open for a few days. During this time manual techniques should be used with caution.

As the patient's condition improves, IMV and CPAP will be used to wean him from the ventilator. Following extubation children over the age of 2 years can be encouraged to use the active cycle of breathing techniques. Huffing and coughing is encouraged with wound support. Use of an incentive spirometer may be helpful in some patients. Ambulation is encouraged as soon as the child's condition allows.

Children under the age of 2 years are often difficult to treat postoperatively as it is not possible for them to cooperate with formal breathing exercises. Treatment may consist of appropriate positioning whilst in bed with encouragement to blow bubbles, etc. Again sitting out in a chair and short walks are important as soon as the condition allows. If secretions are a problem and the patient is unable to clear them effectively suction will have to be used, as described previously.

Following closed heart surgery via a thoractomy children are often ambulant on the first postoperative day. Other physiotherapy techniques may be required if sputum retention is a problem. Particular attention must be given to shoulder movements and posture correction in these patients especially the older child or adolescent.

Transplantation surgery in children

The problems of transplant surgery in children are the same as in adults, that is the availability of compatible donor organs and postoperative rejection (Ch. 15). An additional difficulty is finding a donor organ of a similar size to the recipient.

Rejection is a major problem postoperatively in all forms of transplant. Combination immunosuppressive therapy is given prophylactically to reduce the chance of rejection. However, these drugs have side effects of renal damage, hypertension, growth and developmental effects. The immunosuppressed child is also at great risk of infection.

Heart transplantation

Heart transplants in children are carried out for end-stage cardiomyopathy and congenital heart disease when conventional surgery is not feasible, is too risky or would be ineffective.

Survival rates are 80% at 1 year and 62% at 5 years (Taggart & Dark 1991).

Rejection is monitored by myocardial biopsy, electrocardiography (ECG), and ultrasound.

Heart–lung transplantation

Heart–lung transplants are carried out for end-stage cardiopulmonary disease such as cystic fibrosis or severe irreversible pulmonary hypertension (Eisenmenger's syndrome).

Patients are selected for heart–lung transplantation if their chance of survival is limited but there is some time available to wait for donor organs. Contraindications are mycetoma and previous pleurectomy or pleurodesis (Higenbottam & Whitehead, 1991).

Diagnosis of rejection or chest infection is made by transbronchial biopsy and bronchoalveolar lavage during bronchoscopy.

A problem following heart–lung transplant is the development of obliterative bronchiolitis in about 10–20% of patients (Higenbottam & Whitehead 1991). This is fibrosis of small airways with vascular sclerosis following repeated episodes of rejection, and it may be fatal.

Physiotherapy in heart/heart–lung transplantation. Patients are often admitted for up to a week for assessment prior to selection for heart or heart–lung transplant. During this time the physiotherapist is able to assess fully the respiratory state, build up a relationship with the child and family, and teach postoperative procedures.

Postoperatively, patients are assessed and treatment given as appropriate. Those who have had a heart–lung transplant, particularly patients with cystic fibrosis, are likely to suffer more complications. Below the level of the anastomosis the lungs are denervated and patients are unable to feel the presence of secretions. There may be a problem of thick secretions from the upper respiratory tract gravitating into the lungs.

Patients may be ventilated for only a short time but the chest must be as clear as possible before extubation. Physiotherapy treatment is the same as that following cardiac surgery. Manual hyperinflation should be used with caution because of pleural air leaks, and great care should be taken with suction because of the anastomosis.

Ambulation should be started as soon as the patient's condition allows.

Chest physiotherapy may be required if the patient develops a chest infection and breathing control and positioning may be of value in obliterative bronchiolitis. Physiotherapy may need to be continued at home following discharge.

Liver transplantation

Liver transplantation is used for chronic end-stage liver disease and fulminant hepatic failure. Shortage of paediatric donors means that more and more grafts are reductions of adult livers. In some situations one liver can be used for two patients.

Postoperative complications include bleeding and splinting of the right side of the diaphragm. Patients invariably develop a pleural effusion which is usually right sided but may be bilateral.

Acute rejection is common 5–7 days post-transplant. Some patients develop chronic rejection and require retransplantation (Salt et al 1992).

Physiotherapy. Physiotherapists may have the opportunity to assess these patients preoperatively but often patients with fulminant hepatic failure are operated on as an emergency or are too ill to be seen preoperatively.

Postoperatively, the risk of bleeding in some patients means that handling is kept to a minimum. Patients are assessed regularly and treated as appropriate.

Following extubation, ambulation is encouraged as soon as possible. Large pleural effusions coupled with ascites mean patients are often very breathless and unable to mobilize.

TRAUMA

Accidents are the most common cause of child death after the first year of life; of these 50% are road traffic accidents. Children who have been severely injured may require intensive care and mechanical ventilation, particularly following a head injury.

Head injury

The major effect of head injury is increased intracranial pressure (ICP). Raised ICP can also

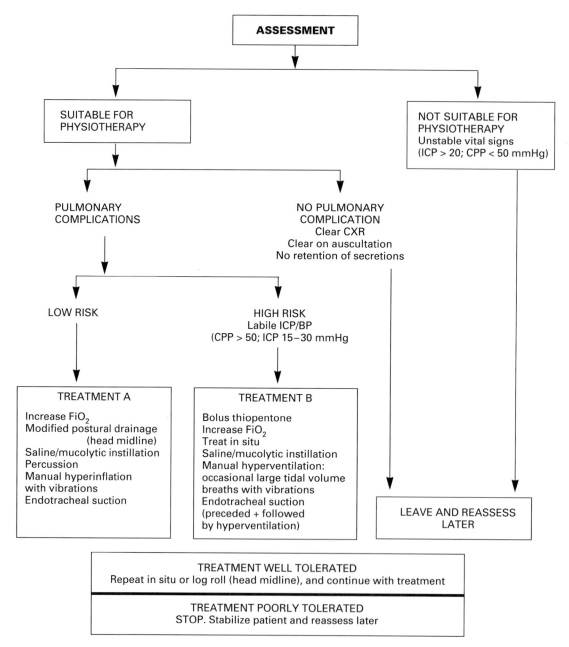

Fig. 13.16   Flow diagram of an approach to chest physiotherapy in children with raised intracranial pressure. Reproduced with permission from Prasad & Tasker 1990 *Physiotherapy* 76 (4): 250

be due to other causes such as space-occupying lesions (tumour, or haematoma) or encephalopathy due to, for example liver failure.

The main aim of management of a child with raised ICP is to keep the child as stable as possible and maintain the cerebral perfusion pressure (CPP). The CPP is the difference between the mean arterial blood pressure and the mean ICP. Normal values for ICP are less than 15 mmHg and for CPP more than 50 mmHg.

Careful assessment is required before any intervention, including physiotherapy and suction.

Maintenance of a clear chest is important to avoid hypoxia which can also increase ICP. It is important to monitor the ICP continuously by means of an intracranial pressure monitor.

The use of drugs such as mannitol or thiopentone before intervention can help reduce acute swings in ICP.

Physiotherapy techniques

These patients are very prone to retention of secretions and lobar collapse as they are often so unstable that no change of position is tolerated. The head down position is generally considered to be contraindicated and any change in position must be carried out with the head maintained in the midline position in relation to the body.

Chest clapping may be better tolerated than vibrations, and manual hyperinflation may be used with careful monitoring (Prasad & Tasker 1990).

Endotracheal suctioning can have severe prolonged effects on ICP (Rudy et al 1986) and great care must be taken to avoid hypoxia.

A protocol for physiotherapy management is shown in Figure 13.16.

CONCLUSION

Children are not just small adults. Their anatomical and physiological differences mean that their need for treatment and the response to it is variable compared with adults. The ability of children to understand and cooperate depends on their age and understanding. It is important for the physiotherapist to be aware of these differences and to adapt treatment so that it is appropriate and effective.

REFERENCES

Barry W, Cockburn F, Cornall R et al 1986 Ribavirin aerosol for acute bronchiolitis. Archives of Disease in Childhood 61: 593–597

Boros S J, Mammel M C, Lewallen P K et al 1986 Necrotising tracheobronchitis, a complication of high frequency ventilation. Journal of Pediatrics 109: 95–100

Byrne W J 1991 Disorders of the umbilical cord, abdominal wall, urachus and omphalomesenteric duct. In: Taeusch H W, Ballard R A, Avery M E (eds) Schaffer & Avery's diseases of the newborn, 6th edn. W B Saunders, Philadelphia

Cordero L, Hon E H 1971 Neonatal bradycardia following nasopharyngeal stimulation. Journal of Pediatrics 78: 441–447

Davies H, Kitchman R, Gordon G, Helms P 1985 Regional ventilation in infancy. Reversal of the adult pattern. New England Journal of Medicine 313: 1627–1628

Dinwiddie R 1990 The diagnosis and management of paediatric respiratory disease. Churchill Livingstone, Edinburgh

Downs J 1989 Endotracheal suction: a method of tracheal washout. Physiotherapy 75: 454

Elliott M J 1987 Congenital heart defects. Surgery 51: 1217–1227

Gandy G H, Roberton N R C 1987 Respiratory problems of the newborn In: Gandy G M, Roberton N R C (eds) Lecture notes on neonatology. Blackwell Scientific, Oxford

Gleeson J G, Price J F 1988 Nebuhaler technique. British Journal of Diseases of the Chest 82: 172–174

Greenough A, Pool J 1988 Neonatal patient triggered ventilation. Archives of Disease in Childhood 63: 394–397

Greenough A, Morley C J, Davis J A 1983 The interaction of the preterm infants spontaneous respiration with ventilation. Journal of Pediatrics 103: 769–773

Greenough A, Morley C J, Wood S, Davies J A 1984 Pancuronium prevents pneumothoraces in ventilated premature infants who actively expire against positive pressure inflation. Lancet i: 1–3

Greenough A, Pool J, Greenall F et al 1987 Comparison of different rates of artificial ventilation in preterm neonates with respiratory distress syndrome. Acta Paediatrica Scandinavica 76: 706–712

Henry R L, Hiller E J, Milner A D et al 1984 Nebulised ipratropium bromide and sodium cromoglycate in the first two years of life. Archives of Disease in Childhood 59: 54–57

Higenbottam T W, Whitehead B 1991 Heart-lung transplantation for cystic fibrosis. Journal of the Royal Society of Medicine 84 (suppl 18): 18–21

Inselman L S, Mellins R B 1981 Growth and development of the lung. Journal of Pediatrics 98: 1–15

Kendall L 1991 Physiotherapy in the paediatric cardiothoracic unit. Association of Chartered Physiotherapists in Respiratory Care Newsletter 19: 19–25

Konig P, Godfrey S 1973 The prevalence of exercise induced bronchial lability in families of children with asthma. Archives of Disease in Childhood 48: 513–518

MacMahon P, Kovar I Z 1990 Neonatal Respiratory Disorders. In: Dinwiddie R (ed) The diagnosis and management of paediatric respiratory disease. Churchill Livingstone, Edinburgh, p 21–56

Mitchell R G 1973 Disorders of the Respiratory Tract. In: Mitchell R G (ed) Ellis and Mitchell disease in infancy and childhood, 7th edn. Churchill Livingstone, Edinburgh, p 291–316

Morley C J 1991 Surfactant treatment for premature babies: a review of clinical trials. Archives of Disease in Childhood 66: 445–450

Muller N L, Bryan A C 1979 Chest wall mechanics and

respiratory muscles in infants. Pediatric Clinics of North America 26 (3): 503–516

O'Callaghan C, Milner A, Swarbrick A 1986 Paradoxical deterioration in lung function after nebulized salbutamol in wheezy infants. Lancet ii: 1424–1425

O'Callaghan C, Milner A, Swarbrick A 1989 Paradoxical bronchospasm in wheezing infants after nebulized preservative-free iso-osmolar ipratropium bromide. British Medical Journal 299: 1433–1434

Prasad A, Tasker R 1990 Guidelines for physiotherapy management of critically ill children with acutely raised intracranial pressure. Physiotherapy 76 (4): 248–250

Price J 1986 Respiratory Disease in Childhood. Association of Paediatric Chartered Physiotherapists Newsletter 39: 19–20

Purcell M 1976 Response in newborn to raised upper airway resistance. Archives of Disease in Childhood 51: 602–607

Reid L 1984 Lung growth in health and disease. British Journal of Diseases of the Chest 78: 113–132

Rodenstein D O, Kahn A, Blum D et al 1987 Nasal occlusion during sleep in normal and near miss for sudden death syndrome in infants. Bulletin European Physiopathologie Respiratoire 23: 223–226

Rudy E B, Baun M, Stone K et al 1986 The relationship between endotracheal suctioning and changes in intracranial pressure: a review of the literature. Reviews in Critical Care 15: 488–494

Sat A, Noble-Jameson G, Barnes N D et al 1992 Liver transplantation in 100 children: Cambridge and King's College Hospital series. British Medical Journal 304: 416–421

Samuels M P, Southall D P 1989 Negative extrathoracic pressure in the treatment of respiratory failure in infants and children. British Medical Journal 299: 1253–1257

Sauve R S, Singual N 1985 Long term morbidity of infants with bronchopulmonary dysplasia. Pediatrics 76: 725–733

Sumner E 1990 Artificial Ventilation of Children In: Dinwiddie R (ed) The diagnosis and management of paediatric respiratory disease. Churchill Livingstone, Edinburgh, p 267–287

Taggart D P, Dark J H 1991 Heart Transplantation in children. British Medical Journal 302: 1035–1036

Thoresen M, Cavan F, Whitelaw A 1988 Effect of tilting on oxygenation in newborn infants. Archives of Disease in Childhood 63: 315–317

Tudehope D I, Bagley C 1980 Techniques of physiotherapy in intubated babies with RDS. Australian Medical Journal 16: 226–228

Vaughan R S, Menke J A, Giacoia G P 1978 Pneumothorax a complication of endotracheal suctioning. Journal of Pediatrics 92: 633–634

Webb M S C, Martin J A, Cartlidge P H T et al 1985 Chest physiotherapy in acute bronchiolitis. Archives of Disease in Childhood 6: 1078–1079

FURTHER READING

Dinwiddie R 1990 Diagnosis and management of paediatric respiratory disease. Churchill Livingstone, Edinburgh

Jordan S C, Scott O 1989 Heart disease in paediatrics, 3rd edn. Butterworths, London

14. Cardiac rehabilitation

Helen McBurney

INTRODUCTION

Since the realization in the 1940s and 1950s that long-term bed rest, the standard medical practice of the times for post-myocardial infarction (MI) patients, was in fact detrimental both physically and psychologically (Levine & Lown 1952, Newman et al 1952), efforts have been made to address these problems. Cardiac rehabilitation, including secondary prevention has become an important part of the management of patients both post-MI and post-coronary artery bypass graft surgery (CABGS).

Goals of cardiac rehabilitation

The major goal of a comprehensive cardiac rehabilitation programme is the achievement of an optimal health status for each patient, and the maintenance of this status, not only physically and psychologically but also in social, vocational and economic terms (Wenger 1986, Mulchahy 1991).

More specific goals of a cardiac rehabilitation or secondary prevention programme may include:

- the limitation of adverse effects of illness
- efficient and effective symptom management
- stratification of risk for a further cardiac event to assist in clinical decision making regarding further treatment
- modification of cardiac risk factors to prevent progression of ischaemic heart disease as far as possible.

In order to achieve both a good functional capacity and a good quality of life, cardiac rehabilitation should not be equated with exercise alone but should also include education and counselling so that patients eventually become responsible for a large part of their own management. Ideally, rehabilitation should begin at the time of admission to hospital and continue after discharge (Mulchahy 1991).

Cardiac rehabilitation team

A comprehensive cardiac rehabilitation programme will include a wide range of skilled health professional staff including: dietician, doctors (cardiologist, junior medical officer, and general practitioner), nurse, occupational therapist, physiotherapist, psychologist and social worker. The patient's support people, family and/or close friends are an important part of any rehabilitation team and can greatly influence outcome.

The larger the team the greater the need for clear, concise communication between staff, patient and support persons to clarify problems, goals, treatment and outcomes.

In a smaller setting a wide range of professional staff may not be available. Overlap in the training of health professionals assists in the provision of quality care. Sometimes it will be necessary for staff to recognize their lack of expertise in a specific area and refer the patient on for specialist assistance. However, as Worcester (1986) observes, not every patient will require the help of every profession.

Role of the physiotherapist

The physiotherapist is primarily concerned with physical aspects of recovery, especially minimizing the deconditioning effects of bed rest and enhancing cardiovascular and musculoskeletal functioning. Initially this will involve assessment, perhaps breathing exercises and assisted or active exercises for some patients, supervised ambulation, stair climbing and other activities. Instruction in home exercise, self-monitoring and provision of activity guidelines are important functions.

The physiotherapist may encourage attendance at an out-patient programme and should report on the patient's physical progress to the team. Worcester (1986) found it appropriate that the physiotherapist should coordinate and conduct the exercise programme, liaising with other staff as required, because of the significant physiological and medical components of a physiotherapist's training. Other aspects of cardiac rehabilitation which may be carried out by the physiotherapist include: relaxation training, investigation of work potential and simulated work testing and, where specifically trained, exercise testing.

RATIONALE FOR CARDIAC REHABILITATION

Early ambulation

Early management of the post-MI patient is based on two conflicting needs, the need for restricted activity to avoid complications and the need for activity to avoid the undesirable effects of bed rest. Levine & Lown (1952) and Newman et al (1952) recognized this problem in their clinical settings and began supervised activity programmes for their post-MI patients, provided they were not suffering any complications.

A randomized controlled trial of early mobilization after acute MI was conducted by Bloch et al (1974). Patients ($n = 154$) were assigned either to an early mobilization group which began supervised activity on day 2 or 3 post-MI, or to a usual hospital care group who underwent 3 weeks of strict bed rest. The authors found no differences in complication rates in the first 6 months, a significant decrease in the duration of hospitalization for the early ambulation group, and significantly greater disability in the control group on follow up. The results of this study confirmed clinical observations of the benefits of early mobilization.

Other authors such as Jelinek et al (1977) confirm that this approach is safe and that fears of exercise having adverse effects such as weakening of the healing myocardium, myocardial rupture or major arrhythmias should be allayed by the number of well designed and positive trials.

Exercise training

In the post-MI and post-CABGS period the natural process of recovery and resumption of normal physical activity will result in some improvement in functional capacity. DeBusk et al (1979) found an increase of one third in exercise tolerance between weeks 3 and 11 post-MI. Training augmented improvement in exercise tolerance by a small amount (DeBusk et al 1979). Lipkin (1991) reported 15–25% increases in exercise tolerance associated with physical training in the short term. Increased maximal oxygen uptake can be achieved in the coronary heart disease patient via the same mechanisms of peripheral adaptation as in normal subjects. Astrand & Rodahl (1986) detail these changes. The principal advantage of training is an increased tolerance for usual activity, which requires a lower percentage of maximal oxygen uptake. In patients with angina pectoris, increases in activity before onset of symptoms are usually noted.

Habitual physical activity has been shown to lower the risk of coronary heart disease in recent large epidemiological studies (Leon et al 1987, Blair et al 1989). Risk factors favourably altered by exercise included blood pressure, weight and blood lipid profiles. Importantly these studies demonstrated that moderate intensity exercise is sufficient to provide significant risk reduction, so that high levels of physical fitness are not necessary for a favourable outcome. In contrast to previous belief it appears that the total weekly energy consumption is more important than the duration and intensity of each individual exercise session.

Another reason often given for exercise training in cardiac rehabilitation is that of improved psychological well being. Newman et al (1952) and Levine and Lown (1952) certainly noted deleterious psychological effects of prolonged bed rest on their subjects and commented that these were lessened by activity programmes. Worcester (1986) advocates exercise programmes for in-patients for psychological benefit. Oldridge & Rogowski (1990) demonstrated an increase in self-efficacy scores associated with a ward ambulation programme for post-MI patients. However, in a long-term study, Stern and Cleary (1982) were unable to demonstrate any difference between their control and exercise groups of post-MI subjects in any psychosocial measures.

Secondary prevention

The evidence that regular exercise reduces the possibility of recurrence of MI, other clinical signs of ischaemic heart disease and associated mortality is not conclusive. Supporting data are provided by Leon et al (1987) who have demon-strated the necessity for long-term moderate exercise in the population at large in order to reduce the risk of coronary heart disease and have shown that current habitual activity level is the important factor. Participation in exercise even at an elite athletic level in the past has little bearing on current risk. Kallio et al (1979) and Hamalainen et al (1989) have used a multiple risk factor intervention approach in two Finnish populations. At follow up the cumulative mortality rate was significantly smaller in the intervention group.

There are no data on morbidity and mortality from controlled clinical trials of the effects of comprehensive cardiac rehabilitation in patients with stable angina or following CABGS. It is hoped that a comprehensive rehabilitation programme will prove to be useful in secondary prevention in these groups, but this remains to be shown.

Education

The current emphasis in health care is on each individual making informed decisions regarding their management and taking responsibility for their own health and care (Doughty 1991, Mulchahy 1991).

Education, especially information regarding smoking, diet, weight, blood pressure and exercise is important for effective secondary prevention (Worcester 1986). To facilitate return to normal living, most patients post-MI or post-CABGS will require some information and guidelines to resume driving, work and other activities. Motivation to comply with advice has been linked to the understanding of illness and the need for risk factor modification (Worcester 1986).

The responsibility for patient education can be shared by all disciplines involved in cardiac rehabilitation (Davidson & Maloney 1985). It is important that advice is consistent and not confusing. Verbal, written and audiovisual material may be used. Worcester (1986) advocates the use of small discussion groups as active involvement achieves better understanding and opportunity for clarification than a lecture format.

The inclusion of partner, family or friend is recommended (Davidson & Maloney 1985, Wenger 1986, Worcester 1986, Mulchahy 1991) as this lessens misunderstandings during conva-lescence and the support of a partner can enhance motivation and adoption of a healthy lifestyle.

Caine et al (1991) found that attention to the quality of information given to CABGS patients, relatives and the community, especially employers, helped to improve outcome. Post-discharge depression, denial or anxiety may make this time especially difficult for the partner and participation in an out-patient programme can support both patient and spouse.

MANIFESTATIONS OF ISCHAEMIC HEART DISEASE

Ischaemic heart disease (IHD) is used synony-mously with the term 'coronary heart disease' and refers to impairment of the cardiac muscle due to imbalance between coronary blood flow and myocardial needs caused by changes in the coronary circulation. (Joint International Society 1979).

The various forms or manifestations of IHD are usually defined separately and include:

- cardiac arrest
- angina pectoris
- myocardial infarction.

Cardiac arrest

This is a sudden event where there is no evidence for any other diagnosis. If resuscitation is not attempted or is unsuccessful then this is usually referred to as sudden death.

Angina pectoris

This is a symptom of myocardial ischaemia, episodic in nature and classically described as central chest or retrosternal pain. Angina can vary considerably from person to person, but usually remains constant in the individual patient (Gazes 1990). Angina may be described according to its location, quality, duration, intensity, and precipitating factors.

Location. Classical angina is retrosternal but it may radiate to or only be felt in the jaw, neck, back, shoulders and arms, more commonly on the left. Differential diagnosis is therefore extremely important in patients presenting with intermittent pain in these areas.

Quality. The sensation of angina is not always described by patients as 'pain'. Common alternatives are discomfort, burning, pressing or a squeezing sensation.

Duration. Angina is intermittent and onset is usually associated with a critical level of physical activity. The feeling may develop gradually and mount in intensity, but subsides quickly with rest or with sublingual nitroglycerin.

Intensity. Angina is often variously described as a 'mild ache', pressing or constricting but is rarely excruciating or intolerable.

Precipitating factors. Angina is usually brought on by an increase in myocardial work so that local oxygen consumption exceeds the supply capacity of the coronary vessels. Exercise is the most common precipitating factor. Some patients may have spontaneous or rest angina which occurs without apparent relation to increased myocardial work and may be due to factors such as coronary artery spasm.

Angina may be classified as 'stable' when the same factor induces the same sensation repeatedly, or 'unstable' when the sensation occurs spontaneously or is occurring with increasing frequency or severity or is caused by a lessening amount of effort.

Myocardial infarction

The clinical diagnosis of acute myocardial infarction (MI) is usually based on the patient history, electrocardiograph (ECG) changes and the elevation of serum enzymes.

History. The pain associated with myocardial infarction is usually similar in location to that of angina but is more severe and prolonged (more than 30 min). It is not relieved by nitroglycerin and may be accompanied by sweatiness, pallor, nausea and vomiting.

ECG. Unequivocal changes involve the development of persistent abnormally large Q waves. The evolution of ST/T wave changes with concomitant enzyme changes is also diagnostic.

Serum enzymes. These are released from irreversibly damaged myocardial cells into the circulation. The rise and fall of serum enzyme levels should be related to the time of cellular injury and is specific for each enzyme measured.

The Joint International Society (1979) states that diagnosis of definite acute MI requires unequivocal ECG changes and/or unequivocal enzyme changes with or without a typical history.

Physical complications. These are many and may include:

1. Rhythm and conduction disturbances—when the conduction system is involved in the MI or if a portion of the myocardium becomes less electrically stable.

2. Heart failure—the consequence of which may be minor or may include pulmonary oedema or shock.

3. Recurrent MI—occurs in 15–20% of MI patients during their initial hospitalization, especially in those who experience unstable angina early post-MI, who have a subendocardial (partial wall thickness) infarct and in those who experience angina and/or breathlessness on early mobilization (Jelinek 1988).

4. Pericarditis (p. 230).

5. Rupture of the myocardial wall—occurs in about 1% of patients and can cause tamponade or a ventricular septal defect. Rupture of papillary muscles may allow valvular regurgitation.

6. Systemic or pulmonary thromboembolism.

Other complications of MI may be anxiety and depression, and/or economic problems due to temporary or permanent loss of earnings.

Cardiac surgery

Many patients with some form of cardiac disorder may undergo cardiac surgery. This may be coronary artery bypass grafts, valvular repair or replacement, or repair of a congenital defect. The early postoperative management of these patients is discussed in Chapter 12.

Many of these patients require ongoing rehabilitation similar in principle to that of any medical cardiac patient in order to make long-term life-style adjustments. There are a few postoperative problems which will need consideration and have important implications for a postoperative programme.

Pain. Because consolidation of the sternum takes 2–3 months, many patients will experience pain in this area for this time. Muscular aches and pain in the chest, shoulders, neck and back, and rib pain are also common. Management should include the use of pain relieving medication, especially prior to activity and continuation of range of movement exercises, until full active range of movement is achieved without pain. Soft tissue techniques such as massage may also be of use.

Fatigue. This is common in the early postoperative period. It is important that there is a balance between activity and rest and a conscious effort should be made to increase activity gradually.

Mood. After discharge from hospital mild depression is common. Most patients will recover spontaneously and find the stimulation of attending a cardiac rehabilitation programme helpful. A few will have a deep and persistent problem requiring professional help.

Visual changes. Blurring of vision may occur postoperatively but should resolve spontaneously over the first few months.

Concentration and memory. These are often poor in the early postoperative phase but should improve slowly.

Constipation. This is not unusual in patients taking some pain relieving medications, but it may cause discomfort and require the use of a laxative.

Palpitations. Many patients are more aware of their heart beat postoperatively as it is often faster for the first few months. Frequent or persistent bouts of palpitations should be reported to the doctor for investigation and management.

Drugs to control the cardiovascular system

Medications involved in the control of the cardiovascular system are too numerous to mention individually, so only those categories of medication which effect exercise are mentioned here.

Beta adrenergic blocking agents

Beta blockers are used to reduce myocardial oxygen demand by decreasing myocardial contractility, heart rate and systolic blood pressure.

Beta blocking medication can be cardioselective and specifically act to inhibit β receptors which mediate cardiac stimulation, or it may be non-selective and act on both β_1 and β_2 receptors so that vascular and bronchial smooth muscle contraction is effected. The selectivity of all beta blocking medications has been noted to be dose related, as the dose increases selectivity decreases. At high doses or with a non-selective beta blocker, bronchospasm and peripheral vasoconstriction may be undesired side effects (Frishman & Teicher 1985).

Beta blockers have been shown to lower heart rate substantially both at rest and at any given exercise intensity. Exercise prescription for a patient on beta blockers should be made with this in mind. The lower heart rate and blood pressure will reduce myocardial oxygen demand and may allow the patient to achieve a higher workload before exertional angina is experienced. However, the peak workload achieved by a patient on beta blockers may be less than without the medication.

Beta blockers reduce myocardial contractility and thus may precipitate or potentiate cardiac failure. As beta blockers vary in duration of action, exercise sessions performed hours after taking medication may result in a greater heart rate response than exercise performed close to the time of taking medication.

Some distressing side effects may be experienced by patients taking beta blockers, including fatigue, bradycardia, impotence and vivid dreams. Sudden cessation of this type of medication can cause rebound phenomena such as reflex tachycardia, hypertension or angina.

Heart rate may not accurately reflect the exercise stress imposed by a given level of work in a patient taking beta blockers. Rating of perceived exertion (RPE) and/or respiratory rate are alternative forms of monitoring.

Nitrates

Nitrates cause dilation of both the arterial and venous circulation by relaxation of smooth muscle in vessel walls and thereby reduce work of the heart by decreased peripheral resistance and decreased venous return. This may allow an improved exercise capacity by increasing the anginal threshold. Nitrates can be used prior to exercise to eliminate or reduce the likelihood of occurrence of angina. Hypotension may occur in patients on nitrates if they cease exercise abruptly, so an effective cool down is important.

Vasodilators

Other vasodilating medications also have the potential to produce post-exercise hypotension if activity is abruptly ceased. Allowance for an adequate cool down should effectively prevent this.

PHYSIOTHERAPY

Assessment

Cardiac rehabilitation may be commenced before a patient with angina experiences any further event, or more often commences during an in-patient stay after an acute MI or CABGS. In any situation some basic assessment is necessary prior to beginning a rehabilitation programme.

Demographic data. These can usually be obtained from the patient's medical record and should include age, address and some social information, especially occupation, interests and the main support person or people who should be included in as much of the cardiac programme as is practicable.

In order to define the scope of cardiac dysfunction, information regarding the cardiac status of the individual should be sought.

Date of cardiac event. This should be considered. In a surgical patient rate of healing of the sternum may alter activities. The question of whether the surgical patient has had any previous, intra- or post operative MI and the functional outcome after this should also be investigated. In a medical patient, some natural recovery of ventricular function will occur with time.

Site of MI. This may affect the outcome and may be roughly mapped out from a consideration of 12-lead ECG traces showing changes post-MI. More detailed mapping of the site of myocardial damage may be obtained from investigations such as radionuclide ventriculography or ^{99}Tn infarct imaging.

Size of MI. This can be estimated from the amount of serum cardiac enzyme elevation in a patient not given thrombolytic therapy.

Current management. At the start of the programme this will include therapy aimed at reduction of cardiac risk factors such as medications, exercise, diet and smoking cessation. Some patients will experience considerable difficulty and stress in undertaking many radical life style changes at one time. These people may need additional support and assistance with many aspects of their management and may find it is better to concentrate on one aspect at a time.

Current signs and symptoms. The signs and symptoms presenting at the time of beginning a programme and the level of activity at which these occur can give a guide to the level at which exercise should be started. In particular, any anginal symptoms (undue breathlessness, pallor, dizziness, coldness and undue perspiration) associated with activity should be noted. It is helpful to have exercise test results to guide exercise prescription, but often these are not available. A record of recent premorbid activity and any limitations to this may be helpful.

Medications. These are frequently prescribed for the management of the cardiovascular system and for any other medical condition of patients involved in a cardiac rehabilitation programme. Some of these medications will have an impact on the cardiovascular, respiratory and/or metabolic response to exercise.

Familiarity with medications enables the physiotherapist to provide a better service through comprehensive evaluation, increased awareness of potential problems or necessary treatment programme modifications related to medication, feedback to the physician regarding the efficacy or side effects of medication changes, patient education to improve compliance and enhanced safety of a treatment programme (Ice 1985).

Occupational and recreational activities. These are important to the individual and should be considered in defining goals for outcome. Jelinek (1988) lists driving a car, sexual activity and occupation as the major concerns of most patients. The demands of these activities may need assessment on an individual basis. Astrand & Rodahl (1986) have established that a work level of 30–40% of maximum aerobic capacity can be sustained for an 8 hour day without symptoms of fatigue.

Current functional level. This needs to be clearly defined at the start of any programme. Subjective and objective information may be used to establish this.

Functional physical capacity was defined by the New York Heart Association (NYHA) on a simple four-class scale assessing symptoms of fatigue, palpitations, breathlessness and angina (Hurst 1974). This is now referred to as the 'Old NYHA scale' (Hurst et al 1990). The criteria for classification of each class are outlined in Table 14.1. Although this classification system was superseded in 1973 by a broader approach, it is often still referred to clinically. The Canadian Cardiovascular Society used a similar four-point scale to describe the amount of effort needed to produce angina. This is outlined in Table 14.2.

Table 14.1 Old New York Heart Association criteria for classification of functional capacity

Class I	Patients with heart disease who have no symptoms of any kind with ordinary physical activity
Class II	Patients who are comfortable at rest but have symptoms with ordinary physical activity
Class III	Patients who are comfortable at rest but have symptoms with less than ordinary activity
Class IV	Patients who have symptoms at rest

Table 14.2 Canadian Cardiovascular Society Classification of angina pectoris

Class 1	Ordinary activity does not cause angina. (Angina may occur with strenuous or prolonged or rapid exertion)
Class 2	Slight limitations to ordinary activity. (Angina with walking or stair climbing rapidly, walking uphill, walking or stair climbing in cold or wind or after a meal)
Class 3	Marked limitation of ordinary activity. (Angina on walking 1–2 blocks on the level or climbing a flight of stairs at normal pace)
Class 4	Inability to carry out physical activity without discomfort. (Angina may be present at rest)

Exercise testing

Formal laboratory exercise testing is considered by many North American authors (e.g. Stang & Lewis 1981) to be mandatory prior to any exercise programme. However, this is not the case in many other countries and other authors such as Miller & Borer (1982) question the value of such tests. In a 1986 survey of Australian hospital practice Worcester found that only 11% of hospitals exercise tested most of their in-patients post-MI and that, in fact, 84% of hospitals tested less than half of their in-patient post-MI population.

The safety of exercise testing as early as 3 days post-MI has been clearly established (Jelinek et al 1977, Miller & Borer 1982). Early exercise testing is advocated to provide both prognostic and therapeutic information. The American College of Sports Medicine (1991) recommends diagnostic exercise testing in the presence of a physician for patients with known cardiac disease in order to make decisions about the need for further evaluation or intervention. Functional exercise testing, with patients remaining on their usual medications, should be used to determine the exercise capacity of patients requiring activity guidelines and exercise prescription.

The risks of testing are considered high in patients with post-MI complications. Absolute contraindications to testing include unstable angina and uncontrolled arrhythmias. In the North American literature a medical decision not to perform an exercise test is an independent factor denoting a high risk of a further cardiac event (DeBusk 1989).

The reliability of an exercise test as a diagnostic tool is compromised when ECG interpretation is difficult, for example in the presence of some dysrhythmias or after a large anterior MI. In this situation the test may provide some useful information regarding exercise capacity, and haemodynamic and respiratory function, but other forms of exercise investigation such as radionuclide ventriculography or echocardiography may be of greater use.

Protocol. In theory, any type of exercise can be used as long as a set reproducible protocol is followed. In practice, the majority of exercise tests are performed on a treadmill or bicycle, beginning at a low level of work and increasing in 2 or 3 min stages. The Bruce protocol (Bruce et al 1973) is commonly used and is given as an example in Table 14.3. A variety of protocols have been developed and may be easily found in texts such as the American College of Sports Medicine (1991). Common criticisms of the Bruce protocol are that the first stage is too hard for many patients and that the jumps in workload are too great between stages. A modification of the Bruce protocol to answer the first criticism is to begin with a stage '1/2' with the treadmill at a speed of 1.7 mph and a slope of 5%, for 3 min.

Treadmill protocols commonly increase both the speed and slope of the machine, bicycle protocols increase workload by increasing resistance against which the subject is pedalling, whilst requiring that rhythm is maintained.

Monitoring of the subject is by continuous ECG, heart rate, blood pressure, symptoms, rating of perceived exertion (RPE) (Table 14.4)

Table 14.3 The Bruce Exercise Test protocol for a treadmill

Stage	Speed (mph)	Slope (%)	Time (min)
1	1.7	10	3
2	2.5	12	3
3	3.4	14	3
4	4.2	16	3
5	5.0	18	3
6	5.5	20	3

Table 14.4 Borg rating of perceived exertion scale

6	
7	Very, very light
8	
9	Very light
10	
11	Fairly light
12	
13	Somewhat hard
14	
15	Hard
16	
17	Very hard
18	
19	Very, very hard
20	

and appearance. Some laboratories will also include the direct measurement of oxygen uptake as a part of their protocol for exercise testing of cardiac patients.

Cessation of an exercise test may be at a predetermined arbitrarily selected end-point, for example a heart rate of 130 beats/min or a set workload, in which case the test is considered submaximal if the subject reaches this point without problems.

Maximal or symptom limited tests require the subject to exercise until unable to continue due to fatigue, breathlessness or angina or the test is stopped by the physician at the expected maximal heart rate or because of ECG abnormalities.

Interpretation of exercise test results is critical to the value of the test as a diagnostic or therapeutic tool. Hare (1990) advocates the use of exercise testing for its effect on patient confidence, especially when implications of the test are discussed with patient and partner.

Reliability, sensitivity and specificity of the test

are jeopardized when insufficient attention is paid to test details. False negative test results are associated with insufficient workload, insufficient number of ECG leads and failure to use all the available information in test interpretation. False positive results are associated with cardiac hypertrophy, an abnormal resting ECG and cardiomyopathy (American College of Sports Medicine 1991).

Information obtained from an exercise test can be compared with normal values for the population where these are available. Bruce (1956) used the concept of 'functional aerobic impairment' to describe the percentage that an individual's functional capacity falls below that expected for age and sex.

Walking tests such as a 6 min walk (p. 60) may be a useful method for quantification of functional capacity in those patients not considered for a formal exercise test because of their level of functional impairment (Lipkin et al 1986b). The reliability of walking tests for cardiac patients is the subject of current investigations.

Desired functional level. This should be discussed realistically with the individual patient, and should be related to premorbid activities and fitness as well as to current level of exercise tolerance. Attainable short-term goals as steps towards the desired outcome will help the patient feel a sense of achievement and progress with any programme. Unrealistic goals such as returning to cross country skiing after a 40 year gap should be discouraged.

Other points. Other points to be included in assessment may relate to other cardiac risk factors such as smoking and obesity or may relate to other medical problems suffered by the patient. In particular, any disability which may affect the ability of the patient to exercise should be clearly documented.

DeBusk et al (1986) suggested that the clinical judgements of physicians regarding the capacity of their patients to safely resume their usual activities after MI are generally correct, but that this judgement can be refined by the use of exercise test results. However, he presented no data to support this statement.

McBurney (1991) presented the results of a study to assess the ability of clinicians to judge physical work capacity of post-MI patients. Ten clinicians working in cardiac rehabilitation were asked to predict exercise test times for patients, using only data available from the medical record. All of the clinicians obtained high positive correlations with the actual exercise test time. Interviews with these clinicians revealed that all had slightly differing decision making strategies but that the most common reference points were: age, date and site or size of infarct, premorbid activity levels, current activity levels and any current symptoms of IHD.

Recording

Database

The individual patient database will be compiled over time as information becomes available. Initial recording should include as much information relating to the preceding assessment points as possible. Analysis of the recorded findings allows an individual treatment plan to be formulated.

Ongoing information

Ongoing notes should include recording of the amount of activity performed in any exercise session, an objective measure of effect such as heart rate or respiratory rate and any other signs or symptoms associated with activity. A baseline or resting level of the parameter selected should be recorded before, during and 2–5 min after cessation of activity.

Home activity diary

The completion of a home exercise diary could assist some patients to continue their programme, and if kept conscientiously is often a good marker of progress.

Treatment

Type of activity

Activities which give the best cardiovascular protection involve regular and rhythmical use of large muscle groups. Such activities include walking, running, swimming, dancing, cycling and rowing. The most common and safest form of exercise is walking.

In order to meet needs associated with daily activities it may be necessary to ensure that some arm exercise is included as part of a whole body exercise programme. Arm exercise has been shown to impose a greater stress on the heart than the same amount of leg exercise (Astrand & Rodahl 1986), so a lesser intensity of arm exercise should be used to be safe and effective.

Large increases in blood pressure have been found in association with isometric activity such as weightlifting and thus sustained and high intensity isometric exercise has been discouraged for cardiac patients. Verrill et al (1992) cite a number of studies in which circuit weight training programmes using isotonic activities have been assessed in patients post-MI and post-CABGS. These programmes have been shown to be safe and effectively to improve muscular strength and endurance.

Frequency, intensity, duration

The frequency, intensity and duration of exercise which should be recommended are factors which have been well investigated over a number of years. The threshold of exercise for cardiovascular protection has been reviewed by Haskell (1985), who concluded that an exercise threshold of about 630 kJ/day is required to decrease the risk of IHD. It appears that regular physical activity is beneficial, but that at high and vigorous levels there are no great gains and an increased risk of injury compared with moderate levels of activity. Leon et al (1987) found that a moderate level of leisure time physical activity was associated with fewer deaths than low levels of activity and with a similar rate of fatality as high levels of activity. Moderate level activity involved the expenditure of an average 6300 kJ/week. This compared with an average of 2100 kJ in the low activity level group.

Common recommendations for exercise to improve and maintain fitness are for a target of exercising 3–5 times per week for a 5–10 min warm up, a 15–60 min training session at 40–85% of functional capacity and a 5–10 min cool down (American College of Sports Medicine

1991). It now appears, however, that these guidelines can be modified. DeBusk et al (1990) found that men completing three 10-min bouts of exercise each day showed the same improvements in fitness as men completing one 30-min bout of exercise per day. Authors such as Haskell (1985) and Leon et al (1987) are also now concentrating on total daily or weekly energy expenditure in exercise.

Goble et al (1991) reported the results of a study in which 308 men were randomly assigned to either an aerobic exercise group or a light exercise group for their 8 week cardiac rehabilitation exercise programme after an anterior MI. The groups were well matched. Aerobic exercise was conducted at a gymnasium three times per week according to the guidelines of the American Heart Association (1979). Light exercise was conducted two times per week in the physiotherapy department and involved flexibility exercises, stationary cycling, stairs, light hand weights and rowing machine activity interspersed with rest periods. Both groups were advised to walk at a comfortable pace for 30 min each day. The effects of the programmes were measured by treadmill exercise test times prior to the start of exercise, at the completion of the 8 week programme and at a 1-year follow up. The only statistically significant difference in exercise capacity was a small and temporary advantage in the aerobic exercise group at the end of the training period. Physical benefits at 1 year were equally well achieved in the light exercise group.

Recommendations for exercise now also include an initial phase involving multiple short bouts of low intensity exercise, distributed throughout the day (American College of Sports Medicine 1991), until the participant is used to the activity and the supervisor is accustomed to his response. It is often necessary to point out to cardiac patients that, although some exercise is good, more is not necessarily better. This may relate to intensity, frequency and/or duration of activity.

Environmental factors may also be important in determining the amount of exercise to be undertaken at any one time, as variables such as wind, terrain, humidity, altitude and temperature extremes are known to affect the body response to exercise.

Intensity of exercise should be monitored and it is appropriate that the patient learns at least one way to do this. Recommended methods are by heart rate, rating of perceived exertion (RPE) or by the use of metabolic equivalents (METs). Heart rate is usually determined by direct measurement from ECG monitoring, radiotelemetry or palpation. In a group situation, palpation of the radial artery and counting the pulse for 15 seconds and then multiplying by 4 is the simplest method. The formula often used clinically (220-Age in years) is not recommended by the American College of Sports Medicine. Several alternative procedures to determine suitable exercise training heart rates are outlined by the American College of Sports Medicine (1991). The use of heart rate to monitor exercise intensity is simple and has the advantage that as exercise tolerance increases the patient will be able to do more before reaching their training heart rate, so that frequent revision of exercise prescription is not necessary.

Monitoring of exercise intensity by RPE has similar advantages and has been found to be a reliable indicator of intensity of effort. Most patients would exercise at the lower end of the 12–16 RPE range.

METs are sometimes used to monitor exercise intensity and rely on the use of tables which give MET values for common activities. Examples are given by the American College of Sports Medicine (1991) and Greenland & Chu (1988). One MET is equal to the resting level of oxygen uptake which is approximately 3.5 ml/kg. min. The use of METs to monitor exercise intensity does not make any allowance for environmental factors and does not allow for body adaptations to exercise so that there is a frequent need to review the level of exercise prescribed in this way.

Phases of recovery

Cardiac rehabilitation is often divided into four periods which are not defined by time. In the past these were defined as: phase I—the period of acute or critical illness usually managed in some form of critical care unit; phase II—the time of in-patient convalescence; phase III—out-patient recovery; and phase IV—long-term maintenance

(Jelinek 1988). In 1990 the American Association of Cardiovascular and Pulmonary Rehabilitation classified phases of rehabilitation as: phase I—hospital in-patient period; phase II—convalescence after hospital discharge; phase III—supervised ongoing rehabilitation; and phase IV—unsupervised ongoing maintenance.

In hospital. In-patient physiotherapy is usually directed at preventing or treating the sequelae of bed rest. This may include techniques to prevent lung collapse, especially in patients with pericarditis, and simple assisted or free range of movement activities. Jelinek (1988) indicates that this phase may last from a few hours to days or weeks.

Activity should be slowly increased and include a graduated exercise and mobilization programme, so that by discharge the patient is able to attend to his own activities of daily living, is ambulant and able to negotiate stairs.

Exercise in this phase can often be directed at negating old wives' tales or myths such as 'reaching your arms above your head will cause death'. A potential outline of in-patient activities is shown in Figure 14.1. Advice for home activity and exercise must be given pre-discharge, and preferably some formal arrangement made for follow up as an out-patient.

After hospital discharge. Continuation of cardiac rehabilitation may be by attendance at an organized education and exercise session one or more times per week for 1–2 months, supplemented by home exercise, or it may be feasible to use a home based exercise training programme such as that studied by Miller et al (1984). Suitable activities include stretches, flexibility and coordination exercises for warm up and cool down and an aerobic component which may utilize one or a combination of activities such as walking, minitrampoline, exercise cycle, and rowing machine (Figs 14.2 and 14.3). Miller et al (1984) found that patients training at home or in a group programme had significant improvements in functional capacity over patients not training or in a control group. Home training patients were monitored twice weekly by telephone.

Long-term continuation of exercise is desirable for stable post-MI and post-CABG patients as well as for the community in general. There are few long-term exercise programmes specific to

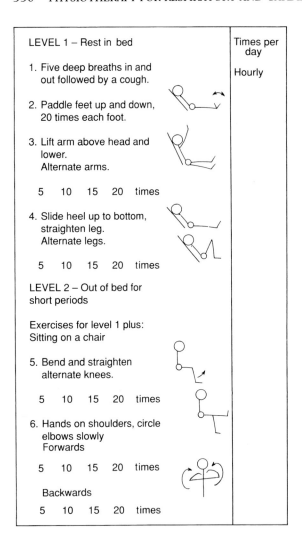

LEVEL 1 – Rest in bed	Times per day
1. Five deep breaths in and out followed by a cough.	Hourly

2. Paddle feet up and down, 20 times each foot.

3. Lift arm above head and lower. Alternate arms.

    5   10   15   20   times

4. Slide heel up to bottom, straighten leg. Alternate legs.

    5   10   15   20   times

LEVEL 2 – Out of bed for short periods

Exercises for level 1 plus:
Sitting on a chair

5. Bend and straighten alternate knees.

    5   10   15   20   times

6. Hands on shoulders, circle elbows slowly
Forwards

    5   10   15   20   times

Backwards

    5   10   15   20   times

Fig. 14.1   Sample in-patient activity sheet (prior to ambulation).

Exercise at a comfortable pace.

Repeat each exercise for:

    30 seconds

    1 minute

    2 minutes

STANDING

1. Legs apart, hand on hips. Bend left knee, straighten. Bend right knee, straighten. Keep trunk upright and facing forward.

2. Hands on shoulders. Turn upper body side to side easy and relaxed to warm up.

3. Quarter squat. Head up, back straight.

4. March on the spot. Lift knees, swing arms.

5. Arm circles forwards
                backwards

FLOOR

6. Bridging. Knees bent, lift bottom. Return to floor.

7. Modified push up - sitting back on to heels then return to floor.

Continue as appropriate.

The floor exercises (6&7) are not suitable for every patient.

Fig. 14.2   Sample out-patient exercise (in addition to a walk).

cardiac patients available. Many people find the stimulus of company assists in long-term motivation to exercise and would benefit from an appropriate community exercise programme.

Supervision

There are many aspects of patient monitoring useful for cardiac patients. Direct visual supervision is difficult in a large group situation, so it is recommended that exercise classes be kept small and be organized so that all participants can be seen.

Telemetry is a useful facility for allowing direct ECG recordings to be made at a central monitor whilst the patient exercises at a distance. The American College of Cardiology recommends this for patients with poor left ventricular function, resting or exercise induced ventricular arrhythmias, decreased systolic blood pressure during exercise, and survivors of cardiac arrest (American College of Cardiology 1986).

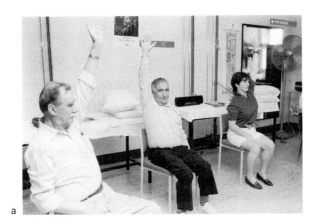

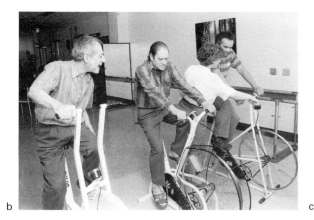

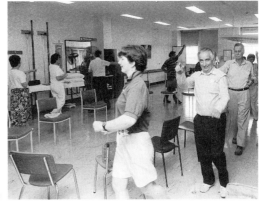

Fig. 14.3 Group out-patient exercise programme. **a** Warm up. **b** Major aerobic activity. **c** Cool down.

Individual supervision may be necessary for patients with special needs or problems, especially those whose functional level is extremely low.

Home exercise has been found to be an acceptable alternative for those unable to attend group activities. Regular telephone contact allows the patient to keep in touch with staff.

Monitoring

The level of exercise achieved in any session is an important part of monitoring and should always be recorded. This might be the distance covered in a given time for walking or the number of repetitions of an exercise.

Signs and symptoms. Signs and symptoms occurring with any level of activity should also be recorded. Angina in particular should be noted, together with the level of activity at which it occurs and, if possible, some objective measure such as heart rate at the time.

Heart rate. Heart rate is known to correlate with activity level (Astrand & Rodahl 1986) and is a useful measure of the stress imposed on the body by exercise. Resting, peak exercise and recovery heart rates associated with activity are useful measures (Fig. 14.4).

Many heart rate monitors are commercially available. Leger & Thivierge (1988) studied the validity and stability of measures from a wide range of monitors and found excellent correlations between ECG and monitors using chest electrodes. Monitors using finger or ear probes were found to be unsatisfactory during exercise.

Should the patient be taught to take his pulse?

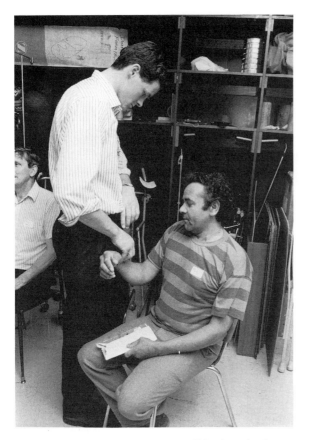

Fig. 14.4 Heart rate monitoring by radial pulse palpation pre- or post-exercise.

Some authors argue that this is mandatory and others suggest that it increases anxiety. Patients who have silent ischaemia certainly need to be able to regulate their exercise level reliably so that their activity is below the ischaemic threshold. Heart rate measurement is one way of doing this. It is quick and easy, reliable and requires only a watch with a second hand.

Rating of perceived exertion (RPE) could be an alternative to this. In patients on beta blocking medications, heart rate response to exercise will be attenuated and other objective measures such as respiratory rate or RPE may be more reliable and sensitive.

Rating of perceived exertion. RPE scales were developed by Borg to rate intensity of exercise. The RPE Scale (Borg 1982) uses 15 grades ranging from 6 to 20 to describe intensity of effort. This scale is shown in Table 14.4 (p. 326).

The RPE scale is simple and practical for clinical use. Gutmann et al (1981) investigated the relationship between RPE and heart rate during exercise testing and training in a group of post-CABG patients. They found that patients perceived exercise similarly at given heart rates, but that with recovery, time and further training the same RPE was given for higher heart rate levels. This finding is consistent with improvement in fitness. Studies cited in Williams & Eston (1989) have found that RPE can be used to control intensity of exercise. A rating of 12–13 is equal to 60–80% of maximal oxygen uptake in most individuals, while 16–17 has been found to correlate to 90%. A general conclusion reached by Williams & Eston (1989) is that the Borg RPE scale is a valid measure of exercise intensity for both indicating and regulating intensity of effort. It is worth noting that it may take several training sessions for an individual to become reliable at regulating his exercise effort by using this scale.

Breathlessness. Breathlessness is normally associated with exercise, especially when the activity is vigorous or prolonged. Respiratory rate is another measure which can be used to assess exercise effort. If the cardiac patient is exercising at a moderate level he should not be so breathless that he is unable to talk. In fact, the ability to answer a simple question verbally is a simple clinical method for assessment of breathlessness.

Blood pressure. Blood pressure usually rises gradually with 'aerobic style' exercise and should not drop dramatically during activity. Monitoring of blood pressure is a part of comprehensive patient monitoring, but is usually only performed at initial in-patient exercise sessions unless there is a problem with stability. If the patient complains of lightheadedness or dizziness his blood pressure should be checked.

Other signs. Pallor, fatigue and excessive perspiration are all signs associated with inability of the heart to maintain adequate cardiac output and should be treated as indicators of poor exercise tolerance.

Crackles. Crackles associated with cardiac failure are also an important sign which should be checked in patients who are extremely breathless with activity but have no respiratory disorder.

Angina. Angina is a major sign of myocardial

insufficiency and if it occurs with activity the patient should stop and rest. If rest is not sufficient to relieve angina then sublingual nitroglycerin should be available for use. Angina occurring with exercise should be documented and discussed with the relevant medical personnel.

Outcome evaluation

Quality of life is not easy to define, but some authors have studied this in relation to cardiac rehabilitation. Measures used by Oldridge et al (1991) included a specifically developed quality of life questionnaire which had 97 items of possible concern to patients. Mortality and work status were monitored and exercise tolerance was measured for a rehabilitation and a control group. The rehabilitation programme was found to accelerate recovery at 8 weeks post-MI but by 12 months all measures had improved significantly in both groups.

Return to work is often used as a marker of cardiac rehabilitation success. There is certainly a question as to whether this is valid as specific interventions to facilitate employment are often not a part of a programme. Hedback & Perk (1987) reported a 5-year follow up of a cardiac rehabilitation programme and found that in patients aged less than 55 more patients in the rehabilitation group returned to work than in the control group. In patients over this age group a large number of other factors were important in the decision to return to work.

The use of medical services by rehabilitation and non-rehabilitation groups has not been studied by many workers. Levin et al (1991) reported a cost analysis of their cardiac rehabilitation programme and found that the rehabilitation programme did not increase the costs of post-MI care as these costs were balanced by a decrease in readmissions for cardiovascular diseases.

Beneficial physiological alterations associated with exercise training have been well documented over many years (Astrand & Rodahl 1986). Objective measures such as exercise heart rate and respiratory rate for a given level of activity decrease with training. Subjective decreases in perceived effort are also reported.

Many of the benefits of cardiac rehabilitation have only been reported in studies with long-term follow up (Hedback & Perk 1987, Levin et al 1991). It appears that long-term follow up is necessary to maintain benefits of a programme and that analysis of effect and costs are best demonstrated in this way.

Effectiveness of education is again an area in which there has been little formal evaluation. Studies on the effects of outcomes from education and studies on the effects of education programmes on both knowledge and behaviour are lacking.

Morbidity and mortality are also frequently used as markers of success in assessment of cardiac rehabilitation programmes. Hedback & Perk (1987) found no difference in mortality between their rehabilitation and their reference groups but the recurrence rate of non-fatal MI and the total cardiac event rate was lower in their intervention group.

Complications of exercise

Adverse effects of exercise are noted within both the normal and cardiac populations. In particular, orthopaedic breakdown is more common in middle aged or older patients and is more likely with frequent or prolonged activity. Adequate warm up and cool down can reduce the incidence of orthopaedic problems.

Cardiovascular complications are less common but serious. Sudden death is defined as unexpected and atraumatic death as that within 6 hours of a normal state of health (Amsterdam 1990). This includes fatality during or within 30 min of concluding exercise.

Haskell (1978) reported the incidence of death during exercise training of cardiac patients as 1 per 212 182 patient-hours. Sudden death during exercise is usually associated with structural heart disease and the usual mechanism is ventricular fibrillation; however, malignant arrhythmias may occur throughout the spectrum of cardiac disease. Haskell noted that many exercise related deaths in cardiac patients occurred with activity in excess of normal exercise and with failure to heed symptoms induced by exercise.

OTHER CONSIDERATIONS

The older patient

There are no specific age related contraindications to joining a cardiac rehabilitation programme. Williams et al (1984a) have demonstrated that the older cardiac population can benefit from an out-patient cardiac exercise programme to the same extent as younger patients.

There are some general considerations which may apply to any population, but are more prevalent in the elderly. Older people may have more than one chronic condition which limits their exercise ability, for example osteoarthritis, peripheral vascular disease or pulmonary disease. Modification of an exercise programme on an individual basis may be necessary.

Landin et al (1985) cite evidence that the older population will have lost work capacity and suggest that 50% of the diminished function in muscle strength and mass, cardiac output and heart rate, respiratory capacity, bone mass and joint flexibility may be attributed to disuse. Stretches, flexibility exercises and range of movement activities should be incorporated as a part of an exercise programme.

Older patients will usually start their cardiac exercise programme at a lower level than their younger counterparts (Williams et al 1984a). This will often necessitate both a lower workload and an interval programme of shorter duration and with longer rest periods. At a lower exercise intensity patients can be encouraged to exercise daily (Williams et al 1984b) in order to encourage improvement without untoward effects.

Older patients can gain significant improvement in functional status with a lower intensity, longer term exercise programme. Wenger and Alpert (1989) suggest that this contributes to the patient's ability to maintain an independent lifestyle.

Cardiac failure

Heart failure is a complex and increasingly prevalent clinical syndrome. The basic cause of the inability of the heart to pump blood at a rate sufficient for the needs of the body may be cardiac or extracardiac in origin. Cardiac disturbances may be related to muscle contractile failure due to ischaemic heart disease, myocarditis or cardiomyopathy, or to disorders causing impaired filling or emptying of the cardiac chambers such as valvular stenosis or regurgitation. Extra cardiac disorders which may cause failure include hypertension, anaemia and thyrotoxicosis. This discussion will focus only on failure due to reduced ability of the myocardium to pump blood. Wenger (1989) points to an increased survival rate after myocardial infarction of patients with ventricular dysfunction and the ageing of the population as two major factors contributing to the increased incidence of cardiac failure.

Reduction in symptoms and improvement in functional capacity are the goals of treatment which Wenger (1989) found were most appreciated by patients. Without these outcomes the prolongation of survival is considered less desirable.

Until the past decade patients with cardiac failure were excluded from cardiac exercise programmes because of concern regarding the risks of exercise related arrhythmias and death and the possibility of further damage to the myocardium (Wenger 1988). Current medical practice as outlined by Shabetai (1988) involves bed rest during an acute unstable phase, with no subsequent limitations on usual physical activity.

Wenger (1988) suggests that the exercise capacity of patients with chronic heart failure is usually limited by breathlessness and/or fatigue, although the mechanisms which cause these limitations are still not clearly understood.

Exercise ability in patients with cardiac failure is widely variable. Franciosa et al (1981) have demonstrated that indices of left ventricular performance such as resting left ventricular ejection fraction do not correlate with exercise capacity in patients with heart failure. In clinical practice some patients with cardiac enlargement and a poor resting left ventricular ejection fraction will be able to perform near normal levels of exercise. In other patients, activities of daily living are a substantial physiological stress causing breathlessness and fatigue.

The physiological exercise responses of patients with coronary artery disease including left ventricular dysfunction have been shown to be identical to those of age matched normals and patients with coronary artery disease without left ventricular dysfunction (Kellerman et al 1988).

Many studies have now demonstrated that exercise training is a safe and effective method of improving functional capacity in patients with impaired ventricular function (Lee et al 1979, Conn et al 1982, Arvan 1988, Sullivan et al 1988). Sullivan et al (1988) found that exercise training induced adaptations in peripheral musculature which contributed to the improvement in exercise ability.

In prescribing exercise for a patient with ventricular dysfunction Mathes (1988) suggested that special consideration must be given to factors such as usual activity level and body weight. General debility may necessitate the initial use of very low level interval training, with the use of exercise such as stationary cycling where carriage of body weight is almost eliminated. In general, the principles of exercise prescription will be the same as those for other cardiac patients. The rate of exercise may determine the limiting symptoms in patients with heart failure. Lipkin et al (1986a) found that fast exercise was usually limited by breathlessness and slower or endurance exercise by fatigue. Fatigue that continues for hours or days after a particular bout of exercise is considered by Dubach and Froelicher (1989), an indicator that the amount of work was excessive either in workload, time or both.

Exercise training at an appropriate level in patients with stable compensated heart failure may have a major impact on quality of life with only a small increase in functional capacity. Patients who require a low level, long-term, small and slow increment exercise programme may be major beneficiaries of cardiac rehabilitation (Dubach & Froelicher 1989), especially if exercise training is combined with other measures to improve symptoms and quality of life such as dietary and vocational advice and instruction in energy conservation techniques.

Valvular heart disease

Some patients with valvular disorders have concomitant coronary artery disease and may benefit from the full range of services offered in cardiac rehabilitation. Other patients with valvular disorders may also benefit from an exercise programme for general fitness, dietary advice or work simplification. Valvular heart disease has not been studied as extensively as coronary artery disease especially with respect to exercise ability; however, some useful information is available.

Mitral stenosis and regurgitation

A decrease in exercise performance has been noted in association with progressively severe mitral stenosis, with good correlation between symptoms of fatigue, weakness and exertional breathlessness, severity of valvular obstruction and decline in exercise tolerance or degree of valvular regurgitation and exercise tolerance (Lutz & Wenger 1985). Carstens et al (1983) performed pre- and post operative exercise studies on 46 patients undergoing mitral valve replacement, 19 undergoing aortic and mitral valve replacement and 17 undergoing mitral valve reconstruction. Their postoperative evaluation generally found marked improvement in symptoms and some improvement in exercise performance. Disturbed haemodynamics persisted 6 months after surgery with elevated pulmonary artery pressures at rest which rose further during exercise and a low cardiac output at rest which failed to increase normally with exertion. The ability to exercise was generally significantly less than that of age matched sedentary control subjects. The extent to which this reflects decreased fitness prior to surgery is unknown.

Aortic stenosis and regurgitation

Patients with severe aortic stenosis are rarely assessed with exercise because of the possibility that exercise-induced syncope and/or sudden cardiac death may occur secondary to an inability to increase stroke volume and an actual or relative decrease in cardiac output with exercise. Results of postoperative evaluation in 49 patients studied by Carstens et al (1983) showed a generally good exercise performance after surgery, although haemodynamics remained abnormal.

Impairment of exercise tolerance often occurs late in the natural history of aortic regurgitation. Krayenbuehl et al (1979) found significant improvement in left ventricular function after aortic valve replacement, with residual impairment being greater in aortic regurgitation than in stenosis or a combination of regurgitation and stenosis. The need for early operative intervention was not demonstrated by Henry et al (1980) in their prospective study of 42 patients.

Sire (1978) reported on 44 patients randomly assigned to either an exercise training or a control group after aortic valve replacement. At 12 months postoperatively the exercise training group had a significantly higher physical work capacity and were much more likely to be in paid employment than their control counterparts.

Double valve surgery

Carstens et al (1983) found that their 19 patients undergoing double valve surgery had an outcome similar to those undergoing mitral valve surgery. A significant improvement in symptoms was accompanied by a small improvement in exercise ability.

Exercise recommendations

A longer-term slow increment exercise programme is indicated for patients following valvular surgery because of their reduced functional ability preoperatively and the continued abnormal haemodynamics, particularly their inability to increase cardiac output with exertion. Goforth & James (1985) have found that a workload of 50% of the patient's maximum is one that nearly all patients with non-coronary heart disease can comfortably perform at the start of exercise training. This is usually achieved by brisk walking. As with patients post-MI, ejection fraction does not correlate with exercise tolerance (Lutz & Wenger 1985).

Congenital heart disease

A large number of cardiac surgical procedures are undertaken to repair congenital heart lesions.

These patients may not require the full range of cardiac rehabilitation services, as they do not have coronary artery disease and many are infants at the time of surgery. However, many can benefit from general health advice and may have specific questions and problems.

In the paediatric population it has been noted that delayed motor development occurs in children with congenital heart defects (Box & Burns 1990). This may be related to the level of hypoxaemia associated with the defect, type of malformation, length of time prior to surgery or congestive heart failure.

Motor developmental delay was noted to persist for 2 or more years by Box & Burns (1990) after corrective surgery in pre-school age children. The older the child at time of surgery, the greater the delay. These authors suggested physiotherapists should be involved in the long-term follow up of children after congenital heart defect repair to minimize motor developmental delays.

Many patients with surgically corrected or repaired congenital heart defects are now adults or approaching adulthood and seek advice on safe and appropriate activity. They may be limited in their ability to perform work by residual deficits, but exercise should be encouraged in this population as part of a healthy lifestyle, and with the knowledge that training will assist in performance improvement.

Perrault & Drblik (1989) have reviewed much of the literature on this topic and found that maximum exercise tolerance after repair of congenital heart disorders is related in particular to three factors: age at time of definitive surgical repair (the younger the better); the severity of any lesions remaining after surgery; and the age of the patient at the time of investigation. While a normal maximal exercise capacity may be attained by some patients after surgical repair they noted some important exercise related differences in function: firstly that near normal exercise capacity does not imply normal exercise haemodynamic responses and secondly that in general there is some variance in exercise capacity when a comparison is made between people with corrected congenital lesions and age matched normals.

Atrial septal defect

Lutz & Wenger (1985) note that even after closure of a large atrial septal defect (ASD) some patients will have a very low functional capacity. No limitations are usually placed on participation in physical activity and sport once the postoperative recovery phase is over. However, a good result is usually achieved with no significant difference in work capacity between patients and age matched controls, especially if surgical correction occurred before 10 years of age.

Pulmonary stenosis

Little information is available on performance after repair of pulmonary stenosis. Early repair is now favoured as this seems to limit the long-term effects of obstruction to right ventricular ejection and thus minimizes right ventricular hypertrophy, hyperplasia and failure (Perrault & Drblik 1989). It appears that patients can safely participate in exercise and sport provided right ventricular function is adequate.

Ventricular septal defect

The haemodynamic consequences of a ventricular septal defect (VSD) are largely determined by its size. Early correction lessens damage to the pulmonary vascular bed. Almost all patients have some ventricular conduction abnormality. Exercise tolerance after VSD repair is very variable and depends on the extent of any residual deficit, arrhythmias and pulmonary vascular resistance (Perrault & Drblik 1989). When pulmonary hypertension is present preoperatively this rarely alters after VSD repair.

Reports on postoperative function cited by Perrault & Drblik (1989) suggest that, while many patients will have a good outcome, in general their exercise tolerance is less than that of age matched controls. Unless residual shunt or arrhythmias are present participation in sport and exercise is encouraged. An exercise test may be useful to identify activity induced arrhythmias. Moller et al (1991) published the results of more than 30-years follow up of 296 patients surviving closure of a VSD. The defect had completely closed in 80% of cases; 59 patients had died. Mortality was associated with high pulmonary vascular resistance (>7 mmHg/1. min. m²), complete heart block and being older than 5 years at the time of operation. Of the patients, 208 rated themselves in NYHA class I for function.

Tetralogy of Fallot

In patients exercising after a repair of Fallot's tetralogy the ability to perform is affected by the amount of residual circulatory deficit and with the severity of changes in left and/or right ventricular function in the preoperative period. In many patients excellent surgical results are obtained, allowing them to live a normal life, symptom and medication free (James et al 1976); however, cardiac output is lower in patients than in age matched normals. A comparable aerobic performance may be found between patients with corrected Fallot's tetralogy and age matched controls, but patients are unable to reach elite standards of performance because of the limitation of exercise cardiac output. Exercise participation should be encouraged at a level allowed by the success of the repair. James et al (1976) recommend a prior exercise test to identify patients who have developed arrhythmias following intraventricular surgery.

Exercise recommendations

In patients with congenital cardiac disorders undergoing exercise training either before or after surgery, special consideration must be given to the existing pathophysiology, keeping in mind that surgical intervention will not restore normal function to the heart. Goforth & James (1985) recommend submaximal activities with long, slow warm up and cool down periods. Training patients to be aware of symptoms and their level of perceived exertion may assist in keeping exercise at a submaximal level.

Compliance

When planning an exercise programme which requires long-term adherence, strategies to maximize compliance must be considered.

In a short-term study of patients after CABGS Shankar et al (1990) found that at 1 month following hospital discharge, self-reports of behaviour with respect to smoking, exercise and diet were consistent with physiological measurements in approximately 50% of subjects.

Oldridge et al (1991) reported a 46.5% drop out rate of post-MI patients from an exercise programme at a 3-year follow up. Investigation of their subject sample showed that those most likely to drop out were smokers and 'blue collar' workers. There was no difference in drop out rate between the high intensity and low intensity exercise programmes.

An earlier study by the same group (Andrew et al 1981) had found that the three main reasons given for lack of compliance were:

- inconvenience (of exercise centre, times, parking)
- poor perception of the exercise programme (fatigue, lack of staff attention and enthusiasm, poor belief in need for exercise for health)
- family and lifestyle factors (interfered with work, spouse negative or indifferent).

From these complaints some potential strategies to improve compliance might include: flexibility in timing of exercise programmes, staffing to meet the needs and interests of the participants, spouse involvement, feedback of improvement to maintain motivation, and the possibility of a home exercise programme.

Cost effectiveness

In a time of economic restraint and burgeoning health care expenditure the costs and effectiveness of any programme should be considered. Doubliet et al (1986) discuss the meaning of the term 'cost effective' as used in medical literature and consider it most appropriate when a procedure has benefits worth the costs involved. In assessing the worth of any programme it is necessary to have well defined and agreed outcome measures.

The assessment of effectiveness of cardiac rehabilitation has involved the use of a number of quite different outcome measures, for example: a decrease in morbidity and/or mortality (Marra et

al 1985, Hamalainen et al 1989), improvement in functional capacity (Greenland & Chu 1988), return to work (Marra et al 1985, Oldridge et al 1991), reduction in risk factors (Hedback et al 1990), change in quality of life (Greenland & Chu 1988, Oldridge et al 1991) and, more recently, the long-term utilization of health care services, especially hospital readmissions (Blodgett & Pekarik 1987, Huang et al 1990), outpatient and local doctor attendances.

The costs of each of these outcomes are difficult to assess in monetary terms as many health care choices are influenced by factors not easily quantified or given a monetary value. The importance and desirability of each of these outcomes also varies from individual to individual, across health care settings and between nations. Equally the patient's perception of costs and benefit should be considered. Is increased survival time worth the necessary effort to the individual?

Some of the beneficial evidence in favour of cardiac rehabilitation has already been presented in this chapter. Counting cost and benefit to the community is a much larger and more difficult issue. The costs associated with a cardiac rehabilitation programme include as a minimum those of the venue, equipment and personnel and to the patient those of their own time and effort.

Many studies of cardiac rehabilitation programmes like Marra et al (1985) have not demonstrated benefits in terms of morbidity and mortality like the studies of Hamalainen et al (1989) and Kallio et al (1979), but they have shown short-term improvement in functional capacity and psychosocial status. Oldridge et al (1988) believe that this is because trials have been too small and have used heterogeneous patient populations. The results of their meta analysis suggest that comprehensive cardiac rehabilitation has a beneficial effect on mortality.

In considering the costs of cardiac rehabilitation, Worcester (1986) suggests that the reduction in indirect costs of cardiac illness (loss of income and social security payments) vastly outweigh the costs of a cardiac rehabilitation programme to the extent that A$100 of indirect cost could be saved for every dollar expended on the direct costs of effective cardiac rehabilitation. Huang et al (1990) found a 38% reduction in rehospitalization costs in his group of post-MI rehabilitation participants compared with a no-rehabilitation group. After adjustment for other factors, participation in an exercise programme was a favourable influence in longer-term cost reduction.

The strongest evidence of the cost effectiveness of cardiac rehabilitation comes from the studies of Hedback and Perk (1987, 1990).

Legal aspects

Cardiac rehabilitation is a recently developed health care service and a diversity of programmes are offered across differing health care settings. Personnel, policies, procedures and methods of operation may differ from programme to programme, and certainly the law differs from country to country and state to state. There are a number of legal issues and concerns which should be addressed by cardiac rehabilitation providers.

Standards of care. Acceptable standards of conduct or of care in cardiac rehabilitation may be established by reference to respected authorities. Professional associations with expressed positions regarding protocols for cardiac rehabilitation programmes include the American Heart Association (1990), the American Medical Association (1981), the American College of Cardiology (1986), the American Association of Cardiovascular and Pulmonary Rehabilitation (1990) and the American College of Sports Medicine (1991). Unfortunately, the standards of these bodies are not uniformly consistent; however, they do provide some guidance for the development of local programme policies and procedures and point to areas of concern.

Policies and procedures. In developing policies and procedures, safe and appropriate patient care should be of paramount concern (Herbert & Herbert 1988). Policies and procedures should be documented in writing with reference to the appropriate professional standards of care. The potential for serious adverse reactions to occur during exercise should alert all concerned to the necessity for and use of protocols.

Staffing. Programme personnel may come from a variety of professional backgrounds. In some countries statutes and laws may define the scope of a profession. Failure to comply with such laws may expose staff to legal action. Exercise prescription is considered in some countries to be a part of medical practice and in this situation exercise can only be prescribed by the physician. In any programme only properly authorized professionals should prescribe exercise. Appropriate monitoring while exercising patients is part of any reasonable standard of care.

Informed consent. Consent to treatment is another area of concern. Many patients enter cardiac rehabilitation with only a vague idea of what is involved and usually give written consent only for procedures such as exercise testing. The American Heart Association (1990) and American College of Sports Medicine (1991) now suggest informed consent be obtained for a cardiac rehabilitation programme, and have developed forms for this purpose.

Shephard (1981) lists the common bases for legal claims against cardiac rehabilitation providers as: failure to detect pre-existing medical abnormalities contraindicating the proposed programme, failure to monitor the patient adequately before, during and after exercise, lack of skill or delay in handling an emergency, lack of equipment, drugs and trained personnel necessary for resuscitation, lack of informed consent and inadequate documentation of procedures.

Legal concerns for cardiac rehabilitation programmes can be minimized by good management practices within the programme.

CONCLUSION

Cardiac rehabilitation is only now being demonstrated to be a cost effective form of management for the cardiac patient. The training of a physiotherapist gives an excellent background for integral involvement in multidisciplinary cardiac rehabilitation. Exercise is an effective and important way of altering cardiac risk factors and of optimizing function for cardiac patients, but should be applied judiciously.

REFERENCES

American Association of Cardiovascular and Pulmonary Rehabilitation 1990 Scientific evidence of the value of cardiac rehabilitation services with emphasis on patients following myocardial infarction—section 1: exercise conditioning component. Journal of Cardiopulmonary Rehabilitation 10: 79–87

American College of Cardiology 1986 Recommendations of the American College of Cardiology on cardiovascular rehabilitation. Journal of the American College of Cardiology 7: 451–453

American College of Sports Medicine 1991 Guidelines for exercise testing and prescription, 4th edn. Lea & Febiger, Philedelphia

American Heart Association Subcommittee on Rehabilitation 1979 Standards for cardiovascular exercise treatment programs. Circulation 59: 1084A–1090A

American Heart Association 1990 Exercise standards: a statement for health professionals from the American Heart Association. Circulation 82: 2286–2322

American Medical Association 1981 Physician-supervised exercise programs in rehabilitation of patients with coronary heart disease. Journal of the American Medical Association 245: 1463–1466

Amsterdam E A 1990 Sudden death during exercise. Cardiology 77: 411–417

Andrew G M, Oldridge N B, Parker J O et al 1981 Reasons for dropout from exercise programs in post coronary patients. Medicine and Science in Sports and Exercise 13: 164–168

Arvan S 1988 Exercise performance of the high risk acute myocardial infarct patient after cardiac rehabilitation. The American Journal of Cardiology 62: 197–201

Astrand P-O, Rodahl K 1986 Textbook of work physiology, 3rd edn. McGraw-Hill, New York

Blair S N, Kohl H W, Paffenbarger R S et al 1989 Physical fitness and all cause mortality a prospective study of healthy men and women. Journal of the American Medical Association 262: 2395–2401

Bloch A, Maeder J P, Haissly J C et al 1974 Early mobilisation after myocardial infarction. A controlled study. American Journal of Cardiology 34: 152–157

Blodgett C, Pekarik G 1987 Program evaluation in cardiac rehabilitation IV: efficiency evaluation. Journal of Cardiopulmonary Rehabilitation 7: 466–474

Borg G V 1982 Psychophysical bases of perceived exertion. Medicine and Science in Sports and Exercise 14: 377–381

Box R C, Burns Y R 1990 The motor performance of preschool aged children after surgery for congenital heart disease. Australian Journal of Physiotherapy 36: 235–242

Bruce R A 1956 Evaluation of functional capacity and exercise tolerance of cardiac patients. Modern Concepts of Cardiovascular Disease 25: 321–326

Bruce R A, Kusumi F, Hosmer D 1973 Maximal oxygen intake and nomographic assessment of functional aerobic impairment in cardiovascular disease. American Heart Journal 85: 546–562

Caine N, Harrison S C W, Sharples L D, Wallwork J 1991 Prospective study of quality of life before and after coronary artery bypass grafting. British Medical Journal 302: 511–516

Carstens V, Behrenbeck D W, Hilger H H 1983 Exercise capacity before and after cardiac valve surgery. Cardiology 70: 41–49

Conn E H, Sanders-Williams R, Wallace A G 1982 Exercise responses before and after physical conditioning in patients with severely depressed left ventricular function. The American Journal of Cardiology 49: 296–300

Davidson D M, Maloney C A 1985 Recovery after cardiac events. Physical Therapy 65: 1820–1827

DeBusk R F 1989 Specialised testing after recent acute myocardial infarction. Annals of Internal Medicine 110: 470–481

DeBusk R F, Houston N, Haskell W et al 1979 Exercise training soon after myocardial infarction. The American Journal of Cardiology 44: 1223–1229

DeBusk R F, Blomqvist C G, Kouchoukos N T et al 1986 Identification and treatment of low risk patients after acute myocardial infarction and coronary artery bypass graft surgery. The New England Journal of Medicine 314: 161–166

DeBusk R F, Stenestrand U, Sheehan M, Haskell W L 1990 Training effects of long versus short bouts of exercise in healthy subjects. The American Journal of Cardiology 65: 1010–1013

Doubliet P, Weinstein M C, McNeil B J 1986 Use and misuse of the term 'cost effective' in medicine. The New England Journal of Medicine 314: 253–256

Doughty C 1991 A multidisciplinary approach to cardiac rehabilitation. Nursing Standard 5: 13–15

Dubach P, Froelicher V F 1989 Cardiac rehabilitation for heart failure patients. Cardiology 76: 368–373

Franciosa J A, Park M, Levine T B 1981 Lack of correlation between exercise capacity and indexes of resting left ventricular performance in heart failure. The American Journal of Cardiology 47: 33–39

Frishman W H, Teicher M 1985 Beta adrenergic blockade; an update. Cardiology 72: 280–296

Gazes P C 1990 Clinical cardiology, 3rd edn. Lea & Febiger, Philadelphia

Goble A, Hare D L, Macdonald PS et al 1991 Effect of early programmes of high and low intensity exercise on physical performance after transmural acute myocardial infarction. British Heart Journal 65: 126–131

Goforth D, James F W 1985 Exercise training in noncoronary heart disease. In: Wenger N K (ed) Exercise and the heart, 2nd edn. F A Davis, Philadelphia

Greenland P, Chu J 1988 Efficacy of cardiac rehabilitation services with emphasis on patients after myocardial infarction. Annals of Internal Medicine 109: 650–663

Gutmann M C, Squires R W, Pollock M L et al 1981 Perceived exertion — heart rate relationship during exercise testing and training in cardiac patients. Journal of Cardiac Rehabilitation 1: 52–59

Hamalainen H, Luurila O J, Kallio V et al 1989 Long term reduction in sudden deaths after a multifactorial intervention programme in patients with myocardial infarction: 10 year results of a controlled investigation. European Heart Journal 10: 55–62

Hare D L 1990 Cardiac rehabilitation. Australian Family Physician 19: 1043–1052

Haskell W L 1978 Cardiovascular complications during exercise training of cardiac patients. Circulation 57: 920–924

Haskell W L 1985 Physical activity and health: need to define the required stimulus. The American Journal of Cardiology 5: 4D–9D

Hedback B E and Perk J 1987 5 year results of a comprehensive rehabilitation programme after myocardial infarction. European Heart Journal 8: 234–242

Hedback B E, Perk J, Engvall J, Areskog N-H 1990 Cardiac rehabilitation after coronary artery bypass grafting: effects on exercise performance and risk factors. Archives of Physical Medicine and Rehabilitation 71: 1069–1073

Henry W L, Bonow R O, Borer J S et al 1980 Evaluation of aortic valve replacement in patients with valvular aortic stenosis. Circulation 61: 814–825

Herbert W G, Herbert D L 1988 Legal aspects of cardiac rehabilitation exercise programs. The Physician and Sports Medicine 16: 105–112

Huang D, Ades P A, Weaver S 1990 Cardiac rehospitalisations and costs are reduced following cardiac rehabilitation. Journal of Cardiopulmonary Rehabilitation 10: 108

Hurst J W (ed) 1974 The heart, 3rd edn. McGraw-Hill, New York

Hurst J W, Schlant R C, Rackley C E (eds) 1990 The heart, 7th edn. McGraw-Hill, New York

Ice D 1985 Cardiovascular medications. Physical Therapy 65: 1845–1851

James F W, Kaplan S, Schwarz D C et al 1976 Response to exercise in patients after total surgical correction of tetralogy of fallot. Circulation 54: 671–679

Jelinek V M 1988 Exercise after myocardial infarction: a practical guide to prescription. Patient Management Jan: 69–80

Jelinek V M, Ziffer R W, McDonald I G et al 1977 Early exercise testing and mobilization after myocardial infarction. The Medical Journal of Australia 2: 589–593

Joint International Society and Federation of Cardiology/World Health Organisation Task Force on Standardisation of Clinical Nomenclature 1979 Nomenclature and criteria for ischaemic heart disease. Circulation 59: 607–609

Kallio V, Hamalainen H, Hakkila J, Luurila O J 1979 Reduction of sudden deaths by a multifactorial intervention programme after acute myocardial infarction. Lancet ii: 1091–1094

Kellerman J J, Shemesh J, Ben Ari E 1988 Contraindications to physical training in patients with impaired ventricular function. European Heart Journal 9 (suppl F): 70–73

Krayenbuehl H P, Turina M, Hess O M et al 1979 Pre- and postoperative left ventricular contractile function in patients with aortic valve disease. British Heart Journal 41: 204–213

Landin R J, Linnemeier T J, Rothbaum D A et al 1985 Exercise testing and training of the elderly patient. In: Wenger N K (ed) Exercise and the heart, 2nd edn. F A Davis, Philadelphia

Lee A P, Ice R, Blessey R, Sanmarco M E 1979 Long term effects of physical training on coronary patients with impaired ventricular function. Circulation 60: 1519–1526

Leger I and Thivierge M 1988 Heart rate monitors: validity stability and functionality. The Physician and Sports Medicine 16: (5) 143–151

Leon A S, Connett J, Jacobs D R, Rauramaa R 1987 Leisure time physical activity levels and risk of coronary heart disease and death. Journal of the American Medical Association 258: 2388–2395

Levin L-A, Perk J, Hedback B 1991 Cardiac rehabilitation — a cost analysis. Journal of Internal Medicine 230: 427–434

Levine S A, Lown B 1952 Armchair treatment of acute coronary thrombosis. The Journal of the American Medical Association 148: 1365–1369

Lipkin D P 1991 Is cardiac rehabilitation necessary? British Heart Journal 65: 237–238

Lipkin D P, Canepa-Anson R, Stephens M R, Poole-Wilson P A 1986a Factors determining symptoms in heart failure: comparison of fast and slow exercise tests. British Heart Journal 55: 439–445

Lipkin D P, Scriven A J, Crake T, Poole-Wilson P A 1986b Six minute walking test for assessing exercise capacity in chronic heart failure. British Medical Journal 292: 653–655

Lutz J F, Wenger N K 1985 Use of exercise testing in noncoronary heart disease. In: Wenger N K (ed) Exercise and heart disease, 2nd edn. F A Davis, Philadelphia

McBurney H 1991 Clinical judgement of fitness in the post myocardial infarct population. Proceedings of the world confederation for physical therapy 11th international congress, Vol II, p 931–933

Marra S, Paolillo V, Spadccini F, Angelino P F 1985 Long term follow up after controlled randomised post MI rehabilitation programme: effects on morbidity and mortality. European Heart Journal 6: 656–663

Mathes P 1988 Physical training in patients with ventricular dysfunction: choice and dosage of physical exercise in patients with pump dysfunction. European Heart Journal 9 (suppl F): 67–69

Miller D H, Borer J S 1982 Exercise testing early after myocardial infarction risks and benefits. The American Journal of Medicine 72: 427–438

Miller N H, Haskell W L, Berra K, DeBusk R 1984 Home versus group exercise training for increasing functional capacity after myocardial infarction Circulation 70: 645–649

Moller J H, Patton C, Varco R L, Lillehei C W 1991 Late results (30 to 35 years) after operative closure of isolated ventricular septal defect from 1954 to 1960. The American Journal of Cardiology 68: 1491–1497

Mulchahy R 1991 Meeting report: twenty years of cardiac rehabilitation in Europe: a reappraisal. European Heart Journal 12: 92–93

Newman B, Andrews M F, Koblish M S, Baker L A 1952 Physical medicine and rehabilitation in acute myocardial infarction. Archives of Internal Medicine 85: 552–561

Oldridge N B, Rogowski B L 1990 Self efficacy and inpatient cardiac rehabilitation. The American Journal of Cardiology 66: 362–365

Oldridge N B, Donner A P, Buck C W et al 1983 Predictions of drop out from cardiac exercise rehabilitation, Ontario exercise-heart collaborative study. The American Journal of Cardiology 51: 70–74

Oldridge N B, Guyatt G H, Fischer M E, Rimm A A 1988 Cardiac rehabilitation after myocardial infarction: combined experience of randomised clinical trials. Journal of the American Medical Association 260: 945–950

Oldridge N B, Guyatt G, Jones N et al 1991 Effects on quality of life with comprehensive rehabilitation after acute myocardial infarction. The American Journal of Cardiology 67: 1084–1089

Perrault H, Drblik S P 1989 Exercise after surgical repair of congenital cardiac lesions. Sports Medicine 7: 18–31

Shabetai R 1988 Beneficial effects of exercise training in compensated heart failure. Circulation 77: 775 – 776

Shankar K, Mihalko-Ward R, Rodell E et al 1990 Methodologic and compliance issues in post coronary bypass surgery subjects. Archives of Physical Medicine and Rehabilitation 71: 1074 –1077

Shephard R J 1981 Ischaemic heart disease and exercise. Croom Helm, London

Sire S 1987 Physical training and occupational rehabilitation after aortic valve replacement. European Heart Journal 8: 1215 –1220

Stang J M, Lewis R P 1981 Early exercise tests after myocardial infarction. Annals of Internal Medicine 94: 814 – 815

Stern M J, Cleary P 1982 The national exercise and heart disease project: long term psychosocial outcome. Archives of Internal Medicine 142: 1093 –1097

Sullivan M J, Higginbotham M B, Cobb F R 1988 Exercise training in patients with severe left ventricular dysfunction: hemodynamic and metabolic effects. Circulation 77: 506 – 515

Verrill D, Shoup E, McElveen G et al 1992 Resistive exercise training in cardiac patients. Sports Medicine 13: 171–193

Wenger N K 1986 Rehabilitation of the coronary patient: status 1986. Progress in Cardiovascular Diseases 29: 181–204

Wenger N K 1988 Left ventricular dysfunction: exercise capacity and activity recommendations. European Heart Journal 9 (suppl F): 63 – 66

Wenger N K 1989 Quality of life: can it and should it be assessed in patients with heart failure. Cardiology 76: 391–398

Wenger N K, Alpert J S 1989 Rehabilitation of the coronary patient in 1989. Archives of Internal Medicine 149: 1504 –1506

Williams J G, Eston R G 1989 Determination of the intensity dimension in vigorous exercise programmes with particular reference to the use of the rating of perceived exertion. Sports Medicine 8: 177–189

Williams M A, Maresh C M, Aronow W S et al 1984a The value of early outpatient cardiac exercise programmes for the elderly in comparison with other selected age groups. European Heart Journal 5 (suppl E): 113 –115

Williams M A, Esterbrooks D J, Sketch M H 1984b Guidelines for exercise therapy of the elderly after myocardial infarction. European Heart Journal 5 (suppl E): 121–123

Worcester M 1986 Cardiac rehabilitation programmes in Australian hospitals. National Heart Foundation of Australia, Woden, Australia

15. Cardiopulmonary transplantation

Catherine E. Bray

INTRODUCTION

The first human cardiac transplant was performed by Dr Christian Barnard and his team at Groote Schuur Hospital, South Africa, in 1967 (Barnard 1968). Despite initial enthusiasm, the problems of acute rejection and infection soon slowed the practice of the procedure. Several units continued with their programmes, gaining valuable clinical experience. However, it was the introduction of cyclosporin A, in the late 1970s, which significantly advanced immunosuppressive therapy and encouraged many centres world-wide to establish and continue heart transplantation programmes. This new age of transplantation also saw the first long-term survivors of heart–lung (Reitz 1982), single lung (Cooper et al 1987) and double lung (Patterson et al 1988) transplantation.

The transplantation of the thoracic organs is now an accepted practice in over 200 centres world-wide. In 1990, a total of 3054 heart, 194 heart–lung, 214 single lung and 60 double lung transplant procedures were registered as being performed on recipients, aged from newborn to 70 years (Kriett and Kaye 1991).

The primary indication for cardiac transplantation is for the relief of severe symptoms in individuals with end-stage dilated cardiomyopathy (Keogh et al 1991). Cardiopulmonary and pulmonary transplantation is increasingly utilized for patients with end-stage pulmonary disease which may or may not be associated with cor pulmonale. The indications for the various forms of cardiopulmonary transplantation are outlined in Table 15.1.

ASSESSMENT

The assessment of potential recipients (which may be done on an out-patient basis) involves a review of the patient's past medical history and the results of previous investigations and interven-

Table 15.1 Indications for cardiopulmonary transplantation

Heart transplantation	Heart–lung transplantation	Lung transplantation	Double lung transplantation
End-stage heart failure as a result of: Postviral cardiomyopathy Ischaemic cardiomyopathy Idiopathic cardiomyopathy Disabling angina with inoperable coronary artery disease	Pulmonary vascular disease, e.g. primary pulmonary hypertension. Eisenmenger's syndrome. Pulmonary parenchymal disease (with non-reversible cardiac dysfunction), e.g. bronchiectasis, cystic fibrosis, sarcoidosis, fibrosing alveolitis, CAL	End-stage fibrotic lung disease, e.g. pulmonary fibrosis, occupational lung disease, sarcoidosis, pulmonary hypertension (with satisfactory/reversible right ventricular function), CAL	An acceptable alternative to heart–lung transplantation for patients with satisfactory right ventricular function and bilateral pulmonary sepsis, e.g. bronchiectasis, cystic fibrosis

CAL, chronic airflow limitation.

tions. Further investigations are carried out to define the following:

- severity of cardiac and/or pulmonary dysfunction
- identification of contraindications (Table 15.2)
- immunological status (ABO group, human leucocyte antigen (HLA) tissue typing)
- previous exposure to potentially complicating infections (cytomegalovirus (CMV), toxoplasmosis, hepatitis B, hepatitis C and methicillin-resistant staphylococcus aureus)
- nutritional status
- psychological status (Keogh et al 1991).

Once accepted for the active waiting list, potential recipients are reviewed every 1–3 months.

THE TRANSPLANTATION PROCESS

Donors

Potential donors have been declared brain dead and have usually been the victims of a head injury or cerebrovascular accident. Table 15.3 outlines the transplant specific donor requirements.

Another source of donor hearts is from heart–lung transplantation. In the 'domino' technique the heart from a patient undergoing heart–lung transplantation is utilized in a heart transplant.

When a potential donor becomes available, the donor hospital notifies a central organ transplant coordinator and provides information on the donor's age, weight and ABO blood grouping. The coordinator in turn contacts the transplant unit(s) that may utilize the organ(s) which are available.

All donor matching involves ABO blood group compatibility. Cardiac donor–recipient matching is done such that the donor weight is no more than 20% below that of the recipient. A positive donor weight advantage is necessary when the recipient's transpulmonary gradient is increased (Keogh et al 1991). Pulmonary donors are matched with the recipient's weight and dimensions of the thoracic cavity.

In the early days of transplantation it was necessary for the donor to be transported to the transplant centre. Today, hearts, heart–lung blocks, lungs and other transplantable organs/tissues are utilized via distant procurement procedures.

Table 15.2 Contraindications to transplantation (procedure specific exclusion criteria)

General	Heart	Heart–lung	Lung
Absolute exclusion			
Irreversible renal dysfunction (except in combined heart–kidney transplantation)	Raised transpulmonary gradient (> 15 mmHg) and/or pulmonary vascular resistance (> 4 mmHg) (patients who are excluded may be reconsidered for heterotopic heart or heart–lung transplantation)	Systemic corticosteroids (retard healing, especially tracheal or bronchial anastomosis)	Right ventricular ejection fraction <25% (patients who are excluded, may be reconsidered for heart–lung transplant)
Irreversible hepatic dysfunction			
Active malignancy			Systemic corticosteroids
Immunodeficiency			
Alcohol/drug abuse			
Morbid obesity			
Relative exclusion			
Active systemic infection		Previous extensive pleural surgery	Previous extensive pleural surgery
Recent pulmonary infarction			
Insulin dependent diabetes mellitus		Malnutrition	Malnutrition
		Immobility	Immobility
Peripheral or cerebrovascular disorders		Cachexia	Cachexia
Psychological instability			

Table 15.3   Donor selection criteria

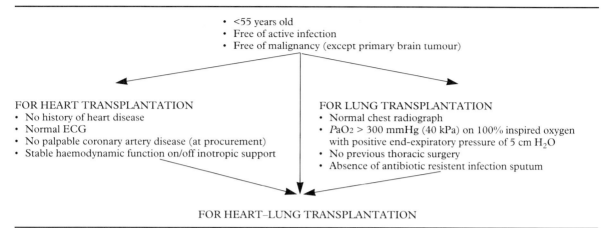

- <55 years old
- Free of active infection
- Free of malignancy (except primary brain tumour)

FOR HEART TRANSPLANTATION
- No history of heart disease
- Normal ECG
- No palpable coronary artery disease (at procurement)
- Stable haemodynamic function on/off inotropic support

FOR LUNG TRANSPLANTATION
- Normal chest radiograph
- PaO_2 > 300 mmHg (40 kPa) on 100% inspired oxygen with positive end-expiratory pressure of 5 cm H_2O
- No previous thoracic surgery
- Absence of antibiotic resistent infection sputum

FOR HEART–LUNG TRANSPLANTATION

Operative procedures

Cardiac transplantation

Orthotopic transplantation. Preparation of the heart (and heart–lung) transplant recipient is similar to that for any patient undergoing cardiac surgery (anaesthesia, median sternotomy and cardiopulmonary bypass). When the donor heart is present in the recipient theatre and has passed a final inspection, the recipient heart is removed, by incising the atria, pulmonary artery and aorta (leaving the posterior walls of both atria, including the sinoatrial (SA) node). The donor heart is sutured in place: the anastomoses joining recipient and donor atria, the pulmonary arteries and finally the aortas (Keogh et al 1986) (Fig. 15.1).

Heterotopic transplantation. Heterotopic transplantation is a less commonly used procedure than orthotopic transplantation. In this 'piggyback' procedure the recipient heart is left in place and the donor heart (connected to the recipient's in parallel by anastomoses made between the two hearts at the atria, pulmonary arteries and aortas) is positioned in the right chest. Both hearts contribute to the cardiac output (Weber 1990).

Heart–lung transplantation

The heart and lungs are excised separately, allowing identification and protection of the

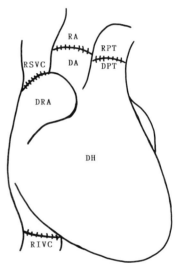

Fig. 15.1   Orthotopic technique: the donor heart following implantation. DH, donor heart; RPT, recipient pulmonary trunk; DPT, donor pulmonary trunk; RA, recipient aorta; DA, donor aorta; RSVC, recipient superior vena cava; DRA, donor right atrium; RIVC, recipient inferior vena cava.

phrenic, recurrent laryngeal and vagus nerves, a most critical part of the procedure. The heart is removed leaving the posterior wall of the right atrium. The left, then right lung is removed (following stapling of the bronchi, to minimize the risk of contaminating the area) and the trachea is divided above the bifurcation. The donor heart–lung block is implanted starting with the tracheal, then the atrial and aortic anastomoses. Ventilation is established (ensuring the patency of the airway anastomosis) and the heart resuscitated (Jamieson 1984) (Fig. 15.2).

Lung transplantation

Single lung transplantation. The procedure commences as a lateral thoracotomy. The recipient's lung is removed and the donor lung positioned in the chest. Cuffs on the left atrium of the donor and recipient heart are joined. The pulmonary artery anastomosis is completed and circulation is restored to the lung, allowing for inspection of the arterial and atrial anastomoses. The bronchial anastomosis is performed and ventilation is resumed (Cooper et al 1987). Cardiopulmonary bypass is made available for the procedure but is rarely needed. The single lung procedure may also involve a small laparotomy via which a pedicle of greater omentum is mobilized, brought upward into the chest and wrapped around the bronchial anastomosis, to restore bronchial artery circulation and improve healing of the anastomosis. Alternatively, bronchial healing may be promoted by the 'telescoping' of the donor and recipient bronchial anastomosis. The latter technique avoids the need for a laparo-

tomy and allows for early mobilization and oral nutrition.

Double lung transplantation. The early experiences of double lung transplantation involved the implantation en bloc of both lungs via a median sternotomy utilizing an omental wrap to secure the tracheal anastomosis (Patterson et al 1988). In an effort to avoid the high incidence of airway complications associated with the original procedure, the technique of two sequential lung transplants via anterolateral, bilateral thoracotomies with transverse sternotomy is now preferred. The procedure of direct revascularization of the bronchial arteries with the internal mammary artery is sometimes used to promote healing (Madden et al 1992). The donor procedure for double lung transplantation allows for the separate excision of the heart, facilitating the utilization of donor organs (Kaiser et al 1991).

Postoperative care

The intensive care area and ward management of the cardiopulmonary transplant patient is similar to that for any patient having undergone cardiac or thoracic surgery. The major differences include drug therapy and the intensive and comprehensive monitoring necessary because of the potential for rejection and infection. The degree and duration of protective isolation of recipients varies considerably between centres. Some units protectively isolate recipients in laminar airflow rooms, while others only require thorough hand washing before contact with the patient.

Rejection of the transplanted organs

The same immune response that protects the body against foreign chemicals and organisms, is also responsible for graft (transplanted organ) rejection. The presence of the transplanted organs triggers the immune system to respond, that is, to reject them. Both humoral (B cell lymphocyte mediated) and cellular (T cell lymphocyte mediated) immune responses may be involved in graft rejection. Rejection may occur at any time following transplantation, but the risk is greatest in the first 10–18 days post-transplantation (Weber 1990).

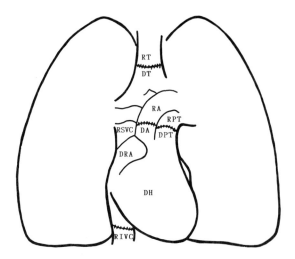

Fig. 15.2 The donor heart–lung block following implantation. DH, donor heart; RPT, recipient pulmonary trunk; DPT, donor pulmonary trunk; RA, recipient aorta; DA, donor aorta; RSVC, recipient superior vena cava; DRA, donor right atrium; RIVC, recipient inferior vena cava; RT, recipient trachea; DT, donor trachea.

Acute rejection

Acute rejection occurs within the first 3 months after transplantation. Most recipients can anticipate two or more episodes of this cell mediated immune response. The patient may be asymptomatic despite a definitive biopsy diagnosis.

In heart recipients it may be associated with: malaise, shortness of breath, peripheral oedema, low grade fever, nausea, vomiting, a voltage drop on ECG and/or an atrial arrhythmia (Keogh et al 1986). Endomyocardial biopsy (using a bioptome, passed down the right internal jugular vein and sampling tissue from the right ventricle) is currently the only way to objectively diagnose rejection. Biopsies are performed routinely on a regular basis for the first year following transplantation, and then only if indicated symptomatically.

A clinical diagnosis of acute lung rejection is usually made from a combination of findings: fever, shortness of breath, increasing infiltrates on chest radiograph, deteriorating gas exchange and lung function, the exclusion of infection and rapid symptomatic improvement with increased immunosuppression (Lawrence 1990) (Fig. 15.3).

To establish a diagnosis of lung rejection (and to identify infection) transbronchial lung biopsy may be utilized. There are, however, intrinsic difficulties in obtaining adequate tissue samples and in performing the procedure on critically ill patients. Transbronchial lung biopsies are carried out on a regular basis and when symptoms necessitate.

Chronic rejection

Chronic rejection occurs over months to years. In the transplanted heart it is characterized by diffuse and rapidly progressing coronary artery disease manifesting in myocardial infarction, congestive heart failure or sudden cardiac death. It is a major factor limiting long-term survival and is seen in approximately 40% of patients 5 years following transplant (Squires 1990). Periodic coronary angiography is utilized for the diagnosis and monitoring of this process.

Obliterative bronchiolitis, associated with lung transplantation, involves an inflammatory process in the small airways which leads to the obstruction

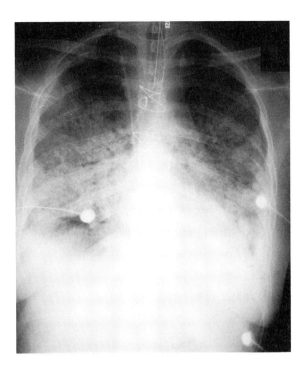

Fig. 15.3   A chest radiograph showing acute pulmonary rejection in a heart–lung recipient.

and destruction of pulmonary bronchioles. It is suggested that obliterative bronchiolitis is the result of 'late' rejection and may be advanced (or even triggered) by respiratory infection. It is one of the major factors influencing long-term survival of heart–lung and possibly lung recipients. Its successful management requires the close monitoring of pulmonary function and aggressive, early immunosuppression augmentation (Theodore et al 1990) (Fig. 15.4).

Immunosuppression

Immunosuppressive therapy is necessary for the rest of the recipient's life. Most maintenance immunosuppressive regimens utilize a combination of two or three drugs. By combining a number of drugs the doses of each can be adjusted to reduce associated side effects (Table 15.4).

Infections

Infection continues to be a complicating and life-threatening feature of transplantation, especially

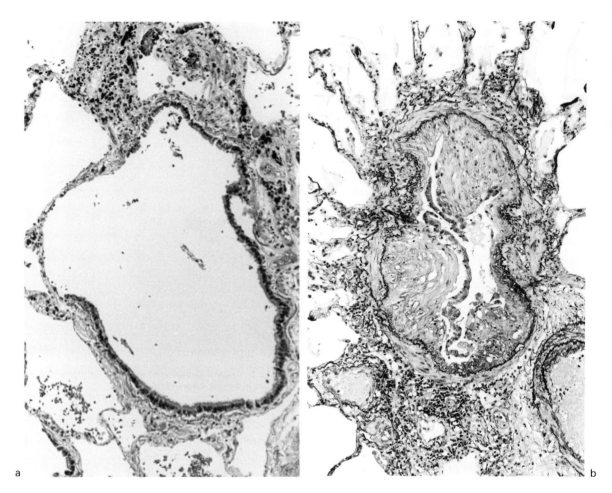

a

b

Fig. 15.4 **a** A normal bronchiole lined by ciliated, columnar epithelium deep to which there is a thin layer of smooth muscle. **b** Obliterative bronchiolitis: nodules of submucosal fibrous tissue have developed elevating the lining mucosa and substantially occluding the lumen.

in the first 3 months following the surgery. High dose immunosuppressive therapy allows for the growth of opportunistic organisms (Table 15.5).

Patients are usually discharged from the hospital to home (if within a 30 minute drive from the unit) or to the hospital accommodation between days 10 and 28 postoperatively. Patients continue to be closely monitored on an outpatient basis, usually for the first 3 months postoperatively. Regular follow up continues until most patients can be reviewed on a 6- to 12-monthly basis. All patients are well informed of the signs or symptoms with which they must contact their carer centre.

SPECIAL CONSIDERATIONS FOR THE PHYSIOTHERAPIST

The key to a successful cardiopulmonary transplant programme is a well informed, communicative, multidisciplinary team. With medical and nursing staff, social worker, pharmacist and dietitian the physiotherapist is vitally involved in the monitoring and education of the recipients, throughout each phase of the transplantation process. To do so effectively, the physiotherapist needs a strong knowledge base, particularly focused on the features of transplantation which will strongly influence the recipient's ability to

Table 15.4 Immunosuppression

Drug	Effect	Side-effects
Maintenance immunosuppression		
Cyclosporine	T-cell suppressor, lesser B-cell effect	Nephrotoxicity, hepatic dysfunction, hirsutism, tremor, hypertension, susceptibility to malignant neoplasms
Azathioprine	Decreases the body's ability to generate T-cells	Bone marrow suppression, hepatic dysfunction, nausea, anorexia
Corticosteroid (prednisolone)	Decreases antibody production and depresses the maturation of T-cells	Water retention, hypertension, gastrointestinal ulceration, altered glucose metabolism, mood changes, osteoporosis
Anti-rejection therapy		
Corticosteroid (methyl prednisolone)	Reverses acute rejection, as above	As above
Antithymocyte globulin	T-cell cytolytic (can be used in prevention)	Fever, rigors, neutropenia, 'serum' sickness
OKT3	For the management of cardiac rejection	Acute pulmonary oedema, fever, rigors, headache, tremor
	T-cell cytolytic	
	Blocks generation and function of T-cells	

Table 15.5 Common infections seen post-cardiopulmonary transplant

Infection	Common manifestation	Management
Bacterial (especially postoperative days 0–7)	Respiratory involvement; bronchial and/or lobar pneumonias	Specific antibiotic therapy
Viral		
Cytomegalovirus (primary or reactivation infection), especially subacute phase	Systemic, gastrointestinal inclusion/ulceration, pneumonitis (especially lung and heart–lung recipients)	Ganciclovir (intravenous, twice daily, 10–14 days; prophylaxis, intravenous, 3 times weekly for donor–recipient cytomegalovirus mismatch)
Herpes (simplex and zoster)	Usual manifestations	Acyclovir
Fungal		
Candida	Oral, oesophageal	Nystatin, Fluconazole, Amphotericin B
Aspergillus	Respiratory	Amphotericin B, Itraconazole
Protozoal		
Pneumocystis carinii	Respiratory	Bactrim (treatment and prophylaxis)
Toxoplasma gondi	Systemic	As above

participate in rehabilitation activities and later to resume employment and leisure activities.

Denervation of the heart/lungs

At rest. Most heart and heart–lung block recipients will have a higher than normal resting heart rate: they lack the inhibitory vagal influence.

The lungs of heart–lung and lung recipients are denervated distal to the tracheal/bronchial anastomosis. As a result, the recipient's ability to cough spontaneously in response to secretions accumulating distal to the anastomosis is impaired.

Exercise. Denervation of the heart, in particular, has significant implications for the exercising of heart and heart–lung recipients. In the normally innervated heart it is changes in heart rate, not stroke volume, which account for the increase in cardiac output in response to dynamic exercise. There is substantial evidence that the denervated heart also increases its cardiac output in response to exercise. It does so early in the activity by increasing its stroke volume (based on the Frank–Starling mechanism). The heart rate of the recipient rises more gradually than that of a normal individual following the commencement of exercise, does not reach a similar peak and slows more gradually once exercise is stopped. This pattern of heart rate response is primarily the result of changing levels of circulating catecholamines, which play an increasingly important role in increasing cardiac output, at high workloads.

It is important to note that, although the transplanted heart does demonstrate compensatory exercise responses, the peak intensity of exercise and the duration of activity may be lower than that of normal individuals. If these limitations are present, it has been suggested that it may be the result of: the donor heart having undergone an ischaemic period and reperfusion, myocyte necrosis as a result of acute rejection episodes, and/or undetected or chronic rejection which is characterized by diffuse coronary artery disease (Squires 1990, Horak 1990).

Denervation also prevents the transmission of pain from any ischaemic area of myocardium (Weber 1990). As a result patients should be advised against unsupervised exercise at high intensities for long periods. This is especially important if angiography indicates the presence of coronary artery disease.

Immunosuppression

It is important that physiotherapists working with transplant recipients are mindful of the effects of immunosuppressive drug therapy, particularly corticosteroids, on the musculoskeletal system. The overall exercise capability of many transplant recipients is limited by peripheral musculoskeletal factors (Kavanagh et al 1988). Drug related myopathy and prolonged periods of inactivity, pre- and postoperatively may be responsible for these limitations.

The contribution of corticosteroids to the process of osteoporosis must also be acknowledged particularly for those patients whose preoperative management, (at any stage) has involved the prolonged use of steroid therapy. Special care when exercising and immediate and thorough investigation of reports of pain (especially back and hip pain) are essential for these patients, especially postmenopausal women and those over 45 years of age.

When prescribing exercise and advising patients on resuming sporting activities, both physiotherapist and patient must be mindful of the inhibiting influence of steroid therapy on healing.

Infection/rejection

When a recipient is diagnosed as being in severe rejection (and provided that his cardiac rhythm and oxygen saturation are stable) his activity should be limited to walking at a slow, comfortable pace within the limits of the ward area. The rehabilitation programme is recommended when the anti-rejection therapy is being reduced and the patient is asymptomatic.

In instances of minimal and moderate rejection or infection, exercise is continued according to the patient's presentation and symptoms. For lung and heart–lung recipients it is of paramount importance to monitor oxygen saturation regularly at rest, and throughout any exercise activities, even when they report no symptoms, but a biopsy has indicated an acute rejection episode. Again, monitoring of the patient's heart rate, rhythm and blood pressure is of importance.

PHYSIOTHERAPY MANAGEMENT

Physiotherapy has always played an important part in cardiopulmonary transplantation. The number of centres carrying out these procedures has expanded over recent years and so has the role of the physiotherapist within these units. Physiotherapy is now an integral part of all stages of the patient's management: at assessment, preoperatively and at both the acute and rehabilitation phases of postoperative care.

Assessment

All patients referred for formal assessment are seen by the physiotherapist. The assessment of potential heart transplant recipients focuses on respiratory history and function, muscle bulk and strength, and previous and current activity levels. At this interview/assessment the physiotherapist may provide advice on dividing fatiguing activities of daily living (ADL) into more easily managed subtasks and outline a programme of gentle stretches and exercises to maintain mobility and strength.

All potential heart–lung and single lung transplant recipients accepted for formal assessment are seen by the physiotherapist who assesses the patient's:

- posture
- breathing pattern (at rest and while mobilizing)
- cervical and thoracic spine mobility
- chest wall mobility
- muscle range and strength (upper limb, trunk, quadriceps, etc.)
- activity/exercise tolerance (including oximetry during a 'self-care' activity and a 6 minute walking test).

The findings are then reviewed with those of other team members in considering if the patient is an appropriate candidate for transplantation.

Preoperative care

The goals in the preoperative period are to:

- establish a good rapport between patient and physiotherapist
- provide each potential recipient with a thorough understanding of his role in transplantation.
- improve and maintain the potential recipient's physical condition
- assist the patient to use his time constructively
- improve the potential recipient's (and support person/s) quality of life, while awaiting transplant.

All patients awaiting heart–lung and lung transplants are included in a conditioning-rehabilitation programme (CRP). Patients living within ready access to the hospital attend the gymnasium one to five times weekly and continue elements of the programme in a home routine. Patients who regularly attend other hospitals for ongoing out-patient treatment are supervised by their own physiotherapist in a modified form of the conditioning programme. Patients who live beyond the reach of regular hospital attendances are worked through a home conditioning programme and are managed and progressed through the work by correspondence with the transplant physiotherapist.

The CRP involves five treatment/training components: patient education, 'aerobic' training, specific muscle training, thoracic mobility techniques and relaxation and stress management techniques. Each of the five components specifically addresses one or more previously identified problems and involves a number of techniques (Table 15.6). The patient's heart rate and rhythm, blood pressure and oxygen saturation are checked before and during the gymnasium activities. Supplementary oxygen is used as appropriate.

The ongoing monitoring of all potential heart–lung and lung recipients is the responsibility of each member of the multidisciplinary team. These patients should be formally team reviewed at regular intervals, appropriate to the rate of their disease progression. If significant deterioration in the potential recipient's functional status and/or physical condition is noted, an intervention strategy involving one or a number of intensive therapies may be devised in an effort to optimize the patient's condition. In particular cases of increasing hypercapnic respiratory failure the application of continuous positive airway pressure (CPAP) or intermittent positive pressure ventilation through a nasal mask during sleep may provide intermittent ventilatory support, reducing inspiratory muscle expenditure and allowing effective participation in preoperative rehabilitation (Carrey et al 1990). Nasogastric or gastrostomy feeding may be of benefit in these instances.

The patients for heart only transplant are not routinely included in the CRP. Those potential recipients, like those accepted for active listing for heart–lung and lung transplantation are reviewed by the physiotherapist and preoperative management includes:

Table 15.6   A conditioning–rehabilitation programme for potential heart–lung and lung recipients

Problems(s) addressed	Management/techniques
Component 1: Patient education Poor quality of life while awaiting transplant	ADL advice Alternative strategies for recreational time Instruct family in massage and relaxation techniques
Fear of intubation/ventilation	Explanation of surgical and intensive care procedures Visit to intensive care unit Talk with (selected) recipients
Poor awareness of patterns of breathing	Review of chest anatomy, muscles of breathing, normal and abnormal breathing patterns Practice in 'isolating'/focusing on specific muscles and patterns of breathing
Component 2: 'Aerobic' training Poor endurance	Treadmill and bicycle ergometer programmes (intermittent work/rest periods) Home walking programme
Component 3: Specific muscle training Muscle weakness	Upper limb/trunk programme Abdominal programme Quadriceps programme Home weight programme
Component 4: Thoracic mobility techniques Preoperative musculoskeletal discomfort and postoperative pain	Soft tissue techniques Joint mobilization for cervical, thoracic, costal and sternal articulations
Component 5: Relaxation and stress management Preoperative respiratory crisis management and postoperative pain management	Relaxation techniques

- explanation of the surgical/intensive care procedures
- visit to the intensive care unit
- explanation/practice of commonly used postoperative physiotherapy techniques
- revision of advice on activities of daily living
- instruction for the support person(s) in general soft tissue massage techniques (for example effleurage, skin rolling and kneading) and the use of a relaxation technique/tape.

The patients are then given an outline of a home programme and are encouraged to practise:

- breathing control and thoracic expansion exercises
- cervical, thoracic and upper limb stretches
- upper limb weight work
- intermittent walking programme (if appropriate for their cardiopulmonary limitations).

Postoperative care

Acute care

The goals for the immediate postoperative period are to:

- assist in weaning patients from mechanical ventilation and in establishing energy cost-efficient patterns of breathing
- encourage and optimize secretion clearance
- establish and progress pre-rehabilitation activities as soon as is appropriate
- promote the patient's independence/self-reliance
- consolidate and extend the information/education component of the preoperative programme.

For the majority of patients, postoperative physiotherapy is started immediately (30 minutes to 1 hour) post-extubation, which is usually 6–12 hours following transfer to the intensive care unit from theatre. There are occasions, however, when it may be necessary for the physiotherapist to be involved before extubation. This may be to facilitate the removal of secretions. More often, the treatment involves techniques of breathing control when a patient, weaning from ventilatory support, is showing signs of distress without obvious fatigue. Well supported positioning, utilization of the stimulation and reassurance of hands-on instruction alternated with shoulder and cervical soft tissue techniques can bring about a change in respiratory pattern and rate, and positively affect arterial blood gases and the haemodynamic status. These tehniques are especially effective when the physiotherapist–patient relationship has been well established in the preoperative period. In some instances it is also appropriate to encourage the patient to utilize the relaxation method he chose and practised in the preoperative conditioning programme.

Initial treatments involve:

- the active cycle of breathing techniques:
  — breathing control
  — thoracic expansion exercises
  — the forced expiration technique
  — gravity assisted positions as appropriate
- assisted limb work, progressing to active, antigravity limb exercise over the first day and as required and appropriate.

The frequency and duration of treatments in the early postoperative days are dependent upon the patient's presentation, needs and progress. Experience suggests that frequent, brief treatments are most beneficial. Thorough and comprehensive monitoring and reassessment of the patient by every health professional involved in the acute care are of paramount importance both to the individual patient and the auditing of the programme as a whole.

It is essential that the physiotherapist assesses and reassesses the patient at each treatment, remembering the vulnerability of the immunosuppressed patient, both to infection and rejection. Subjective and objective assessment findings must be reviewed along with the latest microbiology results, arterial blood gases, chest radiograph, lung function measurements and oxygen saturation at rest and while mobilizing. Any changes, no matter how subtle should be noted and reassessed regularly. Effective communication between staff, particularly surgeon, physician, nursing staff and physiotherapist is essential for optimal patient care.

For heart–lung and lung recipients, gravity-assisted positions for middle/lingula and basal segments are incorporated into their daily treatment during the acute phase. As a result of denervation of the lungs (that is the absence of the recipient's ability to cough spontaneously in response to secretions accumulating distal to the anastomosis) it is essential that the physiotherapist evaluates (and educates the patient to do likewise) that the recipient's effective huff is dry sounding. If the huff is moist sounding, appropriate techniques should be employed to clear the bronchial secretions.

Patients may be sat out of bed (depending on their cardiovascular stability) as early as day 1 postoperatively. Patients usually start mobilizing from bed to chair on day 2 or 3.

Heart–lung and lung recipients (especially the very debilitated patients) may commence a light upper limb weight programme as early as day 3, depending on their wound pain and stability (using weights of 500–750 g).

Patients may be transferred to the ward as early as day 3 or 4 postoperatively. At this stage, patients are usually seen 3 or 4 times daily. Once free to mobilize from the bed area, patients are commenced on stair walking and gentle bicycle ergometer work. Usually on day 3 or 4, soft tissue (Chaitow 1988) and/or joint mobilization techniques (Maitland 1986) are commenced as indicated. These have proven particularly valuable with the single lung recipients whose primary pain after 3 or 4 days appears to be associated with the articulations and muscle groups which have been stressed during surgery.

Should a patient require prolonged ventilatory support or reintubation, his stretching, strengthening and mobilization work is started/continued as appropriate. It would appear that this work is of importance, in many cases, to making an early and lasting break from invasive ventilatory support. Nasal CPAP and/or ventilation may be utilized in the wearing of ventilatory support or in the prevention of reintubation.

Rehabilitation

The primary goals in the rehabilitation phase after transplantation are to:

- improve the patient's physical condition (posture, strength and endurance)
- improve the patient's (and support person(s)) confidence in becoming involved in a full range of activities of daily living and appropriate exercise activities
- nurture realistic expectations for employment, sport and leisure activities
- promote independence in maintaining and monitoring the physical condition.

When the patients are allowed to mobilize from the ward area, they are commenced on a gymnasium based rehabilitation programme. Each patient's programme is tailored to suit his current physical status and is orientated toward his specific goals for employment and recreational pursuits. Even the most debilitated patient is included in the gymnasium programme and his support person(s) are also encouraged to attend and become involved in supervising and encouraging exercise activities and in extending the patient's off-ward activities to include walking out-of-doors and eating 'out'.

In-patients attend the gymnasium 1 or 2 times daily. Out-patients are encouraged to attend the gymnasium 3–5 times weekly, depending upon their condition and distance from the hospital, for a period of 8–12 weeks.

Each patient's gymnasium programme is based on varying times and intensities of work in a number of activities. Activities are introduced gradually according to the patient's physical condition, wound/musculoskeletal discomfort and level of confidence. Table 15.7 outlines the activities/equipment used, their primary purpose(s) and the varying duration of activities that patients are progressed through.

In our experience, the most effective way to determine the appropriate intensity of an activity has been to exercise according to a scale of perceived exertion such as the Borg scale (Borg 1970, Pandolf 1983). Activities are introduced at an intensity such that the patient's subjective description of his level of exertion is 'very light' or 'light'. The intensity is subsequently progressed to levels of exertion described as 'somewhat hard' and 'hard'. The same scale of exertion that is used in this rehabilitation phase is also used in the preoperative conditioning programme and the patient's home-based, maintenance work so that by the time a patient is ready for discharge from the immediate supervision of the gymnasium environment, he is well practised in judging and progressing activity intensity and is encouraged to apply this scaling to his recreational activities and workplace tasks.

Thorough supervision/monitoring of recipients before and while participating in gymnasium activities is of the utmost importance, especially in the early weeks of rehabilitation, while patients are unfamiliar with 'reading' the symptoms often associated with infection/rejection episodes. Prior

Table 15.7   Gymnasium activities utilized in the post-transplant rehabilitation programme

Activity	Purpose	Time/repetitions
Treadmill	Warm up	12 min
Bicycle ergometer	Endurance/aerobic fitness	5–40 min
Multigym	Quadriceps strengthening	12–30 repetitions
Rowing machine	Quadriceps/upper limb/upper trunk strengthening	12–30 repetitions
Weights	Upper limb and shoulder girdle strengthening	1–10 kg, 10–30 repetitions
Minitrampoline	Glutei and lower limb strengthening	1–15 min
'Wobble' boards	Ankle/knee stability	1–5 min

to commencing their gym activities, patients are asked to comment on their ability to cope with activities of daily living and walking and how it compares with their performance in the previous days. Patients are checked for any change in weight, lung function tests (for heart–lung and lung recipients this includes twice daily self-monitoring of peak expiratory flow rate), blood pressure, heart rate and rhythm and resting oxygen saturation. Heart rate and blood pressure (and oxygen saturation for heart–lung and lung recipients) are monitored throughout the gymnasium session. Any uncharacteristic changes in the above parameters are noted as is any decline in a patient's ability to cope comfortably with an activity that previously has been well within his ability. Medical staff in the out-patients clinic are notified and the patient is reviewed and investigated accordingly.

Patient participation in and progression through a rehabilitation programme needs to be flexible and readily modified and 'back tracked' to accommodate the sometimes unpredictable nature of the postoperative course. There will be occasions when patients are unable to exercise:

- immediately following cardiac or transbronchial biopsy (or other 'minor' procedures/ investigations)
- when symptoms and/or a biopsy are indicative of a significant rejection or infection episode.

When exercise can be resumed, it will need to be at a lesser intensity than when the patient last participated in the activities and, as always, progressed considering his presenting condition. This is particularly important if the patient has just completed a course of intravenous steroid therapy and has noted symptoms of myopathy.

Patients who have had heart–lung or lung transplants should be made aware of their vulnerability to respiratory tract infections. The huff can be used as an assessment tool. If secretions are detected the active cycle of breathing techniques should be started and continued until the secretions have cleared.

At 3–6 weeks postoperatively, abdominal and lower back strengthening exercises are added to the work-out. These exercises and some upper limb weight work are outlined in each patient's maintenance programme, which is based on a four times weekly aerobic exercise of the patient's choice, whether it be walking, cycling, swimming or running or a combination of these. Specific stretching/strengthening programmes are also outlined for patients returning to physically demanding employment and sporting activities.

CONCLUSION

Physiotherapy is an integral part of the management of the cardiopulmonary transplant recipient. The role of the physiotherapist has expanded considerably in the last 5 years and the future looks equally exciting. There are also numerous research opportunities available to physiotherapists working with transplant programmes.

The greatest challenge facing cardiopulmonary transplant programmes is the limited number of donor organs available for the ever expanding potential recipient waiting list. An essential part of addressing this dilemma is for units to ensure that maximal effort is made to optimize the physical condition of potential and actual recipients, providing the best possible situation for a successful transplant outcome. Physiotherapy has much to offer these patients and it is essential that the physiotherapist is an active member of the cardiopulmonary transplant team.

Acknowledgements

I would like to acknowledge the assistance of Ms Fiona Brownscombe (Physiotherapist), Ms Maxine Peebles (Secretary) and Drs Peter Macdonald and Stephen Rainer.

REFERENCES

Barnard C 1968 Human cardiac transplantation, American Journal of Cardiology 22: 584–596

Borg G 1970 Perceived exertion as an indicator of somatic stress. Scandinavian Journal of Rehabilitation Medicine 2(3): 92–948

Carrey Z, Gottfried S, Levy R 1990 Ventilatory muscle support in respiratory failure with nasal positive pressure ventilation. Chest 97: 150–158

Chaitow L 1988 Soft-tissue manipulation: a practitioner's guide to the diagnosis and treatment of soft tissue dysfunction and reflex activity. Healing Arts Press, New York

Cooper J, Pearson F, Patterson G, Todd T, Glinsberg R, Goldberg M, DeMajo W 1987 Technique of successful lung transplantation in humans. Journal of Thoracic and Cardiovascular Surgery 93: 173–181

Horak A 1990 Physiology and pharmacology of the transplanted heart In: Cooper D, Novitzky D (eds) The transplantation and replacement of thoracic organs. Kluwer, Lancaster

Jamieson S, Stinson E, Oyer P, Baldwin J, Shumway N 1984 Operative technique for heart–lung transplantation. The Journal of Thoracic and Cardiovascular Surgery 87: 930–935

Kaiser L, Pasque M, Trulock E, Low D, Dresler C, Cooper J 1991 Bilateral sequential lung transplantation: the procedure of choice for double-lung replacement. Annals of Thoracic Surgery 52: 438–446

Kavanagh T, Yacoub M, Mertens D, Kennedy J, Campbeil R, Sawyer P 1988 Cardiorespiratory responses to exercise training after orthotopic cardiac transplantation. Circulation 77(1): 162–171

Keogh A, Baron D, Spratt P, Esmore D, Chang V 1986 Cardiac transplantation in Australia. Australian Family Physician 15(11): 1474–1481

Keogh A, Macdonald P, Chang V, Farnsworth A, Harvison A, Connell J, Jones B, Johnston R, Spratt P 1991 Seven years of heart transplantation in Australia— the St Vincent's Hospital experience. On the Pulse III (2): 2–7

Kriett J, Kaye M 1991 The registry of the International Society for Heart and Lung Transplantation: eighth official report, 1991. The Journal of Heart and Lung Transplantation 10(4): 491–498

Lawrence E 1990 Diagnosis and management of lung allograft rejection In: Grossman R, Maurer J (eds) Clinics in chest medicine. W B Saunders, Philadelphia, vol II(2), p 269–278

Madden B, Hodson M, Tsang V, Radley-Smith R, Khaghani A, Yacoub M 1992 Intermediate-term results of heart-lung transplantation for cystic fibrosis. Lancet 339: 1583–1587

Maitland G 1986 Vertebral manipulation. Butterworths, London

Pandolf K 1983 Advances in the study and application of perceived exersion. Exercise, Sports Science Review 11: 118–158

Patterson G, Cooper J, Goldman B, Weisel R, Pearson F, Water P, Todd T, Scully H, Goldberg M, Ginsberg R 1988 Technique of successful clinical double-lung transplantation. Annals of Thoracic Surgery 43: 626–633

Reitz B 1982 Heart and lung transplantation. Heart Transplantation 1(1): 80–81

Squires R 1990 Cardiac rehabilitation issues for heart transplantation patients. Journal of Cardiopulmonary Rehabilitation 10: 159–168

Theodore J, Starnes V, Lewiston N 1990 Obliterative bronchiolitis In: Grossman R, Maurer J (eds) Clinics in chest medicine. W B Saunders, Philadelphia, vol II(2), p 309–321

Weber B 1990 Cardiac surgery and heart transplantation In: Hudak C, Gallo B, Benz J (eds) Critical care nursing: a holistic approach, 5th edn. J B Lippincott, Philadelphia

FURTHER READING

Cooper D, Novitzky D (eds) 1990 The transplantation and replacement of thoracic organs. Kluwer, Lancaster

Grossman R, Maurer J (eds) 1990 Clinics in chest medicine: pulmonary considerations in transplantation. W B Saunders, Philadelphia, vol II(2)

Kavanagh T, Yacoub M, Mertens D, Campbell R, Sawyer P 1989 Exercise rehabilitation after heterotopic cardiac transplantation. Journal of Cardiopulmonary Rehabilitation 9: 303–310

Keteyian S, Ehrman J, Fedel F, Rhoads K 1990. Heart rate-perceived exertion relationship during exercise in orthotopic heart transplant patients. Journal of Cardiopulmonary Rehabilitation 10: 287–293

Squires R, Allison T, Miller , Gau G 1991 Cardiopulmonary exercise testing after unilateral lung transplantation: a case report. Journal of Cardiopulmonary Rehabilitation 11: 192–196

Vibekk P 1991 Chest mobilization and respiratory function In: Pryor J (ed) Respiratory care. Churchill Livingstone, Edinburgh

16. Spinal injuries

Trudy Ward

INTRODUCTION

The prognosis for the patient sustaining spinal cord injury has until this century remained poor. An unknown Egyptian physician of 2500 BC describing spinal cord injury in the Edwin Smith Papyrus wrote: 'An ailment not to be treated' (Grundy et al 1993). This view continued until the work of Guttman and others encouraged development of special centres throughout the world and saw the problems associated with spinal cord injury at last being addressed, although the mortality from tetraplegia until the 1960s remained at 35% (Grundy et al 1993). Improvements in management at the time of the accident, technological advances in diagnosis and management approaches have contributed to the continuing fall over recent years in mortality and morbidity rates (Hornstein & Ledsome 1986).

The respiratory care of patients with spinal cord injury is examined in this chapter; however, the total management of patients requires a holistic, multidisciplinary approach to ensure effective rehabilitation.

THE MECHANICS OF RESPIRATION

In order to appreciate the effect of spinal cord injury on respiratory function it is necessary first to understand the mechanics of normal respiration. Table 16.1 illustrates the main muscles of respiration and their level of innervation.

Inspiration in the normal subject occurs as a result of the creation of negative intrapleural pressure. This may be achieved by contraction of the diaphragm causing it to descend, or by action of the intercostal muscles at lower lung volumes

Table 16.1 The muscles of respiration

Respiratory muscle	Level of innervation	Respiratory action
Sternocleidomastoid	C1–3	Inspiration
Trapezius	C1–4	Inspiration
Diaphragm	C3–5	Inspiration
Scaleni	C4–8	Inspiration
Intercostals	T1–11	Expiration/inspiration
Abdominals	T2–L1	Expiration

causing an increase in the lateral and anteroposterior diameter of the thorax (Morgan et al 1986). The intercostal muscles also work to stabilize the rib cage against the tendency for paradoxical inward movement caused by contraction of the diaphragm. Further stability is provided by the sternocleidomastoid, scaleni and trapezius muscles which assist the elevation and fixation of the ribs during forced or maximal inspiration, and will probably also act with other muscles in normal quiet respiration to ensure efficient movement of the chest wall (De Troyer & Heilporn 1980).

Expiration is normally a passive process, active muscle contraction being used during more forceful activities such as coughing or sneezing. The abdominals form the major muscles of expiration and also have an important role in maintaining the position of the diaphragm so improving its efficiency. The intercostal muscles also have an expiratory function at higher lung volumes. Coughing and sneezing primarily rely for their powerful and explosive natures on the ability of respiratory muscles to generate sufficient inspiratory volumes, followed by the production of powerful expiration against controlled closure of the glottis (Braun et al 1984). The effectiveness of the cough depends on the linear velocity of the air in the airways. At high lung volumes, clearance will occur principally from the larger airways. At low volumes the effect is more marked in the smaller airways (Brownlee & Williams 1987).

THE EFFECT OF SPINAL CORD INJURY

Following spinal cord injury, the muscles innervated below the level of injury will become weakened or paralysed. The higher the level of injury, the greater the functional consequence on respiration. In addition, injury above T6 can cause disruption of the autonomic nervous system with loss of normal parasympathetic and sympathetic interaction, due to sympathetic paralysis.

Respiratory complications remain a major cause of death and morbidity for the patient with spinal cord injury, especially in the early and intermediate stages (Alvarez et al 1981). Those particularly at risk are:

• Tetraplegic patients
• Patients with thoracic or lumbar lesions with rib or sternal injuries
• Patients with pre-existing lung disease.

For the tetraplegic patient, the ability to produce effective inspiration and cough will be severely impaired. This will be most marked during the phase of spinal shock when muscles below the level of injury are flaccid and the rib cage at its most mobile. Contraction of the diaphragm will therefore result in a marked paradoxical breathing pattern with limited apical expansion. Some improvement may occur as spinal shock resolves and the muscles become hyper-reflexive or spastic (Mansel & Norman 1990). With time the tendons, ligaments and joints of the rib cage stiffen due to decreased active movement. This, together with spasticity, will provide some compensation for loss of intercostal activity in stabilizing the rib cage (De Troyer & Heilporn 1980, Estenne et al 1983).

Transection of the cord above C4 will cause paralysis of the diaphragm, intercostal and abdominal muscles leaving the patient with sternocleidomastoid and trapezius for respiration.

Unaided these are usually incapable of sustaining long-term ventilation, and for survival these patients will require mechanical assistance.

Patients with cervical lesions below C4 will have partial or total diaphragmatic action plus accessory muscles and can be ultimately independent of mechanical ventilation. Paralysis of the intercostal muscles will result in marked changes in the mechanical properties of the lungs as resultant paradoxical breathing (Fig. 16.1) will have a tendency to cause microatelectasis, and chest wall instability will add to the work of breathing. A relatively minor insult to the respiratory system could therefore lead to major respiratory problems (De Troyer & Heilporn 1980). Effective cough for these patients requires the addition of external compression to produce the necessary large positive intrathoracic pressures (Braun et al 1984) and this is discussed later.

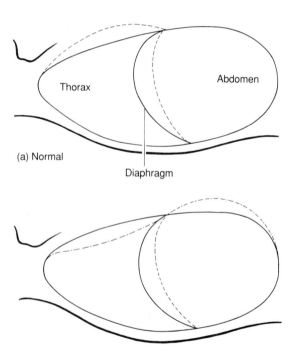

(a) Normal

(b) Paralysis below C5 showing paradoxical movement of the chest wall and abdomen

- - - - - Active movement
— · — Passive movement

Fig. 16.1 Movement of the diaphragm, chest wall and abdomen. **a** Normal. **b** Paralysis below C5.

Patients with thoracic lesions will have some preservation of intercostal function but paralysis of the abdominal muscles. The lower the level of lesion the more inspiratory ability will approach normal values, although paralysis of the abdominal muscles will result in a decrease in potential expiratory effort. Damage below L1 produces little effect on respiratory function.

THE EFFECT OF POSTURE

In the normal subject, mechanisms exist to ensure that adequate ventilation is maintained in all positions. In the supine position, contraction of the diaphragm displaces the abdominal contents without significantly expanding the rib cage, there being greater compliance of the abdomen than the rib cage. In standing, abdominal tone increases to support the abdominal contents, thereby decreasing abdominal wall compliance. Contraction of the diaphragm, intercostal and accessory muscles now cause greater rib cage expansion, resulting in an increase in vital capacity of about 5% (Chen et al 1990).

Positional changes will, however, affect the respiratory function of the tetraplegic patient. In supine, the weight of the abdominal contents force the diaphragm to a higher resting level so that contraction produces greater excursion of the diaphragm. In sitting or standing, the weight of the unsupported abdominal contents increases the demand on the diaphragm which now rests in a lower and flatter position (Alvarez et al 1981, Chen et al 1990), decreasing effectiveness and restricting available excursion for creating negative intrapleural pressure. Chen et al (1990) recorded a 14% drop in predicted vital capacity in the tetraplegic patient on changing position from supine to sitting or standing. It is therefore important with these patients not to assume that ventilation will be sufficient in all positions.

RESPIRATORY ASSESSMENT

Accurate assessment and regular review of the respiratory status of a patient is vital. Initial assessment must be carried out as soon as possible to establish a baseline against which future deterioration or improvement can be monitored.

Assessment procedure is discussed in Chapter 1. For complete assessment of the patient with spinal cord injury, the following details should be considered:

1. Motor and sensory neurological levels.
2. Associated injuries — rib fractures and flail segments are particularly likely in the patient with thoracic spinal injury and these may require modification of treatment techniques. Patients involved in diving accidents may present with the additional respiratory complications of water aspiration. The presence of intra-abdominal trauma or complications such as paralytic ileus, acute gastric dilatation or gastrointestinal bleeding will require modification to the techniques used by the physiotherapist, especially in assisted coughing.
3. Associated lung trauma — common injuries include pneumothorax, haemothorax and pulmonary contusion.
4. Pre-existing lung disease — problems such as asthma or chronic airflow limitation may exist and will be treated as indicated.
5. Presence of ventilatory support.
6. Psychological state — major psychological adjustment is required by the patient with spinal cord injury, not only to the injury itself, but also to the necessary treatment procedures. Sensory deprivation may cause loss of orientation, made worse by enforced immobilization and restricted visual input. Anxiety and interrupted sleep patterns caused by frequent turns and other procedures can result in increased patient confusion and fatigue. These factors will all affect respiratory function and must be considered by the physiotherapist to enable the most effective and appropriate planning of respiratory treatment.
7. Results of the chest radiograph and arterial blood gases, if available.
8. Altered levels of consciousness.
9. Respiratory rate at rest — with normal diaphragm activity the rate remains regular at 12–16 breaths/min. In the presence of a weak or fatiguing diaphragm the rate will increase (Alvarez et al 1981).
10. Assessment of breathing pattern to establish the degree of paradoxical movement or presence of unequal movement of the chest wall.

11. Assessment of diaphragm function, by inspection or palpation of the upper abdomen.

12. Assessment of cough to ascertain effectiveness.

13. Measurement of vital capacity — repeated measurement of vital capacity provides an indication of trends developing in respiratory function, and should be recorded in all the positions in which the patient may be nursed to detect postural variations (Morgan et al 1986). This will be especially pronounced in the presence of unilateral phrenic nerve damage. Values will vary depending on the level of injury. Ledsome & Sharp (1981) observed initial vital capacities of 30% of predicted normal value in C5/C6 patients, rising to 58% at 5 months. The high thoracic patient may be expected to have a vital capacity of around 80% of predicted normal (Bromley 1991). Vital capacity may fall over the first few days post-injury due to factors such as muscle or patient fatigue, respiratory complications, or cord oedema which results in a rise in neurological level. Improvement is usually seen as oedema resolves and respiratory function stabilizes (Ledsome & Sharp 1981, Axen et al 1985). Vital capacity values of 500 ml or less may, in conjunction with clinical assessment, indicate the need for ventilation (Gardner et al 1986).

14. Auscultation of the chest to detect areas of lung collapse, pleural effusion or secretions.

PHYSIOTHERAPY TECHNIQUES

Respiratory management of the patient with spinal cord injury requires the application of the same principles as other respiratory problems; the skills used are discussed in Chapters 7 and 8. The goals of treatment include:

- Clearance of secretions from the lungs
- Improvement in breath sounds
- Increase in lung volumes
- Strengthening of the available muscles of respiration
- Improvement of pulmonary and rib cage compliance
- Education of the patient and his carer.

Treatment may be prophylactic or directed to treat specific problems.

Prophylactic treatment

This will include breathing exercises, modified postural drainage by regular turning and assisted coughing. **Breathing exercises** to encourage maximal inspiration must be established at an early stage, although the absence of sensations below the level of injury may necessitate the use of overbed mirrors to supplement verbal and tactile feedback. Exercises are directed to improve lateral basal and apical chest wall expansion and diaphragmatic excursion, but care must be taken to avoid tiring the diaphragm. Patients with intercostal paralysis, however, are usually unable to perform localized breathing exercises.

Many articles have been written on the reduction of respiratory fatigue and increase in endurance achieved by **respiratory muscle training** (Cheshire & Flack 1978, Gross et al 1980, Hornstein & Ledsome 1986).

Gross et al (1980) used inspiratory muscle training in the form of variable resistance over a 16-week period and reported respiratory improvement in symptoms, endurance and inspiratory muscle strength. It was acknowledged, however, that continuous training would be necessary to maintain improvement, a statement supported by Ledsome & Sharp (1981).

Incentive spirometry enables respiratory training with immediate visual feedback to reinforce success. This can be particularly beneficial for the high tetraplegic patient for whom physical achievement is limited (Cheshire & Flack 1978). The use of incentive spirometry can be useful in involving relatives in respiratory rehabilitation at an early stage.

Intermittent positive pressure breathing (IPPB) can be used in conjunction with other methods of training, although work by Rose et al (1987) concluded that solely increasing lung volumes had no major effect on lung function in stable tetraplegics. IPPB may be useful in increasing inspiratory volume to aid the clearance of secretions in patients with sputum retention and lung collapse, or in enhancing the administration of nebulized drugs in cases of ineffective inspiratory ability.

Glossopharyngeal breathing is another technique that can be used to increase lung volumes and assist secretion clearance (p. 127) in the high tetraplegic. Vital capacity may be increased by as much as 1000 ml (Alvarez et al 1981).

Assisted coughing

Assisted coughing is a vital inclusion in any respiratory programme. Patients may be able to clear sputum from small to large airways, but will need assistance to produce an effective cough for expectoration. Assistance is provided by the application of a compressive force directed in an inwards and upwards direction against the thorax to create a push against the diaphragm, thus replacing the work of the abdominal muscles. Pressure on the abdominal wall alone must be avoided. The sound of the resultant cough is the best indicator of the force required, but care must be taken to avoid movement of any fracture. Pressure directed down through the abdomen must be avoided, especially in the acute patient, due to the possibility of associated abdominal injury, or paralytic ileus.

Various methods of achieving assisted cough are described in the literature (Braun et al 1984, Brownlee & Williams 1987, Bromley 1991), Braun et al (1984) recording a 15% increase in peak expiratory flow using lower thoracic compression. The methods which may be used in the supine patient are illustrated in Figure 16.2.

a If one person is assisting the cough, hands should be placed so that one rests on the near side of the thorax and the other on the opposite side of the thorax, with the forearm resting across the lower ribs. As the patient attempts to cough the physiotherapist pushes inwards and upwards with her forearm and stabilizes the thorax with her hands.

b Alternatively, the hands are positioned bilaterally over the lower thorax and with elbows extended the physiotherapist pushes inwards and upwards evenly through both arms.

c, d In the case of the patient with a large thorax or having particularly tenacious sputum, two people may be required to produce an effective cough.

Care must be taken to avoid movement at the fracture site, and to synchronize the applied compressive force with the expiratory effort of the patient. Once the cough is completed, pressure must be lifted momentarily from the lower ribs, thus enabling the patient to use his diaphragm to initiate the next breath. If there is concern over fracture site stability or the amount of force needed for effectiveness, another person should be used to stabilize the patient by supporting his shoulders on the bed. In the presence of paralytic ileus or internal injury, extreme care must be taken during assisted coughing to avoid the application of pressure over the abdomen. Patients should be encouraged to cough 3–4 times per day, with nursing staff involvement in this process. If possible, patients will be taught self-assisted coughing when in a wheelchair, and relatives will learn how to assist the patient to cough in both lying and sitting.

Abdominal binders have been used on patients with high spinal cord injury for many years, both to minimize the effect of postural hypotension and aid respiration (Goldman et al 1986). Their effect is achieved by providing support to the abdominal contents, decreasing the compliance of the abdominal wall and thereby allowing the diaphragm to assume a more normal resting position in the upright posture (Alvarez et al 1981). Goldman et al (1986) investigated the effect of abdominal binders on breathing in tetraplegic patients, and concluded that in the supine position there was no change, but when sitting there was a trend for improvement in lung volumes. This may help the patient considerably during the early stages of mobilization.

Treatment of the non-ventilated patient with respiratory problems

In the presence of respiratory problems such as retained secretions or lung collapse, sputum clearance is of paramount importance and vigorous, aggressive treatment is often needed. Physiotherapy treatment plans will be determined by ongoing assessment. Unless contraindicated by other complications, postural drainage either with an electric turning bed or manual turn into supported side lying should be used as appropriate. Great care must be taken to maintain spinal alignment and cervical traction throughout

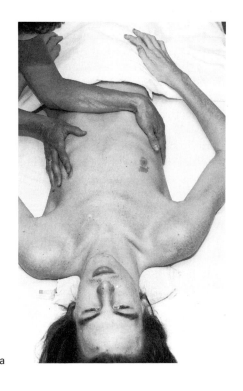

a

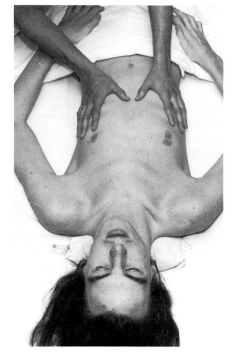

b

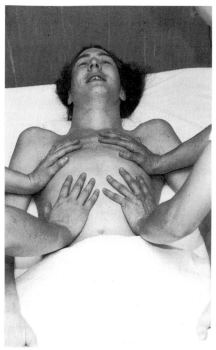

c

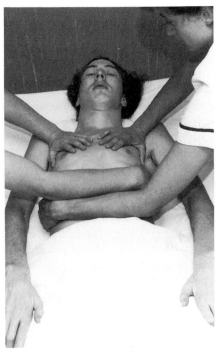

d

Fig. 16.2   Assisted coughing (see text).

treatment. The effect of positioning on lung venti-lation and perfusion must be considered (Ch. 7). Patients should never be left unsupervised during postural drainage in case of sudden sputum mobilization which could cause the patient to choke unless cleared by assisted coughing. Treatment may consist of vibration, shaking and chest clapping as necessary, followed by assisted coughing. 'Little and often' is the general rule as patients will tire quickly, but treatment must be effective, using two physiotherapists if necessary. Where possible, treatment should link in with planned turn times to allow some rest between various procedures.

Nasopharyngeal suction may be used if clear-ance by assisted cough alone is insufficient, but great care must be taken as pharyngeal suction can cause stimulation of the parasympathetic nervous system via the vagus nerve, resulting in bradycardia and even cardiac arrest. Hyper-oxygenation of the patient with 100% oxygen prior to treatment will help minimize this possi-bility (Wicks & Menter 1986), but atropine or an equivalent drug should be available for adminis-tration intravenously should profound brady-cardia occur.

Occasionally, bronchoscopy using a fibreoptic bronchoscope may be necessary to treat cases of unresolving lung or lobar collapse.

Care of the ventilator dependent patient

Mechanical ventilation of the patient with spinal cord injury may be considered in the following circumstances:

1. Injury to the upper cervical spine C1–C3, resulting in paralysis of the diaphragm.
2. Deterioration in respiratory function as a result of oedema or bleeding within the spinal canal causing the neurological level to rise so affecting the diaphragm. Patients are most at risk during the first 72 hours.
3. Respiratory muscle fatigue. Tracheostomy alone may be sufficient as this will reduce the dead space by up to 50% (Bromley 1991).
4. Associated chest or head injuries which require management by elective ventilation.

Insertion of a minitracheostomy may be consid-ered for patients with problems purely of retained secretions (Gupta et al 1989).

Physiotherapy goals for treatment for the venti-lated patient are the same as those for the non-ventilated patient (p. 360). Treatment will include modified postural drainage, vibration and shaking with manual hyperinflation followed by suction to remove secretions. Frequency of treat-ment will be determined by assessment of the respiratory condition, but should not exceed 15–20 minutes. Patients requiring ventilation due to complications from spinal cord injury are often not sedated and a system of communica-tion must be established before physiotherapy is started.

Ventilatory weaning considerations

A significant number of patients can be weaned from mechanical ventilation. In a study by Wicks & Menter (1986) factors which affected the predicted outcome of weaning included:

- Level of neurological injury
- Age less than 50 years
- Vital capacity improvement to 1000 ml.

There are other associated injuries and complica-tions which may affect the results.

Weaning from the ventilator should start as soon as the patient's condition permits and is best performed with the patient supine, allowing the most effective diaphragm function (Mansel & Norman 1990). Weaning must take into account the possibility that the patient's respiratory muscles will have atrophied if ventilation has been prolonged. The goal must therefore be to achieve spontaneous breathing for short periods several times a day to avoid fatigue. Gardner et al (1986) suggested that spontaneous respiratory effort until the patient is tired may result in diaphragmatic fatigue, which may take about 24 hours to recover.

Additional mechanical support may aid the patient during the weaning period, emphasis being placed on psychological support and encouragement during this phase.

For the patient on long-term ventilation, a battery-driven ventilator may be attached to the wheelchair to enable mobility (Fig. 16.3). Home

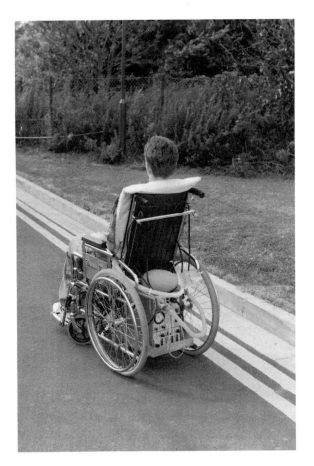

Fig. 16.3   Ventilated patient in a wheelchair.

ventilation may also be a considered option, although planning, education and support must be provided for all involved to achieve successful integration of the patient and his family back into the community.

The ethical dilemmas surrounding the ventilation of the high tetraplegic patient have challenged, and will continue to challenge, medical practice (Gardner et al 1985, Purtilo 1986, Maynard & Muth 1987, Gupta et al 1989). Only the ventilated tetraplegic knows what it is like to be a ventilated tetraplegic, and only his carer knows what it is like to care for him. In one review (Gupta et al 1989) of 21 patients who had required artificial ventilation, 18 stated that they would prefer a further period of continuous ventilation to being allowed to die. Sixteen of the 21 nearest caring relatives indicated that they were glad that their relative had been kept alive by ventilation. The study concluded that patients with spinal cord injury should be ventilated, provided that total emotional, educational and physical support could be given and maintained to all involved. This would seem to be most important.

In a case study, Maynard & Muth (1987) reveal how one individual's request to cease life-supporting ventilation was met. They suggest that 'if rehabilitation is defined as achieving optimal quality of life for people with severe disability then quality must be defined by the disabled individual'. An individual's perception as to what constitutes acceptable quality of life will change over time (Purtilo 1986) and this poses the question of the feasibility of the involvement of the newly injured patient and relatives in the decision regarding ventilation, unable as they are to appreciate the global implications of tetraplegia. However, the patient and his family must be kept fully informed and their views taken into account before any decisions are made (Gardner et al 1985).

Increasingly, the use of resources is questioned. Effective use of resources implies that the best value is obtained, but how should this be assessed and by whom? To withhold treatment from the tetraplegic patient requiring ventilation poses the ethical dilemma of excluding treatment known to be of benefit in sustaining life, but who should assess the cost to the patient? The ethical issues surrounding the high tetraplegic will continue to be debated but, ultimately, whatever is decided to be appropriate for an individual patient, psychological and physical support must be given to all involved (Gardner et al 1985).

Diaphragmatic pacing*.* Phrenic nerve pacing may sometimes be used on selected patients to free them from ventilatory dependence (Miller et al 1990). A paralysed diaphragm can be electronically stimulated if the phrenic nerve is intact and the cell bodies of C3, C4, C5 at the spinal cord viable. Electrodes may be placed to stimulate the phrenic nerve either in the neck or thorax, and are connected to a receiver embedded in the skin of the anterior chest wall. Stimulation is achieved by means of a radio transmitter placed over the receiver. Extensive postoperative training is necessary to increase diaphragmatic endurance, and teach the patient, his family and carers the necessary skills and understanding of the device.

For some patients, phrenic nerve pacing will provide an alternative to the ventilator, although this will remain as an emergency back up. For others, pacing provides selective periods of freedom from mechanical ventilation enabling easier wheelchair mobility and improved psychological status.

CONCLUSION

Greater understanding of the problems of the spinal cord injured patient has led to continuing improvements in morbidity and mortality rates. Respiratory complications can now be managed more effectively as understanding of the problems facing these patients improves. Physiotherapists have, and will continue to have, much to offer in the respiratory care of the patient with spinal cord injury.

REFERENCES

Alvarez S, Peterson M, Lunsford B 1981 Respiratory treatment of the adult patient with spinal cord injury. Physical Therapy 61 (12): 1737–1745

Axen K, Pineda H, Shunfenthal I, Haas F 1985 Diaphragmatic function following cervical cord injury: Neurally mediated improvement. Archive of Physical Medicine and Rehabilitation 66 (April): 219–222

Braun S, Giovannoni R, O'Connor M 1984 Improving the cough in patients with spinal cord injury. American Journal of Physical Medicine 63 (1): 1–10

Bromley I 1991 Tetraplegia and paraplegia. A guide for physiotherapists, 4th edn. Churchill Livingstone, Edinburgh

Brownlee S, Williams S 1987 Physiotherapy in the respiratory care of patients with high spinal injury. Physiotherapy 73 (3): 148–152

Chen C, Lien I, Wu M 1990 Respiratory function in patients with spinal cord injuries: effects of posture. Paraplegia 28: 81–86

Cheshire D, Flack W 1978 The use of operant conditioning techniques in the respiratory rehabilitation of the tetraplegic. Paraplegia 16: 162–174

De Troyer A, Heilporn A 1980 Respiratory mechanics in quadriplegia. The respiratory function of the intercostal muscles. American Review of Respiratory Disease 122: 591–600

Estenne M, Heilporn A, Delhez L, Yernault J-C, De Troyer A 1983 Chest wall stiffness in patients with chronic respiratory muscle weakness. American Review of Respiratory Disease 128: 1002–1007

Gardner B, Theocleous F, Watt J, Krishnan K 1985 Ventilation or dignified death for patients with high tetraplegia. British Medical Journal 291: 1620–1622

Gardner B, Watt J, Krishnan K 1986 The artificial ventilation of acute spinal cord damaged patients: a retrospective study of forty-four patients. Paraplegia 24: 208–220

Goldman J, Rose L, Williams S, Silver J, Denison D (1986) Effect of abdominal binders on breathing in tetraplegic patients. Thorax 41: 940–945

Gross D, Ladd H, Riley E, Macklem P, Grassino A 1980 The effect of training on strength and endurance of the diaphragm in quadriplegia. American Journal of Medicine 68: 27–35

Grundy D, Swain A 1993 ABC of spinal cord injury, 2nd edn. British Medical Journal, London

Gupta A, McClelland M, Evans A, El Masri W 1989 Minitracheostomy in the early respiratory management of patients with spinal cord injury. Paraplegia 27: 269–277

Hornstein S, Ledsome J 1986 Ventilatory muscle training in acute quadriplegia. Physiotherapy Canada 38(3): 145–149

Ledsome J, Sharp J 1981 Pulmonary function in acute cervical cord injury. American Review of Respiratory Disease 124: 41–44

Mansel J, Norman J 1990 Respiratory complications and management of spinal cord injuries. Chest 97(6): 1446–1452

Maynard F, Muth A 1987 The choice to end life as a ventilator dependent quadriplegia. Archives of Physical and Medical Rehabilitation 68: 862–864

Miller J, Farmer J, Stuart W, Apple D 1990 Phrenic nerve pacing of the quadriplegic patient. Journal of Thoracic and Cardiovascular Surgery 99: 35

Morgan M, Silver J, Williams S 1986 The respiratory system of the spinal cord patient. In: Bloch R, Bashaum M (eds) Management of spinal cord injuries. Williams and Wilkins, Baltimore

Purtilo R 1986 Ethical issues in the treatment of chronic ventilator dependent patients. Archives of Physical and Medical Rehabilitation 67: 718–721

Rose L, Geary M, Jackson J, Morgan M 1987 The effect of lung volume expansion in tetraplegia. Physiotherapy Practice 3: 163–167

Wicks A, Menter R 1986 Long-term outlook in quadriplegic patients with initial ventilator dependency. Chest 3: 406–410

17. Care of the dying patient

B. Wendy Burford   Stephen J. Barton

INTRODUCTION

Palliative care is the essence of care for many people with respiratory conditions because so many of these diseases are disabling and incurable. It is to be emphasized that it is the disease itself which is terminal and not the patient; because the disease is in the terminal phase this does not mean the withdrawal of appropriate treatment. To maintain contact with the patient, by a short visit, when it is no longer appropriate to continue active interventions is important to the patient, carer and physiotherapist.

Throughout the disease process it is important to maintain a holistic approach, the physical symptoms are often glaringly obvious but other components are often forgotten by the professionals. Good symptom control takes into account the physical, social, psychological and spiritual aspects affecting both the patient and those caring for them (Fig. 17.1).

PSYCHOLOGICAL FACTORS

The psychological factors of the disease process reverberate around the patient, relatives and the staff involved. For both the patient and the carer

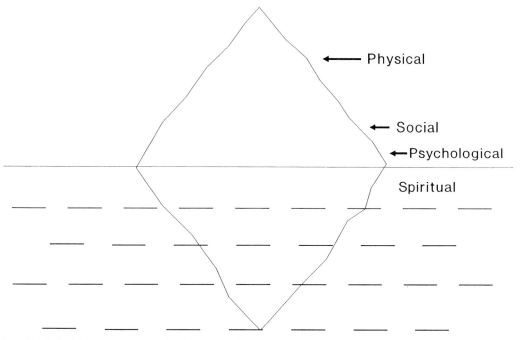

Physical

Social

Psychological

Spiritual

Fig. 17.1 'An iceberg' demonstrates how health care professionals perceive the physical, social, psychological and spiritual needs of patients.

the grieving process begins with the diagnosis of a life threatening condition. The patient anticipates lack of function and the thought of leaving the family, 'How will they cope without me?'. The family tree (Fig. 17.2) can be used to show who is important to the patient and if they have faced a significant loss before.

It is important to recognize that an understanding of the psychological aspects of dying is as important as the understanding of the physiological changes that are occurring within the dying patient.

When a patient and the family have been given the diagnosis of a terminal illness, and learn that the emphasis of treatment will now be aimed at palliative care and the effective control of symptoms, to allow for quality of life instead of a cure, the grieving process begins.

Effective care of the dying patient lies in the approach of the different members of the health care team's ability to understand the problems faced by each individual patient and family, and then to initiate the appropriate actions.

The stages of the grieving process described below can occur at any time and in any order (Fig. 17.3).

Denial

After the initial shock that the patient has a

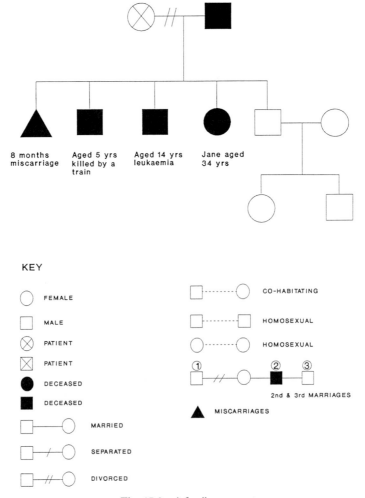

8 months miscarriage   Aged 5 yrs killed by a train   Aged 14 yrs leukaemia   Jane aged 34 yrs

KEY

○ FEMALE

□ MALE

⊗ PATIENT

⊠ PATIENT

● DECEASED

■ DECEASED

□—○ MARRIED

□—/—○ SEPARATED

□—//—○ DIVORCED

□------○ CO-HABITATING

□------□ HOMOSEXUAL

○------○ HOMOSEXUAL

① □—//—○—② ■—③ □
2nd & 3rd MARRIAGES

▲ MISCARRIAGES

Fig. 17.2 A family tree.

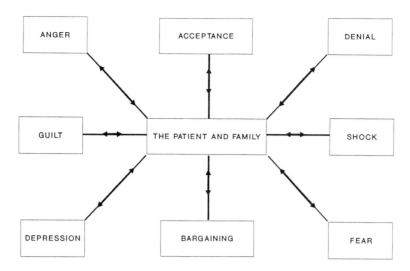

Fig. 17.3   The psychological components of terminal care.

terminal illness, the denial phase begins. 'There must be some mistake', 'They don't really mean me', or 'They must have someone else's results'. This behaviour continues in the hope that if it is denied long enough it will eventually go away, or the result will change.

It is a coping mechanism that we all use at some time during our life to protect ourselves from something unpleasant. It is even harder to accept the news of a terminal disease if one has a sense of well being and one's physical condition is not yet compromised by symptoms. For example, some newly diagnosed lung cancer patients present to their general practitioners with a cough that is not resolving or responding to conventional antibiotic therapy. The chest radiograph shows a mass, and subsequent fibreoptic bronchoscopy confirms that there is a tumour present. Cytology confirms small cell (oat cell) lung cancer. It is even harder for patients to accept that without treatment their life expectancy is approximately 3 months and with treatment probably between 12 and 18 months, especially if they are still able to lead a near normal lifestyle.

Shock

No matter how much preparation is given before confirmation of bad news, it can still surprise and shock when given. The two most common

reactions seen in hospital are the hysterical and inconsolable, or the numbing and emotionless response. Of these two responses the hysterical reaction is often the easier to deal with, once the patient and family are through the initial stage. Working with them it is possible to build up a relationship of mutual trust and respect and to help them come to terms with the future and what it may hold.

With the latter of the two responses, it may be impossible to help the patient until they have let down the barriers that they are using to protect themselves. It will inevitably be a long process trying to win the patient's and relatives' confidence and so helping them face up to the future.

Anger

Anger may be felt by many people during the terminal phases of a person's life, varying from the patient to the immediate members of the family. Their reactions will be as diverse as their reasons for trying to understand what is happening.

The patient or relatives may initially become angry with the doctor or nurse when informed of the diagnosis, and although this anger is directed at them it should not be taken personally. It is usually an automatic response when given information that one cannot cope with. It may also be a reflection on the person's coping ability that they have to retaliate when faced with a situation that is alien to them. Often patients become angry and frustrated as the illness progresses, due to a loss of their physical ability and independence, becoming more dependent on the carer either in the home or in hospital. It is therefore very important that both the patient and carer should be involved in all decisions made with regard to medical and nursing management and so help to retain autonomy of care.

The family may become angry and highly critical of the treatment and care being offered to their loved one. This anger may be as a result of their own feelings of guilt and inadequacy and inability to cope with the fact that their partner is actually going to die and leave them alone, and it is this fear that is presenting itself as anger.

Many parents when faced with the death of one of their children will initially respond with anger — anger at God for allowing this to happen, anger at the medical profession for not doing enough to help, and anger at each other for allowing this to happen by not caring enough.

Guilt

Guilt is an emotion common to all involved in the life of a terminally ill patient. The patients themselves may feel a sense of guilt for becoming a burden on their family. The burden may be physical because they are no longer able to look after themselves, or it may be financial, especially if they are the main bread winner of the family. They may have feelings of guilt that they will eventually be leaving their partner to cope alone after they have gone.

The carers will often feel guilty if they are unable to cope with the patient in the community, and hospital admission is required. They often see this as letting their loved one down. There may also be feelings of guilt on the part of the family that they are being left behind and will have to cope.

Depression

Depression is the emotion that everyone expects to see at some time in someone faced with the prospect of dying. Depression can present in different forms and has many components that need to be considered. These vary from feelings of melancholia and somatic complaints to feelings of deep despair and suicidal tendencies.

The more common symptoms are changes in behaviour, with the person becoming withdrawn, having reduced concentration, loss of interest and increased irritability, for example laughter and the noise of children are no longer welcomed with a tolerant smile but arouse irritation and frustration. There may be changes in the sleep pattern which consist of early morning waking rather than difficulty in getting off to sleep. This can lead to insomnia which is highly resistant to hypnotics and, although the answer is in treatment of the underlying depression, the patient and the family cannot see this and often demand more powerful drugs.

Changes in appetite are commonly associated with depression and in mild cases compulsive eating may be witnessed with the patient helping himself to 'tit-bits from the biscuit tin'. Generally appetite is diminished and weight loss is more common, and in severe cases it can be dramatic.

Somatic complaints are multiple and range from the common tension symptoms, such as pain in the head, back and neck. The tension can manifest itself locally or can be very generalized.

Fear

Fear is a natural component of terminal care, and the uncertainty that people face. It may only be a temporary feeling or it can remain with the patient and family until the end. Usually this feeling can be overcome by a little thought on the part of the doctor and the nurse. Quite often a simple explanation of any procedures that are about to be performed will suffice to help and reassure the patient and carer. Honest and realistic answers to any of their questions will help reassure the patient and reinforce what is happening and what to expect.

Bargaining

Bargaining is a mental process that many people will experience when faced with a terminal disease. For example, the patient with lung cancer who promises to give up smoking if it will buy more time, or the frequent saying 'If only the doctor had done something earlier'. This process is often associated with feelings of guilt and will be faced by both the patient and the family.

Acceptance

Acceptance is the final stage of the grieving or bereavement process, it is the coming to terms with, the resolution of one's emotions or the resolving of conflicts. It is only when this phase is reached that patients can be at peace with themselves, accepting and preparing for death, a death with dignity. To allow for this to happen, all components have to be equal and when this equilibrium between physical symptoms and psychological state is balanced, then a peaceful death can follow.

PHYSICAL FACTORS

Respiratory conditions which physiotherapists may see in the terminal care stage include lung cancer, cystic fibrosis, emphysema and cryptogenic fibrosing alveolitis. The period between the time of diagnosis of a terminal condition and the stage of terminal care varies from years to several weeks. Most patients with cystic fibrosis will have lived with the knowledge that their life expectancy is limited, but for patients with lung cancer the diagnosis will probably be a shock to them and to their families.

There are different types of lung cancer and these include squamous cell carcinoma, adenocarcinoma, large cell and small cell carcinoma. Half of the lung cancers arise peripherally, but the others are situated more centrally, proximal to a segmental bronchus and are less often resectable. The cell type will be identified by histological or cytological investigation and will influence the treatment the patient will receive. Of all cases presenting, only about 25% are suitable for surgery. The majority of patients who develop lung cancer have a relatively poor prognosis (Mountain 1986).

Psychologically, patients who are found to have an inoperable tumour may find it difficult to accept that no 'active' treatment is offered whilst they remain asymptomatic. Radiotherapy in the treatment of lung cancer is primarily palliative but is reserved for the control of symptoms, that is haemoptysis, bone pain or nerve pain, superior vena caval obstruction, breathlessness (intraluminal radiotherapy), dysphagia, cough, spinal cord compression, lymphangitis and cerebral metastases.

With small cell (oat cell) carcinoma there is usually evidence of disease elsewhere in the body at the time of diagnosis which therefore excludes surgery. The overall prognosis is very poor but the tumour does respond for a time to chemotherapy and/or radiotherapy.

Symptom control in lung cancer

Pain

Pain is the symptom most feared both by the patient and carer and once a diagnosis of cancer is made physical pain is the symptom which they all anticipate, although one-third of patients with cancer do not experience any physical pain (Twycross & Lack 1990).

Pain is influenced by our physical, social, psychological and spiritual attitudes. Pain is whatever the patient says it is. It is individual and is affected by the patient's previous experience of pain, and there are racial and cultural differences. Patients often fear the process of dying rather than death itself and it is important to emphasize that measures can be taken to control physical pain in the majority of patients.

Analgesics should be given on a regular basis, there is no place for 'as required' analgesia in the situation of chronic pain. The aim is to ensure that the patient is pain free and this can only be achieved by the regular administration of drugs, often in combination. Pain should be assessed regularly and adjustments made to the analgesia.

It is important to gain the patient's trust and confidence and to restore their sense of worth, well being and self esteem, thereby enabling them to feel more relaxed. Some patients find this by utilizing complementary therapies, for example aromatherapy, reflexology, gentle massage and relaxation techniques (possibly including a relaxation tape). Time spent with the patient allaying their fears will often enable a reduction in the amount of analgesia required.

Bone pain. This is usually the result of metastatic deposits (this may present as a pathological fracture and may require surgery). Radiotherapy as a single treatment is often very beneficial for bone pain. A non-steroidal anti-inflammatory agent combined with an opiate drug may control the pain.

Nerve pain. This is caused by the invasion or destruction of nerve fibres, for example superior sulcus tumours (Pancoast tumour). These tumours grow in the apex of the lung and invade the brachial plexus. Mesotheliomas are tumours usually occurring in patients who have had exposure to asbestos. They grow in the pleura and cause intractable chest wall nerve pain.

Nerve pain can be difficult to control and is often opiate resistant. Drugs which may be helpful are tricyclic agents, anticonvulsants, corticosteroids and local anaesthetic congener drugs such as Flecainide. Nerve blocks may be attempted and transcutaneous electrical nerve stimulation may bring some relief to this type of pain.

Liver pain. This is caused by metastases invading the liver capsule. This pain responds to corticosteroids.

Headaches. These may be caused by raised intracranial pressure from cerebral metastases. Corticosteroids and cranial irradiation will relieve this symptom.

Muscle spasm. This may be experienced following convulsions if the patient has cerebral metastases. Muscle relaxants may be administered.

Drugs for the control of chronic pain must be given regularly (Fig. 17.4):

- Mild analgesics—paracetamol, aspirin
- Moderate analgesics—codeine phosphate, dihydrocodeine (DF 118), co-proxamol
- Strong analgesics—morphine, diamorphine, methadone.

There is no minimum or maximum amount of opiate which can be given. Co-analgesics frequently have to be used. The advent of the syringe driver, which delivers a controlled regular amount of drug, has made it possible for many patients with terminal illness to be nursed at home until their death.

Nausea

Nausea may be a side effect of chemotherapy or a result of the administration of opiates. It may also

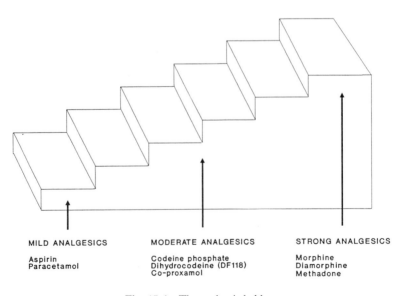

MILD ANALGESICS

Aspirin
Paracetamol

MODERATE ANALGESICS

Codeine phosphate
Dihydrocodeine (DF118)
Co-proxamol

STRONG ANALGESICS

Morphine
Diamorphine
Methadone

Fig. 17.4 The analgesic ladder.

be caused by severe constipation, electrolyte imbalance, or a raised intracranial pressure. Some patients obtain relief of nausea from antiemetic drugs and steroids. Dexamethasone may help to reduce a raised intracranial pressure. (Cold fizzy drinks eg. ginger ale may be tolerated by the nauseated patient.)

Breathlessness

Positioning the patient plays a very important part and the high side lying position can be of great assistance to the breathless patient (Fig. 8.2, p. 114). Many patients prefer sitting upright in an armchair and may wish to sleep in the armchair at night. Some find resting on a pillow across a small table helpful (Fig. 8.6, p. 117).

Oxygen therapy is usually of no value except psychologically for the patient with terminal malignant disease and sets up yet another physical barrier between the patient's family/carer.

Occasionally when a tumour is causing tracheal obstruction heliox, a mixture of helium (79%) and oxygen (21%), is sometimes used to relieve respiratory distress (p. 156).

Opiate drugs can be helpful in the relief of breathlessness and may be administered either orally or by subcutaneous infusion. An anxiolytic may be of use, for example Valium. Nebulized morphine has been shown to relieve breathlessness in some patients with severe chronic lung disease (Young et al 1989).

Superior vena caval obstruction

Superior vena caval obstruction is caused by the spread of a tumour into the mediastinum or by enlarged lymph nodes. Pressure on the superior vena cava leads to oedema in the face, neck and arms. The patient may complain of difficulty breathing, headaches and feeling faint when he bends down. Stridor may be present.

Urgent treatment is necessary and radiotherapy is probably the most effective except for patients with small cell carcinoma who usually respond to chemotherapy. Opiate and corticosteroid drugs may alleviate breathlessness. The head of the bed may be raised in an attempt to reduce the facial oedema during the night.

Death rattle

This noise is produced by the movement of secretions in the hypopharynx in association with the inspiratory and expiratory phases of respiration. This is heard in patients who are too weak to expectorate. Repositioning the patient is often effective in reducing the sound for both patient and family. Oropharyngeal suction is unpleasant for the patient, particularly if conscious, and is usually ineffective. Hyoscine may be given by subcutaneous injection. If the patient is unconscious and the syringe driver is being used, the administration of hyoscine subcutaneously is the treatment of choice and can be combined with diamorphine.

Physiotherapy

The physiotherapist may have been involved with the patient throughout his illness and there will be a stage when most physical treatment techniques are inappropriate, but it is important that the physiotherapist maintains contact with the patient and his family during the terminal stages. Positioning the patient for comfort and relief of breathlessness, and assisting the patient to clear a plug of sputum may be beneficial. Even if the physiotherapist feels she is achieving very little, the patient would feel abandoned if her visits stopped.

SOCIAL FACTORS

Social factors affect the total well being of the patient. The patient may be concerned about his inability to work and the financial implications which may affect the whole family. This can cause depression and it is important that the patient is aware of the social benefits to which he is entitled. Industrial claims can be instigated if it is an industrial related disease, for example mesothelioma. A social worker should be available and good communication among the multidisciplinary team will lead to more effective treatment.

The patient may fear rejection by family, friends and colleagues and this may lead to social isolation. As the disease progresses the patient experiences a loss of libido and those who have received cytotoxic chemotherapy become sterile. This has implications for family life.

The control of symptoms enables a more socially acceptable lifestyle. Family and friends should be included in the decision making and care of the patient both at home and during hospitalization. This helps the carers to cope when death occurs.

SPIRITUAL CARE

To help a patient attain or maintain peace of mind it is important to be aware that the patient's personal value system may have been shaken as a result of the illness. 'It may be that the person's concept of God or his understanding of the spiritual dimensions of his life are stunted; that religious ceremonies are neither meaningful, nor supportive, nor a source of strength to him' (Kitson 1985).

Sensitive listening may enable the patient to express his fears, hopes and conflicts. The lack of a firm commitment to a religion does not mean that the patient does not have spiritual requirements. Religious practices should be observed and patients and families are usually happy to explain practices which are unfamiliar to members of the multidisciplinary team of carers. Ministers and religious leaders should be available.

RESPONDING TO THE DYING PATIENT AND HIS RELATIVES

It is important to be natural and to spend time with the dying patient. You do not have to talk all the time, but give the patient an opportunity to express his fears and anxieties. Patients often ask questions which are uncomfortable to answer.

Am I going to die? The patient will put this question to the person he trusts, and an honest reply is being sought. The response 'Do you think you are?' gives the patient the chance to vocalize his fears and opens up an opportunity for you to say 'Yes, but I don't know when' and to ask them if they are afraid. Many patients say they are not afraid of death but of the process of dying.

When am I going to die? This is always difficult because we cannot predict the answer. We can say 'Yes, you are very sick but we do not know when you are going to die'.

All questions should be handled very sensitively. Sit with the patient and do not rush away. It is not appropriate to tell the patient not to worry, but listen to their fears and anxieties. You cannot say that you know how they are feeling because we all have individual ways of coping.

Tell the nurse who is looking after the patient about the type of questions you have been asked. Return to the patient later in the day as this will allow them to ask you more questions if they wish and shows that you are offering them support at a difficult time.

How am I going to die? This is a question frequently asked by dying patients. Always be honest. Ask the patient how he feels he might die. This allows him to express his fears.

Many breathless patients lie awake at night, afraid to go to sleep in case they do not wake up. It is often the fear of dying alone, without anyone noticing, that keeps them awake. During the day there are people around. Breathless patients need reassurance that they are not going to suffocate and that drugs can be given to relieve symptoms.

If good symptom control is maintained the patient should die quite peacefully.

How to approach relatives before and after a death

The relatives should be kept informed of the patient's deteriorating condition and should be encouraged to participate in the care of the patient as much as they wish. In stressful situations we all behave differently and it is important to allow relatives to express their worries and fears. Many adults have never seen anyone die except on films or television where death is often portrayed as being frightening.

The staff should explain to the relatives how they think a patient will die, that the breathing will get slower and eventually stop. Following the patient's death the relatives should have the opportunity to stay with the patient until they feel ready to leave.

It is important to acknowledge what has happened. This may be verbally by saying how sorry you are to hear of the patient's death. Non-verbal communication can be very comforting. A gentle touch on the arm can convey more than a list of platitudes.

Support for staff

Staff need the opportunity to talk through the problems they are experiencing when working with the dying patient. This helps the individual to cope with their feelings and physiotherapists should be sensitive to these needs. It is particu-larly difficult when patients are young or in the same age group as the professional.

Many dilemmas have arisen for staff working with patients who are terminally ill but awaiting transplantation. When the patient's physical condition is deteriorating, what would normally be considered appropriate management may be withheld in anticipation of donor organs becoming available.

It is important that the patient is able to live until he dies. 'We cannot judge a biography by its length, by the number of pages in it; we must judge by the richness of the contents... Sometimes the "unfinisheds" are among the most beautiful symphonies' (Frankl 1964).

REFERENCES

Frankl V 1964 Man's search for meaning. Hodder & Stoughton, Bury St Edmunds, Suffolk
Kitson A 1985 Spiritual care in chronic illness. In: McGilloway O, Myco F (eds) Nursing and spiritual care. Harper & Row, London, ch 11, p 145
Mountain C F 1986 A new international staging system for lung cancer. Chest 89: 225S–233S

Twycross R, Lack S 1990 Therapeutics in terminal cancer, 2nd edn. Churchill Livingstone, Edinburgh, p 11
Young I, Daviskas E, Keena V A 1989 Effect of low dose nebulised morphine on exercise endurance in patients with chronic lung disease. Thorax 44: 387–390

FURTHER READING

Buckman R 1988 I don't know what to say. Papermac (Macmillan), London
Hoogstraten B, Addis B J, Hansen H et al (eds) 1988 Lung tumours. Springer-Verlag, Berlin
Kübler Ross E 1970 On death and dying. Macmillan, New York
Lugton J 1987 Communicating with dying people and their relatives. Austen Cornish/Lisa Sainsbury Foundation, Great Britain

McGilloway O, Myco F (eds) 1985 Nursing and spiritual care. Harper & Row, London
Murray Parkes C 1986 Bereavement studies of grief in adult life, 2nd edn. Penguin, Harmondsworth
Souhami R, Tobias J 1986 Cancer and its management. Blackwell Scientific, Oxford

18. Hyperventilation

Diana M. Innocenti

INTRODUCTION

Hyperventilation is a 'physiological response to abnormally increased respiratory "drive" which can be caused by a wide range of organic, psychiatric and physiological disorders, or a combination of these' (Gardner & Bass 1989). It is a state of breathing in excess of metabolic requirements resulting in a lowering of the alveolar partial pressure of carbon dioxide (PACO$_2$) and arterial partial pressure of carbon dioxide (PaCO$_2$). 'Hyperventilation' is synonymous with 'hypocapnia'.

Acute hyperventilation has been recognized for many generations. It results in paraesthesiae, cramps, lightheadedness and unconsciousness. The disorder of chronic hyperventilation is less well accepted as a clinical entity, although it has been described since 1864 under various names (e.g. muscular exhaustion of the heart, soldier's heart, effort syndrome). It was first described as the hyperventilation syndrome in 1937 (Kerr et al 1937).

Unfortunately, episodes of stress or acute symptoms relating to an episode of hyperventilation (which are inappropriately interpreted by the patient) may develop into the chronic syndrome if they are not recognized and managed sensitively at the time. Some patients do not have a 'first attack' but experience an insidious onset of symptoms over several years.

Patients may attend a succession of clinics, presenting with increasingly alarming symptoms. If organic disease is not found and the symptoms persist, anxiety supervenes and stimulates further hyperventilation. This cycle is perpetuated by physiological and/or psychological causes or the formation of new habitual patterns. If the hyperventilation continues the chemoreceptors in the respiratory centre will eventually reprogramme to a low carbon dioxide trigger level.

SIGNS AND SYMPTOMS

Hypocapnia induces vascular constriction resulting in decreased blood flow. The respiratory alkalosis associated with hyperventilation causes a lowering of calcium ions in the plasma which precipitates hyper-irritability of motor and sensory axons (Macefield & Burke 1991). Fluctuations in PaCO$_2$ can have a destabilizing effect on the autonomic system resulting in a sympathetic dominance (Freeman & Nixon 1985). The patients are often in a state of arousal. It has been shown (Folgering et al 1983) that the mean urinary excretion of adrenaline in a group of hyperventilators was three times as high as in a group of normals. Altered patterns of breathing may cause musculoskeletal dysfunction with subsequent pain. Some patients present with a constant level of hypocapnia which drops further as a result of trigger mechanisms. Others present with normal resting levels of carbon dioxide but with episodic lowering of the PaCO$_2$ to a level that precipitates symptoms (Table 18.1).

CAUSES OF HYPERVENTILATION

It is essential for the physiotherapist to distinguish between the chronic hyperventilation syndrome and hyperventilation which has a specific cause. It is therefore necessary to ensure that the patient has been suitably investigated to

Table 18.1   Commonly reported signs and symptoms can be loosely grouped into systems

System	Symptoms/signs
Cardiovascular	Palpitation Chest pain (pseudoangina) Peripheral vasoconstriction
Gastrointestinal	Dysphagia Dyspepsia Epigastric pain Diarrhoea
General	Exhaustion Lethargy Weakness Headache Sleep disturbance Excessive sweating Disturbance of concentration and memory Anxiety Panic attacks Phobic states 'Depersonalization'
Musculoskeletal	Muscle pains Tremors Involuntary contractions Cramps Tetany (rarely)
Neurological	Paraesthesiae Lack of coordination Dizziness Disturbance of vision and hearing Syncope (rarely)
Respiratory	Breathlessness 'Air hunger' Excessive sighing Chest pain Bronchospasm

Table 18.2   Some causes of hypocapnia

Drugs	Drug ingestion (causing acidosis or respiratory dyskinesia) Alcoholism
Organic disorder	Anaemia Asthma Chronic severe pain Central nervous system disorders Diabetes mellitus Pneumonia Pulmonary embolus Pulmonary oedema (left ventricular failure)
Physiological	Altitude Pyrexia Pregnancy Luteal phase of the menstrual cycle
Psychiatric	Depression Anxiety

eliminate any underlying disease or disorder. Some causes of hypocapnia are listed in Table 18.2.

PERSONALITY

Why do some people respond to physiological and environmental stimuli by habitual hyperventilation? Ventilation is controlled by chemoreceptors in the medulla, mechanoreceptors in the muscles, joints and lung tissue and may also be influenced by the cerebral cortex. Probably the main stimulus to breathing is the response of the respiratory centre to carbon dioxide. One hypothesis is that the sensitivity of these centres is personality linked (Clark & Cochrane 1970). The type of person who presents with a chronic hyperventilation syndrome tends towards the perfectionist personality, one who functions at a high level of arousal to achieve self-set high expectations and unrealistic time frames and one who tends to be constantly active in mind and body (until as a result of the symptoms some patients become physically unfit and may become chronic invalids).

BREATHING PATTERNS

The breathing pattern commonly related to the chronic hyperventilation syndrome is predominantly upper thoracic. The accessory muscles are seen to be working. The respiratory rate and volume are often extremely irregular and the pattern interspersed with sighs (Fig. 18.1).

The patterns vary widely from gross upper thoracic movement with sternomastoid action at a rate of 50 breaths/min, to a near-normal rate and volume and minimal upper thoracic movement. The degree of lower thoracic movement and abdominal movement also varies from almost nil to normal.

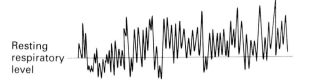

Resting
respiratory
level

Fig. 18.1 Diagrammatic representation of a typically
irregular pattern taken from a spirometry trace.

The patterns vary with each patient and within
the daily time span of each patient. The only
constant feature in hypocapnia is that the patient
moves more air than that which is required by the
metabolic rate. There does not seem to be a strict
correlation between the abnormality of the
breathing pattern, the depression of $PaCO_2$ and
the severity and type of symptoms. It has been
recorded that $PaCO_2$ can be raised by the use of
metoprolol (a beta blocker) with no effect on the
subjective symptoms (Folgering et al 1983).

However, subjective symptomatic improvement, improved exercise tolerance, fitness and an
improved quality of life resulting from re-
education of the breathing pattern and patient
involvement in the control of responses to the
environment, are positive enough to continue
with this form of physiotherapy.

TREATMENT

Treatment is directed towards re-education of the
breathing pattern. A conscious control of rate,
volume and regularity of the breathing cycle
devised to raise $PaCO_2$ by a small measure is
taught and practised. A predominantly relaxed,
passive abdominal movement (reflecting the
movement of the diaphragm) is preferred and
movement directed away from the upper thorax.
This in turn may help to induce physical and
mental relaxation. The treatment described here is
based on a simple understanding of the respiratory
cycle and of conscious control of the breathing
pattern. Relaxation is often aided by a regular,
slow pattern of breathing. It may be necessary with
some very tense patients to practise a relaxation
technique before, during or after the breathing
control. The long-term goal is to decrease ventilation sufficiently to raise the resting $PaCO_2$.

In the short-term, until the new pattern of
breathing becomes the natural, constant, unconscious, spontaneous method of breathing, the
patient will continue to experience episodes of
symptoms. These symptoms may be related to
certain recognizable situations, stress or exercise.
It is necessary to control the breathing pattern at
these times and/or take 'first aid' measures of
breath holding or rebreathing expired carbon
dioxide. In time, with reassurance and perseverance, it should be possible to prevent intermittent
dropping of $PaCO_2$ by identifying the trigger
situations and practising precautionary measures.

THE ASSESSMENT

The assessment should include:

- history
- signs and symptoms
- personality
- physical examination
- it may be helpful to include a provocation test.

History

It is helpful to elicit when the patient was first
aware of symptoms and the response to them.
The first awareness may have been an acute
'attack', for instance driving home on the
motorway on a Friday night after a stressful week
and experiencing dizziness, tingling in the limbs
and central chest pain. The response to this could
be that of believing it to be a heart attack. This
would be very understandable, especially if a
member of the family had recently died of
coronary disease. The anxiety would stimulate the
respiratory rate further and the symptoms would
increase— possibly to the point of admission to
the nearest accident and emergency department.

Misrepresentation of the symptoms of an acute
short-term episode of stress may cause a natural
response to be transformed into a pattern of
inappropriate responses in daily life.

Signs and symptoms may not present so
dramatically. Commonly there is a history of
glandular fever or a prolonged viral illness or
fever. The patient never fully recovers and many
of the listed signs and symptoms supervene. A

great emotional reaction such as the death of a spouse, close relative or friend, family breakdown, frightening experience or prolonged emotional pressure may be recognized as the trigger point on close and sensitive questioning.

Family history

Have parents, siblings or more distant relatives experienced similar symptoms, allergy, cardiac or respiratory disease?

Childhood history

General health, including illness patterns (especially respiratory problems), physical ability and exercise tolerance, should be recorded.

History of premature birth, oxygen therapy or artificial ventilation immediately after birth are incidents which are increasingly reported.

History of chronic pain should be noted as this may be the underlying cause (Glynn et al 1981).

Hypermobility syndrome may have an effect on the ventilation due to abnormally compliant lungs and hypermobility of the thoracovertebral joints.

Signs and symptoms

These should be recorded, listed and numbered in order of severity and/or occurrence and concern.

Assessment of personality

A detailed analysis of the personality is neither possible nor necessary in this setting. However, a simple assessment may be made by noting the posture, facial expression, demeanour of the hands, manner in which the history is given and the patient's emotional responses and reactions to the situations related in the history.

One patient may be overtly obsessive and perfectionist and obviously reacting against the uncertainties of life, whilst another may be superficially tranquil, masking the underlying burden of troubles and emotions which are being carried. These usually come spilling out when sensitively invited to give a history.

Physical examination

With the chest unclothed note is made of:

1. The shape of the chest (including any physical deformity).

2. The pattern of breathing, i.e. the place of movement, size, regularity and rate of breathing. The physiotherapist should have a watch with a second hand available so that the breathing rate per minute can be recorded. The patient should not be informed at this stage of the rate per minute, as the re-education will take place at the level of the individual breath or phase of breath and a knowledge of the greater time scale can be damaging.

3. The findings from auscultation.

Provocation test

The test is done (Hardonk & Beumer 1979) using end tidal $P_{A}CO_2$ recordings. The patient is requested to hyperventilate for 3 minutes to drop the alveolar $P_{A}CO_2$ by at least 1.33 kPa (10 mmHg). The rate of recovery is recorded. If recovery is less than 2/3 of the former resting level after 3 minutes, the test is recorded as positive diagnosis of hyperventilation. However, about 1/4 of normals show this phenomenon.

The apparatus for this test may not be available in the respiratory function unit, but it is possible to use a modified form without $P_{A}CO_2$ recording in the physiotherapy department.

This test is made with the patient dressed and sitting comfortably. The patient is requested to breathe as deeply and as quickly as possible for 3 minutes and asked to take note of any symptoms which may occur during or after the test. These will be discussed and recorded when the procedure has been completed. The physiotherapist may have to encourage the process, as it becomes very tiring. Some patients cannot maintain the effort for 3 minutes. The time and course of recovery is recorded. If the patient is very distressed a rebreathing bag may be used to hasten the recovery.

The ensuing discussion will include any symptoms which occurred and whether they were recognized as personal symptoms or new experiences. The relationship between hyperventilation and the stimulated signs and symptoms becomes evident. This is a useful pretreatment procedure for patients who do not accept that the symptoms which are experienced are related to the method of breathing. The use of a rebreathing bag to hasten recovery and to depress symptoms also helps the patient to accept the link of hyperventilation and subsequently depressed carbon dioxide levels, with symptoms.

TREATMENT PLAN

The treatment plan will be agreed after discussion of symptoms and findings. The patient must highlight the greatest problem areas, related if possible to lifestyle and expectations.

Treatment in the short term (to control symptoms) and in the long term (spontaneously to maintain a corrected pattern of breathing) will be described and agreed.

Agreement will also be sought to look constructively at the activities of the day and to try to identify possible factors influencing the onset of symptoms. It is usually not difficult to obtain a firm commitment to take responsibility for the home treatment programme, as the patients are only too delighted to find a rationale for their problems and the recognition that it is possible to help themselves.

A fitness programme may be discussed at this stage, but it will not be introduced until later in the plan.

BREATHING EDUCATION

The most comfortable position for learning breathing awareness is lying with suitable support. Most people with chronic hyperventilation do not have respiratory disease and therefore can lie flat without distress. The suggested position is supported with one or two pillows under the head and a pillow under the knees (Fig. 18.2). The knee pillow helps to prevent tension in the abdominal muscles and thus enables a natural passive abdominal movement during the respiratory cycle. For patients who find that this position is uncomfortable or that it precipitates breathlessness or a feeling of vulnerability another position should be found. Usually sitting with adequate support is acceptable.

Recognition of the relationship of body movements to the flow of air in breathing is the

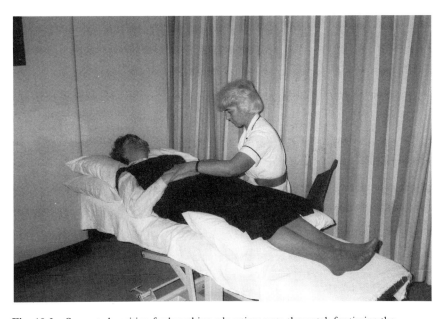

Fig. 18.2 Suggested position for breathing education: note the watch for timing the breathing pattern.

first step of awareness. Sensory input is increased if the patient rests both hands on the abdomen. The physiotherapist lightly covers them with her hands. This light contact helps to bond the physiotherapist–patient relationship and allows the physiotherapist to feel, as well as observe, the movements related to the breathing cycle.

A simple description of respiration is given, relating the flow of air in and out, to the chest, diaphragmatic and abdominal movements. The transfer of oxygen and carbon dioxide should be described in lay terms so that the patient can relate this knowledge to the symptoms, which are secondary to the falling carbon dioxide levels.

Tuition and discussion will continue in this position until the physiotherapist is satisfied that the patient has grasped the basic information. Generally the patient has relaxed more as the interaction has been a distraction from excess self-awareness.

Having had the breathing described the patient is asked to close the eyes and try to concentrate on what is happening with regard to the breathing. It may be necessary for the physiotherapist to relate what is happening. Care must be taken not to direct the pattern but merely to describe it:

- 'You are now breathing in and now you are breathing out'
- 'Your abdomen is swelling and now your abdomen is falling back to rest'.

At this early stage it is necessary for the patient to relate air movement with the associated body movement and to recognize that as the air moves 'in' the body moves 'out', and vice versa.

As soon as one becomes conscious of one's breathing there is a natural feeling of discomfort. Breathing is naturally reflex and subconscious. When it is brought into the consciousness, as it has to be for re-education, there is a discomfort which has to be recognized and at the same time disregarded. Re-education has to take place within this forum.

The patient is then asked to concentrate on the 'in breath' and notice when and how it starts and finishes. The attention is then transferred to the 'out breath' and note taken of the beginning and end of this phase. Particular note should be taken of the end of the phase when the breath gently stops spontaneously. The spontaneous rest point is then described and recognized as the natural rest point in the breathing cycle and the patient is helped to feel it as a relaxation place and not a place of tension. Some work may be done regarding general relaxation into this place of 'no movement'. Most patients can accept this experience and begin to recognize it as a welcome rest.

In order to recognize the full breathing capacity it is helpful to stop the breath at the upper point of the tidal volume and then to request a continuation of inspiration until full inflation is achieved. In this way it is possible to experience the inspiratory capacity. Similarly, the expiratory reserve can be experienced by breath holding at the bottom of the tidal volume and then to exhale entirely by using all the expiratory muscles.

Having practised these two manoeuvres the patient will also recognize that the relaxed tidal volume is relatively easy compared with the muscle work needed above and below the tidal flows. Patients may be able to use this information to enable recognition of when an increase in the work of breathing may indicate an increased tidal volume and onset of symptoms.

BREATHING PATTERN RE-EDUCATION

The initial education and breathing awareness training is followed by re-education of the components that have been identified as being disordered. These components are:

- flow rate
- tidal volume
- regularity
- place of movement.

The new breathing cycle may be of two or three phases, depending on the patient's ability and body preference.

Method

The two-phase cycle would consist of a gentle inspiration followed by a slow expiration which consciously trickles the air out to use up a longer time period. In a three-phase cycle the natural rest point at the end of expiration is used and extended. A gentle inspiration is followed by an easy (passive) expiration which naturally changes into the rest period which is extended until the next inspiration is gently initiated. Care has to be taken not to extend this rest to the point of a gasping inspiration.

By this stage the patient and physiotherapist will be aware of the size, speed and rhythm of the breathing pattern. The physiotherapist will describe these components and clarify with the patient what changes need to be made. A change of volume, speed of flow, regularity and/or place of movement may be required. One component, a combination, or all of these may need to be changed.

As most patients who hyperventilate have a predominantly thoracic movement, this needs to be changed to a gentle passive movement of the abdominal wall. Some patients find it extremely difficult to obtain any abdominal movement and it may be necessary to spend several treatment sessions using different word combinations and different manual pressures on the chest and abdomen until a more relaxed abdominal movement is achieved. Large or forced movements must be discouraged. Any increase in ventilation will increase or precipitate symptoms. In general, most patients manage to recognize what is needed to change from a thoracic *in and up* pattern to an abdominal *in and down* pattern. A new pattern must be found by gradual and patient work. It will be very individual. Guidance can be given breath by breath and phase by phase, relating which movement is good and which incorrect, thus reinforcing correct patterns of volume and movement which will of course be smaller and slower and more regular.

This decrease in ventilation will raise the $PaCO_2$. The higher level is uncomfortable at first. The patient is helped to accept the sensation of unease or discomfort if the sensation is described, discussed and understood.

It can be experienced by directed breath holding and should be recognized when the breathing pattern is being changed. It is necessary to experience this sensation at a minimal level while practising the corrected pattern. The decrease of ventilation should not create an unacceptably strong sensation. This would increase anxiety. It should be barely perceptible and acceptable. By maintaining the controlled pattern for as long as possible the respiratory centre can be re-programmed to trigger inspiration at a higher level of carbon dioxide. The re-programming is similar to that of patients with ventilatory insufficiency in chronic obstructive disease. An imperceptible increase in $PaCO_2$ over a period of time causes the respiratory centre to accept higher levels before triggering inspiration.

If the desire to breathe becomes too great to contain, simple swallowing may ease the discomfort. If this is not sufficient, a slow, controlled deep breath may be taken. To compensate for moving this large volume of air a longer period of time must be used. It is helpful to hold the breath after expiration for a count of five or six (2–3 seconds). In a normal subject the $PaCO_2$ drops as the result of a deep breath and takes 3–4 minutes to return to normal if no compensatory measures are taken. Patients need to learn of this phenomenon and to use the knowledge positively by compensating for deep breathing or sighing by breath holding (preferably at the point of expiration) for a count of five or six.

The stretch reflexes in the joints and muscles of the chest wall probably also play a part in the sensation of unease as the patterns of movement are altered.

Once a pattern has been found that fulfils the change criteria and suits the patient, it must be reinforced in the patient's mind. Some are able to recognize the pattern without external help, others find it difficult to recognize the time scale required. The correction in time may be helped by the physiotherapist guiding, by counting monotonously, the time span of the phases of each breath. The possibilities are many and individual. They may progress from *In out in out in* . . . to a slower more natural pattern of *In and out two three four and in and out two three* . . . (Fig. 18.3). The use of a tape recorder, to capture the counting of the pattern during a treatment session, may help the patient to practise more effectively at home.

The patient should learn to control the breathing pattern in sitting, standing, walking, during and after exercise and at times of stress

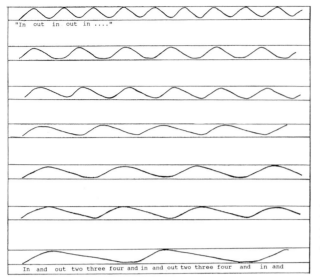

"In   out   in   out   in ...."

In and out two three four and in and out two three four   and in and

Fig. 18.3   Some suggested breathing patterns demonstrating a regular small tidal volume with various flow rates and rest periods.

and risk. It may be necessary to practise these activities during treatment sessions. Natural breathlessness will occur on exercise and should be recognized. If it does not subside within an acceptable time span, tuition may be needed to help with the control by changing one component at a time. First slow the rate, then decrease the volume, then slow the rate, etc., until control is achieved.

Treatment sessions will take approximately 1 hour. Out-patients will need to attend weekly at first. As the patient progresses the sessions will become less frequent. Some patients need only two or three sessions; others 12 or 14 spaced out over 12 or 18 months. At the time of discharge it is important for the patient to know where to telephone for advice and review if necessary. In-patients will probably be treated daily at first, with sessions being spaced as soon as possible to allow the patient responsibility for practice.

COMPENSATORY PROCEDURES IN THE SHORT TERM

The old habit (irregularity, deep breaths or frequent sighs) may precipitate symptoms. One first-aid measure is a conscious compensation for the movement of a large volume of air by breath holding (p. 383). This is so planned that a natural size of breath is subsequently possible.

Intermittent breath holding is a useful manoeuvre to practise throughout the day. It is not anticipated by a deep breath, rather the breathing cycle is stopped anywhere in the cycle for a count of two or three or such time that does not provoke a larger inspiration to follow. It can be practised and linked to simple everyday activities until it becomes a conditioned reflex.

The hypothesis of this manoeuvre is to raise the $PaCO_2$ minimally and regularly to help to prevent the dropping of carbon dioxide to symptomatic levels due to overventilation and slow recovery times.

PLANNED REBREATHING

It has been recorded that paper bag rebreathing may carry the hazard of hypoxia (Callaham 1989). However, poorly programmed rebreathing in acute hyperventilators who may have undiagnosed cardiac or respiratory conditions should not rule out the careful, controlled use of rebreathing therapy for chronic hyperventilators. There is a small group of people who cannot control the breathing pattern when it is most needed. There may be many reasons for this. One reason is that the low $PaCO_2$ has an effect on memory programming and recall. If the $PaCO_2$ can be raised by rebreathing, the patient becomes more clear headed and can then remember the breathing control programme.

At times of acute distress or inability to control the disordered breathing, a bag of 25 cm × 30 cm minimum may be used as a rebreathing apparatus. The bag must be shaken out so that it is full of room air. The open end of the bag is placed loosely over the nose and mouth allowing free passage of air between face and bag. The patient should breathe freely within the bag (Fig. 18.4). Rebreathing of the expired gases takes place thus raising the $PaCO_2$.

After approximately 6 – 8 breaths the bag must be removed from the face, shaken out and refilled with fresh room air. The procedure should continue with regular shaking of the bag until the hyperventilation, are house bound and unable to do household and personal routines. The face mask may be worn for the duration of the task. The $PaCO_2$ is artificially raised by the rebreathing function of the mask. The vent holes are left open so that room air can be drawn in to maintain sufficient oxygen concentration (Fig. 18.5).

The face mask may be the short-term therapy of choice for patients who are terminally ill or who hyperventilate with anxiety. It is unwise to use bags or masks too freely as some patients become dependent on the aid and never learn self-control. They should only be used when the patient's personality and situation is understood and when all other avenues have been investigated.

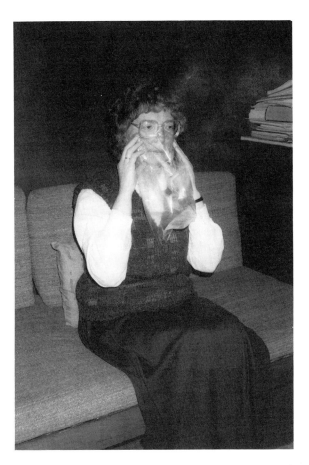

Fig. 18.4 Rebreathing from a bag.

acute presenting symptoms subside or until the patient is capable of controlling the breathing pattern effectively. For safety reasons the rebreathing bag must only be used in the sitting or standing position and *never* in lying. Should the patient lose consciousness the bag would fall away from the face and not remain in situ with the risk of asphyxia.

Rebreathing only raises the $PaCO_2$ during the procedure and, if the breathing pattern is not changed, it would fall back when rebreathing ceased. The purpose of the procedure is to raise the carbon dioxide sufficiently to enable conscious control of the breathing pattern.

An ordinary oxygen mask with large holes, as used for inhalation therapy, may be used for patients who are unable to control the breathing sufficiently at certain times or who, as a result of

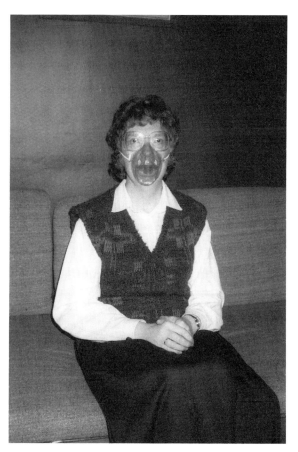

Fig. 18.5 Rebreathing from a mask.

SPEECH

Many patients report that speaking and singing stimulate the symptoms. Advice and training in breath control during these activities may be needed to smooth and slow the speech pattern and to regulate gentle, small inspirations at punctuation points.

HOME PROGRAMME

Therapy is directed towards re-educating the breathing pattern, not to breathing exercises. Practice sessions should be as many and for as long as possible. Using a practical approach an acceptable programme must be worked out by the physiotherapist and the patient. At first it may only be possible to practise for 5 minutes twice a day, but three or four sessions for 20–30 minutes is obviously more beneficial. Many patients find that as their lifestyle changes, more time can be made available for breathing control and relaxation sessions.

It is good to start the day with a period of conscious control of breathing. It is suggested that 10–15 minutes is spent in practice before rising in the morning. Travelling by bus or train is time well spent in conscious breathing control. Car drivers can use constructively the time while waiting at traffic lights. Coffee, lunch and tea breaks could afford a few minutes of practice. Fifteen or twenty minutes should be put aside when returning home from work or shopping to relax and practise breathing control. It is worth spending this time after a working day to allow the body to equilibrate. The evening can be more enjoyable when not fighting symptoms. The last period of practice can be done having retired to bed using the favourite sleeping position.

Compensatory breath holding, intermittent breath holding and general physical and mental relaxation should become part of the normal day. If risk situations are suspected, a period of breathing control before the event is encouraged.

People who have presented with hyperventilation syndrome are probably always at risk. They must therefore remember to practise breathing control before risk situations such as flying, travelling to a high altitude, heat and periods of prolonged excitement or stress.

EXERCISE AND FITNESS PROGRAMMES

As a result of the disordered breathing pattern, many patients have been unable to exercise and have become unfit, thus compounding the problem. Slowly graded exercise schemes can be compiled. These may need to start with very simple movements two or three times only. The progression must be carefully graded, and to err on the slow side is preferable to advancing too quickly. Impatience for progress may cause decline rather than improvement. Swimming is an excellent form of free exercise which encompasses general movement synchronized with the breathing.

GROUP THERAPY

Some centres arrange self-help groups for exercise, relaxation and discussion. These sessions can be beneficial after an individual pattern of breathing control has been mastered and the patient is progressing to control in exercise. At a later stage fitness training can be carried out in a group, although it should never be competitive. Each person should be following an individual programme.

These group sessions must be monitored carefully to ensure that they are not used for 'swapping symptoms'. With careful guidance they can help to give confidence.

CONCLUSION

Patience and perseverance of physiotherapist and patient is necessary for the long term re-education of the breathing pattern, which aims at slowly increasing the resting $PaCO_2$ to more normal levels. The chosen pattern should eventually become the new, unconscious, constant method of breathing.

Chronic habitual hyperventilators are often gifted and interesting people who are generally highly motivated and compliant towards treatment. A high proportion of sufferers are helped by a systematic, individual treatment programme and by an intelligent and sympathetic approach to the syndrome. The condition is a challenging one for the physiotherapist and the patient's improvement is pleasing.

In recent years more recognition has been given to the syndrome. There are many phenomena which are not yet understood and there are many areas inviting research. Work is currently in progress in a few centres which is offering a greater understanding of the physiological complexities.

REFERENCES

Callaham M 1989 Hypoxic hazards of traditional paper bag rebreathing in hyperventilating patients. American Emergency Medicine 18(b): 622–628

Clark T J H, Cochrane G N 1970 Effect of personality on alveolar ventilation in patients with chronic airways obstruction. British Medical Journal 1: 273–275

Folgering H, Ruttern H, Rouman Y 1983 Beta-blockade in the hyperventilation syndrome. A retrospective assessment of symptoms and complaints. Respiration 44(1): 19–25

Freeman L J, Nixon P G F 1985 Chest pain and the hyperventilation syndrome: some aetiological considerations. Postgraduate Medical Journal 61: 957–961

Gardner W N, Bass C 1989 Hyperventilation in clinical practice. British Journal of Hospital Medicine 41(1): 73–81

Glynn C J, Lloyd J W, Folkard S 1981 Ventilatory response to intractable pain. Pain 11(2): 201–211

Hardonk H J, Beumer H M 1979 In: Vinker P J, Bruyn G W (eds) The handbook of clinical neurology. North Holland, Amsterdam, vol 38, p 309–360

Kerr W J, Dalton J W, Bliebe P A 1937 Some physical phenomena associated with the anxiety states and their relation to hyperventilation. Annals of Internal Medicine 2: 961–962

Macefield G, Burke D 1991 Paraesthesiae and tetany induced by voluntary hyperventilation. Brain 114: 527–540

FURTHER READING

Lewis B I 1959 Hyperventilation syndrome. A clinical and physiological evaluation. California Medicine 91: 121–126

Lum L C 1976 The syndrome of habitual chronic hyperventilation. Modern Trends in Psychosomatic Medicine 3: 196–229

Tenny S M Lamb T W 1965 Physiological consequences of hypoventilation and hyperventilation. Handbook of Physiology. American Physiology Society, Bethesda, Maryland, sect 3, vol 2, p 979–1003

19. Asthma in adults, and the *Aspergillus*

Barbara A. Webber   Jennifer A. Pryor

ASTHMA IN ADULTS

The British Thoracic Society (1993) describes asthma as 'a common and chronic inflammatory condition of the airways whose cause is not completely understood. As a result of inflammation the airways are hyperresponsive and they narrow easily in response to a wide range of stimuli. This may result in coughing, wheezing, chest tightness, and shortness of breath and these symptoms are often worse at night. Narrowing of the airway is usually reversible, but in some patients with chronic asthma the inflammation may lead to irreversible airflow obstruction'. The wide range of stimuli include both physical and chemical agents, for example cold air, exercise and smoke.

The British Thoracic Society (1993) also describes the characteristic pathological features of asthma which 'include the presence in the airway of inflammatory cells, plasma exudation, oedema, smooth muscle hypertrophy, mucus plugging, and shedding of epithelium. These changes may be present even in patients with mild asthma when they have few symptoms'.

The *pathogenesis of asthma* is complicated and with research the understanding of the underlying mechanisms is changing (Barnes & Holgate 1990). Proposed mechanisms include mast cell activation, and the release of inflammatory mediators, many of which are pharmacological bronchoconstrictors, for example histamine, prostaglandins, leukotrienes and platelet activating factor (PAF).

Classification

There are several clinical classifications of asthma owing to the complex nature of the condition. Patients with asthma may be classified as being atopic or non-atopic. *Atopic* subjects have raised serum levels of total IgE antibody and specific IgE antibody in response to inhaled allergens such as grass pollens, house dust mite, aspergillus, dog and cat danders. *Non-atopic* subjects do not have elevated total IgE levels in their serum. Skin tests with allergens are negative and no specific IgE antibody to such allergens is found in the serum.

There is more likely to be a familial link in atopic subjects than non-atopic ones, but it is possible that atopy and asthma are inherited independently (Stark 1990, Barnes & Holgate 1990).

Both non-specific and specific agents can provoke asthmatic reactions in atopic and non-atopic subjects. Non-specific agents include: upper respiratory tract infections, emotional factors, exercise, cold air, cigarette smoke and non-antigenic dusts. Specific agents include drugs, for example aspirin, and occupational agents such as isocyanates and epoxy resins (occupational asthma).

'Extrinsic' and 'intrinsic' are other terms often used in the classification of asthma. Inhaled allergens are likely to provoke symptoms in extrinsic asthma and unlikely to provoke symptoms in intrinsic asthma. Extrinsic atopic asthma is found in subjects who have other features of atopy, for example hay fever or eczema, but several types of occupational asthma can be categorized as extrinsic non-atopic. Intrinsic asthma is usually of late onset (adult life) in subjects who are non-atopic and have no evidence of an extrinsic cause.

Asthma in some subjects is provoked by exercise (*exercise-induced asthma*). This does not usually develop until the exercise has ceased, but in more severe cases it will develop during exercise. There are many hypotheses regarding the mechanism behind exercise-induced asthma. One is that it is related to loss of heat and/or water from the respiratory tract which may stimulate mediator release causing acute bronchoconstriction (McFadden 1981, Anderson et al 1982, Lee et al 1983).

Clinical features of asthma

Clinical features include: wheeze, breathlessness, 'tightness' of the chest, and cough which occurs particularly at night and is often paroxysmal. The features of asthma may be episodic or persistent.

Episodic asthma. This may range from mild episodes of wheeze, cough and breathlessness to an acute severe attack. A diurnal variation of symptoms is a common feature. The severe attack is recognized by tachycardia (a pulse rate of more than 110 beats/min), pulsus paradoxus (an inspiratory fall in systolic blood pressure of more than 10 mmHg), difficulty in completing sentences without pausing for breath, central cyanosis, and severe breathlessness — often with the patient sitting forward gasping for breath—which if not treated leads to exhaustion. The breath sounds during an attack would initially be wheezy. The 'silent chest' (greatly reduced breath sounds) represents minimal movement of air and is a sign of very severe asthma. This lack of wheeze must not be misinterpreted.

Persistent asthma. With persistent asthma there is little relief from symptoms and there may or may not be diurnal variations. A possible diagnosis in a patient with persistent asthma is that of allergic bronchopulmonary aspergillosis (p. 395).

Investigations

Assessment. Subjective findings on interview may reveal a family history of asthma or atopy. Other subjective and objective findings are discussed in Chapter 1.

Measurement of airflow obstruction. The peak expiratory flow (PEF) meter can be used to observe patterns of airflow obstruction over time.

Several patterns have been recognized (Turner-Warwick 1977): the 'brittle' asthmatic, the 'morning dipper' and the 'irreversible' asthmatic. Serial recordings of PEF either at home or in hospital should be taken at least on getting up in the morning and before going to bed at night. For comparative purposes it is essential that the times of day at which the recordings are taken remain approximately the same and that drugs are taken at a similar time of day with respect to the PEF recordings. A common feature of asthma is the worsening of airflow obstruction during the night. Using a peak flow chart the relationship of the recordings to the patient's predicted value is immediately recognizable and the response to a bronchodilator can be recorded (Fig. 19.1a). The 'brittle' asthmatic shows a chaotic pattern of peak flow recordings (Fig. 19.1b). These vary from normal to that of severe airflow obstruction within a 24 hour period and stabilization of the condition is difficult.

With 'irreversible' asthma some patients demonstrate long periods of irreversible airflow obstruction, but with reversibility after the introduction of corticosteroids. Other patients never reach their predicted peak flow values but show quite marked fluctuations (25% or more) within a 24 hour period. In addition to their predicted PEF value being marked on the chart it is useful to note the patient's recent known best value. Some irreversible asthmatics show no reversibility in PEF or FEV_1, but respond to treatment by demonstrating an increase in FVC (Fig. 19.1c).

Occupational asthma may be detected by a gradual fall in PEF during the working week with an increase during the weekends and holiday periods.

Other useful measurements of airflow obstruction are FEV_1 and the FEV_1/FVC ratio. Measurements of lung volume are of limited value in the diagnosis and management of asthma, but on occasions changes in FVC or residual volume account for improvement or deterioration in symptoms which are not detected by changes in FEV_1 or PEF.

Arterial blood gases. Blood gas analysis is important in all asthmatic patients, admitted to hospital or an emergency department, with a deterioration in their condition (British Thoracic

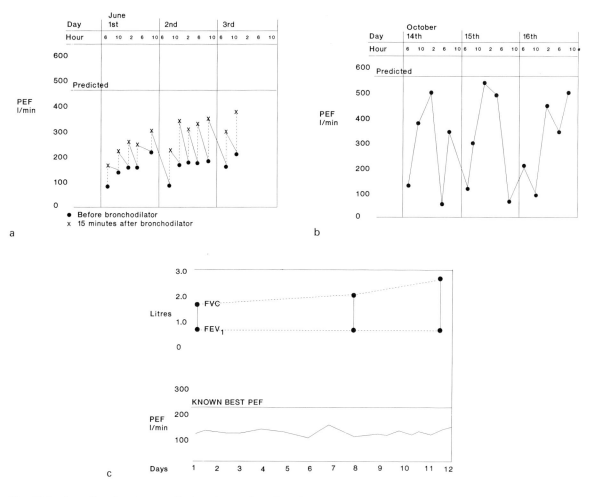

Fig. 19.1   Lung function charts. **a** Peak expiratory flow chart demonstrating bronchodilator response. **b** 'Brittle asthmatic'. **c** 'Irreversible asthmatic' with gradual improvement in FVC.

Society 1993). A respiratory alkalosis is a feature of acute severe asthma. Hypoxaemia develops as a result of bronchoconstriction which causes a ventilation–perfusion ($\dot{V}/\dot{Q}$) imbalance. Hyperventilation initially produces a low $PaCO_2$. A rise in $PaCO_2$ is a very serious sign of exhaustion and impending respiratory failure.

Chest radiograph. Hyperinflation is a characteristic of severe asthma, but the chest radiograph is also necessary to exclude a pneumothorax or pneumomediastinum. Signs of segmental or lobar collapse or patchy shadows due to pneumonic consolidation may be evident.

Sputum. Sputum is usually mucoid but may be mucopurulent. In asthma associated with infection the sputum should be cultured to identify infecting organisms. The presence of eosinophils in the sputum is common in asthma and large numbers of eosinophils will give the sputum an opaque appearance and may colour it yellow or green. This must not be misinterpreted as an infection. Another feature of sputum in asthma is the presence of bronchial casts (Curschmann's spirals).

Haematology. Blood eosinophilia is common in atopic asthma, but may also occur in some non-atopic subjects. Total IgE levels in the serum are raised in atopic asthmatics.

Skin-prick tests. Solutions containing various antigenic materials can be pricked into the dermis of the forearm and a positive response is indicated when a weal of more than 2 mm diameter is present after 10–20 min.

Bronchial challenge tests. Non-specific chemicals, histamine or metacholine can be used to investigate airway hyperreactivity. Patients with asthma react to these agents at lower concentrations than do normal subjects, but false-positive results may be obtained. Bronchial provocation tests may be carried out in the investigation of occupational allergens.

An exercise provocation test may be used to identify asthma. PEF measurements are taken before (until a stable baseline is achieved), during and after running on a treadmill. The recordings are taken at 2-min intervals during exercise, at 1 min intervals for the first 5 min after stopping exercise and then at 10, 15, 20 and 30 min from the end of exercise. If the recording is still falling a further recording is made at 60 min. A fall of more than 10% several minutes after the end of exercise is characteristic of asthma (Cramer 1992). This protocol is based on exercise studies in normal subjects and subjects with asthma reviewed by Godfrey et al (1973).

Another test for airway hyperreactivity is the cold air test where responsiveness to the inhalation of cold air is measured (Assoufi et al 1986).

Medical management

The goals of medical management are to abolish symptoms, to restore normal or near-normal lung function and to minimize the risk of a severe attack. There is a wide variation in the presentation of asthma. There are asthmatics who have only occasional mild attacks, some who have acute severe episodes and others with chronic persistent asthma. In the management of asthma, specific agents known to be precipitating factors should be avoided where possible.

Drug therapy includes bronchodilators (β_2 agonists, anticholinergics, xanthines), and anti-inflammatory agents (corticosteroids, sodium cromoglycate) (British Thoracic Society 1993). Some patients will be well controlled on inhaled β_2 agonists and inhaled corticosteroids alone, while others will require additional oral preparations. The drug and the device used for delivery must be carefully selected for each individual and adequate training should be provided to ensure maximal benefit and minimal side-effects.

Patients should have a relevant understanding of asthma and be educated in the management of their own treatment (Brewis 1991). It is important that the patient realizes the action of each drug and continues to use the preventative drugs (e.g. corticosteroids) even when feeling well. Patients should be able to recognize signs which indicate that their asthma is worsening. Regular twice daily recordings of peak expiratory flow in a diary card will provide objective measurements as many patients are otherwise unaware of a gradual deterioration. Many patients will be trained by their doctor to initiate or increase either doses of inhaled corticosteroids alone or inhaled and oral corticosteroids under specified circumstances.

In patients with exercise-induced asthma, wheezing can often be prevented using an inhaled β_2 agonist 10–15 min before exercise.

Acute severe asthma

This is potentially life threatening and treatment should begin immediately with high concentration oxygen therapy, high doses of β_2 agonists and high doses of systemic steroids. Intravenous aminophylline may be given, but serum theophylline concentrations must be measured. Antibiotics are only indicated if there is evidence of an infection. Patients who do not respond to the initial intensive treatment regimen may require mechanical ventilation. If patients with severe asthma are not admitted to hospital they need close supervision for several days.

Physiotherapy

The physiotherapist should reinforce the advice given to the patient by the doctor regarding asthma management. With improvements in the drug management of asthma the role of the physiotherapist has changed and the emphasis is now on education and prevention.

Problems experienced by patients with asthma include breathlessness and wheeze, reduced exercise tolerance, an irritating cough and sometimes excess bronchial secretions, and lack of understanding of the nature of asthma and its management. The specific problems of each individual will be identified on assessment and the goals of treatment and the treatment plan can be established.

Breathlessness and wheeze

On assessment, airflow obstruction is monitored using a peak flow meter and this provides an opportunity to ensure that the technique of using the meter is correct (Fig. 19.2). If inhaled drugs are due to be taken the physiotherapist should supervise and assess the patient's technique. A placebo device may be used if a dose of the drug is not due at this time. If it becomes apparent that the patient cannot manage to inhale from the prescribed device, the physiotherapist should suggest an effective alternative.

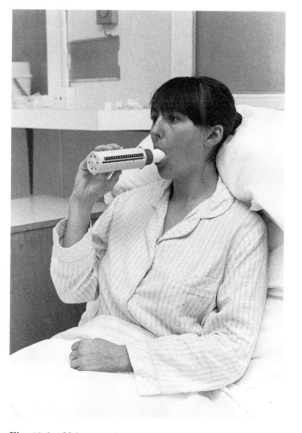

Fig. 19.2 Using a peak expiratory flow meter.

This is also an opportunity for the physiotherapist to ascertain the patient's understanding of his asthma, the drugs he has been prescribed and his knowledge of their effects which will influence compliance. Further education should be provided if necessary.

The physiotherapist will have observed the patient's breathing pattern and breathing control can be either reinforced or introduced. The use of breathing control in the high side lying position is often helpful during episodes of breathlessness. Patients who are chronically breathless benefit from breathing control in the other positions of rest and when walking up slopes and stairs (p. 113).

Exercise

Normal physical activities should be encouraged for patients with asthma including normal sports and games at school and college, and a sport of interest for an adult. Exercise-induced asthma can usually be controlled by the subject by taking his prescribed inhalers 10–15 min before exercise. A survey of school teachers' understanding of asthma and sports and games, highlighted the need for education in this area to increase active participation of pupils with asthma in exercise at school (Bevis & Taylor 1990).

Excess secretions

Not all patients will have excess secretions, but some including those whose attack may have been precipitated by an upper respiratory tract infection will have excess secretions. In these patients techniques to clear secretions should be included in the treatment plan. Treatment using the active cycle of breathing techniques has been shown to improve lung function in a treatment session in patients with asthma (Pryor & Webber 1979).

During productive periods patients should use these breathing techniques after taking their inhaled bronchodilators. Treatment in the sitting position is often sufficient, but sometimes more benefit may be gained by using the side lying position.

Acute severe asthma

In acute severe asthma the physiotherapist may assist in the treatment of the problems of breathlessness and wheeze. Nebulization of bronchodilators will probably have been prescribed as this technique allows the inhalation of the drug over a longer period of time than when a metered dose inhaler is used. Bronchodilatation should occur during the period of inhalation and a progressively greater fraction of the drug, as reflected by plasma levels, can reach the lungs (Shenfield 1974). Peak flow recordings should be taken before and approximately 15 min after the end of the inhalation.

It may be the physiotherapist who positions the patient comfortably and encourages relaxation of the upper chest and shoulders during inhalation of the nebulized drugs (Fig. 19.3). The combination of positioning and breathing control may reduce the effort of breathing.

The delivery of bronchodilator drugs via an intermittent positive pressure breathing (IPPB) device may occasionally be indicated in some exhausted patients to relieve the work of breathing (Fig. 19.4). There is no evidence of a greater bronchodilator effect using IPPB when compared with a nebulizer (Webber et al 1974), but there is evidence of a reduction in the work of breathing when using IPPB (Ayres et al 1963). The possibility of a pneumothorax or pneumomediastinum must be excluded by the chest radiograph before IPPB is instigated.

It is inappropriate to attempt to mobilize and clear excess bronchial secretions until bronchodilatation has begun and either the huff or cough has become productive of sputum.

When it is indicated, the active cycle of breathing techniques can initially be used in the high side lying position. Emphasis should be given to the pauses for relaxation and breathing control after a single huff. The physiotherapist should be cautious with chest shaking in a patient who has been on long-term steroids where osteoporosis may have developed.

Occasionally, mechanical ventilation is indicated in patients with acute severe asthma, but there may not be an indication for physiotherapy until the patient is extubated and breathing spontaneously. If there is adequate bronchodilatation and audible crackles indicate the loosening of excess bronchial secretions, physiotherapy may be appropriate. Following the inhalation of a bronchodilator via the endotra-

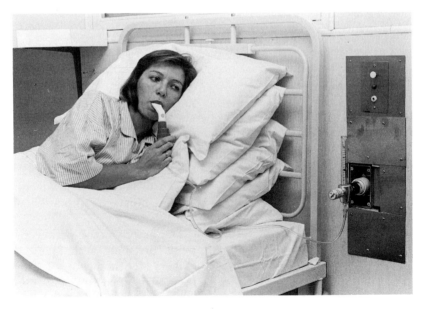

Fig. 19.3 Inhalation of nebulized bronchodilator.

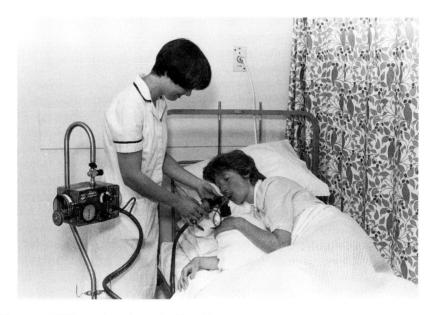

Fig. 19.4   IPPB to reduce the work of breathing during inhalation of nebulized bronchodilator.

cheal tube manual hyperinflation may be tried, but if after suction the airway pressure has risen manual hyperinflation should not be repeated at this stage. The instillation of 2–5 ml normal saline (0.9%) before manual hyperinflation may be of value.

Following extubation bronchodilators may be given by nebulizer or IPPB, and after bronchodilatation the mechanical effect of IPPB may be used to loosen the tenacious cast-like secretions.

Ambulation should be encouraged as soon as possible together with the use of breathing control. If the patient is to be weaned off nebulized bronchodilators the alternative device must be demonstrated to be equally effective. Patients who are on nebulized bronchodilators will probably also be taking inhaled corticosteroids by metered dose inhaler or powder device and the effectiveness of the technique of inhalation should have been observed. For those patients using nebulized drugs at home a simpler device may be equally effective during the day time which facilitates a more normal life-style.

Before discharge, the medical team including the physiotherapist should be confident that the patient is capable of self-management of his asthma which includes an understanding of his condition, the drugs he is taking and their effects, and a written plan by which he can adjust his treatment according to variations in his PEF recordings. He should also be familiar with the use of breathing control for episodes of breathlessness and the techniques to clear secretions when necessary.

Evaluation of physiotherapy

The effects of physiotherapy can be measured by a decrease in breathlessness and airflow obstruction, an increase in exercise tolerance and a decrease in cough especially at night. In the acute severe patient with asthma there will also be an improvement in arterial blood gas tensions.

ASPERGILLUS

Aspergillus is a common fungus producing airborne spores which can cause various pulmonary disorders. Many atopic asthmatic patients are sensitive to *Aspergillus fumigatus* and a few of these develop the complication of *allergic bronchopulmonary aspergillosis*.

Allergic bronchopulmonary aspergillosis

In allergic bronchopulmonary aspergillosis (ABPA) there is a local immune reaction against the fungus but no invasion of lung tissue. The fungus grows in mucus plugs which may be brownish in colour and hard and sticky.

ABPA is characterized by asthma, chronic productive cough and obstruction of the proximal bronchi with mucus plugs. Bronchiectasis often develops distal to these obstructions and is therefore more proximal than most other forms of bronchiectasis.

The diagnosis is made on the combination of asthma, eosinophilia of blood and sputum, positive skin test to *Aspergillus fumigatus*, precipitins to *Aspergillus* in the blood and transient shadowing on the chest radiograph due to areas of lung collapse. The shadows tend to disappear from one place and to reappear in another over a period of weeks or months.

Medical management

This usually includes high dose corticosteroids and bronchodilators to control episodes of acute asthma and lower doses of corticosteroids are continued as maintenance therapy. Current antifungal agents are ineffective, but new drugs are being evaluated.

Physiotherapy

The patient's problems will include breathlessness and wheeze, tenacious bronchial secretions and reduced exercise tolerance. The treatment for breathlessness, wheeze and reduced exercise tolerance is similar to that for asthma, but there is a greater emphasis on the clearance of secretions to try to prevent or minimize the development of bronchiectasis.

On assessment, the appropriate gravity-assisted positions are identified. Bronchodilators should precede physiotherapy and may be given either by nebulizer or IPPB. IPPB is useful to assist in loosening secretions and heated humidification may be of value before treatment. In patients who have had long-term corticosteroid treatment

where osteoporotic changes may have occurred, care must be taken if chest shaking or compression is indicated, but chest wall support is probably more appropriate.

Evaluation of physiotherapy

Effective physiotherapy will be indicated by a clearing of the shadows on the chest radiograph. If the patient has expectorated large plugs of tenacious sputum he will feel 'much better' and his PEF, FEV_1 and FVC may improve dramatically. In patients with smaller plugs of sputum the improvements in lung function will be more gradual. Effective treatment will also lead to a reduction in breathlessness and an increase in exercise tolerance.

Aspergilloma

An aspergilloma, a form of mycetoma, is the fungal colonization of a pre-existing cavity within the lungs which may have resulted from such conditions as tuberculosis, pulmonary infarction, lung abscess or bronchiectasis.

Haemoptysis is a characteristic feature of an aspergilloma, but there will be additional signs and symptoms relating to the underlying condition. The haemoptysis may be slight or severe. The chest radiograph shows an opacity with a crescent of air (halo) which separates the fungus ball from the wall of the cavity.

Medical treatment is usually not indicated unless haemoptysis is severe. Consideration for pulmonary resection is frequently complicated by poor respiratory reserve due to pre-existing lung disease. Other treatments have included systemic antifungal agents, bronchial artery embolization and antibiotic therapy, but with limited success.

Physiotherapy

A physiotherapy problem will not be directly related to the aspergilloma, but the patient may present with physiotherapy problems relating to the underlying condition. Occasionally the physiotherapist may be asked to give inhaled nebulized antifungal agents.

Invasive aspergillosis

Invasive aspergillosis is invasion of the lung parenchyma by a species of aspergillus. It is most often seen in immunocompromised patients. Intravenous antifungal agents are administered, but physiotherapy would only be indicated for treatment of the underlying condition.

REFERENCES

Anderson S D, Schoeffel R E, Follet R et al 1982 Sensitivity to heat and water loss at rest and during exercise in asthmatic patients. European Journal of Respiratory Diseases 63: 459 – 471

Assoufi B K, Dally M B, Newman Taylor A J, Denison D M 1986 Cold air test: a simplified standard method for airway reactivity. Clinical Respiratory Physiology 22: 349 – 357

Ayres S M, Kozam R L, Lukas D S 1963 The effects of intermittent positive pressure breathing on intrathoracic pressure, pulmonary mechanics and the work of breathing. American Review of Respiratory Disease 87: 370 – 379

Barnes P J, Holgate S T 1990 Asthma: pathogenesis and hyperreactivity. In: Brewis R A L, Gibson G J, Geddes D M (eds) Respiratory medicine. Baillière Tindall, London, ch 17.3, p 558 – 603

Bevis M, Taylor B 1990 What do school teachers know about asthma? Archives of Disease in Childhood 65: 622 – 625

Brewis R A L 1991 Patient education, self-management plans and peak flow measurement. Respiratory Medicine 85: 457– 462

British Thoracic Society 1993 Guidelines on the management of asthma. Thorax 48 (2) Supplement: S1–S24

Cramer D 1992 Personal communication, Department of Clinical Physiology, Royal Brompton Hospital

Godfrey S, Silverman M, Anderson S D 1973 Problems of interpreting exercise-induced asthma. Journal of Allergy and Clinical Immunology 52: 199–209

Lee T H, Assoufi B K, Kay A B 1983 The link between exercise, respiratory heat exchange, and the mast cell in bronchial asthma. Lancet i: 520 – 522

McFadden E R 1981 An analysis of exercise as a stimulus for the production of airway obstruction. Lung 159: 3 –11

Pryor J A, Webber B A 1979 An evaluation of the forced expiration technique as an adjunct to postural drainage. Physiotherapy 65: 304 – 307

Shenfield G M 1974 The assessment of sympathomimetic bronchodilator drugs. MD thesis, University of Oxford

Stark J E 1990 Asthma: clinical features and investigation. In: Brewis R A L, Gibson G J, Geddes D M (eds) Respiratory medicine. Baillière Tindall, London, ch 17.6, p 619 – 644

Turner-Warwick M 1977 On observing patterns of airflow obstruction in chronic asthma. British Journal of Diseases of the Chest 71: 73 – 86

Webber B A, Shenfield G M, Paterson J W 1974 A comparison of three different techniques for giving nebulised albuterol to asthmatic patients. American Review of Respiratory Disease 109: 293 – 295

FURTHER READING

Clark T J H, Godfrey S (eds) 1983 Asthma, 2nd edn. Chapman & Hall, London

Crompton G K 1990 Bronchopulmonary aspergillosis. In: Brewis R A L, Gibson G J, Geddes D M (eds) Respiratory medicine. Baillière Tindall, London, ch 26.1, p 1035 –1050

20. Bronchiectasis, primary ciliary dyskinesia and cystic fibrosis

Barbara A. Webber   Jennifer A. Pryor

BRONCHIECTASIS

'Bronchiectasis' is the term used for chronic dilatation of one or more bronchi (Cole 1990). This leads to impaired drainage of bronchial secretions, usually with persistent infection of the affected lobe or segment.

The cause of bronchiectasis may be congenital, for example primary ciliary dyskinesia, cystic fibrosis, sequestrated lung segments or bronchomalacia. Pertussis, measles, tuberculosis and pneumonia may also cause bronchiectasis, but with early medical intervention the incidence following these conditions has fallen. Bronchiectasis may complicate hypogammaglobulinaemia because of the patient's reduced capacity to resist bacterial infection. Other causes include allergic bronchopulmonary aspergillosis (p. 395) and obstruction of a bronchus by a tumour, mucus plug or an inhaled foreign body where persistent secondary infection in the distal airways leads to dilatation and distortion of the bronchi.

The bronchial wall damage with destruction of cartilage and alteration in the normal ciliated epithelium is a result of the inflammatory process. The bronchial circulation may show widespread anastomoses with varicosities and there is an increase in mucus secreting glands.

Clinical features of bronchiectasis include cough, purulent sputum, wheeze, haemoptysis, breathlessness, chest pain (pleuritic), malaise, fever, weight loss, finger clubbing (rare in bronchiectasis unassociated with cystic fibrosis), crackles and wheezes over the affected areas, signs of consolidation and collapse with a superimposed infection and purulent rhinosinusitis including post-nasal drip.

There is a rare form of bronchiectasis known as 'dry' bronchiectasis which may be a consequence of pulmonary tuberculosis or a type where the patient has recurrent haemoptyses, but no infected secretions.

There are more specific signs and symptoms which occur with primary ciliary dyskinesia and cystic fibrosis which are discussed later in this chapter.

Investigations for bronchiectasis include:

- *Assessment* using subjective and objective findings are discussed in Chapter 1
- *The chest radiograph* may be normal but there may be signs of thickened bronchial walls (tramlining), crowding of vessels with loss of volume and cyst-like shadows with fluid levels
- *High resolution computed tomography* is now an important diagnostic tool in bronchiectasis and the invasive technique of bronchography is rarely used
- *Sputum specimens* for examination and culture to identify the microorganisms and their sensitivity to antibiotics, and for cytological examination to exclude malignant disease
- *Bronchoscopy* should be considered if a foreign body or tumour is suspected
- *Lung function tests*
- *Serum immunoglobulins* will detect patients with hypogammaglobulinaemia
- *Serum precipitins test* may identify allergic bronchopulmonary aspergillosis and would be carried out following positive skin tests to *Aspergillus*
- *Sweat test* to exclude cystic fibrosis
- *Nasomucociliary clearance test* or lung clearance

studies using radioaerosol methods to exclude cilial defects.

Medical management

This includes antibiotics and sometimes bronchodilator drugs. Topical medication may be indicated for chronic mucopurulent rhinosinusitis and the recommended technique for inhaled, topical deposition of drugs is in the head down and forward position to encourage entry of the drops to the ethmoid and maxillary sinuses (Wilson et al 1987).

A general practitioner may provide the patient with a prescription for an antibiotic which he can start immediately an infective episode occurs. Where there is an immunoglobulin deficiency, replacement therapy should be given in an attempt to prevent further lung damage. Surgical resection would only be considered if the bronchiectasis is localized. In very severe widespread bronchiectasis with respiratory failure, lung transplantation may be considered.

Bronchography

The instillation of a radio-opaque medium is no longer widely used as an investigative procedure. When it is used for patients with probable bronchiectasis, physiotherapy would help to clear the airways before the bronchogram and to assist the clearance of the contrast medium immediately after.

Much of the contrast medium will either be expectorated spontaneously or absorbed from the peripheral airways into the bloodstream, but where the peripheral airways are blocked, as in bronchiectasis, physiotherapy can assist in the clearance of the medium.

It is important that patients have nothing to eat or drink for at least 3 hours after a bronchogram when the effect of the local anaesthetic will have worn off. If the procedure has been performed through the cricothyroid membrane, the patient should apply pressure over the cricothyroid cartilage during huffing or coughing for at least 6 hours to avoid the possibility of subcutaneous (surgical) emphysema.

Physiotherapy

The patient's problems with which the physiotherapist can help include excess bronchial secretions and breathlessness.

Excess bronchial secretions

Following assessment the affected areas of the lung can be determined. It is important that the patient understands the pathology of the condition and the reasons for treatment. Clinically, effective physiotherapy will reduce the episodes of superimposed infection and may help to minimize further lung damage.

The active cycle of breathing techniques in gravity-assisted positions as indicated on assessment, are used. Self-treatment is introduced with or without self-chest clapping accompanying the thoracic expansion exercises and self-chest compression may be combined with huffing (Fig. 20.1). It is likely that a minimum of 10 min in any one productive position will be necessary and the end-point of treatment must be recognized by self-assessment, that is two consecutive cycles where effective huffs are dry sounding and non-productive. The sitting position may be adequate for patients with minimal secretions.

Regular daily treatment is essential but the number of times in a day will vary between individuals and must be increased during episodes of superimposed infection. For many patients treatment once a day is sufficient. Some patients find their chest is 'dry' at the beginning of the day and it is important that the time for treatment is when their chest is most productive, but also a time that is compatible with their life-style to encourage compliance with treatment.

Patients using gravity-assisted positions for the lower and middle zones may find a full length postural drainage frame (Fig. 20.2) comfortable and convenient for treatment.

Elderly or frail patients may benefit from assistance, by a relative or other carer, with chest clapping and shaking during the thoracic expansion exercises. Careful instruction needs to be given by a physiotherapist.

It is important that the physiotherapy

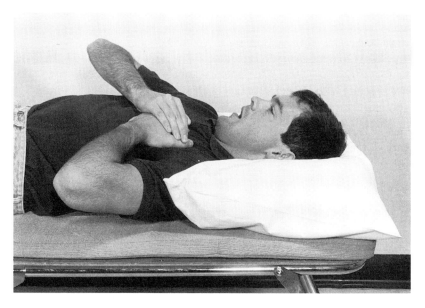

Fig. 20.1   Self-treatment — huff with chest compression.

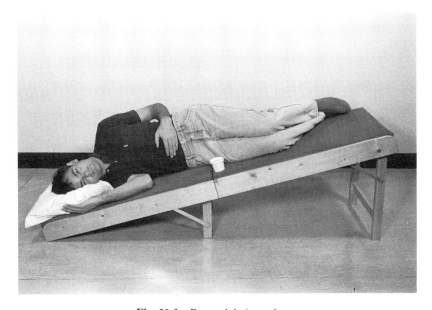

Fig. 20.2   Postural drainage frame.

techniques and positions for treatment are reassessed at intervals. Currie et al (1986) recommend a regular review. Most patients should be reassessed within 3 months of initial instruction and at least annually thereafter.

Encouragement to exercise will not only assist in the mobilization of bronchial secretions but will also improve general physical fitness.

Breathlessness

Some patients with bronchiectasis also demonstrate a degree of bronchospasm and will benefit from the inhalation of a bronchodilator before physiotherapy to clear secretions. Instruction in the use of an appropriate device for drug delivery is important.

It is the minority of patients with bronchiectasis who complain of breathlessness, and for these patients the rest positions to relieve breathlessness, and breathing control in walking and stair climbing should be included in the treatment programme.

Acute exacerbation of infection

Patients may be admitted to hospital with an acute exacerbation of their chest infection. The patient will probably be expectorating an increased amount of more purulent sputum and may be febrile, dehydrated and breathless. Haemoptysis is not uncommon and pleuritic chest pain may be present. The most severely affected may be in respiratory failure.

It is likely that mechanical adjuncts will be required in addition to the active cycle of breathing techniques to assist in the clearance of excess bronchial secretions. A nebulized bronchodilator and/or high humidification before treatment may help in the mobilization of tenacious secretions.

Intermittent positive pressure breathing (IPPB) could help both in the clearance of secretions and in the relief of the work of breathing. There are patients who many years ago received the more radical treatment of resection of more than one lobe and by the time they reach middle age they have very poor respiratory reserve. A superimposed infection in these patients may precipitate respiratory failure. Modified positioning, for example side lying or high side lying, combined with IPPB may be an effective form of treatment in minimizing the effort of clearing secretions (p. 135).

Following resection of lung tissue the anatomy of the bronchial tree may alter and the traditional positions for drainage of segments of the remaining lobes may be unsuitable. The physiotherapist should try varying positions until the optimal ones are found.

Pleuritic chest pain would contraindicate chest clapping and shaking, but periodic continuous positive airway pressure could be considered (p. 139).

The presence of blood streaking in the sputum is not a contraindication to physiotherapy and treatment should be continued. If there is frank haemoptysis physiotherapy should be temporarily discontinued, but resumed as soon as the sputum is only mildly blood stained to avoid retention of old blood and mucus. Before discharge from hospital it is important that the patient is able to take the responsibility for his treatment and is confident with the positions and techniques required to continue regularly at home. If a bronchodilator has been prescribed this would be given before treatment and a few patients with bronchiectasis may be prescribed nebulized antibiotic drugs which should be inhaled after clearance of secretions. If a patient is on the waiting list for lung transplantation, a preoperative rehabilitation programme should be established and postoperative treatment would be as outlined in Chaper 15.

Evaluation of physiotherapy

Effective treatment will be recognized by a decrease in quantity of sputum, absence of fever, improvements in spirometry, a reduction in breathlessness and an increase in exercise tolerance. Improvements in oxygen saturation and blood gas tensions may also be apparent.

PRIMARY CILIARY DYSKINESIA

Primary ciliary dyskinesia (PCD) is an autosomal recessive inherited condition with a frequency of between 1 in 15 000 and 1 in 30 000 (Cole 1990). It affects the cilia resulting in recurrent infections in the nose, ears, sinuses and lungs, and abnormalities in sperm motility may cause infertility in males.

Kartagener is frequently associated with the syndrome in which there is a triad of lung infections, dextrocardia and situs inversus (Kartagener 1933). Abnormalities of the cilia were later identified and not all these patients had dextracardia or situa inversus. The condition then became known as 'immotile cilia syndrome', but with the discovery of a range of cilial abnormalities both in beat frequency and ultrastructure and the knowledge that not all cilia are immotile, the term 'primary ciliary dyskinesia' was adopted (Greenstone et al 1988).

Pneumonia may be the presenting feature in infants, but the early signs in children may be a loose cough, runny nose and recurrent upper and lower respiratory tract infections with or without wheeze. Frequently the child has hearing problems associated with secretory otitis media (glue ear).

Specific investigations which would clarify the diagnosis of PCD would include the nasal mucociliary clearance test (Stanley et al 1984) and photometric determination of ciliary beat frequency (Rutland & Cole 1980). A sweat test will exclude the diagnosis of cystic fibrosis.

Medical management

Early diagnosis is important as early treatment will minimize lung damage. Antibiotic therapy may be indicated for upper and lower respiratory tract infections, the insertion of grommets may be necessary to control the accumulation of fluid in the middle ear and occasionally hearing aids may be used to assist hearing. Nasal douching may help to keep the nose clear.

Physiotherapy

Daily physiotherapy if introduced at the time of diagnosis becomes a way of life for the child. It is important that parents detect signs of infection early: a child may be lethargic, 'off colour' and feel abnormally hot. Physiotherapy treatment should be increased during infective episodes and parents must understand that it is not only antibiotics which will cope with an infection.

Owing to the cilial defect, secretions are most likely to collect in the dependent areas: the lower lobes and often the middle lobe and lingula. The middle lobe which may be situated on the left side, due to situs inversus, is more commonly affected than the lingula. The goal of treatment should be to assist clearance of secretions from the dependent parts of the lungs using gravity-assisted positions and the active cycle of breathing techniques. Even if the chest is dry sounding and non-productive the parents should be shown the positions for the middle lobe (Fig. 20.3), lingula and lateral segments of the lower lobes, and encouraged to use these positions for drainage

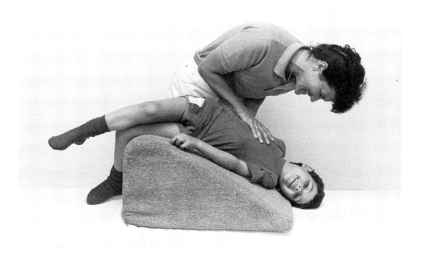

Fig. 20.3 Assisted treatment for the right middle lobe.

daily. A child should be encouraged to blow his nose regularly.

Huffing games can be introduced from the age of 2 years and by the age of 8 or 9 years the child can begin to do some of the treatment himself and gradually become independent. Sports and other active exercises should be encouraged. Even with grommets in place children can enjoy swimming (Pringle 1992).

Very occasionally, nasopharyngeal suction may be indicated in the infant when it is impossible to clear nasal and bronchial secretions by any other means.

Regular assessment of techniques, remotivation of the patient and support for the parents is an important aspect of physiotherapy. It is probable that chronic lung damage will be minimized if physiotherapy is continued on a regular basis.

Evaluation of physiotherapy

In the young patient with primary ciliary dyskinesia effective treatment in the stable condition will be recognized by the presence of only minimal coughing on exertion. During an infective episode signs and symptoms of effective treatment include a reduction in shortness of breath and coughing, and a reduction in wheeze and fever if either or both had been present.

In addition in the older patient a constant volume of sputum would be expectorated while stable, and during an episode of infection an increased volume of expectorated sputum should decrease with effective treatment.

CYSTIC FIBROSIS

Cystic fibrosis is the most frequent cause of suppurative lung disease in Caucasian children and young adults and is characterized by chronic pulmonary disease, pancreatic insufficiency and increased concentrations of electrolytes in the sweat (Høiby & Koch 1990).

Cystic fibrosis is an autosomal recessive condition most commonly found in Caucasian populations and occurring in approximately 1 in 2 500 live births. It has been identified in populations with origins in Europe, the Middle East and the Indian subcontinent. It is much less common in African and Oriental races (Royal College of Physicians 1990).

Carriers of the cystic fibrosis gene show no signs of cystic fibrosis, but if both parents carry the abnormal gene each child born has a theoretical 1 in 4 chance of acquiring the condition at conception.

When the condition was first described by Anderson (1938), life expectancy was less than 2 years, but with increased recognition of the disease especially in its milder forms and improved treatment the mean survival has become 27–30 years of age (Batten 1988) and the oldest known patient was 68 years at the time of diagnosis (van Biezen et al 1992).

The cystic fibrosis defect lies on chromosome 7 and the gene was identified in 1989 (Rommens et al). Genes are made from the chemical deoxyribonucleic acid (DNA) and some pieces of DNA code for protein. The faulty gene in cystic fibrosis codes for the transmembrane conductance regulator (CFTR). The abnormality in this protein leads to changes in ion transport (McBride 1990) producing changes in the nature of the mucous and serous secretions produced by the exocrine glands and cells of the respiratory system and digestive tract. The mucus is abnormally viscid and the secretions abnormally concentrated.

Diagnosis can be made by measuring the amount of sodium in the sweat and a concentration of more than 70 mmol/l is diagnostic of cystic fibrosis (Hodson et al 1983).

Water moves across biological barriers by osmosis, provided the barriers are permeable to water. In the normal airways there is absorption of sodium ions and a secretion of chloride ions through the respiratory epithelium. In cystic fibrosis sodium absorption from the airways is exaggerated and chloride secretion into the airways is blocked (Cuthbert 1991). This results in less water moving from the respiratory epithelium to the airways. The excessive transport of sodium ions from the airways to the respiratory epithelium with the consequent absorption of fluid may reduce the sol layer of the mucus and result in the deposition of thick, viscid mucus in the cilia. These deposits are difficult to dislodge and provide an excellent breeding ground for viruses and bacteria.

The lungs in people with cystic fibrosis are structurally normal at birth, but the tenacious bronchial secretions are difficult to clear and frequently become infected. Infection stimulates further mucus secretion and a generalized obstructive, suppurative cycle is set up. Repeated infections cause bronchiolitis, mucus impaction and cyst formation eventually leading to bronchiectasis and fibrosis (Fig. 20.4). The cycle of infection and inflammation impairs ciliary function and reduces mucus clearance. As the pulmonary disease progresses chronic hypoxia leads to pulmonary hypertension and cor pulmonale and it is the severity of the pulmonary disease that determines morbidity and mortality (Penketh et al 1987).

There is a broad spectrum of presenting signs and symptoms in cystic fibrosis and this may be a reflection of the many gene variants which have been identified. Many patients are diagnosed early in life with signs and symptoms related either to the respiratory or gastrointestinal systems.

Prenatal screening may be undertaken if there is a known family history of cystic fibrosis and these tests are becoming more reliable.

In the neonate, meconium ileus is the most common presenting feature occurring in about 10–15% of cases. Signs of intestinal obstruction may occur within 24 hours of birth. The infant fails to pass meconium after birth because the bowel is obstructed by sticky inspissated intestinal contents, but in milder cases there may only be delay in the passing of meconium. Three or four weeks after birth a sweat test should be performed in infants with meconium ileus to clarify the diagnosis as this condition can occur in infants who do not have cystic fibrosis.

Another common presenting sign in infants and young children is a voracious appetite and failure to thrive due to malabsorption from the alimentary tract.

Abnormalities in ion transport in the pancreas lead to inflammation and later fibrosis of the acinar portion of the gland and to hyposecretion of the major digestive enzymes secreted by the pancreas. The presenting symptom is steatorrhoea, the passing of characteristically fatty and offensive stools. Pancreatic steatorrhoea is often accompanied by abdominal discomfort and distension. In some patients steatorrhoea is not a presenting feature or may be mild.

The complication of diabetes mellitus in the older patient may possibly result from progressive fibrosis of the pancreas. Another feature occurring in a small number of adults is liver damage which starts as focal biliary fibrosis and may progress to portal hypertension and occasionally hepatic failure. A few patients develop gastro-oesophageal reflux.

Meconium ileus equivalent (MIE) is a form of small intestinal obstruction occurring in some adults with cystic fibrosis. It causes abdominal distension and discomfort, vomiting and constipation, and should not be confused with appendicitis.

Most males with cystic fibrosis are infertile due to the lack of development of the vas deferens and epididymis. Most women have normal or near normal fertility, but puberty may be delayed.

Arthritis or hypertrophic osteoarthropathy

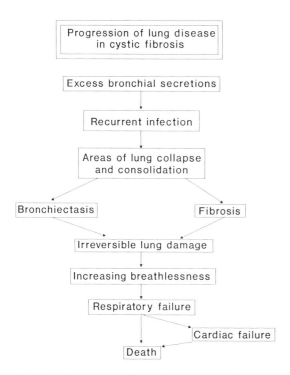

Fig. 20.4 Progression of lung disease in cystic fibrosis.

causing painful swelling of one or more joints is a well recognized feature.

The respiratory signs and symptoms vary. Some patients may be asymptomatic for many years, others may have a dry cough and later a persistent cough with purulent sputum. The organisms most commonly isolated are *Staphylococcus aureus*, *Haemophilus influenzae* and *Pseudomonas aeruginosa*, and an increasing prevalence of *Pseudomonas cepacia*. Haemoptysis is common and usually mild, although episodes of frank haemoptysis may occur. A wheeze is sometimes present, and patients may be breathless on exertion. With increasing breathlessness appetite becomes poor and the patient loses weight. Chest pain may be associated with an exacerbation of a bronchopulmonary infection or a pneumothorax.

Most patients develop finger clubbing and with more severe disease may become cyanosed. The chest radiograph is usually normal at birth and an early change is bronchial wall thickening, particularly in the upper zones. As the disease progresses, overinflation of the lungs may occur with ill-defined nodular shadows, numerous ring and parallel line shadows indicating bronchial wall thickening and bronchiectasis (Fig. 2.16, p. 44). Crackles and wheezes may be heard on auscultation. Some patients develop nasal polyps, these may grow rapidly and are frequently recurrent. They may be related to chronic sinus infection.

Pulmonary function tests will initially show signs of obstruction, but with advanced disease a restrictive pattern may be superimposed on the obstructive defect and a diffusion abnormality will also become apparent. As the disease progresses ventilation/perfusion imbalance occurs leading to hypoxaemia, pulmonary hypertension and cardiac failure.

Asthma is as common in patients with cystic fibrosis as it is among the normal population. Many cystic fibrosis patients have a positive skin test to *Aspergillus fumigatus*. It is often seen in the sputum, but allergic bronchopulmonary aspergillosis, although uncommon, will be recognized by recurrent wheezing, deteriorating chest symptoms and fleeting fluffy shadows on the radiograph.

The clinical features related to the alimentary, respiratory and reproductive systems and to the sweating mechanism are illustrated in Figure 20.5. Although there is an ion transport defect in cystic fibrosis the intracellular mechanisms involved have not yet been defined, but are the subject of intense research.

Investigations for cystic fibrosis are similar to those for bronchiectasis, but would also include pancreatic function studies and tests for faecal fat.

Medical management

Antibiotics are used to treat infections and may be given orally, intravenously or by inhalation. *Pseudomonas aeruginosa* is often resistant to oral antibiotics. Patients needing frequent or prolonged antipseudomonal treatment may require implantable intravenous access devices as thromboses may occur when long-term access is via peripheral veins. Selected patients can use these devices at home (Stead et al 1987).

Patients with deteriorating lung function and persistent pseudomonal infection often benefit from inhalation of nebulized antibiotic drugs (Hodson et al 1981) following physiotherapy to clear secretions. These are usually inhaled twice daily.

Some patients benefit from the inhalation of bronchodilator drugs. Steroids may be indicated if asthma or allergic bronchopulmonary aspergillosis complicate cystic fibrosis.

There is little evidence to support the use of mucolytic agents such as *N*-acetylcysteine (Parvolex). These compounds are thought to reduce sputum viscosity, but may induce bronchospasm and should only be used with caution.

N-acetylcysteine is, however, of benefit either orally or by enema in the treatment of meconium ileus equivalent. Meconium ileus in the neonate usually requires surgery to relieve the obstruction.

An energy intake of at least 15% more than the normal daily recommended diet (Batten 1988) is essential to allow for malabsorption and the increased metabolic requirements during infection and to maximize muscle bulk and function. Supplements of fat soluble vitamins and vitamin K are usually necessary in addition to pancreatic

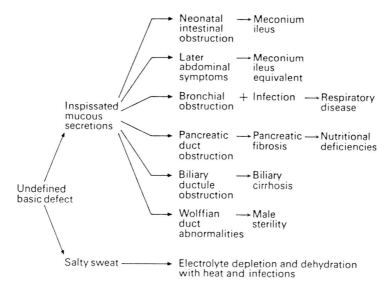

Fig. 20.5 Chief clinical consequences of the undefined basic abnormality in cystic fibrosis. (Reproduced with permission from Goodchild MC, Dodge JA 1985 Cystic fibrosis — manual of diagnosis and management, 2nd edn, Baillière Tindall, London.)

enzymes which should be taken with all meals and snacks.

When nasal obstruction by polyps is incomplete a corticosteroid nasal spray may be tried. Complete obstruction is unusual and polypectomy may be indicated.

Haemoptysis will usually stop spontaneously, but if bleeding is severe and prolonged embolization of the bronchial artery to the affected lobe would be considered (Batten & Matthew 1983).

Pneumothorax can occur spontaneously in the older patient. It may absorb without treatment, but if it persists or increases in size an intercostal drain will probably be inserted. Surgical intervention is withheld if possible, in case transplantation is to be considered in the future. If necessary oversewing of the bleb and a localized pleurodesis may be performed.

Heart–lung transplantation has been successfully carried out in patients with end-stage lung disease (Smyth et al 1991), but careful assessment and optimal management is essential and there is a limited availability of donor organs. Nasal intermittent positive pressure ventilation may be indicated for some patients on the waiting list for transplantation (Hodson et al 1991).

In the end-stage of cystic fibrosis, right ventricular failure is treated using diuretics and long-term oxygen therapy. To allay anxiety and to reduce breathlessness morphine or one of its derivatives is a useful treatment.

There are indications of exciting new developments in the management of cystic fibrosis, but these (for example, gene therapy) are in the early stages. The inhalation of recombinant human deoxyribonuclease (DNase), a new type of mucus dissolving agent, may reduce the viscosity of cystic fibrosis sputum by acting on the DNA in purulent lung secretions (Hubbard et al 1992, Hodson et al 1993). This may have implications for physiotherapy management.

Physiotherapy

Parents of an affected child and the older patients need to have an understanding of cystic fibrosis and the treatment that is indicated. The presenting problems of each patient will vary, and within each patient will fluctuate from a chronic stable state to an acute changing state. An exacerbation of a bronchopulmonary infection will produce changes which can be detected by accurate assessment of the signs and symptoms. Other relevant problems can also influence the cardiorespiratory system, for example the abdominal pain of meconium ileus equivalent. Other features of cystic fibrosis, arthropathy or unstable diabetes for example, will affect the physiotherapist's treatment plan.

The patient's problems with which the physiotherapist can help include excess bronchial secretions, reduced exercise tolerance and breathlessness.

Excess bronchial secretions

Bronchial secretions may be minimal or excessive. The infant at the time of diagnosis may be asymptomatic. Most paediatricians recommend introducing physiotherapy at this time and, if physiotherapy becomes an accepted part of life, compliance will probably be better than if physiotherapy is introduced at a later stage. A close bonding usually develops between the parents and the child. It is important that both parents are involved and to include the siblings in the care of the affected child so that they do not feel left out.

In the infant in the absence of specific radiological signs drainage of the apical segments of the upper lobes is included as the infant will spend much of his time lying down. The position is sitting upright on the parent's lap with the head and shoulders supported (Fig. 20.6). Other recommended positions are lying on each side with the chest tilted downwards, the infant supported on the parent's lap and thighs (lateral segments of the lower lobes (Fig. 20.7). By rolling the infant slightly backwards towards the supine position the right middle lobe and lingula can be drained.

The techniques of positioning, chest clapping and chest vibrations will assist the mobilization of secretions and stimulate coughing. For the infant, chest clapping is performed using the first three fingers of one hand slightly elevating the middle finger and should always be done over a layer of clothing. Treatment should be undertaken before feeds and for 5–10 min twice a day, for example sitting up and then positioning the infant for the lower lobe and middle zone of either the right or

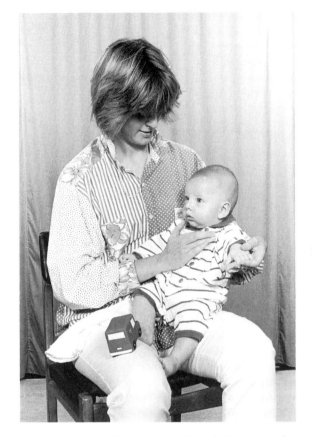

Fig. 20.6 Position for treatment of the apical segments of the upper lobes. (Reproduced with permission of the Royal Brompton Hospital.)

left lung, the other side being treated during the second session of the day.

When the child begins to walk the apical segments can be omitted from treatment, but it is then important to include the anterior segments of the upper lobes. The posterior segments of the upper lobes will probably be drained while the child is leaning forward playing with his toys.

If an infant or child has specific radiological signs, chest clapping in the appropriate gravity-assisted positions (p. 126) should be used. Treatments may need to be more frequent and if tolerated, of slightly longer duration.

Treatment even at a young age should be fun. The young child can be bounced up and down on his parent's knees and another exercise which is fun for the family is the 'upside down piggy back' (Fig. 20.8). Laughing will also stimulate coughing

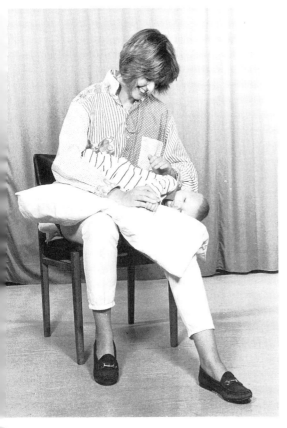

Fig. 20.7   Position for treatment of the lateral segment of the right lower lobe. (Reproduced with permission of the Royal Brompton Hospital.)

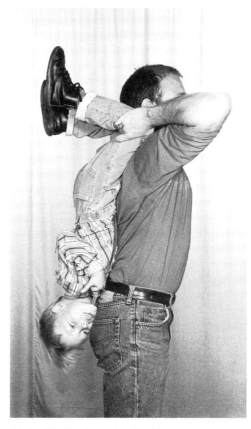

Fig. 20.8   'Upside down piggy back'.

and the minitrampoline can be introduced (Fig. 20.9).

From the age of 2 years, 'huffing' games can be started, for example blowing pieces of cotton wool or tissue using a tube in the mouth. The whole family can be involved in these games (Fig. 20.10). From about 3 years of age the child can be encouraged to take deep breaths during the periods of chest clapping, but this should be for no more than three or four breaths before pausing for a period of breathing control. The parents should now understand that treatment is no longer passive but is the active cycle of breathing techniques (p. 116).

Babies and small children will swallow their bronchial secretions, but as soon as possible expectoration should be encouraged. Learning to blow the nose is important to keep the upper airways clear.

By the age of 8 or 9 years the child can begin to do some of the treatment himself and gradually learn to be independent of his parents for periods of time. This will give his parents confidence that he will be able to continue his treatment when away from home staying with friends.

The adolescent often prefers to take full responsibility for his physiotherapy treatment and this should continue throughout adult life, although there are some patients who are too frail to manage completely on their own. Modified gravity-assisted positions should be considered for patients with gastro-oesophageal reflux.

Infants are treated on their parents' knees, but as the child grows older and if the head down position is indicated he can lie over a wedge of foam (Fig. 20.11) or pillows. A tipping frame supporting the whole body is more comfortable for the older patient (Fig. 20.2). Paroxysms of

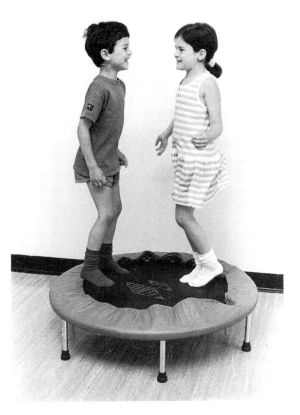

Fig. 20.9 Exercise on the minitrampoline.

coughing are exhausting and ineffective. They should be minimized by emphasizing breathing control. When control is gained, one or two huffs combined with breathing control will be more effective in the clearance of secretions.

The physiotherapist should be involved with the change in techniques from infancy to adulthood. Assessment and reassessment of the patient's condition are essential for the necessary changes in treatment to be recognized and implemented.

The frequency and duration of treatment will vary. When secretions are minimal, treatment once a day may be sufficient but additionally some form of exercise should be encouraged. Many patients will require treatment two or three times a day, but the programme should be realistic and allow for other normal activities. If a session is required in the middle of the day this can probably be done in a sitting position at school, college or work.

Treatment is usually more effective if no more than three positions are used, as a minimum of 10 min in any one productive position is recommended. Although the cause is unknown the upper lobes are frequently the most severely affected and it is important to consider the

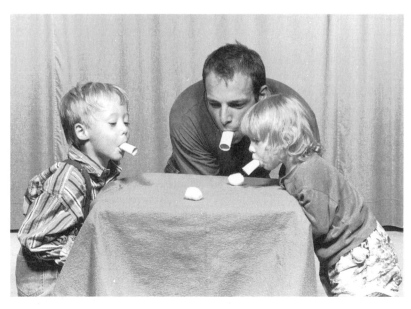

Fig. 20.10 Huffing games.

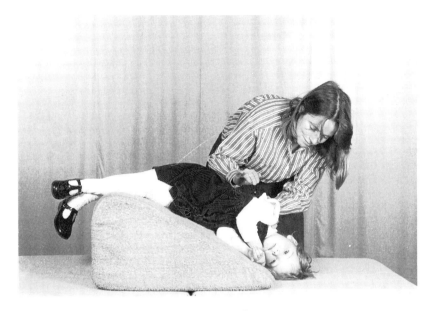

Fig. 20.11   Foam wedge for treatment.

anterior and posterior segments of the upper lobes when assessing the patient and planning treatment.

Inhalation of drugs. Bronchodilator drugs may be prescribed and these should be inhaled before treatment to clear secretions. In some patients the airflow obstruction is partially reversible with bronchodilators. Zach et al (1985) suggest that bronchodilators may increase airway wall instability, but there is no evidence to support this when the active cycle of breathing techniques is used after the inhalation of β-adrenergic bronchodilators (Pryor et al).

Another possible effect of β-adrenergic drugs is an increase in cilial action (Wood et al 1975) and this may improve mucociliary clearance.

Normal saline (0.9%) or hypertonic saline (3–7%) (Pavia et al 1978, Sutton et al 1988) may be inhaled before physiotherapy to assist in clearance of secretions. If hypertonic saline is used a test dose should be given with recordings of PEF or FEV_1 before and 5 min after inhalation to identify any increase in airflow obstruction.

Mucolytic agents, for example N-acetylcysteine (Parvolex), should be used with caution. A reduction in sputum viscosity does not necessarily produce an increase in expectoration of sputum and bronchospasm may be induced.

Aerosol antibiotics (p. 145) should be inhaled after secretions have been cleared. Spirometry is necessary before and after the initial dose to detect any increase in airflow obstruction. If this should occur the effect is usually minimized by the inhalation of a bronchodilator before treatment.

Exercise

Exercise should play an important part in the management of cystic fibrosis to improve general physical fitness. It has been shown to improve cardiorespiratory fitness and muscle endurance (Orenstein et al 1981), to reduce breathlessness (O'Neill et al 1987) and to improve self esteem and promote a feeling of well being (Stanghelle et al 1988). Exercise increases mucociliary clearance, but it is less effective in the clearance of bronchial secretions than the active cycle of breathing techniques (Salh et al 1989).

When the diagnosis of cystic fibrosis is made, if practical, it is a good idea for the family to take up some form of exercise that they will all enjoy. Children should take part in normal school games when possible and adults should be encouraged to take some form of enjoyable exercise regularly (Fig. 20.12). In the winter months when outdoor sports may not be appropriate a stationary bicycle (Fig. 20.13) is often useful to provide a progressive exercise programme.

Exercise capacity can be assessed by measuring maximum oxygen uptake (VO_2Max) using a bicycle ergometer test. A progressive exercise programme should be based on a work load to achieve 50–60% of VO_2Max. If formal exercise testing is not available, 50% of peak work capacity (PWC) can be used as the starting point for exercise (Dodd 1991).

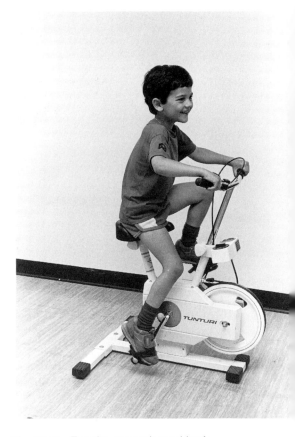

Fig. 20.13   Exercise on a stationary bicycle.

The PWC (in watts (W)) can be calculated using a bicycle ergometer. The patient starts cycling at a low wattage, for example 10–12 W, and this is increased by 10 W each minute until the patient can cycle no further. In patients with cystic fibrosis the limiting factor to exercise may be either breathlessness or muscle fatigue. The workload reached in this test approximates the PWC. Oxygen saturation and heart rate should be monitored. Many of these patients will tolerate a low oxygen saturation (SaO_2).

In patients with advanced pulmonary disease who desaturate during exercise, supplemental oxygen has been shown to increase exercise tolerance and aerobic capacity, and it can reduce exercise-related arterial oxygen desaturation (Marcus et al 1992). The long-term effects of oxygen desaturation and, therefore, the place of oxygen therapy in chronic pulmonary disease remains controversial (Coates 1992).

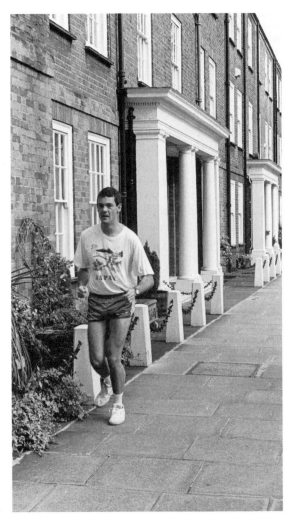

Fig. 20.12   Jogging.

Exercise should be discontinued if a patient develops a fever, as his metabolic requirements will be increased during this period. A patient who has exercise-induced asthma should remember to inhale his bronchodilator before starting exercise. When exercising a patient who has a small pneumothorax, or following a recent pneumothorax or haemoptysis, the physiotherapist should monitor the signs and symptoms during an exercise session.

In the occasional patient with osteoarthropathy exercise may be contraindicated during a period of acute joint involvement. The patient with diabetes should maintain an adequate sugar level during increased physical activity and a sweet drink or biscuit before exercise may be all that is required. Salt depletion may occur if exercising in hot weather or when in a hot climate, and salt supplements may be needed.

Posture and trunk mobility exercises should be encouraged to try to maintain flexibility of the thoracic cage. Manual therapy techniques may increase thoracic mobility in patients with cystic fibrosis and may improve lung function (Vibekk 1991).

Some patients exercise after postural drainage, either because they are too breathless to exercise until they have cleared their secretions or because they find it more socially acceptable to be coughing less while participating in social sports. Other patients prefer to exercise before physiotherapy. Bilton et al (1992) could find no objective difference in sputum expectoration when exercise either preceded or followed physiotherapy.

Breathlessness

The use of breathing control when walking up stairs and hills should be introduced when breathlessness on exertion becomes noticeable. An irritable cough at night or breathlessness may be minimized by the use of the high side lying position (Fig. 20.14) and other rest positions are often of value to reduce breathlessness.

Acute exacerbation of a bronchopulmonary infection

Signs of an acute exacerbation include an increase in the volume and purulence of sputum, breathlessness, fever, a deterioration in lung function, possible pleuritic chest pain and a reduction in exercise tolerance.

An increase in the duration and frequency of physiotherapy treatments will be indicated and the patient will require assistance with chest clapping, shaking (Fig. 20.15) and compression. The pauses for breathing control may need to be

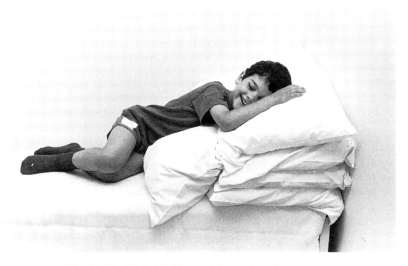

Fig. 20.14   High side lying position for breathlessness.

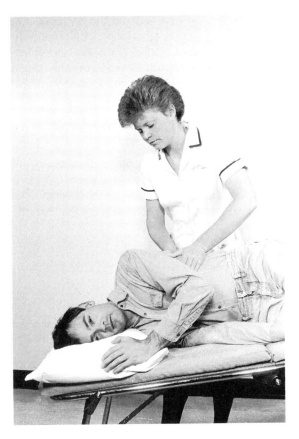

Fig. 20.15 Assisted treatment. (Reproduced with permission of the Royal Brompton Hospital.)

lengthened and treatment should be discontinued before the patient becomes too tired. It may not be possible to reach the 'end-point' (p. 121) of treatment at this stage. There are such wide variations in pathology, and signs and symptoms, that for the inexperienced physiotherapist it is very difficult to know when to discontinue a treatment session. As a rough guide, a treatment at this stage is likely to take 20–30 min.

If oxygen therapy has been prescribed this should be continued throughout treatment. When secretions are very tenacious high humidification should be considered either continuously with oxygen therapy or for 10–15 min before physiotherapy (p. 149).

Other adjuncts may be indicated, for example intermittent positive pressure breathing (IPPB) to reduce the work of breathing and to assist in the clearance of secretions. If the patient has had a

recent pneumothorax or a history of recurrent pneumothoraces IPPB is probably contraindicated. Periodic continuous positive airway pressure (PCPAP) may be the adjunct of choice if the patient is having difficulty clearing secretions because of pleuritic chest pain or chest pain due to a rib fracture.

Nasal intermittent positive pressure ventilation (NIPPV) may be used to improve ventilation particularly overnight and the physiotherapist may be involved in introducing the patient to the ventilator. By adjustment of the settings it is possible to continue NIPPV while carrying out physiotherapy, but it may be more appropriate to disconnect the patient from NIPPV and to use the active cycle of breathing techniques alone or an IPPB device with a mouthpiece.

Complications of cystic fibrosis

Haemoptysis. Blood streaking of sputum is a frequent occurrence in patients with cystic fibrosis and there is no indication to alter the physiotherapy regimen. In cases of frank haemoptysis it is appropriate to discontinue physiotherapy temporarily until the bleeding begins to settle. Positioning may need to be modified and chest clapping withheld, but it is important to restart treatment as soon as possible to avoid the accumulation of old blood in the airways and retention of sputum.

If severe haemoptysis persists a fibreoptic bronchoscopy may be undertaken to identify the bleeding point and embolization of the bronchial artery may be carried out (Batten & Matthew 1983). Following embolization, physiotherapy should be resumed without delay.

Pneumothorax. A small pneumothorax is not a contraindication to chest physiotherapy, but if during treatment the patient becomes more breathless or complains of chest pain the doctor should be notified immediately as it is possible that the pneumothorax could have increased in size.

A larger pneumothorax will require an intercostal drain and physiotherapy should be withheld until the drain has been inserted. Analgesia will probably be required before treatment and the patient's usual physiotherapy regimen should be continued, but chest clapping may be unnecessary and may cause discomfort.

If the air leak persists and surgical intervention is undertaken, it is essential that physiotherapy is restarted as soon as the patient is awake postoperatively. Adequate analgesia and high humidification will assist the clearance of secretions.

Allergic bronchopulmonary aspergillosis. In addition to the purulent secretions of cystic fibrosis there is mucus plugging caused by allergic bronchopulmonary aspergillosis (ABPA). Wheezing is also common. Treatment should include nebulized bronchodilators and the active cycle of breathing techniques. Intermittent positive pressure breathing may be indicated.

Implantable venous access devices. These devices allow many patients to have intravenous antibiotic therapy at home, but it must be remembered that physiotherapy should also be increased during an exacerbation of a bronchopulmonary infection. Chest clapping over the site of the implanted device is uncomfortable and should be avoided, but all other techniques can be used.

Pregnancy. Pregnancy is not a complication in itself, but in the later stages of pregnancy the respiratory system is compromised and lung function will be reduced. Gravity-assisted positions will need to be modified and side lying or high side lying may be the positions of choice for physiotherapy.

The reduction in lung function continues for some time after the birth, especially if the patient has had an anaesthetic and caesarian section. Intensive physiotherapy is important throughout this stage.

Transplantation. The physiotherapist should be involved both before and after heart–lung or lung transplantation. Before transplantation the patient's exercise ability will be very limited but he should have an exercise programme to optimize muscle and cardiovascular function. Postoperatively an extensive rehabilitation programme is essential to gain maximum benefit and improved quality of life (Ch. 15, p. 343).

Following heart–lung or double lung transplantation the lungs are denervated below the tracheal anastomosis with loss of all pulmonary innervation except postganglionic efferent nerves (Hathaway et al 1991). It is probably not neces-

sary for daily physiotherapy to be continued except during episodes of chest infection, but a daily self-assessment should include one or two effective huffs. When a huff which has been dry sounding and non-productive becomes crackly, breathing exercises should be restarted for a period of time until the lungs are clear.

Terminal care. The physiotherapist has an important role in the life of patients with cystic fibrosis and it is inappropriate to withdraw support in the terminal stages even though our treatment may no longer be effective. Assistance can be given with positioning the breathless patient to make him as comfortable as possible. Occasionally adjuncts such as IPPB and PCPAP can be used to assist the clearance of secretions from the upper airways, but care must be taken to use these adjuncts only as a part of physiotherapy treatment and not as a form of pseudo-ventilation.

The active cycle of breathing techniques is modified and will probably consist of encouraging a few deep breaths, long periods of breathing control and supported huffing either in high side lying or sitting leaning forward. The expectoration of one or two plugs of sputum can be a great relief to the patient. Nasotracheal suction is not indicated as it would serve no useful purpose at this stage. Morphine or one of its derivatives will help to relieve anxiety and breathlessness.

Evaluation of physiotherapy

In the patient in a stable condition, the daily weight or volume of sputum expectorated should remain approximately constant with effective physiotherapy and medical management. During an acute exacerbation effective treatment would be indicated by a reduction in sputum.

Lung function is another indicator of improvement in response to treatment of an acute exacerbation, but in long-term studies measurements of lung function must be viewed carefully as most of these will increase as the child grows older. As breathlessness is reduced exercise tolerance will increase.

Appetite will return and weight will be gained as fever subsides and breathlessness is reduced. Activities of daily living and absenteeism from school or work can also be used as indicators.

Continuity of care

Continuous assessment and reassessment of these patients is essential for effective management. The patient's needs will change as he progresses from infancy through school, college, university and work, but the emphasis is on leading as normal a life as possible while making time to include regular physiotherapy. It is the knowledge and understanding of the condition and the effects of physiotherapy which will influence patient compliance through these stages (Passero et al 1981, Hames et al 1991). Parents and patients should be involved in the planning of home programmes and realistic programmes can then be established.

Although the majority of parents and, when he is older, the patient himself can take the responsibility for physiotherapy treatments, it is essential that there is a regular review of the techniques by a physiotherapist. This also provides an opportunity to update the techniques and to discuss any

problems. There are times when the parents or patient are unable to cope effectively on their own and the need for assistance during these periods should be recognized and help should be arranged.

If the patient is treated at both a local hospital and a specialist cystic fibrosis unit, communication between physiotherapists is essential to avoid confusion about treatment.

The physiotherapist must remember that she is a part of a multidisciplinary team and she must be aware of the role of the other members. Good communication within the team is essential.

In caring for the patient with cystic fibrosis the physical care is important, but the psychological effects on both the family and the patient must also be considered. Many countries have cystic fibrosis associations which offer encouragement and support for patients and their families. In spite of the frequently high demands of treatment the majority of adult patients with cystic fibrosis are in full-time employment and take an active part in community life.

REFERENCES

Anderson D H 1938 Cystic fibrosis of the pancreas and its relation to celiac disease: clinical and pathological study. American Journal of Disease in Childhood 56: 344–399

Batten J 1988 Cystic fibrosis in adolescents and adults. In: Proceedings of the 10th international cystic fibrosis congress. Excerpta Medica, Hong Kong

Batten J C, Matthew D J 1983 The respiratory system. In: Hodson M E, Norman A P, Batten J C (eds) Cystic fibrosis. Baillière Tindall, London, ch 6, p 126–127

Bilton D, Dodd M E, Abbot J V, Webb A K 1992 The benefits of exercise combined with physiotherapy in the treatment of adults with cystic fibrosis. Respiratory Medicine 86: 507–511

Coates A L 1992 Oxygen therapy, exercise, and cystic fibrosis. Chest 101: 2–4

Cole P J 1990 Bronchiectasis. In: Brewis R A L, Gibson G J, Geddes D M (eds) Respiratory medicine. Baillière Tindall, London, Ch 18, p 726–759

Currie D, Munro C, Gaskell D, Cole P J 1986 Practice, problems and compliance with postural drainage: a survey of chronic sputum producers. British Journal of Diseases of the Chest 80: 249–253

Cuthbert A W 1991 Abnormalities of airway epithelial function and the implications of the discovery of the cystic fibrosis gene. Thorax 46: 124–130

Dodd M E 1991 Exercise in cystic fibrosis adults. In: Pryor J A (ed) Respiratory care. Churchill Livingstone, Edinburgh, p 27–50

Greenstone M, Rutman A, Dewar I et al 1988 Primary ciliary dyskinesia: cytological and clinical features. Quarterly Journal of Medicine New Series 67(253): 405–430

Hames A, Beesley J, Nelson R 1991 Cystic fibrosis: what do patients know and what else would they like to know? Respiratory Medicine 85: 389–392

Hathaway T, Higenbottam T, Lowry R, Wallwork J 1991 Pulmonary reflexes after human heart-lung transplantation. Respiratory Medicine 85 (suppl A): 17–21

Hodson M E, Penketh A R L, Batten J C 1981 Aerosol carbenicillin and gentamicin treatment of pseudomonas aeruginosa infection in patients with cystic fibrosis. Lancet ii: 1137–1139

Hodson M E, Beldon I, Power R et al 1983 Sweat tests to diagnose cystic fibrosis in adults. British Medical Journal 286: 1381–1383

Hodson M E, Madden B P, Steven M H et al 1991 Non-invasive mechanical ventilation for cystic fibrosis patients — a potential bridge to transplantation. European Respiratory Journal 4: 524–527

Hodson M E et al 1993 DNase . . . (in press)

Høiby N, Koch C 1990 Pseudomonas aeruginosa infection in cystic fibrosis and its management. Thorax 45: 881–884

Hubbard R C, McElvaney N G, Birrer P et al 1992 A preliminary study of aerosolized recombinant human deoxyribonuclease I in the treatment of cystic fibrosis. New England Journal of Medicine 326: 812–815

Kartagener M 1933 Zur pathogenese der Bronchiektasien. Beitrage zur Klinik der Tuberkulose 83: 489–501

Marcus C L, Bader D, Stabile M W et al 1992 Supplemental oxygen and exercise performance in patients with cystic fibrosis with severe pulmonary disease. Chest 101: 52–57

McBride G 1990 More progress in cystic fibrosis. British Medical Journal 301: 627

O'Neill P, Dodd M, Phillips B et al 1987 Regular exercise and reduction of breathlessness in patients with cystic fibrosis. British Journal of Diseases of the Chest 81: 62–69

Orenstein D M, Franklin B A, Doershuk C F et al 1981 Exercise conditioning and cardiopulmonary fitness in cystic fibrosis. Chest 80: 392–398

Passero M A, Remor B, Salomon J 1981 Patient-reported compliance with cystic fibrosis therapy. Clinical Pediatrics 20: 264–268

Pavia D, Thomson M L, Clarke S W 1978 Enhanced clearance of secretions from the human lung after the administration of hypertonic saline aerosol. American Review of Respiratory Disease 117: 199–203

Penketh A R L, Wise A, Mearns M B et al 1987 Cystic fibrosis in adolescents and adults. Thorax 42: 526–532

Pringle M B 1992 Swimming and grommets. British Medical Journal 304: 198

Pryor J A, Webber B A, Warner J O, Hodson M E The Flutter VRP1 as an adjunct to chest physiotherapy in cystic fibrosis (in press)

Rommens J M, Iannuzzi M C, Kerem B et al 1989 Identification of the cystic fibrosis gene: chromosome walking and jumping. Science 245: 1059–1065

Royal College of Physicians 1990 Cystic fibrosis in adults. Recommendations for care of patients. Royal College of Physicians, London, p 1

Rutland J, Cole P J 1980 Non-invasive sampling of nasal cilia for measurement of beat frequency and study of ultrastructure. Lancet ii: 564–565

Salh W, Bilton D, Dodd M, Webb A K 1989 Effect of exercise and physiotherapy in aiding sputum expectoration in adults with cystic fibrosis. Thorax 44: 1006–1008

Smyth R L, Higenbottam T, Scott J, Wallwork J 1991 The current state of lung transplantation for cystic fibrosis. Thorax 46: 213–216

Stanghelle J K, Winnem M, Roaldsen K et al 1988 Young patients with cystic fibrosis: attitude toward physical activity and influence on physical fitness and spirometric values of a 2-week training course. International Journal of Sports Medicine 9: 25–31

Stanley P, MacWilliam L, Greenstone M et al 1984 Efficacy of a saccharin test for screening to detect abnormal mucociliary clearance. British Journal of Diseases of the Chest 78: 62–65

Stead R J, Davidson T I, Duncan F R et al 1987 Use of a totally implantable system for venous access in cystic fibrosis. Thorax 42: 149–150

Sutton P P, Gemmell H G, Innes N et al 1988 Use of nebulised saline and nebulised terbutaline as an adjunct to chest physiotherapy. Thorax 43: 57–60

van Biezen P, Overbeek S E, Hilvering C 1992 Cystic fibrosis in a 70 year old woman. Thorax 47: 202–203

Vibekk P 1991 Chest mobilization and respiratory function. In: Pryor J A (ed) Respiratory care. Churchill Livingstone, Edinburgh, p 103–119

Wilson R, Sykes D A, Chan K L et al 1987 Effect of head position on the efficacy of topical treatment of chronic mucopurulent rhinosinusitis. Thorax 42: 631–632

Wood R E, Wanner A, Hirsch J, Farrell P M 1975 Tracheal mucociliary transport in patients with cystic fibrosis and its stimulation by terbutaline. American Review of Respiratory Disease 11: 733–738

Zach M S, Oberwaldner B, Forche G, Polgar G 1985 Bronchodilators increase airway instability in cystic fibrosis. American Review of Respiratory Disease 131: 537–543

FURTHER READING

Brewis R A L, Gibson G J, Geddes D M (eds) 1990 Respiratory medicine. Baillière Tindall, London

Dinwiddie R 1990 The diagnosis and management of paediatric respiratory disease. Churchill Livingstone, Edinburgh

Hodson M E, Geddes D M (eds) Cystic fibrosis. Chapman & Hall, London (in press)

21. Immunosuppression or deficiency

Denise Hills

INTRODUCTION

The ability of an individual to remain healthy requires the cooperation and interaction of a very sensitive series of components, all designated to protect the host. Undifferentiated stem cells (originating from bone marrow) specialize into two major defence systems. These are the cellular and the humoral immune systems.

The cellular system

Cell-mediated immunity is made up of T lymphocytes (T cells) which are derived from the thymus and then migrate to the lymph nodes and spleen. When stimulated, some of these cells migrate via the blood stream into affected tissue where they interact with foreign material. The key to the cell-mediated immune system is the T-helper cells (T_4 cells), one of the T lymphocytes (Weir 1977), which process foreign antigen presented to them by macrophages and stimulate the appropriate cytotoxic cell lines (killer cells, CD8 cells), and B lymphocytes (B cells) to mount a response against all foreign cells or viruses with the same antigen make-up. These cells attack foreign material, both individually and in conjunction with macrophages (phagocytic cells). Phagocytic cells are either fixed in tissues, for example in the spleen, bone marrow, lung, liver (reticuloendothelial system), or in the circulation, that is the monocytes and polymorphonuclear neutrophils. This system helps to guard primarily against viral, fungal and protozoal invasion as a first line of defence, along with circulating humoral factors.

The humoral system

The humoral immune system consists of B lymphocytes which produce immunoglobulins (antibodies), i.e. IgG, IgA, IgM, IgD and IgE. These immunoglobulins, found in serum, tissue fluids and secretions, develop an affinity for harmful agents during primary infection and they retain this affinity during subsequent infections. The immunoglobulin pool is made up of approximately 75% IgG (found in vascular and intervascular spaces), 15% IgA (in saliva, tears, colostrum, intestinal and bronchial secretions) and 10% IgM (in intravascular spaces). The remainder is made up of IgD found on the surface of B lymphocytes, and IgE on the membrane of mast cells where it interacts with allergens in allergic individuals.

Should any aspect of the complex host immune system be deficient or suppressed, the response elicited to a particular infective agent may be ineffective, leaving the host open to overwhelming and possibly life threatening infection.

Classification of immune deficient states

There are many different congenital immunodeficiency syndromes in existence, usually rare and of little clinical importance to the physiotherapist. More frequently, the physiotherapist in a general hospital will be involved with patients suffering from immunodeficiency or suppression secondary to malignancies, immunosuppressive drugs, chronic disease and, increasingly, human immunodeficiency virus (HIV) infection. These states of immunodeficiency are listed in Table 21.1, however, of greater importance is the understanding of the overall type of deficiency, cellular, humoral or mixed, which in each case may be associated with certain patterns of infection (Table 21.1).

Infective agents

The immunosuppressed or deficient individual may be infected by a range of organisms varying from the more common pathogens, for example *Haemophilus influenzae*, to opportunistic infections which are only pathogenic in the presence of severe immune dysfunction, of which *Pneumocystis carinii* is an example (Table 21.2). Cell-mediated defects leave the host susceptible to infection from viruses, fungi, mycobacteria and protozoa, in contrast to humoral system defects, which are associated with infection by bacteria. Mixed defects will show the complete range of susceptibility, causing a complex clinical situation.

Presenting problems

The severity and extent of the presenting problems will depend on the degree of defect from which the patient suffers. In the Swiss-type agammaglobulinaemia, for example, survival is rarely beyond the second year of life due to overwhelming viral and bacterial infection. The most frequently affected site in immunosuppressed or deficient states is the respiratory tract, with sinusitis and pulmonary infections often recurrent and persistent. Bronchiectasis is a common complication of repeated pulmonary infections; however, abscess and cavity formation, empyemas and pleural effusions may occur.

Otitis media is a frequent complication and skin infections may also be present (bacterial or viral).

Gastrointestinal infections and resultant malabsorption may cause generalized weakness and

Table 21.1   Immunodeficiency states with major types of immune defect

Immunodeficient state	Immune defect	Site*
Congenital		
Swiss-type agammaglobulinanaemia (AGGA)	Immature stem cells	M
Bruton-type AGGA	Immature B cells	H
Di George syndrome	Immature T cells	C
Immunodeficiency with ataxia talangiectasis	Immature T cells	C
Wiskott–Aldrich syndrome	Inability to respond to polysaccharide antigens	H
Partial defects, e.g. types I, III, V and VI dysimmunoglobulinaemia	Altered antibody levels	H
Infections		
HIV/AIDS	T-helper cell destruction	C
Leishmaniasis, malaria	Organism suppresses stem cell function	M
Malignancies		
Lymphomasarcoma	Defective T cells and defective B cell function	M
Hodgkin's disease		
Chronic lymphocytic leukaemia		
Iatrogenic		
Immunosuppressive drugs, e.g. corticosteroid and cytotoxic drugs	Suppressed T cell and B cell function	M
Irradiation therapy		
Organ transplants		
Spleenectomy	Loss of phagocytic activity	M
Other		
Diabetes mellitus	Reduced neutrophil function	M
Uraemia	Reduced lymphocyte function	M
Malnutrition	Reduced T cell and phagocytic activity	C
Chronic disease	Reduced cell proliferation and response	M

*C, cellular immune defect; H, humoral immune defect; M, mixed defect.

Table 21.2   Common opportunistic pathogens with their main clinical features, found in immunocompromised patients

Pathogen	Characteristics
Bacteria	
Streptococcus pneumoniae	Pulmonary: lobar pneumonia, empyema
	Meningitis
	Septic arthritis
	Pericarditis
	Septicaemia
	Otitis media
	Sinusitis
Staphylococcus aureus	Bronchopneumonia
	Abscess formation
	Osteomyelitis
	Endocarditis
	Septic arthritis
	Skin infection
Streptococcus pyogenes	Consolidation with or without pleural disease
	Septicaemia
Klebsiella pneumoniae	Bronchopneumonia with or without abscess, possible septicaemia
Pseudomonas aeruginosa	Common nosocomial infection, e.g. burns, skin sites, central lines, focal with or without septicaemia
Haemophilus influenzae	Bronchopulmonary disease
	Sinusitis
	Otitis media
	Septic arthritis
Legionella pneumophilia	Interstitial pneumonia
Escherichia coli	Colitis with or without septicaemia
Salmonella	Colitis—not self-limiting
Fungi	
Candida albicans	Dermatological
	Oral, oesophageal, bronchial in AIDS
	Disseminated infections in neutropenic patients
Cryptococcus neoformans	Interstitial pneumonitis with haematological spread to meninges, liver, spleen
	Localized at a site as cryptococcoma
Aspergillus funigatus	Necrotizing bronchopneumonia
	Intracavitary fungal growth
	Invasive spread to tissues
	Generalized dissemination
Histoplasmosis	Dermatological
	Disseminated
	Pulmonary with or without cavitation
Nocardia asteroides	Pulmonary: solitary or widespread consolidation
	Disseminated to brain
	Dermatological
Mycobacteria	
Mycobacterium tuberculosis	Pneumonitis
	Systemic
Atypical mycobacteria e.g. *Mycobacterium avium* intracellulare	Low grade disseminated infection pulmonary
Viruses	
Cytomegalovirus	Pneumonitis with patchy diffuse infiltrates
	Enteritis
	Chorioretinitis
Herpes simplex/herpes zoster	Dermatological
	Pulmonary
	Neurological

Table 21.2   *(contd)*

Pathogen	Characteristics
Protozoa	
Pneumocystis carinii	Diffuse interstitial pneumonia
Toxoplasma gondii	Disseminated disease
	Interstitial pneumonitis
	Cerebral abscess, encephalopathy, meningoencephalitis

emaciation. Mobility may be affected by septic arthritis and osteomyelitis, secondary to bacterial infection.

The neurological system does not escape susceptibility, and problems may include meningitis, encephalitis and mental deterioration, peripheral nerve lesions, myelopathy, neuropathy, space-occupying lesions and demyelinating diseases.

The result is that the physiotherapist is often faced with a patient who has multiple, complex problems presenting separately or concurrently. This complexity is highlighted by the acquired immune deficiency syndrome (AIDS) patient, for example, who, as the immune deficiency increases (reflected by decreasing T_4-helper cell levels) shows progressive and fairly unpredictable presentation of increasingly severe infections over all body systems. This can be a challenge for the medical staff, who need to isolate infections and instigate specific treatment regimens to combat each infection to maximal effect.

PHYSIOTHERAPY

The problems a physiotherapist may encounter in this group of patients are many and varied, offering a challenge not only in the short-term problem solving, but also in the achievement of long-term goals which may be very complex.

The physiotherapist should make a detailed assessment of the patient to identify physiotherapy problems and to plan the treatment programme. Accurate documentation will assist in the long-term management of this group of patients, allowing trends to be recognized. The physiotherapist must also be aware of the patient's social situation, occupation, hobbies and functional needs so that treatment goals can be

agreed with the patient. The treatment of physiotherapy problems caused by immunosuppression or deficiencies in children must be modified appropriately.

The following are some of the problems the physiotherapist may find on examination and be required to deal with in patients with immunosuppression or deficiency.

Respiratory problems

In immune deficiency states the respiratory system is the most frequently affected site.

Breathlessness

The degree of breathlessness may vary from breathlessness on exertion to that occurring even at rest, dependent on the extent of the pathology. The main causes include hypoxaemia, pleural effusions, pneumothorax and pneumonia. Pneumocystis carinii pneumonia (PCP) is a major life threatening infection in AIDS patients which causes progressive severe hypoxaemia and breathlessness (Fig. 21.1).

Positioning can be used to optimize ventilation and perfusion. The pattern of breathing control should be encouraged and the use of rest positions, for example high side lying and forward lean sitting.

When hypoxaemia is a major cause of the breathlessness, oxygen therapy is likely to be used. If a venturi system is not used, or a high oxygen concentration is necessary (e.g. 60% and above), high humidity should be considered.

The medical management may include the use of continuous positive airway pressure (CPAP) via a full face mask or nasal mask at approximately 5–10 cmH$_2$O if patients have not responded to

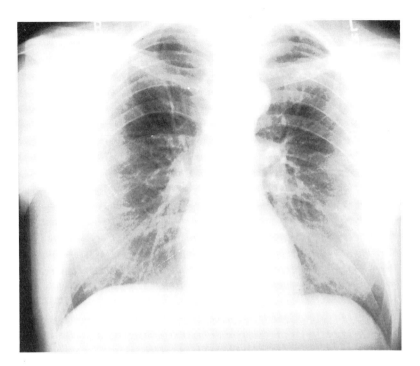

Fig. 21.1   Chest radiograph showing bilateral interstitial shadowing, a classic indication of PCP.

oxygen therapy alone. CPAP has been demonstrated to increase the PaO_2 and decrease breathlessness in cases of PCP in AIDS patients (Kesten & Rebuck 1988, Miller & Mitchell 1990, Miller & Semple 1991), but patients need to be monitored closely.

Patients with suspected PCP who suffer from progressive breathlessness, hypoxaemia and a dry cough may be referred for sputum induction to assist in the diagnosis. Sputum induction involves the nebulization of hypertonic saline (3 – 5%) inhaled from an ultrasonic nebulizer (Fig. 21.2) or efficient jet nebulizer. The mode of action of the hypertonic saline is unclear. Several studies (Bigby et al 1986, Leigh et al 1989) advocate the use of strict protocols to avoid contamination of the sample. The patient may be requested to be 'nil by mouth' overnight, and thorough brushing of the teeth, tongue and gums with rinsing the mouth using large quantities of water or normal saline is important to clear oral debris. The nebulized hypertonic saline should be inhaled for up to 20 minutes, during which time the patient is encouraged to huff and cough until an adequate sample is obtained. Occasionally a sample may be unobtainable.

The sensitivity of sputum induction using an ultrasonic nebulizer ranges from 28 to 94.7% (Bigby et al 1986, Leigh et al 1989, Miller et al 1991) and there is a possibility of serious side effects such as the rapid development of life threatening pleural effusion if a small effusion is already present (Nelson et al 1990). Other adverse effects include breathlessness, nausea and bronchoconstriction (Miller et al 1991). If there is a negative response from sputum induction, fibreoptic bronchoscopy would probably be undertaken. The higher sensitivity of the procedure of bronchoscopy and its minimal side effects have led to its preferred use in some centres (Miller et al 1990).

Excess secretions

This problem is usually caused by a bacterial chest infection or pneumonia. The use of the

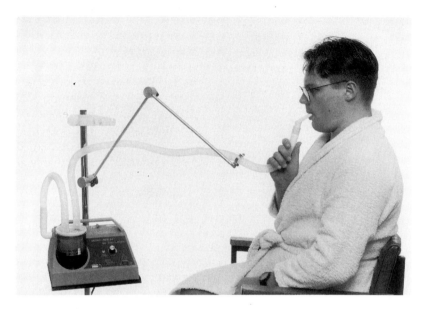

Fig. 21.2   An induced sputum procedure using the Devilbiss Ultra-neb 99 ultrasonic nebulizer.

active cycle of breathing techniques, possibly combined with positioning, vibrations and chest clapping will help to clear excess secretions. The patient should be encouraged to continue the active cycle of breathing techniques as necessary to maintain a clear chest.

Pain

Chest pain may occur in association with pneumonia (pleurisy) or as a result of a chest drain in situ for the treatment of a pneumothorax or pleural effusion. Chest pain may result in a shallow, rapid breathing pattern. Adequate analgesia is essential to allow the patient to breathe more normally and to use the active cycle of breathing techniques. This will reduce the possibility of subsegmental lung collapse and secretion retention as a secondary complication.

Prophylaxis and education

In all immunosuppressed or deficient patients a heightened awareness of developing infection is an asset. Patients can be taught to recognize signs

of respiratory infection, giving them the opportunity not only to report early for medical treatment, but also allowing them to begin self-treatment, for example their breathing exercises, at an early stage. It is useful for patients who develop frequent, recurrent pulmonary infections to be taught the technique of self-postural drainage using the active cycle of breathing techniques and to have these techniques reviewed at regular intervals to ensure effectiveness. Patients who suffer from bronchiectasis will be required to carry out postural drainage at home, on a daily basis, to help prevent further infections.

An area of prophylaxis in which the physiotherapist may become involved is that of supervising or administering nebulized pentamidine isethionate to HIV/AIDS patients to prevent the occurrence of PCP. Pentamidine persists within the lung for long periods of time (Conte & Golden 1988) and therefore two to four weekly dose intervals are appropriate (Leoung et al 1990, Smith et al 1991). The technique involves the administration of a solution of pentamidine dissolved in sterile water, delivered to the patient via an efficient nebulizer and exhalation system (Smaldone et al 1991). In practice, the nebulizer should produce a particle size of $2-5$ μm (maximizing deposition to the alveolar region of the lungs). The exhalation of droplets into the room should be prevented by using a one-way valve system and wide bore tubing out of the window, or an exhalation filter. The efficacy and benefits of this form of prophylaxis have been documented (Smith et al 1991). Side effects are nearly always minimal and local. These may include bronchospasm, increased salivation, cough, unpleasant taste, nausea and a sore throat. The use of a nebulized bronchodilator before the nebulized pentamidine may help to keep the bronchospasm to a minimum (Smith et al 1988). This treatment can be administered as an outpatient procedure, or the patient may be taught to carry out the treatment at home.

Musculoskeletal problems

Pain

Joint and bone pain occur with osteomyelitis and septic arthritis and in these instances contractures could occur as a result of badly positioned limbs, particularly during periods of bed rest. Correct positioning is essential to maintain joint range and muscle extensibility. Joint splinting may be necessary during acute episodes for comfort and to decrease the likelihood of contractures. Ice packs applied to the affected area may help to decrease the pain.

Severe Kaposi sarcoma lesions on the lower limbs in AIDS patients may result in extensive oedema which may cause pain. Patients are inclined to draw their legs up into the flexed position, providing the ideal posture for the development of hip and knee flexion contractures. Advice and explanation on elevation, circulatory exercises and the use of intermittent compression therapy via pumps such as the Multicom pressure therapy unit (Talley Medical Equipment Ltd, UK) may be of some value to help decrease oedema and pain. This should be combined with compression in the form of an elastic lymphoedema stocking to help prevent reoccurrence of the oedema (Badger 1987) and daily passive/active exercise and stretches must also be included in the treatment programme.

Wasting and weakness

Malabsorption is a frequent complication of gastrointestinal infections, chemotherapy or malnutrition. The resultant wasting and weakness can be extremely debilitating, not only in the acute presentation but also as a chronic illness. This will have an effect on physiotherapy regimens as the patient's overall level of tolerance of a physical treatment may be lowered. It is necessary to allow for lethargy and fatigue and to include a generalized exercise programme in the treatment sessions to help build up muscle bulk and strength. The exercise programme should be progressive, and continual reassessment is necessary to judge the correct amount and variety of exercise needed. Imaginative use of equipment both on the ward and in a physiotherapy gymnasium will help to capture and maintain the patient's interest. Advice on on-going exercises and local facilities, for example swimming pools, to continue appropriate levels of activity following discharge is important to reinforce independence and self-care.

Altered tone and coordination

Neurological manifestations of immunosuppression or deficiency are many and varied and may not always fit a predictable pattern. The physiotherapist must treat problems such as spasticity, flaccidity and ataxia as they affect each individual. The techniques the physiotherapist may use are many and varied, but the overall goal should be one of maximal functional gain to achieve the best possible quality of life for each individual.

Mobility

Mobility may be affected not only by weakness, wasting and neurological problems, but also by other complications such as joint contractures. During any episode of immobility it is essential to include the use of passive movements, active-assisted, active or resisted exercises and stretches for the joints and muscles. Where contractures already exist, the use of serial splinting and hold – relax proprioceptive neuromuscular facilitation techniques may help to regain some range of movement in combination with strengthening exercises.

Assessment and provision of walking aids is an important part of achieving and maintaining safe mobility.

Where mobility is limited by breathlessness on exertion, for example in severe bronchiectasis or acute PCP, patients can be taught breathing control on walking and on stair climbing.

Psychological problems

Physiotherapy students rarely receive tuition in counselling. It is important to develop these skills to give the physiotherapist a better understanding and ability to deal more effectively and confidently with the complex emotions and reactions displayed by patients, particularly those with chronic illness and terminal disease. The psychological support that can be provided by offering adequate time and using effective listening skills, can be invaluable to the patient and very rewarding to the physiotherapist.

Immunosuppressed or deficient patients who are suffering from HIV/AIDS may require more support than other groups as they may feel socially rejected and have guilt attached to their illness. This isolation may be compounded by estrangement from their family if they are homosexual or intravenous drug users. Other issues such as risks to employment and insurance,

reinforce the need for confidentiality of the diagnosis and mean that supportive resources in the form of friends and colleagues may be minimal. It is useful for physiotherapists to be aware of appropriate organizations that are available for patients to contact for help or advice.

INFECTION CONTROL

An area of great importance is infection control. Every hospital should have a policy or document on infection control with reference to the prevention of transmission of HIV and hepatitis B virus and guidelines for the use of barrier or isolation nursing in severely immunocompromised individuals. The philosophy and clinical application of universal precautions for infection control is one of the most effective in protecting staff from transmission by 'unknown' carriers of HIV and the hepatitis B virus, and it also addresses the issue of confidentiality. It aims to treat every patient equally and without prejudice (Mullen et al 1989).

CONCLUSION

Immunosuppressed or deficient patients form a challenging group for the physiotherapist. The patients' problems are often complex, but accurate assessment and effective treatment procedures can lead to exciting and rewarding improvements in their quality of life.

REFERENCES

Badger C 1987 Lymphoedema: management of patients with advanced cancer. The Professional Nurse (January): 100–102

Bigby T D, Margolskee D, Curtis J L et al 1986 The usefulness of induced sputum in the diagnosis of Pneumocystis carinii pneumonia in patients with the acquired immunodeficiency syndrome. American Review of Respiratory Disease 133: 515–518

Conte J E, Golden J A 1988 Concentrations of aerosolized pentamidine in bronchoalveolar lavage in patients with AIDS. The Journal of Infectious Diseases 157(5): 985–989

Kesten S, Rebuck A S 1988 Nasal continuous positive airway pressure in *Pneumocystis carinii* pneumonia. Lancet (17 Dec.): 1414–1415

Leigh T R, Hume C, Gazzard B et al 1989 Sputum induction for diagnosis of Pneumocystis carinii pneumonia. Lancet (22 July): 205–206

Leoung G S, Feigal D W, Montgomery A B et al 1990 Aerosolized pentamidine for prophylaxis against

Pneumocystis carinii pneumonia. New England Journal of Medicine 323: 769–775

Miller R F, Mitchell D M 1990 Management of respiratory failure in patients with the acquired immune deficiency syndrome and Pneumocystis carinii pneumonia. Thorax 45: 140–146

Miller R F, Semple S J 1991 Continuous positive airway pressure ventilation for respiratory failure associated with Pneumocystis carinii pneumonia. Respiratory Medicine 85: 133–138

Miller R F, Semple S J G, Kocjan G 1990 Difficulties with sputum induction for diagnosis of Pneumocystis carinii pneumonia. Lancet 335: 112

Miller R F, Kocjan G, Buckland J et al 1991 Sputum induction for the diagnosis of pulmonary disease in HIV positive patients. Journal of Infection 23: 5–15

Mullen R J, Baker E L, Bell D M et al 1989 Guidelines for prevention of transmission of human immunodeficiency virus and hepatitis B virus to health-care workers and public-safety workers. Morbidity and Mortality Weekly Report 38 (suppl 6): 1–37

Nelson M, Bower M, Smith D et al 1990 Life-threatening complication of sputum induction. Lancet 335: 112–113

Smaldone G C, Vinciguerra C, Marchese J 1991 Detection of inhaled pentamidine in health care workers. The New England Journal of Medicine 325 (12): 891–892

Smith D E, Herd D A, Gazzard B G 1988 Reversible bronchoconstriction with nebulised pentamidine. Lancet ii: 905

Smith D E, Hills D A, Harman C et al 1991 Nebulized pentamidine for the prevention of Pneumocystis carinii pneumonia in AIDS patients: experience of 173 patients and a review of the literature. Quarterly Journal of Medicine 79(291): 619–629

Weir D 1977 Immunology—an outline for students of medicine and biology, 4th edn. Churchill Livingstone, Edinburgh, Ch 4, p 79–81

FURTHER READING

Braunwald E, Isselbacher K J, Petersdorf R G et al (eds) 1987 Harrison's principles of internal medicine, 11th edn. McGraw-Hill, New York, part 3, sections 1–9

Hughes W T 1977 Infections in the compromised host. Advances in Internal Medicine 22: 73–96

Pratt R 1991 AIDS, a strategy for nursing care, 3rd edn. Edward Arnold, London

Weir D 1977 Immunology—an outline for students of medicine and biology, 4th edn. Churchill Livingstone, Edinburgh

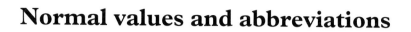

Normal values and abbreviations

NORMAL VALUES

	Heart rate (beats/min)	Respiratory rate (breaths/min)	Blood pressure (mmHg)
Pre-term infants	120–140	40–60	70/40
Full-term infants	100–140	30–40	80/40
1–4 years	80–120	25–30	100/65
Adults	60–100	12–16	95/60–140/90

Conversion tables

1.0 kPa = 0.133 mmHg		pH = 9 – log [H$^+$] where [H$^+$] is in nmol/L	
kPa	mmHg	pH	[H$^+$]
1	7.5	7.52	30
2	15.0	7.45	35
4	30	7.40	40
6	45	7.35	45
8	60	7.30	50
10	75	7.26	55
12	90	7.22	60
14	105	7.19	65

Arterial blood

pH	7.35–7.45 [H$^+$] 45–35 nmol/L
PaO_2	10.7–13.3 kPa (80–100 mmHg)
$PaCO_2$	4.7–6.0 kPa (35–45 mmHg)
HCO_3^-	22–26 mmol/l
Base excess	−2 to +2

Venous blood

pH	7.34–7.42
PO_2	5.0–5.6 kPa (37–42 mmHg)
PCO_2	5.6–6.7 kPa (42–50 mmHg)

Ventilation/perfusion

Alveolar – arterial oxygen gradient A – aPO_2:
Breathing air   0.7–2.7 kPa (5–20 mmHg)
Breathing 100% oxygen   3.3–8.6 kPa (25–65 mmHg)

Pressures

		mmHg	kPa
Right atrial (RA) pressure	Mean	−1 to + 7	−0.13 to 0.93
Right ventricular (RV) pressure	Systolic	15–25	2.0–3.3
	Diastolic	0–8	0–1.0
Pulmonary artery (PA) pressure	Systolic	15–25	2.0 – 3.3
	Diastolic	8–15	1.0–2.0
	Mean	10–20	1.3–2.7
Pulmonary capillary wedge pressure (PCWP)	Mean	6–15	0.8–2.0

Pressures (*contd*)

Central venous pressure (CVP)		3–15 cmH$_2$0
Intracranial pressure (ICP)		<10 mmHg (<1.3 kPa)
Peak inspiratory mouth pressure (*Pi*Max)	Male	103–124 cmH$_2$O (age dependent)
	Female	65–87 cmH$_2$O (age dependent)
Peak expiratory mouth pressure (*Pe*Max)	Male	185–233 cmH$_2$O (age dependent)
	Female	128–152 cmH$_2$O (age dependent)

Blood chemistry

Albumin	37–53 g/l
Calcium (Ca^{2+})	2.25–2.65 mmol/l
Creatinine	60–120 µmol/l
Glucose	4–6 mmol/l
Potassium (K$^+$)	3.4–5.0 mmol/l
Sodium (Na$^+$)	134–140 mmol/l
Urea	2.5–6.5 mmol/l
Haemoglobin (Hb)	14.0–18.0 g/100 ml (men)
	11.5–15.5 g/100 ml (women)
Platelets	150–400 $\times$ 10^9 /l
White blood cell count (WBC)	4–11 $\times$ 10^9 /l
Urine output	1 ml/kg/h

ABBREVIATIONS

A–aDO$_2$	alveolar–arterial oxygen gradient
A–a*P*O$_2$	alveolar–arterial oxygen gradient
ABPA	allergic bronchopulmonary aspergillosis
ADH	antidiuretic hormone
ADL	activities of daily living
AF	atrial fibrillation
AIDS	acquired immune deficiency syndrome
ALS	advanced life support
AP	anteroposterior
ARDS	adult respiratory distress syndrome
ARF	acute renal failure
ASD	atrial septal defect
ATN	acute tubular necrosis
ATPS	ambient temperature and pressure saturated
BIVAD	biventricular device
BLS	basic life support
BP	blood pressure
BPD	bronchopulmonary dysplasia

BSA	body surface area
BTPS	body temperature and pressure saturated
Ca^{2+}	calcium
CO$_2$	carbon dioxide
CABG	coronary artery bypass graft
CAD	coronary artery disease
CAL	chronic airflow limitation
CAVG	coronary artery vein graft
CBF	cerebral blood flow
CF	cystic fibrosis
CFA	cryptogenic fibrosing alveolitis
CFTR	cystic fibrosis transmembrane conductance regulator
CLD	chronic lung disease
cm	centimetre
CMV	controlled mandatory ventilation
CMV	cytomegalovirus
CO	cardiac output
COAD	chronic obstructive airways disease
CPAP	continuous positive airway pressure

CPP	cerebral perfusion pressure		HCO_3^-	bicarbonate
CPR	cardiopulmonary resuscitation		Hct	haematocrit
CRF	chronic renal failure		HD	haemodialysis
CRP	conditioning rehabilitation programme		HDU	high dependency unit
			HFJV	high frequency jet ventilation
CSF	cerebrospinal fluid		HFO	high frequency oscillation
CT	computed tomograph		HFPPV	high frequency positive pressure ventilation
CV	closing volume			
CVP	central venous pressure		HIV	human immunodeficiency virus
			HLT	heart lung transplantation
dl	decilitre		HME	heat and moisture exchanger
DLCO	diffusing capacity for carbon monoxide		Hz	hertz
DNA	deoxyribonucleic acid		IABP	intra-aortic balloon pump
DNR	do-not-resuscitate		ICP	intracranial pressure
DVT	deep vein thrombosis		ICU	intensive care unit
			Ig	immunoglobulin
$ECCO_2R$	extracorporeal carbon dioxide removal		IHD	ischaemic heart disease
			IMV	intermittent mandatory ventilation
ECG	electrocardiograph		in	inches
ECMO	extracorporeal membrane oxygenation		IPPB	intermittent positive pressure breathing
EIA	exercise-induced asthma		IPPV	intermittent positive pressure ventilation
EPP	equal pressure point			
ERV	expiratory reserve volume		IPS	inspiratory pressure support
$ETCO_2$	end-tidal carbon dioxide		IVH	intraventricular haemorrhage
FEF_{50}	forced expiratory flow at 50% of forced vital capacity		JVP	jugular venous pressure
FEF_{75}	forced expiratory flow at 75% of forced vital capacity		K^+	potassium
			KCO	coefficient of gas transfer
FET	forced expiration technique		kg	kilogram
FEV_1	forced expiratory volume in 1 s		kJ	kilojoule
FG	French gauge		kPa	kilopascal
FiO_2	inspired oxygen concentration		kVp	kilovoltage
FRC	functional residual capacity			
ft	feet		L	Litre
FVC	forced vital capacity		l	litre
			LAP	left atrial pressure
g/dl	gram per decilitre		LED	light emitting diode
g	gram		LVAD	left ventricular assist device
GCS	Glasgow coma scale		LVF	left ventricular failure
GPB	glossopharyngeal breathing			
GTN	glyceryl trinitrate		m	metre
			μm	micrometre $(10^{-6}m)$
h	hour		MAP	mean arterial pressure
H_2O	water		MCH	mean corpuscular haemoglobin
Hb	haemoglobin		MCV	mean corpuscular volume

MDI	metered dose inhaler	PCPAP	periodic continuous positive airway pressure
MEF_{50}	maximal expiratory flow at 50% of forced vital capacity	PCV	packed cell volume
MEF_{75}	maximal expiratory flow at 75% of forced vital capacity	PCWP	pulmonary capillary wedge pressure
		PD	peritoneal dialysis
METS	metabolic equivalents	PD	postural drainage
MHz	megahertz	PDA	patient ductus arteriosus
MI	myocardial infarction	Pdi	transdiaphragmatic pressure
MIE	meconium ileus equivalent	PE	pulmonary embolus
min	minute	PEEP	positive end expiratory pressure
ml	millilitre	PEF	peak expiratory flow (rate)
mm	millimetre	PEFR	peak expiratory flow rate
MMAD	mass median aerodynamic diameter	PeMax	peak expiratory mouth pressure
		PEP	positive expiratory pressure
mmHg	millimetres of mercury	pH	hydrogen ion concentration
mmol	millimole	PIE	pulmonary interstitial emphysema
ms	millisecond	PIF	peak inspiratory flow
MVV	maximum voluntary ventilation	PIFR	peak inspiratory flow rate
		PiMax	peak inspiratory mouth pressure
n	number	PIP	peak inspiratory pressure
Na^+	sodium	PND	paroxysmal nocturnal dyspnoea
NEPV	negative extrathoracic pressure ventilation	POMR	problem orientated medical record
		PTB	pulmonary tuberculosis
NICU	neonatal intensive care unit	PTcCO_2	transcutaneous carbon dioxide tension
NIPPV	nasal intermittent positive pressure ventilation	PTFE	polytetrafluoroethylene
nm	nanometre	PVC	polyvinyl chloride
nmol	nanomole	PVH	periventricular haemorrhage
NSAID	non-steroidal anti-inflammatory drug	PVR	pulmonary vascular resistance
		PWC	peak work capacity
O_2	oxygen	$\dot{Q}$	blood flow
OB	obliterative bronchiolitis		
OHFO	oral high frequency oscillation	RAP	right atrial pressure
		R_{AW}	airway resistance
PA	posteroanterior	RBC	red blood cell
PaO_2	partial pressure of oxygen in arterial blood	RDS	respiratory distress syndrome
		REM	rapid eye movement sleep
PAO_2	partial pressure of oxygen in alveolar gas	ROP	retinopathy of prematurity
		RPE	rating of perceived exertion
$PaCO_2$	partial pressure of carbon dioxide in arterial blood	RSV	respiratory syncitial virus
		RV	residual volume
$PACO_2$	partial pressure of carbon dioxide in alveolar gas	RVF	right ventricular failure
PAP	pulmonary artery pressure	s	second
PAWP	pulmonary artery wedge pressure	SA	sinoatrial
PCA	patient controlled analgesia	SaO_2	arterial oxygen saturation
PCD	primary ciliary dyskinesia	S_{GAW}	specific airway conductance
PCP	pneumocystis carinii pneumonia		

SIMV	synchronized intermittent mandatory ventilation	VO_2	oxygen consumption
SOB	shortness of breath	VO_2Max	maximum oxygen consumption
SVO_2	mixed venous oxygen saturation	V_A	alveolar ventilation/alveolar volume
SVC	superior vena cava	VAD	ventricular assist device
		VAS	visual analogue scale
TcO_2	transcutaneous oxygen	VC	vital capacity
$TcCO_2$	transcutaneous carbon dioxide	V_D	dead-space ventilation
TGA	transposition of the great arteries	$\dot{V}_E$	minute ventilation
TLC	total lung capacity	V/Q	ventilation/perfusion ratio
TLCO	transfer factor in lung of carbon monoxide	VSD	ventricular septal defect
		V_T	tidal volume
TV	tidal volume		
		W	watt
$\dot{V}$	ventilation	WBC	white blood count
		WCC	white cell count

Index

Abdominal binders, 361
Abdominal distension, 127, 298
  children, 140, 285–286, 287
    Entonox contraindication, 162
    reduction in lung volume, 199,
      205–206
      management, 206
Abdominal exercises, 248
Abdominal hernias, 245–246
  incisional, 246
  strangulated, 246
Abdominal muscles
  in expiration, 15, 357
  spinal cord injury effects, 358, 359
Accessory inspiratory muscles, 14–15
Acetylcysteine
  cystic fibrosis, 406, 411
  nebulizer inhalation, 147
Acid-base balance
  blood gases, 54, 55, 76
  carbon dioxide carriage, 54
Acidosis
  metabolic, 76
    arterial blood gases, 76–77
    following cardiac surgery, 260
    hyperventilation/Kussmaul
      breathing, 10, 14, 77
    treatment, 77
    ventilatory response, 219
  respiratory, 77
Acquired immune deficiency syndrome
    (AIDS) see Human
    immunodeficiency virus (HIV)
    infection/AIDS
Active cycle of breathing techniques,
    116, 118–121, 184, 223
  applications, 121–127
  asthma, 215, 393, 394
    acute attack, 303
  bronchiectasis, 400, 402
  bronchitis
    acute, 225
    chronic, 225–226
  with chest compression see Chest
    compression
  with chest shaking see Chest shaking
  with chest vibrations see Chest
    vibration
  children, 288, 308, 314

chronic airflow limitation, 218
collapse (atelectasis), 205
  pertussis-associated, 305
cystic fibrosis, 409, 415
emphysema, 226
fibrotic lung conditions, 212, 218
following fractured femur in elderly,
  247
forced expiration technique, 119–121
Guillain–Barré syndrome, 271
immunodeficient patients, 424
ineffective cough, 224
lobectomy patients, 253–254
lung abscess, 227
myasthenia gravis, 270
pneumonia, 227
position, 121
  see also Gravity-assisted positions
postoperative, 203
  cardiac surgery, 261, 262, 314
  cardiopulmonary transplantation,
    353, 355
  children, 308, 314
preoperative instruction, 203, 243
primary ciliary dyskinesia, 403
pulmonary oedema with infection,
  227
respiratory muscle weakness, 213
revision of technique, 121–122
self treatment, 121
thoracic expansion exercises, 116,
  118–119
treatment session end-point, 121
Acupuncture, 229
Acute Physiology and Chronic Health
  Evaluation II (APACHE II),
  237
Adenovirus bronchiolitis, 303
Adrenaline, advanced life support,
  96–97
Adult respiratory distress syndrome
  (ARDS), 83, 276–277
  acid-base status, 77
  cardiac catheterization, 71
  clinical features, 276
  extracorporeal carbon dioxide
    removal, 87
  gas exchange impairment, 219
  imaging, postoperative, 41–42

with inhalational burns, 275–276
management, 219
mechanical ventilation, 85
pathology, 276
physiotherapy, 277
precipitating factors, 276
pulmonary oedema, 209
Advanced life support, 96–97
  airway, 96
  breathing, 96
  circulatory support, 96
  defibrillation/sternal thump, 97
  drugs, 96–97
  electrocardiogram (ECG), 97
Advanced multiple beam equalization
  radiography (AMBER), 24
Aerosol particles, 142
  deposition in bronchial tree, 142
Agammaglobulinaemia, Swiss-type,
  420
Air bronchogram, 31
Air compressors
  domiciliary nebulization, 147
  patient education, 184
Air embolism, 70–71, 91, 219
Air trapping, chest radiography, 31
Airflow limitation, chronic
  acid-base status, 77
  breathlessness, 215–218
    bronchospasm, 217
    causes, 215–216
    exercise programme, 166
    management, 216–218
    type A (pink puffer), 216
    type B (blue bloater), 216
  with cardiac failure, 220
  Chronic Respiratory Questionnaire
    (CRQ), 59
  hyperinflation, 215, 216
    signs, 216
  inguinal hernia, 246
  mechanical ventilation, 85
  mucus secretions viscosity, 150
  nebulized bronchodilators, 145, 148
  pulsus paradoxus, 10
  risk of cardiac/respiratory arrest, 93
  thoracic imaging, 45–46
Airway function tests, 48–51
  in children, 57–58

Airway function tests (*contd*)
  flow–volume curves, 48, 49
  peak expiratory flow (PEF), 48, 49, 51
  spirometry (FEV1 and FVC), 48–49
Airway obstruction
  flow–volume curve, 49
  spirometry, 48–49
  ventilatory failure, 54
  wheezes, 18
Airway suction, 159–162
  catheter size, 159, 162
  children, 289
    cardiac surgery, 313, 314
  Guillain–Barré syndrome, 271
  head injured patients, 269, 270
  inhalational burns, 276
  intubated patient, 159–160
  manual hyperinflation, 157
  minitracheostomy, 161–162
  monitoring, 160
  myasthenia gravis, postoperative
    care, 270
  poliomyelitis, 273
  saline instillation, 160, 162, 289
  sputum specimen, 160
  tetanus, 272
  tracheal epithelial damage, 159
  vacuum pressure, 159
  see also Tracheal suction
Alanine aminotransferase (ALT), 78
  ischaemic hepatitis, 79
Alcohol abuse, 241
Alkaline phosphatase (ALP), 78
Alkalosis
  metabolic, 77
    ventilatory response, 219
  respiratory, 77
Allergic bronchopulmonary
    aspergillosis, 390, 395, 396
  bronchiectasis, 45, 224, 396, 399
  with cystic fibrosis, 406, 415
  medical management, 396
  physiotherapy, 396
Alveolar ventilation, 53
Ambulation, early
  asthma, severe acute, 395
  cardiac rehabilitation, 320
  fractured femur in elderly, 247
  laparoscopic cholecystectomy, 244
  postoperative, 242, 243
    aortic aneurysm, 265
    cardiac surgery, 261, 314
    children, 309, 314
    lobectomy, 254
    lower limb vascular reconstructive
      surgery, 265
    pelvic surgery, 248
Aminophylline, 392
Amniotic fluid embolus, 219
Amputation, lower limb, 265
Anaemia
  breathlessness, 5
  causes, 75
  cyanosis, 12
  eye examination, 12

haemoglobin (Hb), 75
mean corpuscular volume (MCV),
  75
Anaerobic threshold, 60
Anaesthesia, epidural, 238
Anaesthesia, general, 238
  with alcohol abuse, 241
  bronchial secretion effects, 238
  cough reflex failure, 223
  diabetes mellitus, 241
  lung function impairment, 57, 238
  postoperative pulmonary collapse,
    41
  reduction in lung volume, 199, 200
Anaesthesia, local, 238
  with rib fracture, 265
Anaesthesia, regional, 238
Anaesthesia, spinal, 238
Analgesia, 162–164
  administration routes, 229
  head injured patients, 269
  inhalational burns, 275, 276
  lung cancer, 371–372
  measurement of efficacy, 229
  nebulized drugs, 146–147
  patient controlled (PCA), 229
  penetrating chest injury, 267
  postoperative *see* Postoperative pain
    relief
  rib fracture, 265
  sputum retention, 223
Anatomical variants, posteroanterior
    radiograph, 29
Angina, 7, 229–230, 322
  anxiety, 173
  Canadian Cardiovascular Society
    classification, 325
  duration, 322
  during cardiac rehabilitation
    programme, 331, 332–333
  exercise electrocardiogram, 64
  exercise tolerance, 221
  intensity, 322
  location, 322
  management, 259
  precipitatng factors, 322
  quality, 322
  stable, 229, 322
  unstable, 229, 322
    intra-aortic balloon pump, 88
Angiography, 64–65
Anterolateral thoracotomy incision,
  252
Anteroposterior (AP) radiograph, 23,
  30
Antibiotic therapy
  acute epiglottitis, 306
  bronchiectasis, 400, 402
  bronchiolitis, 304
  chronic airflow limitation, 217
  chronic lung disease
    (bronchopulmonary dysplasia),
    301
  collapse (atelectasis), 205
  cystic fibrosis, 406, 411

implanted venous access devices,
  415
fibrotic lung conditions, 212
infection with gas exchange
  impairment, 219
nebulized, 144, 145–146, 402, 406,
  411
  associated airflow obstruction, 146
  solutions, 146
pertussis, 305
pneumonia, 227
  children, 305
preterm/low birth weight infants, 295
primary ciliary dyskinesia, 403
sputum retention, 223
Anticholinergic therapy, 302, 392
Anticholinesterases, 270
Anticoagulants
  deep vein thrombosis, 242
  pulmonary embolism, 220
Antifungal agents, nebulized, 146
Antihypertensive agents, 6
α_1-Antitrypsin deficiency, 216
Anxiety
  breathlessness, 173, 221
  cardiorespiratory patient, 173–174,
    221
  postoperative, 241, 242
Aortic aneurysm, 127, 264
  dissection, 230, 264
  postoperative physiotherapy,
    264–265
  surgery, 264
Aortic stenosis/regurgitation, 309, 313
  heart sounds, 19
  surgery, 313
    exercise performance following,
      335–336
Aortopulmonary window, 28
Apnoea, 14
  neonate/infants, 282, 283, 284
Arm exercises
  cardiac rehabilitation, 328
  following aortic aneurysm surgery,
    265
  lobectomy patients, 254
  thoracoplasty patients, 257
Arrhythmias, 73
  electrocardiography, 64
    monitoring, 72, 74
  following cardiac surgery, 260
  following lung surgery, 256
  hypo/hyperkalaemia, 78
  postoperative cardiac pacing, 11
  pulse deficit, 10
  risk of cardiac arrest, 93
Arterial blood gases, 54–55
  acid-base balance, 55
    metabolic acidosis, 76–77
  interpretation, 20, 76–77
  oxygen therapy monitoring, 153
  postoperative oxygen saturation, 202
Arterial blood pressure monitoring, 70
Arterial cannulation, 11
  catheter insertion, 70

complications, 70
invasive monitoring, 69, 70
Arterial embolisation, 26, 27
Arteriography
bronchial, 26–27
pulmonary, 26
Ascites
cardiac failure, 220
reduction in lung volume, 206
Aspartate aminotransferase (AST), 78
cardiac enzyme estimation, 79
with ischaemic hepatitis, 78
Aspergilloma, 396–397
Aspergillus, 395–397
allergic bronchopulmonary
aspergillosis, 45, 224, 390, 395,
396, 399, 406, 415
aspergilloma, 396–397
invasive aspergillosis, 397
Aspiration
with drug overdose, 274
head injured patients, 269
intensive care patient, 9
postoperative imaging, 41
recurrent cough, 6
Aspirin, 372
Assessment, 3–22, 199
apparatus, 11–12
arterial blood gases, 20
blood pressure, 10
body temperature, 9–10
body weight, 10–11
breathing pattern, 14
breathlessness, 5–6
chest auscultation, 17–20
chest movement, 14–15
chest observation, 13–16
chest pain, 7
chest radiographs, 20
cough, 6
cyanosis, 12
exercise tolerance, 19–20
eyes, 12
fever, 7
functional limitation, 8–9, 19–20
general observation, 9
hands, 12
headache, 8
heart rate, 10
jugular venous pressure, 12–13
objective, problem orientated
medical records (POMR), 9–20
palpation, 15–16
peripheral oedema, 8, 13
pulse rate, 10
respiratory rate, 10
spirometry, 20
sputum, 6–7, 19
subjective, problem orientated
medical records (POMR), 5–9
test results evaluation, 20
wheeze, 7
Asterixis (flapping tremor), 213
Asthma
acid-base status, 77

active cycle of breathing techniques
121
acute severe attack, 303, 390, 392,
394–395
adult, 389–397
airflow limitation
chronic, 45
measurement, 390
monitoring, 393
airway function tests, 48, 49, 51
domiciliary/occupational PEF
measurement, 49
allergic bronchopulmonary
aspergillosis, 390, 395, 396
anxiety, 173
atopic/non-atopic, 389
breathlessness, 6, 215, 393, 394
exercise programme, 166
paroxysmal nocturnal dyspnoea, 6
brittle, 390
bronchial secretions clearance
impairment, 226, 393
bronchospasm, 215
chest radiograph, 45
chest wall pain, 228
children, 301–303
acute attack, 303
cause, 302
management, 302–303
pathology, 302
physiotherapy, 303
classification, 389–390
clinical features, 389, 390
episodic, 390
persistent, 390
with cystic fibrosis, 406, 413
exercise-induced, 215, 303, 389–
390, 393
management, 392
extrinsic/intrinsic, 389
gas exchange impairment, 54
intermittent positive pressure
breathing (IPPB), 136, 138,
141
investigations, 390–392
airflow obstruction measurement,
390
arterial blood gases, 390–391
assessment, 390
bronchial challenge tests, 391–392
chest radiograph, 391
cold air test, 392
exercise provocation test, 392
haematology, 391
skin-prick tests, 391–392
sputum, 391
irreversible, 390
mechanical ventilation, 85
medical management, 392
morning dipper, 390
nebulized bronchodilators, 145, 148,
149
nebulized corticosteroids/
prophylactic drugs, 145
nocturnal cough, 6

occupational, 390
pathogenesis, 389
pathological features, 389
patient education, 392, 393
pectus carinatum (pigeon chest),
14
periodic continuous positive airway
pressure (PCPAP), 141
physiotherapy, 392–395
evaluation, 395
postoperative respiratory
complications, 240
preventive advice, 199
provocative agents, 389
St George's Questionnaire, 59
wheeze, 18, 393, 394
Ataxic breathing, 14
Atelectasis *see* Collapse of lung tissue
Athletes, heart rate, 10
Atrial fibrillation, 73
pulse deficit, 10
Atrial septal defect (ASD), 309, 310
surgery, 258, 310
exercise tolerance following, 337
Atrioventricular septal defect, 310
Atropine, advanced life support, 96
Audit, 22
Autogenic drainage, 132
Autohaler, 143
Axonotmesis, 268
Azygo-oesophageal recess line, 29
Azygos vein enlargement, 29

Barotrauma, ventilator-induced, 41,
42, 86
Baseline dyspnoea index, 195
Basic life support, 94–96
airway, 94–95
breathing, 95–96
circulation, 96
one-rescuer, CPR 96
two-rescuer, CPR 96
Bennett ventilators, 136
Bereavement process, 367–371
Beta$_2$ agonists
asthma, 303, 392
mucociliary clearance stimulation,
222
nebulized bronchodilators, 145
Beta blocking agents, 73
advanced life support, 97
cardiovascular effects, 10, 323–324
cough, 6
monitoring level of exercise, 332
side effects, 324
Bicarbonate, plasma, 76, 77
Bicycle ergometry
cardiac rehabilitation, 326
cardiopulmonary transplantation
postoperative care, 353
cystic fibrosis, 412
lobectomy patients, 254
Bilirubin plasma levels, 78
Biochemical investigations, 76–79
normal values, 432

Biopsy, lung
  fluoroscopic/CT guidance, 25, 38
  open, 255
  percutaneous needle, 26, 38
Bird ventilator, 135, 136, 137, 139
Birth asphyxia, 293, 296
Blalock–Taussig shunt, 259, 311
Blood cultures, 79
Blood gases
  asthma, 390–391
  bronchiolitis, 304
  normal values, 431
  see also Arterial blood gases
Blood glucose, 78
Blood pressure, 10
  following cardiac surgery, 259, 261
  measurement, 10
  monitoring, 67, 68
    cardiac rehabilitation exercise
      programme, 332
    invasive, 69, 70–71
    neonate/children, 292
  normal values, 431
Blue bloater (type B) chronic airflow
    limitation, 216, 217
Body mass index (BMI), 10–11
Body temperature
  children, 284
  monitoring, 67–68
  objective assessment, 9–10
  preterm/low birth weight infants, 295
Body weight
  daily weight, 11
  objective assessment, 10–11
Bomb blast injuries, 267
Bonchial lavage, children, 289
Bordetella pertussis, 304
Borg rating of perceived exertion
    (RPE) scale, 214, 326, 332
  cardiac rehabilitation exercise
      programme monitoring, 329,
      332
  cardiopulmonary transplantation
      rehabilitation, 354
Bradycardia, 10
  infants, 283, 284
Bradypnoea, 10
Brain damage
  breathing patterns, 14
  complicating cardiac surgery, 261
  following cardiopulmonary
      resuscitation, 93, 97
  head injury, 268–269
Breath sounds
  bronchial, 17–18
  diminished, 18
  normal, 17
  vesicular, 17
Breath-actuated pressurized inhaler,
    143
Breathing control, 113–116, 184
  asthma, 215, 303, 393, 395
  breathlessness, 115, 116, 221
  bronchiectasis, 402
  bullous emphysema, 256

cardiac failure, 221
cardiopulmonary transplantation
    postoperative care, 353
  children, 288, 303
  chronic airflow limitation, 217
  cystic fibrosis, 409, 410, 413
  definition, 113
  exercise tolerance effect, 116
  fibrotic lung conditions, 212, 218
  immunodeficient states, 426
  lung cancer management, 253
  pleural disorders, 218
  pneumonectomy patients, 256
  positions facilitating, 115–116
  preoperative instruction, 243
  teaching patient, 113–114
Breathing exercises
  chest injury, 267
  children, 288
  hyperventilation syndrome,
      381–382
    home therapy, 386
  postoperative
    aortic aneurysm surgery, 264
    cardiac surgery, 261
    pneumonectomy, 255
  spinal cord injury, 360
Breathing pattern assessment, 14
Breathlessness, 213–221
  allergic bronchopulmonary
      aspergillosis, 396
  anxiety, 173
  asthma, 390, 393, 394
  baseline dyspnoea index, 195
  breathing control, 115, 116, 221
  bronchiectasis, 401–402
  bronchospasm, 215
  cardiac failure, 220–221
  cardiopulmonary rehabilitation
    exercise programme, 166–167,
      332
    outcome, 165
  chronic airflow limitation, 215–218
  cystic fibrosis, 406, 413
  definition, 214
  duration, 5
  exercise tolerance, 19
  fear/anxiety, 221
  fibrotic lung conditions, 218
  immunodeficient states, 422–423,
      426
  impaired gas exchange, 219
  length-tension inappropriateness
      theory, 214
  lung cancer, 253, 373
  lung function tests, 214
  obesity, 205
  orthopnoea, 6
  oxygen cost diagram, 195
  paroxysmal nocturnal dyspnoea, 6
  pathophysiology, 5
  pleural disorders, 207, 218
  pulmonary embolism, 219–220
  pulmonary oedema, 211
  quantification, 195, 214–215

respiratory muscle weakness, 212,
    218–219
  visual analogue scale, 219
  severity, 5
    New York Heart Association
        grading, 6
  subjective assessment, 5–6
Bronchi, posteroanterior radiograph,
    28
Bronchial challenge tests, 392
Bronchial rupture, 266
Bronchial secretions clearance,
    221–228
  active cycle of breathing techniques,
      116, 118, 119, 223
    gravity-assisted positions, 126
  allergic bronchopulmonary
      aspergillosis, 396
  asthma, 393, 394
    childhood, acute attack, 303
  bronchiectasis, 400–401
    with acute exacerbation of
        infection, 402
  chest clapping, 123
  children, 288–289, 303, 305, 317
  chronic airflow limitation, 217–218
  ciliary clearance mechanism, 222
  cough/expectoration in clearance,
      222
  cystic fibrosis, 408–411
  Flutter VRP1, 134
  glossopharyngeal breathing, 132
  Guillain–Barré syndrome, 271
  head injury, 269
    in children, 317
  humidification, 150, 152
  immunodeficient patients, 423–424
  impairment, 222–228
    see also Sputum retention
  inhalational burns, 276
  intermittent positive pressure
      breathing (IPPB), 136, 138, 139
  lobectomy patients, 254
  lung cancer management, 253
  manual hyperinflation, 157
  with multiple trauma, 268
  myasthenia gravis, 270
  periodic continuous positive airway
      pressure (PCPAP), 141
  pneumonectomy patients, 255
  poliomyelitis, 273
  positioning patient, 103–104
  positive expiratory pressure (PEP)
      technique, 132–134
  postoperative, 203
    cardiac surgery, 261
  spinal cord injury, 360–361
  tetanus, 272–273
Bronchial tree trauma, 266
Bronchiectasis, 399–402
  active cycle of breathing techniques,
      121
  allergic bronchopulmonary
      aspergillosis, 45, 224, 396, 399
  bronchial arteriography, 27

bronchial secretions clearance
  impairment, 224–225
  stimulation, 222
bronchography, 400
causes, 399
chest radiograph, 43
chronic mucopurulent rhinosinusitis,
  399, 400
clinical features, 399
computed tomography, 26, 43, 45
cough, 6
pain-associated inhibition, 224
with cystic fibrosis, 224, 225, 406
immunodeficient patients, 420, 424,
  426
inspiratory crackles, 18
investigations, 399–400
medical management, 400
mucus secretions viscosity, 150
physiotherapy, 400–402
  acute exacerbation of infection,
    402
  breathlessness, 401–402
  evaluation, 402
  excess bronchial secretions,
    400–401
  postoperative respiratory
    complications, 240
  thoracic imaging, 43–45
  topical medications, 400
Bronchiolitis, 303–304
  causal agents, 303
  clinical features, 304
  management, 304
  pathology, 303–304
  physiotherapy, 304
Bronchitis, acute, 225
Bronchitis, chronic
  active cycle of breathing techniques,
    121
  acute exacerbation, 225–226
  airway function, 48, 49
  bronchial secretions clearance
    impairment, 225–226
  cardiopulmonary rehabilitation
    exercise programme, 166
  cough, 6
    ineffective, 223
    pain-associated inhibition, 224
  nasotracheal suction, 161
  oral high frequency oscillation
    technique, 135
  postoperative respiratory
    complications, 41, 240
  reactive depression, 174
  sputum retention, 223
  see also Airflow limitation, chronic
Bronchoalveolar lavage, 79
Bronchodilators
  allergic bronchopulmonary
    aspergillosis, 396
  asthma, 215, 302, 303, 392
    severe acute, 394, 395
  bronchiectasis, 400, 402
  bronchiolitis, 304

bronchitis, acute, 225
bronchitis, chronic, 226
chronic airflow limitation, 217
chronic lung disease
  (bronchopulmonary dysplasia),
  301
cystic fibrosis, 406, 411, 415
heart rate response, 10
inhalational burns, 275, 276
intermittent positive pressure
  breathing (IPPB) delivery, 136,
  138, 141
lobectomy patients, 254
nebulized, 144, 145, 415
  response studies for assessment,
    148–149
  solutions, 145
  sputum retention, 223
  tremor, 12
Bronchography, 400
Bronchopleural fistula, 256
Bronchopneumonia, 226
Bronchopulmonary dysplasia see
  Chronic lung disease
Bronchopulmonary nomenclature, 127
Bronchoscopy
  bronchiectasis, 399
  immunodeficient patients, 423
Bronchospasm
  anxiety, 173
  asthma, 215
  breathlessness, 215
  with chronic airflow limitation, 217
  inhalational burns, 275, 276
  management, 215
  wheezes, 18
Bruce Exercise Test protocol, 326
Bubble-through humidifiers, 152, 154
Bullous emphysema, 45, 46
  surgery, 256
Bupivacaine, 238
Burns, inhalational, 274–276
  adult respiratory distress syndrome
    (ARDS), 275–276
  analgesia, 275, 276
  chemical injury, 274
  Curling's ulcer, 243
  heat injury, 274
  hypoxia, 274–275
  medical management, 275–276
  nutritional support, 275
  physiotherapy, 276
  pneumonia, 274, 276
  restrictive pulmonary dysfunction,
    275

Calcium antagonists, 97
Calcium chloride, 97
Candidiasis prevention, 143
Cape Minor ventilator, 139
Carbenicillin, 146
Carbon dioxide
  arterial blood values, 431
  carriage in blood, 54
  elimination, 101

retention, 12, 101
  chronic bronchitis, 226
  ineffective cough, 223
  with sputum retention, 223
  ventilatory response, 219
Carbon monoxide poisoning, 275
Carbon monoxide transfer test
  (TLCO), 53
Cardiac arrest, 93, 322
  exercise programme-associated,
    333
  preventable deaths, 93
  recognition, 94
  resuscitation see Cardiopulmonary
    resuscitation
  risk situations, 93
Cardiac catheterization, 64
  congenital heart disease, 310
Cardiac enzymes, 79
Cardiac failure
  breathlessness, 220–221
  cardiac rehabilitation, 334–335
  causes, 220, 334
  cystic fibrosis, 407
  definition, 62
  downward chest tilted position
    contraindication, 127
  electrocardiogram (ECG), 64
  exercise tolerance, 221
  fatigue, 220, 221
  heart size, 43, 62
  heart sounds, 19
  imaging, 31, 62
    postoperative, 42–43
    supine, 42
  jugular venous pressure, 13
  management, 221
  nocturnal cough, 6
  orthopnoea, 220–221
  paroxysmal nocturnal dyspnoea
    (PND), 220–221
  peripheral oedema, 13
  pleural effusion, 43, 207
    management, 208
    reduction in lung volume, 220
  preoperative care, 240
  pulmonary oedema, 43, 220
  with respiratory muscle weakness,
    220
  wheeze, 7
Cardiac function, 61–65
  assessment
    cardiac catheterization, 64–65
    electrocardiography, 64
  electrical, 64
  haemodynamic, 64–65
  patient mobilization effect, 105
Cardiac imaging, 62–63
  ejection fraction measurement, 63
  radiography
    lateral view, 29
    posteroanterior view, 28
Cardiac output
  following cardiac surgery, 260
  measurement, 65, 71

Cardiac pacing, postoperative
    apparatus, 11
    radiographic check of wires, 40
Cardiac rehabilitation, 165–167, 262,
        319–339
    aims, 165
    cardiac drug effects, 323–324, 325
    with cardiac failure, 334–335
    cardiac risk factor reduction, 324, 327
    cardiopulmonary transplantation
        postoperative care, 354–355
    clinician assessment of work
        capacity, 327
    compliance, 337–338
    complications of exercise, 333
    with congenital heart disease,
        repaired, 336–337
    cost effectiveness, 338–339
    current functional level estimation,
        325–327
        Canadian Cardiovascular Society
            scale, 325
        exercise testing, 325–327
        Old New York Heart Association
            criteria, 325
    desired functional level, 327
    early ambulation, 320
    education, 321
    exercise training, 166–167, 320–321
        with beta adrenergic blocking
            agents, 323–324
        with nitrates, 324
        with vasodilators, 324
    following cardiac surgery, 323
    goals, 319
    group activities, 167
    informed consent, 339
    legal aspects, 339
    occupational/recreational activities,
        325
    in older patient, 334
    outcome evaluation, 165, 333, 338
    physiotherapy, 319–320, 324–333
        assessment, 324–327
        following hospital discharge,
            329–330
        in hospital, 329
        monitoring level of exercise,
            331–333
        recording, 327, 331
        treatment, 327–329
    policies/procedures, 339
    psychological support, 321
    recovery phases, 329–333
    secondary prevention, 321
    staffing, 339
    standard of care, 339
    team approach, 319
    with valvular heart disease, 335–336
    very sick patient, 165–166
Cardiac reserve estimation, 65
Cardiac risk factors
    reduction with rehabilitation
        programme, 324, 327
Cardiac surgery, 258–262, 323

activity following discharge, 262
cardioplegia, 259
cardiopulmonary bypass, 258, 259
children
    postoperative physiotherapy,
        313–314
    postoperative pulmonary
        hypertensive crises, 314
    preoperative physiotherapy, 313
complications, 260–261
    cardiovascular, 260
    cerebral injury, 261
    renal failure, 260–261
    respiratory, 260
    wound, 261
incisions, 259
physiotherapy, 261–262
postoperative lung function, 202,
    205
postoperative management, 259–260,
    323
postoperative observations, 261
Cardiac tamponade, 323
    blunt chest injury, 266
    complicating cardiac surgery, 260
    complicating central catheter
        placement, 40
    multiple trauma, 267
Cardiogenic shock
    cardiac catheterization, 71
    intra-aortic balloon pump, 88
Cardioplegia, 259
Cardiopulmonary bypass, 258, 259
    cerbral injury following, 261
    weaning
        intra-aortic balloon pump, 88
        ventricular assist device, 89
Cardiopulmonary rehabilitation,
        165–167
Cardiopulmonary resuscitation, 93–98
    advanced life support, 96–97
    basic life support, 94–96
    basic principles, 95
    Do-not-resuscitate (DNR) order, 98
    ethical aspects, 98
    hypothermic patients, 98
    neurological outcome, 93, 97
    stopping, 97–98
    witholding criteria, 97
Cardiopulmonary transplantation,
        343–355
    central coordination procedures, 344
    children, 314–315
    cough reflex following, 349, 353
    donor-recipient matching, 344
    donors, 344–345
    exercise response following, 349–350
    heart/heart-lung denervation,
        349–350
    immunosuppression, 314, 347, 348,
        349, 350
    infection complicating, 347–348,
        349, 350, 355
    multidisciplinary team approach, 348
    physiotherapy, 350–355

postoperative care, 346, 352–355
    acute care, 352–354
    rehabilitation, 354–355
preoperative care, 351–352
    conditioning-rehabilitation
        programme, 351, 352
recipient assessment, 343–344, 351
rejection, 346–347, 350, 355
    acute, 347
    chronic, 347
    diagnosis, 347
Cardiothoracic ratio, 28
Cardiovascular medications, 323–324
Cardiovascular support, 9, 88–89
    intra-aortic balloon pump, 88
    ventricular assist device, 88–89
Cardioversion, electrical, 79
Ceftazidime, 146
Cell-mediated immunity, 419
Censuses, research, 192
Central venous catheter, 11, 70
    complications, 70–71
    radiographic check of position, 40
Central venous pressure (CVP)
    following cardiac surgery, 259, 260
    monitoring, 11, 70
        catheter insertion, 70
        intensive care patient, 11
    normal values, 432
Cerebellar disease, 14
Cerebral aneurysm, 127
Cerebral oedema, 127
Cerebral perfusion pressure (CPP)
    measurement, 72
    monitoring in head injured patients,
        269
Chest auscultation, 17–20
    breath sounds, 17–18
    crackles, 18
    heart sounds, 19
    infants/children, 285
    pleural rub, 18–19
    vocal resonance, 19
    wheezes, 18
Chest clapping, 122–124
    bronchiectasis, 400
    children
        acute asthma, 303
        cardiac surgery, 313, 314
        head injury, 317
        pneumonia, 305
        postoperative, 309
    contraindications, 124
    cystic fibrosis, 408, 409, 413
    hypoxaemia, 123, 124
        oximeter monitoring, 124
    immunodeficient patients, 424
    pertussis-associated lobar collapse,
        305
    self treatment, 122
    spinal cord injury, 363
    with thoracic expansion exercises,
        123, 124
Chest compression, 125–126
    cystic fibrosis, 413

with manual hyperinflation, 157
myasthenia gravis, 270
self-treatment, 125
Chest observation, 13–15
palpation, 15–16
paradoxical breathing, 15
percussion, 16
shape, 13–14
surface landmarks, 13
surgical emphysema, 15–16
vocal fremitus, 16
Chest pain, 8, 228–230
chest wall, 164, 228, 246, 255, 262
immunodeficient patients, 424
management, 228–229
non-respiratory, 229–230
angina, 229–230
aortic dissection, 230
gall bladder disease, 230
neuromuscular, 230
oesophageal, 230
peptic ulcer disease, 230
pericarditis, 230
pleural pain, 228
subjective assessment, 7
tracheobronchial tree, 228
Chest percussion, 16, 127
children, 286
chronic lung disease
(bronchopulmonary dysplasia),
301
meconium aspiration, 296
Chest radiography, 23–25
advanced multiple beam equalization
radiography (AMBER), 24
asthma, 391
bronchiectasis, 399
cardiac failure, 31, 42–43, 62
cardiac imaging, 62
cavitating pulmonary lesions, 39
collapse (atelectasis), 32–33
consolidation, 31–32
decreased density hemithorax, 36–37
documentary information, 30
elevation of diaphragm, 37
evaluation, 20
factors influencing quality, 24–25
intensive care patient, 24
interpretation, 30–31
patient rotation, 31
projection, 30
review areas, 31
state of expiration/inspiration, 31
supine versus erect position, 30–31
kyphoscoliosis, 43
normal chest, 27–31
common anatomical variants, 29
lateral view, 29–30
posteroanterior view, 27–29
opaque hemithorax, 36
phosphor plate, 24, 25
pleural disease, 37–38
pneumothorax, 35
portable films, 23
pulmonary mass, 38

pulmonary nodule, 38–39
views, 23
Chest shaking, 124–125, 126
bronchiectasis, 400
bronchitis, chronic, 226
children, 286
cough reflex impairment, 223, 224
cystic fibrosis, 413
drug overdose, 274
Guillain–Barré syndrome, 271
head injured patients, 269
with manual hyperinflation
treatment, 126
myasthenia gravis, postoperative
care, 270
poliomyelitis, 273
self-treatment, 125
spinal cord injury, 363
tetanus, 272
with thoracic expansion exercises, 124
Chest shape, 13–14
Chest surface landmarks, 13
Chest trauma, 265–267
blunt, 265–266
mechanical ventilation, 85
cardiac enzymes, 79
penetrating, 266–267
see also Chest wall trauma
Chest vibration, 124–125, 126
children, 286
cardiac surgery, 314
cystic fibrosis, 408
head injured patients, 269
immunodeficient patients, 424
with manual hyperinflation, 126
self-treatment, 125
spinal cord injury, 363
with thoracic expansion exercises,
124
Chest wall
movement assessment, 14–15
muscle function tests, 51–53
posteroanterior radiograph, 29
respiratory function, 51
surgery, 256–257
Chest wall deformity
intermittent positive pressure
breathing (IPPB), 139
nasal intermittent positive pressure
ventilation (NIPPV), 85
postoperative respiratory
complications, 240
Chest wall pain, 7, 224, 228
lobectomy patients, 255
manual therapy techniques, 164
postoperative, 246
cardiac surgery, 262
Chest wall trauma
management, 208
mobility exercises, 208
paradoxical breathing, 15
pneumothorax, 208
Cheyne-Stokes respiration, 14
cardiac failure, 221
Chlormethiazole, 241

Cholecystectomy, 243–244
laparoscopic, 244
open, 244
physiotherapy, 244
postoperative complications, 244
Chronic obstructive airways disease
(COAD) see Airflow limitation,
chronic
Chronic Respiratory Questionnaire
(CRQ), 59
Ciliary clearance mechanisms, 222
Clinical trials, 191
Closed-chest cardiac massage, 96
one-rescuer CPR, 96
two-rescuer CPR, 96
Clotting profile, 76
Coagulation disorders
risk of physiotherapy, 76
seriously ill patients, 76
surgical risk, 240
Coarctation of aorta, 309, 312–313
surgery, 259, 261, 313
Codeine phosphate, 372
Coefficient of gas transfer (KCO), 53
Cold air test, 392
Collapse of lung tissue
with asthma, 45
causes, 203
chest radiography, 32–33
left lower lobe, 34–35
left upper lobe, 34
right lower lobe, 34
right middle lobe, 33–34
right upper lobe, 33
with closed intercostal drainage, 250
continuous positive airway pressure
(CPAP), 83, 140, 141
goal of physiotherapy, 205
infants/children, 282
lobar, 203
acute consequences, 203, 205
clinical signs, 203, 205
gas exchange impairment, 219
infection, 205
pertussis, 305
spinal cord injury, 361, 363
longstanding in medical patient, 205
management, 205
manual hyperinflation, 157
opaque hemithorax, 36
postoperative, 140, 201, 203
cardiac surgery, 260, 261
cholecystectomy, 244
gastrectomy, 245
imaging, 41
pulmonary embolism, 43
reduction in lung volume, 199, 203,
205
respiratory distress syndrome, 294
segmental, 83, 203
with sputum retention, 222
subsegmental, 140, 141, 244, 245
chest injury, 267
inspiratory crackles, 18
tracheal deviation, 15

Colostomy, 244–245
Colporrhaphy, 248
Comatose patient
  body positioning, 105
  chest compression, 126
Communication, 173, 175–179
  attitudes, 176
  cultural factors, 177
  dying patient, 374
    relatives, 374
  emotional factors, 177
  ethical aspects, 179
  extraneous interference, 177
  eye contact, 177, 178
  facial expression, 178
  facilitators, 177–178
  factors detracting from effectiveness,
    176–177
  Guillain–Barré syndrome, 271
  importance, 178–179
  language-related factors, 177
  model, 175–176
  positioning, 177–178
  posture/gesture, 178
  purposes, 176
  recall, 178
  skills, 176–177
  touch, 178
Compliance, 184–185
  cardiac rehabilitation, 337–338
Computed tomography (CT), 25–26
  bronchiectasis, 43, 45, 399
  cavitating pulmonary lesions, 39
  hilar/mediastinal lymph node
    enlargement, 38
  hyperlucent lung, 37
  indications, 26
  kyphoscoliosis, 43
  lung abscess, 39
  mesothelioma, 37–38
  pulmonary nodule, 38
Conditioning-rehabilitation
    programme, cardiopulmonary
    transplantation, 351, 352
Congenital abnormalities
  of lung, 298
  neonatal intensive care, 293, 296–298
Congenital central hypoventilation
    (Ondine's curse), 299
Congenital heart disease, 309–313
  cardiac catheterization, 310
  echocardiography, 310
  with excessive pulmonary blood flow,
    309, 310
  with inadequate pulmonary blood
    flow, 309, 310–312
  with increased pressure, 309,
    312–313
  motor developmental delay, 336
  postoperative physiotherapy,
    313–314
  post-repair exercise tolerance,
    336–337
  prenatal diagnosis, 309
  preoperative physiotherapy, 313

Consciousness level
  Glasgow Coma Scale, 9, 237, 268,
    269
  intensive care patient, 9
Consent, 179
  cardiac rehabilitation, 339
  in research studies, 194
Consolidation, lung
  aspiration pneumonia, 41
  bacterial pneumonia, 226
  causes, 32
  chest radiography, 31–32
  following cardiac surgery, 260
  gas exchange impairment, 219
  percussion of chest, 16
  pulmonary embolism, 43
  vocal fremitus, 16
  vocal resonance, 19
Continuous positive airway pressure
    (CPAP), 83–84
  cardiac failure, 221
  cardiac surgery in children, 314
  chronic lung disease
    (bronchopulmonary dysplasia),
    301
  collapse (atelectasis), 205
  continuous flow, 84
  demand flow, 84
  immunodeficient patients, 422–423
  inhalational burns, 275
  laryngotracheobronchitis, acute
    (croup), 306
  in neonate, 299
  ventilatory failure during sleep, 56
Controlled mandatory ventilation
    (CMV), 84
Co-proxamol, 372
Cor pulmonale, 8, 13, 43
  cardiac catheterization, 71
  type B (blue bloater) chronic airflow
    limitation, 216, 217
Coronary angiography, 64
Coronary artery bypass graft surgery
    (CABGS), 258, 259
  rehabilitation following see Cardiac
    rehabilitation
  respiratory complications, 260
Corticosteroid therapy
  allergic bronchopulmonary
    aspergillosis, 396
  asthma, 15, 302, 303, 392
    severe acute, 395
  chronic lung disease
    (bronchopulmonary dysplasia),
    301
  cystic fibrosis, 406, 407
  fibrotic lung conditions, 212
  musculoskeletal adverse effects, 350,
    355
  nebulized drugs, 145
  pain relief, 372
  peripheral oedema, 8, 13
Costochondritis (Tietze's syndrome),
    228
Costophrenic angle, 29

Cough, 222
  asthma, 390
  children, 288–289
  patient mobilization effect, 105
  reflex, 222
  respiratory muscle function, 357–358
  subjective assessment, 6
  see also Bronchial secretions
    clearance
Cough fracture, 6
Cough reflex failure, 223–224
  bypassing upper airway, 224
  CNS depression, 223–224
  drug overdose, 274
  elderly patient, 224
  glossopharyngeal/vagal nerve
    damage, 224
  laryngectomy, 224
  pain, 224
  respiratory muscle weakness, 224
  spinal cord injury, 358, 360
    management, 361, 363
  vocal cord paralysis, 224
Counselling, 175, 179–182
  confidentiality, 181
  contract, 181
  definition, 180
  immunodeficient patients, 426
  mastectomy patients, 246
  non-possessiveness, 180–181
  orientation to action, 181
  physiotherapist's role, 181–182
  positive regard, 180
  willingness to yield control, 181
Crackles
  chest auscultation, 18
  during cardiac rehabilitation exercise
    programme, 332
Creatine kinase (CK), 79
Creatinine serum levels, 78
Crepitations see Crackles
CROP index, 86
Croup see Laryngotracheobronchitis,
    acute
Cryotherapy, 229
Cryptogenic fibrosing alveolitis, 371
Curling's ulcer, 243
Cushing's ulcer, 243
Cyanosis assessment, 12
Cyclosporin A, 343
Cystic fibrosis, 307, 404–416
  active cycle of breathing techniques,
    120, 121
  with allergic bronchopulmonary
    aspergillosis, 406, 415
  with asthma, 406, 413
  breathlessness, 166, 406, 413
  bronchial secretions, 404–405
    clearance, 225, 408–411
  bronchiectasis, 43, 44, 224, 225,
    399, 405, 406
  bronchopulmonary infection, acute
    exacerbation, 413–414, 415
  chest clapping, 123
  complications, 414–415

continuity of care, 416
DNase nebulizer inhalation, 147, 407
exercise programme, 166, 411–413
  minitrampoline, 408
exercise tolerance with pulmonary disease, 412
fertility, 405
finger clubbing, 12
Flutter VRP1 technique, 134
forced expiration technique, 120
gene therapy, 407
genetic aspects, 404
haemoptysis, 414
health education, 183
heart–lung/lung transplantation, 315, 407, 415
implanted venous access devices, 415
incidence, 404
inhalation of drugs, 411
  antibiotics, 146
ion transport abnormality, 225, 404, 405, 406
liver disease, 405
manual therapy techniques, 164
meconium ileus, 298, 405, 406
meconium ileus equivalent, 405, 406
medical management, 406–407
mucus secretions viscosity, 150
nasal polyps, 406, 407
nutrition, 406–407
oral high frequency oscillation technique, 135
osteoarthropathy, 405–406, 413
pain-associated cough reflex inhibition, 224
pancreatic disease, 405, 413
periodic continuous positive airway pressure (PCPAP), 141
physiotherapy, 407–416
  changes in treatment from infancy to adulthood, 408–410
  evaluation, 415
  self treatment, 409
pneumothorax, 407, 413, 414–415
positive expiratory pressure (PEP) technique, 133
  high-pressure, 133
postoperative respiratory complications, 240
pregnancy, 415
prenatal screening, 405
preoperative preparation, 308
prognosis, 404
psychosocial aspects
  anxiety, 173
  defence mechanisms, 174
  family relationships, 174
  stigmatization, 174
  support, 416
pulmonary pathology, 405
respiratory signs/symptoms, 406
salt supplements, 413
self-help groups, 184

sweat test, 404, 405
terminal care, 371, 415
Cystocele repair, 248

Daily weight, 11
Database, POMR, 3–5
Dead space ventilation, 53
Death rattle, 373
Decortication of lung, 258
Decubitus radiographs, 23
  elevation of diaphragm, 37
  pleural disease, 37
  postoperative/critically ill patient, 39
Decubitus ulcer, 247
Deep vein thrombosis
  diagnosis, 242
  after fractured femur in elderly, 247
  postoperative patient, 242–243
    cardiac surgery, 260
    pelvic surgery, 248
  predisposing factors, 242
  prophylaxis, 243
  treatment, 242
Defence mechanisms, 174
Defibrillation, 97
Dehydration
  bronchitis, chronic, 226
  jugular venous pressure, 13
Depression, 174
  breathlessness, 221
  with heart disease, 221
  postoperative, 241
    cardiac surgery, 323
Desferrioxamine, 97
Dextrocardia, 402
Diabetes mellitus
  acid-base balance, ventilatory response, 219
  glucose monitoring, 78
  ketoacidosis, 76–77
  surgery, 241
Dialysis
  with continuous haemofiltration, 90
  general principles, 89
  haemodynamic problems, 89, 91
  hypoxaemia, 89, 91
  infection susceptibility, 91
  mechanical problems, 91
  peritoneal see Peritoneal dialysis
  see also Haemodialysis
Diamorphine, 372
Diaphragm
  measurement of respiratory function, 52, 212
  neonate/infants, 283
  normal breathing movements, 14, 15, 51, 357
  positions facilitating contraction during inspiration, 115
  posteroanterior radiograph, 28–29
  spinal cord injury effects 358, 360
  surface landmarks, 13
  trauma, 262, 267
Diaphragm elevation
  imaging, 37

postoperative pulmonary collapse, 41
pulmonary embolism, 43
Diaphragm weakness/paralysis, 218
  breathlessness, 218
  diaphragmatic pacing, 219
  lung function abnormalities, 212
  orthopnoea, 212
  paradoxical breathing, 15
  positioning, 219
  quantification, 212
Diaphragmatic breathing see Breathing control
Diaphragmatic hernia
  associated lung hypoplasia, 296, 297
  diagnosis, 296
  incidence, 296
  surgical correction, 297
Diaphragmatic pacing, 219
  spinal cord injury, 364–365
Diazepam, 241, 271
Dietary supplements, postoperative, 241
Differential count, 76
Dihydrocodeine (DF 118), 372
Disability measurement, 59–61
Discharge summary, POMS, 3, 22
Diskhaler, 143
Disseminated intravascular coagulopathy (DIC), 76
Diuretics
  cardiac failure, 221
    preoperative care, 240
  chronic lung disease (bronchopulmonary dysplasia), 301
  end-stage cystic fibrosis, 407
  pulmonary oedema, 211
  type B (blue bloater) chronic airflow limitation, 217
DNase inhalation therapy, 147, 407
Domiciliary nebulizer system, 147–148
  air compressors, 147
  bronchodilator response assessment, 149
  in childhood, 143
Domiciliary oxygen therapy, 155
  chronic lung disease (bronchopulmonary dysplasia), 301
  portable oxygen cylinders, 155–156
Domiciliary suction with tracheostomy, 160
Domiciliary visit, 247
Doppler ultrasound
  deep vein thrombosis, 242
  echocardiography, 62
Double lumen endotracheal tube, 252
Down's syndrome, 310
Drug allergies, 5
Drug history, 5
Drug overdose, 274
  ventilatory failure, 54
Dry powder inhalers, 142–143
Dying patient, 367–375

Dying patient (*contd*)
 communication
  patient-carer, 374
  relatives, 374–375
 cystic fibrosis, 415
 holistic approach, 367
 physical factors, 371–373
 physiotherapy, 373
 psychological factors, 367–371
  acceptance, 371
  anger, 369–370
  bargaining, 370–371
  denial, 368–369
  depression, 370
  fear, 370
  guilt, 370
  shock, 369
 social factors, 373–374
 spiritual care, 374
 staff support, 375

Echocardiography, 25
 cardiac imaging, 62
  cross sectional/two dimensional, 62
  Doppler ultrasound, 62–63
 congenital heart disease, 310
Ejection fraction measurement, 63, 65
Elastic stockings
 deep vein thrombosis
  postoperative prevention, 243
  treatment, 242
 HIV infection/AIDS with Kaposi
  sarcoma, 425
Elderly patient
 cardiac rehabilitation, 334
 cough reflex inhibition, 224
 deep vein thrombosis, 242
 fractured femur, 247
 lung function, 57, 58
  following anaesthesia, 57
 postoperative mental changes, 241
 postoperative pneumonia, 227
 postoperative renal function
  impairment, 243
 postoperative respiratory
  complications, 202, 240
Electrocardiogram (ECG), 64
 advanced life support, 97
 exercise testing, 64
  cardiac rehabilitation, 326, 327
 monitoring, 72–74
  exercise in cardiac rehabilitation,
   330
  heart rate, 68
  neonatal/paediatric, 292
 myocardial infarction, 322
 preoperative, 240
Electrolytes, 77–78
Emphysema
 airway function, 48, 49
 imaging, 45
 bronchial secretions clearance, 226
 bullae, 45, 46
  Entonox contraindication, 162
 cardiopulmonary rehabilitation

exercise programme, 166, 167
congenital/acquired in neonate, 298
diminished breath sounds, 18
gas exchange impairment, 53
hyperinflation, 14
ineffective cough, 223
positioning of patient, oxygen
 transport effect, 108
postoperative respiratory
 complications, 41, 240
psychosocial aspects, 174
spontaneous pneumothorax, 258
surgical, 15–16
 blunt chest injury, 266
 following lung surgery, 256
terminal care, 371
vocal resonance, 19
see also Pulmonary interstitial
 emphysema
Empyema
 decortication of lung, 258
 intercostal drainage, 251
 management, 208
 reduction in lung volume, 207
 thoracoplasty, 256
End-tidal CO_2 monitoring, 67, 69
Endotracheal intubation
 advanced life support, 96
 airway suction, 159–160
 aspiration of gastric contents, 41
 check of tube position, 40
 drug overdose, 274
 end-tidal CO_2 monitoring, 69
 Guillain–Barré syndrome, 271
 head injured patients, 269–270
 humidification of inspired air, 160
 ineffective cough, 223
 inhalational burns, 275
 laryngotracheobronchitis, acute
  (croup), 306
 myasthenia gravis, 270
 neonatal/paediatric tubes, 291
 poliomyelitis, 273
 respiratory distress prevention in
  preterm/low birth weight
  infants, 293, 294
Endotracheal suction, 159–160
 head injured children, 317
 ineffective cough, 224
 lobectomy patients, 254
Enteral feeding, postoperative, 241
Entonox
 contraindications, 162
 Guillain–Barré syndrome, 271
 inhalational burns, 275
 with intermittent positive pressure
  breathing (IPPB), 136–137
 for manual hyperinflation, 157
 pain relief, 162–163, 229
 side effects, 163
 storage conditions, 163
Epiglottitis, acute, 306
Equal pressure points, 119
Erect position

haemodynamic effects, 103
lung volume effects, 103
Erythromycin, 305
Ethical committees, 194
Examination, physical, POMR
 database, 5
Exchange transfusion, preterm infant,
 295
Exercise programmes
 asthma, 393
  childhood, 303
 breathlessness with fear/anxiety, 221
 cardiac failure, 221, 334, 335
 cardiac rehabilitation, 166–167, 320,
  324–325, 327–333
 cardiac surgery, 262, 336
 cardiopulmonary transplantation,
  349–350, 354, 355
 chest wall trauma, 208
 chronic airflow limitation, 217
 chronic cardiopulmonary
  dysfunction, 108, 109
 components, 106, 109
 coronary risk factors, 320
 cystic fibrosis, 411–413
 hyperventilation syndrome, 386
 immunodeficient patients, 425
 with intercostal tube drainage, 208
 ischaemic heart disease secondary
  prevention, 321
 lobectomy patients, 254–255
 mobilization of critically ill patient,
  106
 mucociliary clearance effect, 222
 primary ciliary dyskinesia, 404
 psychological well being, 320–321
Exercise provocation test, asthma, 392
Exercise testing
 anaerobic threshold, 60
 cardiac disease, 60
 cardiac rehabilitation, 320, 325–327
  contraindications, 326
  protocol, 326
  reliablility/sensitivity/specificity,
   326–327
 chronic cardiopulmonary
  dysfunction, 108, 109
 lung function assessment, 59–61
  field testing, 60–61
  laboratory estimation, 59–60
  questionnaires, 59
  walking tests, 59, 60
 maximum performance limitation, 60
 maximal work load assessment, 60
 maximum oxygen uptake (VO_2Max)
  assessment, 60
 pneumonectomy, preoperative
  assessment, 255
Exercise tolerance, 19–20
 allergic bronchopulmonary
  aspergillosis, 396
 asthma, 215
 breathing control, 116
 cardiac failure, 221, 334
 chronic airflow limitation, 216

congenital heart disease, repaired, 336–337
fibrotic lung conditions, 218
measurement, 215
reduced, 213–221
shuttle test, 20
six minute walk test, 20
valvular heart disease, 335–336
Exompholos (ompholocele), 297–298
Expiration, prolonged, 14
External intercostal muscles, 14
Extracorporeal carbon dioxide removal, 87
Extracorporeal membrane oxygenation (ECMO), 87
neonatal intensive care, 299
Extrapulmonary air imaging, postoperative, 42
Eye assessment, 12
Eye contact, 177, 178

Face mask
intermittent positive pressure breathing (IPPB), 137, 138
oxygen therapy, 154
Facial expression, 178
Fat embolus, 219
Femoral hernia, 245–246
Femur fracture, elderly patients, 247
Fever (pyrexia), 9–10
children, 284
metabolic demand, 10
microbiological investigations, 79, 80
subjective assessment, 7
Fibrin degradation products (FDPs), 76
Fibrinogen, 76
Fibrinolysis, 242
Fibrosing alveolitis, 53, 54
Fibrotic lung conditions
breathing pattern, 218
breathlessness, 218
causes, 212
exercise tolerance reduction, 218
inspiratory crackles, 18
lung function abnormalities, 212
management, 212
postoperative respiratory complications, 240
reduction in lung volume, 200, 211–212
Finger clubbing, 12, 207, 406
Flail segment, 15
blunt chest injury, 266
Flow–volume curves, 48, 49
Fluid balance assessment, 11
Fluid intake, 150
Fluid replacement therapy, 275
Fluoroscopy, 25
Flutter VRP1, 134
Forced expiration technique, 119–121
cardiopulmonary transplantation postoperative care, 353
children, 120
cystic fibrosis, 120

pain relief, 162
preoperative instruction, 243
Forced expiratory volume in 1 Second (FEV$_1$), 48, 51
Forced vital capacity (FVC), 48, 51
Foreign body inhalation
bronchiectasis, 399
chest radiography, 31
children, 306–307
clinical features, 306–307
management, 307
physiotherapy, 307
collapse (atelectasis), 32
wheezes, 18
Forward lean sitting, 115
Forward lean standing, 115
Free radical scavengers, 97
Full blood count, 75
Functional limitation assessment
objective, 19–20
subjective, 8–9
Functional residual capacity (FRC), 51
with abdominal distension, 205
general anaesthesia effect, 200
postoperative patients, 242
immediate postoperative period, 201
supine position effects, 56, 103

Gall bladder disease, 230
Gamma-glutamyl transferase (GGT), 78
Gas exchange
alveolar ventilation, 53
dead-space ventilation, 53
impairment
breathlessness management, 219
pulmonary causes, 53–54
measurement, 53–54
carbon monoxide transfer test (TLCO), 53
coefficient of gas transfer (KCO), 53
Gastrectomy, 245
Gastro-oesophageal reflux, 127, 230
Gastroschisis, 297–298
Gastrostomy feeding, 241
Glasgow Coma Scale, 9, 237, 268
head injured patients, 269
Glaucoma from nebulizer delivered drugs, 144
Glossopharyngeal breathing (GPB), 127–128, 130–132
contraindications, 132
GPB vital capacity measurement, 130
poliomyelitis, 274
spinal cord injury, 360–361
Glossopharyngeal nerve damage, 224
Goals, POMR, 3, 21
Gravity-assisted positions, 126–127, 128, 129
allergic bronchopulmonary aspergillosis, 396
bronchiectasis, 400

cardiopulmonary transplantation postoperative care, 353
children, 287
asthma, acute attack, 303
cardiac surgery, 313
pneumonia, 305
chronic lung disease (bronchopulmonary dysplasia), 301
collapse (atelectasis), 205
pertussis associated, 305
cystic fibrosis, 408, 409, 415
ineffective cough, 223, 224
meconium aspiration, 296
primary ciliary dyskinesia, 403
spinal cord injury, 360, 361, 363
Guedel airway, 95
Guillain–Barré syndrome, 93, 270–271, 272
clinical features, 270–271
communication system, 271
lung function abnormalities, 212
management, 271
physiotherapy, 271
respiratory muscle function tests, 52
Gynaecological surgery, 247–248

Haematological investigations, 75–76
Haemodialysis, 89, 261
continuous forms, 89
conventional, 89
hypotension/hypoxaemia complicating, 89
vascular access, 89
Haemofiltration, 261
continuous arterio-venous (CAVH), 90
continuous arterio-venous with dialysis (CAVHD), 90
continuous with dialysis, 90
continuous veno-venous (CVVH), 89–90
continuous veno-venous with dialysis (CVVHD), 90
Haemoglobin (Hb)
interpretation, 75
measurement, 54, 75
in oxygen carriage, 54
oxygen dissociation curve, 54
Haemophilia, surgical risk, 240
Haemophilus influenzae
acute epiglottitis, 306
acute exacerbation of chronic bronchitis, 225
bronchiectasis, 225
cystic fibrosis, 225, 406
immunodeficient patient, 420
pneumonia, 305
complicating pertussis, 305
Haemopneumothorax, 266
with penetrating chest injury, 266
Haemoptysis, 6–7
aspergilloma, 396
bronchial arteriography, 27
bronchiectasis, 225, 402

Haemoptysis (*contd*)
  cystic fibrosis, 225, 414
  downward chest tilted position
    contraindication, 127
  IPPB/PCPAP contraindication, 141
Haemothorax, 207
  blunt chest injury, 265–266
  following cardiac surgery, 260
Haleraid, 142
Hands, objective assessment, 12
Head box, 153, 291, 299, 304
  chronic lung disease
    (bronchopulmonary dysplasia),
    301
  respiratory distress prevention in
    preterm/low birth weight infants,
    293
Head down position
  children, 287
  head injured patients, 269
  oxygen transport effect in
    emphysema, 108
  postoperative patients, 261, 263
Head injury, 268–270
  aspiration prevention, 269–270
  brain damage, 268–269
  children, 315–316
    intracranial pressure, 315–316, 317
    physiotherapy, 317
  downward chest tilted position
    contraindication, 127
  intracranial pressure monitoring,
    269, 317
  with multiple trauma, 268
  physiotherapy, 269–270
  rehabilitation, 270
  skull fracture, 269
  unconscious patient, 270
Head and neck surgery, 264
Headache
  morning, 8, 213
  subjective assessment, 8
Health education, 175, 182–185
  cardiac rehabilitation, 321
  chronic airflow limitation, 217
  definition, 183
  goals, 183
  immunodeficient patients, 424–425
  patient compliance, 184–185
  physiotherapist's role, 184–185
  scope, 183–184
  in treatment plan, 21
Health promotion, 182–183
  definition, 182
  health education *see* Health
    education
  health protection, 183
  preventive aspects, 182
Heart rate
  exercise response
    with beta adrenergic blocking
      agents, 324
    cardiac rehabilitation, 329
    cardiopulmonary transplantation,
      350

infants, 284
  monitoring, 67, 68
    cardiac rehabilitation exercise
      programme, 329, 331–332
  normal values, 431
  objective assessment, 10
  physiotherapy effects, 68
Heart sounds, 19
Heart transplantation, 259
  children, 314–315
  contraindications, 344
  denervation of heart, 349–350
  'domino' technique, 344
  donor requirements, 345
  endomyocardial biopsy, 347
  heterotopic transplantation
    procedure, 345
  indications, 343
  orthotopic transplantation
    procedure, 345
  preoperative management, 351–352
  recipient assessment, 351
  rejection
    acute, 347
    chronic, 347
  see also Cardiopulmonary
    transplantation
Heart trauma, 267
Heart-lung transplantation
  children, 315
  contraindications, 344
  cystic fibrosis, 407, 415
  denervation of heart-lung, 349–350,
    353, 415
  donor requirements, 345
  heart donation, 344
  indications, 343
  obliterative bronchiolitis following,
    315
  preoperative conditioning-
    rehabilitation programme, 351,
    352
  preoperative monitoring, 351
  procedure, 345–346
  recipient assessment, 351
  rejection, 347
  see also Cardiopulmonary
    transplantation
Heat/moisture exchangers, 150–151
Heated water bath humidifiers, 150
Heimlich manoeuvre, 94
Heimlich valve, 251
Heliox, 156–157, 373
Hemithorax
  chest radiography, 36–37
    decreased density, 36–37
    opaque, 36
Heparin, 242, 243
Hepatitis B virus, 426
Hepatitis, ischaemic, 78
Hernia
  cough associated, 6
  repair, 245–246
Herniorrhaphy, 245
Herpes zoster (shingles), 230

Hiatus hernia, 262
  surgery, 262–263
High altitude, 54
High risk surgical patient, 199
High side lying
  breathing control, 115
  breathlessness
    asthma, 393, 394
    cystic fibrosis, 413
  bronchial secretions clearance, 126
  bronchiectasis, acute exacerbation,
    402
  intermittent positive pressure
    breathing, 137
  lung cancer patient, 373
  respiratory muscle
    weakness/paralysis, 219
High frequency jet ventilation (HFJV),
  87–88
  neonatal intensive care, 299–300
High frequency oscillation (HFO), 301
  neonatal intensive care, 299–300
High-pressure positive expiratory
  pressure, 133–134
Hilar mass, computed tomography, 26,
  36
Hilum
  lateral radiograph, 29
  posteroanterior radiograph, 28
Histoplasmosis, 38
History, POMR database, 4
  drug, 5
  family, 5
  medical, 4
  social, 5
Holistic approach, 367
Hoover's sign, 15
Horner's syndrome, 12
Huffing technique *see* Forced
  expiration technique
Human immunodeficiency virus (HIV)
  infection/AIDS, 419, 422
  contractures prevention, 425
  health education, 183
  infection control, 426
  Kaposi sarcoma, 425
  nebulized pentamidine, 424–425
  Pneumocystis carinii pneumonia, 422
    prophylaxis, 424–425
  psychological support, 426
Humidification, 149–153
  allergic bronchopulmonary
    aspergillosis, 396
  asthma, bronchospasm management,
    215
  bronchial secretions clearance, 150
  bronchiectasis, 402
  bronchiolitis, 304
  bronchitis, chronic, 226
  chest injury, 267
  chronic airflow limitation, 217
  chronic lung disease
    (bronchopulmonary dysplasia),
    301
  ciliary activity effect, 150

collapsed lung tissue (atelectasis), 205
cystic fibrosis, 414
delivery to patient, 152–153
hazards, 153
head injured patients, 270
ineffective cough, 223, 224
inhalational burns, 275, 276
intubated patient, 160
laryngectomy, 263
laryngotracheobronchitis, acute
(croup), 306
lobectomy patients, 253–254
methods, 150–152
bubble-through humidifiers, 152,
154
heat/moisture exchangers, 150–151
heated water bath humidifiers, 150
nebulizers, 151–152
steam inhalations, 152
systemic hydration, 150
neonate/children, 291, 299
in normal airway, 149
oesophagectomy, 263
oxygen concentrator, 155
with oxygen therapy, 152, 154
Humidity adaptor, 153, 226
Humoral immunity, 419
Hydrotherapy, 274
Hyperbilirubinaemia, 78
Hypercapnic respiratory failure, 219
cardiovascular effects, 213
central nervous system effects, 213
respiratory muscle weakness, 213
signs, 213
type B (blue bloater) chronic airflow
limitation, 216
Hyperkalaemia, 78
Hypernatraemia, 78
Hypertension
blood pressure, 10
downward chest tilted position
contraindication, 127
heart sounds, 19
Hyperthyroidism, 5
Hypertonic saline
mucociliary clearance stimulation,
222
nebulizer inhalation, 147
sputum induction, 423
Hyperventilation, 377
metabolic acidosis, 77
with pulmonary embolism, 220
respiratory alkalosis, 77
Hyperventilation, chronic
(hyperventilation syndrome), 5,
6, 377
assessment, 379–381
breath holding manoeuvre, 383, 384,
386
breathing awareness, 382
breathing education, 381–382
breathing pattern re-education,
382–384
breathing patterns, 378–379, 380
causes, 377–378

exercise/fitness programmes, 386
group therapy, 386
history, 379–380
home therapy, 386
personality, 378
assessment, 380
physical examination, 380
planned rebreathing, 384–385
provocation test, 380–381
signs/symptoms, 377, 380
speech patterns, 386
treatment, 379
treatment plan, 381
Hypogammaglobulinaemia, 224, 399,
400
Hypokalaemia, 78
metabolic alkalosis, 77
Hyponatraemia, 78
Hypopnoea, 14
Hypotension
blood pressure, 10
postural, 10
Hypoxaemia
chronic airflow limitation, 216
fibrotic lung conditions, 218
lobar collapse, 203, 205
risk of cardiac arrest, 93
with sputum retention, 223
Hypoxia
infants/children, 283, 284
ventilatory response, 219
Hysterectomy, 247, 248

Ileostomy, 244
Ileus, 77
Immobilization
bed-rest deconditioning, 103
fractured femur in elderly, 247
lung volume effects, 103
obese patients, 240
oxygen transport effects, 109
peripheral oedema, 13
prevention of negative effects, 99, 109
reduction in blood volume, 103
risks, 107
cardiac/respiratory arrest, 93
Immune system, 419
Immunodeficient states, 419–426
breathlessness, 422–423, 426
sputum induction, 423
bronchiectasis, 224, 399, 400
classification, 419–420
education, 424–425
excess secretions, 423–424
infection susceptibility, 420
mobility, 422, 425–426
neurological problems, 422, 425
opportunistic pathogens, 420, 421
physiotherapy, 422–426
prophylactic, 424–425
presenting problems, 420, 422
psychological problems, 426
septic arthritis/osteomyelitis, 422
pain relief, 425
weakness/wasting, 420, 425

Immunoglobulins, 419
Immunosuppression
cardiopulmonary transplantation,
347, 348, 349, 350
fibrotic lung conditions, 212
musculoskeletal adverse effects, 350
Inappropriate ADH secretion, 78
Incentive spirometry, 141–142
in children/adolescents, 142, 288
postoperative, 308
collapse (atelectasis), 205
following chest deformity surgery,
257
spinal cord injury, 360
Incisional hernia, 246
Incisional site, 238, 239
postoperative respiratory
complications, 241
thoracotomy, 252
Incremental threshold loading, 53
Incubators, 291
preterm/low birth weight infants, 295
Influenza
bronchiolitis, 303
impaired mucociliary clearance
following, 225
pneumonia, 80
Inguinal hernia, 245, 246
Inhaled drugs, 142–149
asthma, severe acute, 395
pressurized aerosol/dry powder
inhalers, 142–143
see also Nebulizer inhalation
Initial plan, POMR, 3, 21
Inspiratory muscle training, spinal cord
injury, 360
Inspiratory pressure support (IPS),
84–85
Inspiratory/expiratory time (I/E) ratio,
14
Intensive care unit (ICU), 237
central venous pressure monitoring,
11
communication, 177
daily weight, 11
feelings of patient, 174, 237
general observation, 9
head injury, 269
indications for admission, 237
intracranial pressure monitoring, 11
neonatal *see* Neonatal intensive care
unit
non-invasive monitoring, 67
nursing observations, 67
paediatric equipment, 289–292
patient assessment, 237
physiotherapy, 238
pulmonary artery pressure
monitoring, 11
risk of cardiac arrest, 93
thoracic imaging, 39–43
support/monitoring apparatus,
39–41
vascular access lines, 11
Intercostal drainage, 11–12

Intercostal drainage (contd)
  ambulation, 250, 254
  chest wall pain, 228
  closed, 248–251
    air leak/fluid drainage, 250
    clamping of tube, 250
    failure, 250, 251
    obstruction/leakage of tubing, 250, 251
    portable devices, 250, 251
    water seal drainage systems, 249
  haemothorax, 266
  lobectomy, 253, 254
  lung resection, 256
  oesophagectomy, 263
  open, 248
  pleural disorders, 208
  pneumothorax, 257–258, 265
  postoperative patient, 242
  removal of drains, 250, 251
  thoracic surgery, 248–251
Intercostal indrawing, 15
Intercostal muscles
  respiratory function, 51, 357
  spinal cord injury effects, 358, 359
Intercostal nerve block, 265
Intercostal neuritis, 164
Intermittent mandatory ventilation
    (IMV), 84
  cardiac surgery in children, 314
  chronic lung disease
    (bronchopulmonary dysplasia),
    301
  in neonate, 299
Intermittent positive pressure breathing
    (IPPB), 135–139
  air-mix control, 136–137
  allergic bronchopulmonary
    aspergillosis, 396
  asthma, severe acute, 394, 395
  breathing circuit, 137
  bronchiectasis, 402
  bronchitis, chronic, 226
  bronchodilator delivery, 141
  with chest wall deformity, 139
  in children, 138
  collapse (atelectasis), 205
  contraindications, 140–141
  cystic fibrosis, 414, 415
  effects, 141
  Entonox pain relief, 163
  with face mask, 137, 138
  flow control, 136
  following removal of tracheostomy
    tube, 159
  Guillain–Barré syndrome, 271
  indications, 141
  ineffective cough, 223, 224
  with inhalational burns, 276
  with nebulizer, 136
  oxygen as driving gas, 155
  patient treatment, 137–139
  position, 137
  postoperative, 243
    aortic aneurysm surgery, 264–265

cardiac surgery, 261
  lobectomy, 253
  lung surgery, 256
  myasthenia gravis, 270
  preparation of apparatus, 137
  respiratory muscle weakness, 213
  respiratory training with tetrapelgia,
    360
  sensitivity, 136
Intermittent positive pressure
    ventilation (IPPV)
  with drug overdose, 274
  inhalational burns, 275
  intra/postoperative lung function
    effects, 200
  laryngotracheobronchitis, acute
    (croup), 306
  manual hyperinflation, 157
  myasthenia gravis management, 270
  poliomyelitis, 273
Internal intercostal muscles, 15
Interstitial lung disease, 6
Interstitial pneumonitis, 226
Interstitial pulmonary oedema
  cardiac failure, 43
    postoperative, imaging, 42–43
Intra-aortic balloon pump, 88
  cardiac failure, 221
  complications, 88
  following cardiac surgery, 260
  indications, 88
  radiographic check of position, 40
Intracranial pressure (ICP)
  monitoring, 69, 72
    children, 317
    complications, 72
    head injured patients, 269
    intensive care patient, 11
  normal values, 432
Intracranial pressure (ICP), raised
  children, 287, 315–316
    monitoring, 317
  head injury, 268, 269, 315–316
  lung cancer, 372, 373
  physiotherapy-associated, 72
Intravascular oxygenation (IVOX), 87
Investigations
  interpretation, 75–80
    biochemistry, 76–79
    haematology, 75–76
    microbiology, 79–80
  POMR database, 5
Ipratropium bromide, 144, 148
Ischaemic heart disease
  arrhythmias, 73
  with cardiac failure, 334–335
  chest pain, 229
  coronary angiography, 64
  exercise electrocardiogram, 64
  exercise tolerance reduction, 221
  exercise training in prevention,
    320–321
  manifestations, 321–323
  postoperative respiratory
    complications, 240

risk factors, effects of exercise, 320
Jaundice
  eye examination, 12
  intensive care unit, 79
  physiological in preterm/low birth
    weight infants, 295
Jet nebulizers, 143–144
  in children, 144
  dead volume, 144
  drug dosages, 144
  with face mask, 144
  flow rate, 144
  for humidification, 151–152
  position, 144
  sputum induction, 222, 423
Joint contractures prevention
  burns patients, 276
  Guillain–Barré syndrome, 271
  immunodeficient states, 425
  with multiple trauma, 268
  poliomyelitis, 273, 274
Jugular venous pressure, 12–13

Kartagener's syndrome, 307, 402
  bronchiectasis, 224
Kerley B lines, 43, 62
Kernicterus, 295
Kinetic beds/chairs, 107–108
Klebsiella pneumoniae
  bronchiectasis, 224
  cavitating pulmonary lesions, 39
  lung abscess, 227
Kussmaul's respiration, 14,
    77
Kyphoscoliosis, 14
  chest radiography, 31
  computed tomography, 43
  intermittent positive pressure
    breathing (IPPB) technique, 139
  thoracic imaging, 43
Kyphosis, 14

Lactate dehydrogenase (LDH), 78
  cardiac enzyme estimation, 79
Laparoscopic surgery, 244
Laryngeal carcinoma, 263
Laryngeal dysfunction
  cough, 6
  nasotracheal suction, 161
Laryngeal oedema, 274
Laryngectomy, 263–264
  cough reflex inhibition, 224
  postoperative communication, 263
  tracheostomy, 263
Laryngotracheobronchitis, acute
    (croup), 305–306
  physiotherapy, 306
Lateral radiograph, 23
  collapse (atelectasis), 33–35
  emphysema, 45
  normal chest, 29–30
Left atrial pressure
  estimation, 71
  following cardiac surgery, 260
  monitoring, 71–72

Left ventricular preload estimation, 71
Leg exercises
    following fractured femur in elderly, 247
    pelvic surgery, 248
    pulmonary embolism, 220
Lifting techniques, postoperative
    aortic aneurysm surgery, 265
    gynaecological surgery, 248
    hernia repair, 246
Lignocaine
    advanced life support, 97
    nebulizer inhalation, 146
    spinal/epidural anaesthesia, 238
Limb movements
    following cardiac surgery, 261
    following cardiopulmonary transplantation, 353
Linear tomography, 23, 25
    cavitating pulmonary lesions, 39
Liver function tests, 78–79
Liver transplantation, 315
Lobectomy, 253–254
    chest drainage, 253, 254
    chest wall pain, 255
    lung cancer, 253
    lung function following, 57
    physiotherapy, 253–255
    sleeve resection, 253
    wound support, 254
Lordotic view, 23
Low birth weight infant
    causes of low birth weight, 293
    infection, 294, 295
    jaundice, 295
    neonatal intensive care, 293
        problems, 293–294
    nutrition, 296
    periventricular haemorrhage/leucomalacia, 294–295
    pneumonia, 294
    pulmonary haemorrhage, 296
    respiratory distress, 293–294
    temperature control, 295
    ventilation, 298
Lower limb ischaemia, 265
Lung abscess
    bronchial secretions clearance, 227
    Entonox contraindication, 162
    imaging, 39
    IPPB/PCPAP contraindication, 141
Lung biopsy, 25, 26, 38, 255
Lung cancer, 252–253
    breath sounds, 18
    breathlessness, 373
    collapse (atelactasis), 32
    consolidation, 32
    death rattle, 373
    haemoptysis, 7
    IPPB/PCPAP contraindication with bronchial tumour, 141
    lobectomy, 253
    nausea, 372–373
    non-surgical treatment, 253
    pain relief, 371–372

persistent pneumonia, 227
physiotherapy, 373
    following relief of airway obstruction, 253
    lobectomy, 253–254
    vocal cord palsy, 253
pleuritic pain, 228
presenting symptoms, 369
prognosis, 371
recurrent laryngeal nerve involvement, 253
risk factors, 252
superior vena caval obstruction, 373
symptom control, 371–373
terminal care, 371
TNM staging system, 252–253
Lung cysts, neonatal, 298
Lung decortication, 258
Lung development, 281–282
    functional aspects, 57, 283–284
Lung disease, chronic (bronchopulmonary dysplasia)
    neonatal complicating ventilatory support, 300–301
    physiotherapy, 301
    treatment, 301
Lung function tests, 47–61
    age-associated effects, 57–58
    arterial blood gases, 54–55
    bronchiectasis, 399
    calibration of equipment, 48
    chest wall/respiratory muscles, 51–53
    in children, 57
    disability measurement, 59
    exercise testing, 59–61
    functional residual capacity (FRC), 51
    gas exchange, 53–54
    growth effects, 57–58
    interpretation, 58–59
    oxygen carriage, 54–55
    physical properties of lung, 51
    posture effects, 56–57
    principles, 48
    respiratory failure, 56
    spirometry, 20
    thoracic surgery effects, 56
Lung surgery, 251–256
    bronchopleural fistula complicating, 256
    bullous emphysema, 256
    cardiac arrhythmias complicating, 256
    double lumen endotracheal tube, 252
    incision, 252
    intercostal drainage, 256
    lobectomy, 253–254
    lung function impairment, 57
    phrenic nerve palsy following, 256
    pleural effusion following, 256
    pneumonectomy, 255–256
    postoperative complications, 256
    segmentectomy, 255

surgical emphysema following, 256
    wedge resection, 255
Lung transplantation, 402
    contraindications, 344
    cystic fibrosis, 415
    denervation of lung, 349–350, 353, 415
    donor requirements, 345
    double lung transplant, 343, 346
    indications, 343, 400
    preoperative conditioning-rehabilitation programme, 351, 352
    preoperative monitoring, 351
    procedure, 346
    recipient assessment, 351
    rejection, 347
        obliterative bronchiolitis, 347
        transbronchial lung biopsy, 347
    see also Cardiopulmonary transplantation
Lung trauma, 266
Lung volume measurement, 51
Lung volume reduction, 199–213
    causes, 199–200
Lungs
    blood vessels, 28
    fissures, 28
        accessory, 29
        lateral view, 29
    lobes, 28
    posteroanterior radiograph, 28
    segments, 28
Lymphocytes, 419
Lymphoedema of arm, post-mastectomy, 246–247

McGill pain questionnaire, 195, 196
Macrocytosis, 75
Magnetic resonance imaging (MRI), 26
    cardiac, 62, 63
Malnutrition
    in alcoholics, 241
    body mass index (BMI), 11
    immune depression, 11
    postoperative respiratory complications, 240–241
    infection, 202, 227
    preoperative correction, 241
    respiratory function, 10, 11
Manchester repair, 248
Manual hyperinflation, 157–158
    adult respiratory distress syndrome (ARDS), 277
    airway suction, 157
    asthma, severe acute, 395
    cardiac surgery, 261
        in children, 313
    with chest compression, 157
    with chest shaking/vibrations, 126
    children/infants, 158, 287–288, 313, 317
    contraindications, 158
    with drug overdose, 274
    Entonox pain relief, 163

Manual hyperinflation (*contd*)
  Guillain–Barré syndrome, 271
  head injury, 269, 317
  ineffective cough, 224
  inhalational burns, 276
  monitoring, 158
  with multiple trauma, 268
  myasthenia gravis, postoperative
    care, 270
  poliomyelitis, 273
  position, 157
  with saline instillation, 158, 269
  sedation, 157
  spinal cord injury, 363
  tetanus, 272
  weaning from ventilator, 159
Manual therapy skills, 164
  contraindications, 164
  following cardiac surgery, 262
Marcaine, 146
Mastectomy, 246–247
  physiotherapy, 246–247
  simple/radical, 246
Maximum expiratory pressure
    (*Pe*Max), 52
Maximum inspiratory pressure
    (*Pi*Max), 52
Maximum oxygen uptake (VO₂Max)
  exercise test, 19
  laboratory measurement, 60
Maximum voluntary ventilation
    (MVV), 53
Mean corpuscular haemoglobin
    (MCH), 75
Mean corpuscular volume (MCV), 75
Mechanical ventilation *see* Respiratory
    support
Meconium aspiration, 293, 296, 300
Meconium ileus, 298, 405, 406
Meconium ileus equivalent, 405, 406
Mediastinal chest drain, 259
Mediastinal mass
  computed tomography, 26
  percutaneous needle biopsy, 26
Mediastinal shift
  with closed intercostal drainage,
    250
  complicating central catheter
    placement, 40
  following pneumonectomy, 255
  pleural effusion, 207, 218
  tension pneumothorax, 208, 265
  tracheal deviation, 15
Mediastinum
  lymph node enlargement, 38
  radiography, 24, 27–28
  vascular injury, 266
Mesothelioma, 37–38
Metabolic equivalents (METs), 329
Metastases, pulmonary, 38, 39
Metered dose inhaler (MDI) *see*
    Pressurized aerosol (metered
    dose) inhalers
Methadone, 372
Microbiological investigations, 79–80

blood cultures, 79
  sputum/tracheal aspirate, 79–80
  swabs, 80
  urine, 80
Microcytosis, 75
Mind maps, 188, 189
Minitracheostomy
  airway suction, 161–162
  ineffective cough, 223, 224
  inhalational burns, 275
  lobectomy, 254
  oesophagectomy, 263
  pneumonectomy, 255
  spinal cord injury, 363
Mobilization of patient
  kinetic beds/chairs, 107–108
  oxygen transport effects, 99
    with acute cardiopulmonary
      dysfunction, 101–102, 105–108
    assessment, 105–106, 110
    with chronic cardiopulmonary
      dysfunction, 108–109
    exercise programme, 106, 109
    monitoring, 106
    physiological rationale, 105
  postoperative
    aortic aneurysm surgery, 264
    cardiopulmonary transplantation,
      353
Monitoring, 67–74
  arterial catheterization, 70
  blood pressure, 67, 68, 69, 70–71,
    292, 332
  body temperature, 67–68
  cardiac rehabilitation exercise
    programmes, 329, 331–332
  central venous pressure (CVP), 11,
    70–71
  electrocardiogram (ECG), 68,
    72–74, 292, 330
  end-tidal CO₂, 67, 69
  heart rate, 67, 68
  intracranial pressure, 69, 72, 317
  complications, 72
  head injured patients, 269
  intensive care patients, 11
  invasive, 69–72
    inaccuracies, 69
  left atrial pressure, 71–72
  neonate/children, 292, 317
  non-invasive, 67–69
  nursing observations, 67
  observation of apparatus, 11–12
  oxygen saturation, 67, 68–69
    oxygen therapy monitoring, 153
  pulmonary capillary wedge pressure
    (PCWP), 71
  radiographic check of catheter
    position, 40
  respiratory rate, 67, 68, 332
  transcutaneous *P*O₂/*P*CO₂, 67, 69
Morphine, 147, 217, 223, 372, 407, 415
Mouth-to-mouth respiration, 96
Movement, active/passive

burns patients, 276
  children, 289
  following cardiac surgery, 323
  Guillain–Barré syndrome, 271
  immunodeficient states, 425
  multiple trauma, 268
  poliomyelitis, 273
  tetanus, 272
Mucociliary clearance, 222
  postoperative patient, 201
Mucolytic agents inhalation, 147
Mucus plugs
  asthma, 45, 226
  breath sounds, 18
  children, 289
  collapse (atelectasis), 32
  postoperative, 41
Mucus secretion, 221
  clearance *see* Bronchial secretions
    clearance
  composition, 222
  inhalation anaesthesia response,
    238
  viscosity, 150
Multiple trauma, 267–268
  blunt injuries, 267
  penetrating injury, 267
  physiotherapy, 268
  priorities in management, 267
Myasthenia gravis, 270
Mycobacterium tuberculosis
  bronchiectasis, 224
  lung abscess, 227
Mycoplasma
  impaired mucociliary clearance
    following infection, 225
  pneumonia, 80, 305
Myocardial contusion, 266
Myocardial infarction, 322–323
  cardiac arrest risk, 93
  cardiac catheterization, 71
  cardiac enzymes, 79
  chest pain, 229
  complications, 322–323
  electrocardiogram (ECG), 64, 322,
    324
    post-infarction exercise ECG, 64
  exercise testing following, 325–327
    contraindications, 326
  history, 322, 324
  intra-aortic balloon pump support,
    88
  management, 259
  psychological complications, 323
  pulmonary oedema, 209, 211
  recurrence, 322
  rehabilitation *see* Cardiac
    rehabilitation
  serum enzymes, 322, 324
  site/size, 324
Myocardial ischaemia
  angina pectoris, 7
  electrocardiogram (ECG), 64
  see also Ischaemic heart disease
Myopathies, 51

Nasal cannulas
  chronic lung disease
    (bronchopulmonary dysplasia),
    301
  oxygen therapy, 154
Nasal continuous positive airway
    pressure, 260
Nasal flaring, 285
Nasal intermittent positive pressure
    ventilation (NIPPV), 85
  chronic airflow limitation, 85
  cystic fibrosis, 414
  domiciliary use, 85
  nocturnal ventilatory failure, 56
  respiratory muscle weakness, 213
  sputum retention management, 223
Nasogastric tube feeding, 11–12
  bronchiolitis, 304
  postoperative patient, 241, 242, 244,
    245, 263
  preterm infants, 296
Nasopharyngeal airway (nasal prong), 291
  low birthweight infants, 299
Nasopharyngeal suction, 160
  bronchitis, chronic, 226
  children/neonate, 289
  consent, 179
  drug overdose, 274
  head injured patients, 269
  ineffective cough, 223, 224
  oesophagectomy, 263
  pneumonectomy, 255
  poliomyelitis, 273
  primary ciliary dyskinesia, 404
  spinal cord injury, 363
    bradycardia complicating, 363
Nasotracheal intubation, 306
Nasotracheal suction, 161
  bronchitis, chronic, 226
  contraindications, 161
  with drug overdose, 274
  ineffective cough, 223, 224
  position, 161
Nebulizer inhalation, 143–148, 184
  antibiotics in cystic fibrosis patients,
    406, 411
  asthma
    children, 302, 303
    severe acute, 394, 395
  bronchodilator response studies,
    148–149
  domiciliary, 143, 147–148, 149
  humidification, 151–152
  indications for use, 145–147
  jet nebulizers, 143–144
  oxygen as driving gas, 154–155
  pentamidine in AIDS patients,
    424–425
  sputum induction, 423
  ultrasonic nebulizers, 145, 148
Negative extrathoracic pressure
    ventilation (NEPV)
  chronic lung disease
    (bronchopulmonary dysplasia),
    301

neonatal intensive care, 299
Negative pressure ventilation, 85
  poliomyelitis, 273
Neonatal intensive care unit
  blood pressure monitoring, 292
  complications of ventilatory support,
    300–301
    bronchopulmonary
      dysplasia/chronic lung disease,
      300–301
    pneumothorax, 300
    pulmonary interstitial emphysema,
      300
    retinopathy of prematurity, 300
    subglottic stenosis, 300
  congenital abnormalities, 293,
    296–298
  electrocardiographic (ECG)
    monitoring, 292
  endotracheal tubes, 291
  equipment, 289–292
  handling, 293
  headbox, 291
  humidifiers, 291
  incubators/radiant warmers, 291
  indications for admission, 292
  infants with perinatal problems, 293,
    296
  low birth weight infant, 293–296
  nasal prong (nasopharyngeal tube),
    291
  parent-infant bonding, 293
  phototherapy unit, 291
  physiotherapy, 292–298
  preterm infants, 293–296
  respiratory monitoring, 292
  transcutaneous carbon dioxide
    monitors, 292
  transcutaneous oxygen monitors, 292
  ventilation, 290–291, 298–301
    conventional positive pressure
      ventilation, 298–299
    extracorporeal membrane
      oxygenation, 299
    high frequency jet ventilation
      (HFJV), 299–300
    high frequency oscillation (HFO),
      299–300
    indications, 298
    mechanical ventilators, 290–291
    negative extrathoracic pressure
      ventilation, 299
    patient-triggered, 299
    respiratory distress syndrome, 293,
      294
    retinopathy of prematurity
      prevention, 299
Neonate
  intensive care see Neonatal intensive
    care unit
  nasopharyngeal suction, 289
  pneumonia, 305
  position for oxygenation, 287
  REM sleep, 283
  respiratory assessment, 284

respiratory distress see Respiratory
    distress syndrome
Neurofibromatosis, 43
Neurological disorders
  Cheyne–Stokes respiration, 14
  nasotracheal suction, 161
Neuromuscular disorders, 270–274
  breathlessness, 5
  nasal intermittent positive pressure
    ventilation (NIPPV), 85
  risk of cardiac arrest, 93
Neurophysiological facilitation
    technique, 268
Neuropraxia, 268
New York Heart Association (NYHA)
    scale, 6, 215, 325
Night sweats, 7
Nimodipine, 97
Nitrates, cardiovascular effects, 324
Nitroglycerin, 333
Nocturnal carbon dioxide retention
  morning headache, 8
  respiratory muscle weakness,
    212–213
Non-steroidal anti-inflammatory drugs
    (NSAIDs), 229
  bone pain in lung cancer, 372
  pneumonia, 227
Non-verbal communication, 175,
    176–178
Nutrition
  bronchiolitis, 304
  chronic airflow limitation, 217
  pertussis, 305
  preterm/low birth weight infants, 296
  respiratory muscle weakness, 219
Nutritional support
  inhalational burns, 275
  postoperative, 241

Obesity
  body mass index (BMI), 11
  breathlessness, 205
  chest expansion palpation, 15
  deep vein thrombosis, 242
  gallstones, 244
  hernias, 245, 246
  percussion note, 16
  postoperative respiratory
    complications, 11, 41, 202, 227,
    240
  reduction in lung volume, 205–206
  respiratory function, 10, 11, 205
    following anaesthesia, 57
    postoperative, 202
  risk of cardiac arrest, 93
  type B (blue bloater) chronic airflow
    limitation, 216
Obesity hypoventilation syndrome, 206
Oblique radiograph, 43
Obliterative bronchiolitis, following
    lung/heart–lung transplantation,
    315, 347
Observational research, 190
Obstructive sleep apnoea, 56

Oesophageal atresia with tracheo-oesophageal fistula, 297
Oesophageal cancer, 263
Oesophageal pain, 230
Oesophageal spasm, 230
Oesophageal tear, 230
    penetrating chest injury, 267
Oesophagectomy, 263
Ompholocele see Exompholos
Ondine's curse see Congenital central hypoventilation
Open lung biopsy, 255
Opiate analgesia, 229
    lung cancer pain relief, 372, 373
    postoperative
        breathing patterns, 202
        in children, 308
Oral contraceptives, 242
Oral high frequency oscillation (OHFO), 134–135
Orogastric feeding, preterm infants, 296
Oropharyngeal airway, 161
    with multiple trauma, 268
Oropharyngeal suction, 160, 161
    poliomyelitis, 273
Orthopnoea, 6
    diaphragm weakness, 218
    pulmonary oedema, 211
    respiratory muscle weakness, 212
Osteoporosis, 247
Otitis media
    immunodeficient patient, 420
    primary ciliary dyskinesia, 403
Outcome audit, 22
Outcome evaluation, 21
Oxygen concentrator, 155, 184
Oxygen consumption estimation, 71
Oxygen cost diagram, 195, 214
Oxygen delivery estimation, 53–54, 71
Oxygen dissociation curve, 54
Oxygen saturation
    chest physiotherapy effects, 68
    measurement, 54–55
    monitoring, 67, 68–69
        oxygen therapy, 153
    normal values, 431
Oxygen therapy, 83, 153–157
    asthma, acute attack, 303, 392
    bronchiolitis, 304
    bronchitis, chronic, 226
    cardiac failure, 221
    chronic airflow limitation, 216–217
        long term, 217
        type B (blue bloater), 216, 217
    chronic lung disease (bronchopulmonary dysplasia), 301
    collapse (atelectasis), 205
    cystic fibrosis, 407, 414
    domiciliary, 155–156, 301
    drug overdose, 274
    fibrotic lung conditions, 212
    fixed performance device, 153–154
    gas exchange impairment, 219

with humidification, 152, 154, 226
immunodeficient patient, 422
inhalational burns, 275
inspired phased delivery system, 156
with intermittent positive pressure breathing device, 155
laryngotracheobronchitis, acute (croup), 306
monitoring, 153
nebulizers, 154–155
oxygen concentrator, 155
with portable oxygen, 155–156
    patient assessment, 156
pulmonary embolism, 220
respiratory muscle weakness, 213
sputum retention, 223
toxicity, 86
by transtracheal catheter, 156
variable performance device, 154
Oxygen transport, 54
    with cardiopulmonary dysfunction, 101
    haemoglobin oxygen saturation measurement, 54
    improvement by positioning/mobilization of patient, 99
    pathway, 99–101
    tests, 54–55

Paediatrics, 281–317
    abdominal distension, 285–286
    acute epiglottitis, 306
    acute laryngotracheobronchitis (croup), 305–306
    asthma, 301–303
    bronchiolitis, 303–304
    childhood respiratory disease, 301–307
    comparisons with adult
        anatomical aspects, 282–283
        physiological aspects, 283–284
    congenital heart disease/cardiac surgery, 309–315, 336–337
    cystic fibrosis see Cystic fibrosis
    equipment, 289–292
    hernias, 245, 246
    inhaled foreign body, 306–307
    intensive care see Neonatal intensive care unit
    lung development, 281–282
    pertussis, 304–305
    physiotherapy techniques, 286–289
    pneumonia, 305
    primary ciliary dyskinesia, 307
    psychological aspects, 281
        parental stress, 281
    respiratory assessment, 284–286
        auscultation, 285
        barrel shaped thoracic cage, 285
        discussion with carers, 284
        examination, 284–285
        investigations, 284
        medical notes, 284

nursing charts, 284
observations, 285, 286
respiratory distress
    behaviour/appearance, 285
    grunting, 285
    head bobbing, 285
    nasal flaring, 285
    neck extension, 285
    recession, 285
    stridor, 285
    tachypnoea, 285
surgery, 307–309
transplantation procedures, 314–315
trauma, 315–317
    head injury, 315–316
ventilation, 301
    in neonate/infant see Neonatal intensive care unit
Pain
    cough reflex inhibition, 224
    measurement scales, 195–196, 229
        McGill pain questionnaire, 195, 196
        visual analogue scales, 196
    see also Chest pain
Palpation, 15–16
    chest expansion, 15–16
    trachea, 15
Pancoast's tumour, 372
    hand muscle wasting, 12
Paracetamol, 372
Paradoxical breathing, 15
    flail chest, 266
    Hoover's sign, 15
    spinal cord injury, 358, 359
Parainfluenza virus bronchiolitis, 303
Paralysed patient
    active cycle of breathing, 126
    body positioning, 105
    glossopharyngeal breathing, 130
    joint contractures prevention, 199
Paraspinal line, 29
Paroxysmal nocturnal dyspnoea, 6
    cardiac failure, 220–221
    pulmonary oedema, 211
Partial thromboplastin time, 76
Patient controlled analgesia (PCA), 241
Peak expiratory flow (PEF), 48, 49, 51
    asthma assessment, 390, 393
Peak expiratory mouth pressure, normal values, 432
Peak inspiratory mouth pressure, normal values, 432
Pectus carinatum (pigeon chest), 14
    surgery, 257
Pectus excavatum (funnel chest), 14
    chest radiography, 31
    surgery, 257
Pelvic floor exercises, 248
Pelvic tilting, 248
Pentamidine
    AIDS patients, 424–425
    nebulized, 144, 146
Percutaneous needle biopsy, 26

complications, 38
CT/fluoroscopic guidance, 38
pulmonary mass, 38
pulmonary nodule, 38
Percutaneous transluminal coronary
    angioplasty, 259
Pericardial chest drain, 259
Pericardial constriction, 71
Pericardial effusion, 64
Pericarditis
    chest pain, 7, 230
    electrocardiogram (ECG), 64
Perinatal problems, neonatal intensive
    care, 293, 296
Periodic continuous positive airway
    pressure (PCPAP), 139–140
    bronchiectasis, acute exacerbation,
        402
    chest injury, 267
    in children, 140
    collapse (atelectasis), 140, 205
    contraindications, 140–141
    cystic fibrosis, 414
    effects, 141
    humidification, 139
    indications, 141
    with inhalational burns, 276
    position, 140
    postoperative, 203, 243
        aortic aneurysm surgery, 264
        cardiac surgery, 261
        lobectomy, 253
    treatment regimen, 140
Peripheral nerve injury, 268
Peripheral oedema
    cardiac failure, 220
    objective assessment, 13
    subjective assessment, 8
Peritoneal dialysis, 89, 90, 261
    complications, 90
    pleural effusion, 206, 207
    reduction in lung volume, 206
Periventricular haemorrhage, 294–295
Periventricular leucomalacia, 295
Persistent ductus arteriosus (PDA),
    309, 310
Pertussis, 304–305
    bronchiectasis, 224
    bronchopneumonia, 305
    clinical features, 304–305
    management, 305
    physiotherapy, 305
Pethidine, 308
Phlebography, 242
Phosphor plate radiography, 24, 25
    postoperative/critically ill patient, 39
Phototherapy, preterm infants, 295
Phototherapy unit, 291
Phrenic nerve palsy, 256, 299
Pink puffer (type A) chronic airflow
    limitation, 216
Platelet count, 75, 76
Pleural cancer, 228
Pleural disorders
    breathlessness, 218

imaging, 37–38
management, 208–209, 218
reduction in lung volume, 199,
    206–209
Pleural effusion
    breathlessness, 218
    cardiac failure, 43, 62, 220
    causes, 207
    clinical features, 207
    drainage, 25
    following liver transplantation, 315
    following lung surgery, 256
    imaging, 23, 62
    lung function effects, 207
    opaque hemithorax, 36
    percussion of chest, 16
    pulmonary embolism, 43
    reduction in lung volume, 206–207
    tracheal deviation, 15
    ultrasonography, 23, 25
    vocal fremitus, 16
    vocal resonance, 19
Pleural rub, 18–19
Pleural surgery, 257–258
Pleurectomy, 258
Pleuritic chest pain, 7, 228
    pneumonia, 226, 227
    TENS pain relief, 164
Pleurodesis, 258
Pneumococcus pneumonia, 305
Pneumoconiosis, 39
Pneumocystis carinii 420, 422
    nebulized pentamidine, 146
    sputum induction for diagnosis, 423
Pneumomediastinum
    complicating asthma, 45
    postoperative imaging, 42
    with surgical emphysema, 15, 16
Pneumonectomy, 255–256
    lung function following, 57
    mediastinal position maintenance,
        255
    physiotherapy, 255–256
    preoperative assessment, 255
Pneumonia
    acid-base status, 77
    bronchial secretions clearance,
        226–227
    bronchopneumonia, 226
    cavitating pulmonary lesions, 39
    children, 305
    classification, 226
    community acquired, 80
    consolidation, 32, 226
    continuous positive airway pressure
        (CPAP), 83
    empyema, 207
    gas exchange impairment, 54
    with inhalational burns, 274, 276
    interstitial pneumonitis, 226
    lobar, 32, 226
    mechanical ventilation, 85
    microbiological investigations, 79–80
    persistent with bronchial carcinoma,
        227

pleuritic pain, 226, 227, 228
postoperative, 227
    imaging, 42
preterm/low birth weight infants, 294
ventilator patients, 80
Pneumoperitoneum, 244
Pneumothorax
    blunt chest injury, 265
    breathlessness, 218
    causes, 35
    chest radiography, 35
    complicating asthma, 45
    complicating central catheter
        placement, 40
    complicating emphysema, 46
    cystic fibrosis, 407, 413, 414–415
    Entonox contraindication, 162
    following cardiac surgery, 260
    imaging in postoperative/critically ill
        patient, 39
    intercostal drainage, 251
    IPPB/PCPAP contraindication, 140
    lung volume reduction, 208
    neonate, 300
    percussion note, 16
    pleuritic pain, 228
    reduction in lung volume, 208
    spontaneous, 208
        formation mechanisms, 257–258
        intercostal drainage, 258
        management, 258
        recurrence, 258
    with surgical emphysema, 266
    tension, 35, 41, 208, 250, 265, 267,
        300
    tracheal deviation, 15
    vocal fremitus, 16
    vocal resonance, 19
Poliomyelitis, 273–274
    clinical features, 273
    management, 273
    physiotherapy, 273–274
    residual paralysis, 273
    respiratory function effects, 51
    respiratory muscle paralysis, 273
Pollutants, atmospheric
    lung cancer risk, 252
    mucociliary clearance effect, 222
Polycythaemia
    causes, 75
    cyanosis, 12
    eye examination, 12
    haemoglobin (Hb) measurement, 75
Portable oxygen cylinders, 155–156
Portable radiography, 23
    pneumothorax, 35
    postoperative/critically ill patient, 39
Positioning
    bronchiectasis, acute exacerbation,
        402
    cardiopulmonary transplantation
        postoperative care, 353
    cystic fibrosis, 408
    drainage of pulmonary secretions,
        103–104

Positioning (*contd*)
  gravity-assisted *see* Gravity-assisted
      positioning
  head injured patients, 269
  immunodeficient patients, 424
    with septic arthritis/osteomyelitis,
        425
  kinetic beds/chairs, 107–108
  lung cancer patient, 253, 373
  with multiple trauma, 268
  oxygen transport effects, 99, 110
    with acute cardiopulmonary
        dysfunction, 101–105
    assessment, 104, 110
    with chronic cardiopulmonary
        dysfunction, 108
    physiological rationale, 102–104
    progression of stimulus, 105
    treatment planning, 104–105, 110
  poliomyelitis, 273
  postoperative, 242, 243
    aortic aneurysm surgery, 264
    cardiac surgery, 261, 313, 314
    children, 313, 314
    lobectomy, 253
  prevention of negative effects of
      immobilization, 109
  respiratory muscle weakness, 219
Positive end expiratory pressure
    (PEEP), 84, 86
  adult respiratory distress syndrome
      (ARDS), 276, 277
  barotrauma, 41, 86
  chest radiography, 41
  with manual hyperinflation, 157
Positive expiratory pressure (PEP),
    132–134
  high-pressure, 133–134
Positive pressure ventilation,
    conventional
  in neonate, 298–299
    weaning from ventilator, 299
Posteroanterior (PA) radiograph, 23, 30
  collapse (atelactasis), 33–35
  normal anatomy, 27–29
Posterolateral thoracotomy incision,
    252
Postherpetic neuralgia, 164
Postoperative air leaks, 141
Postoperative pain relief, 202, 203,
    229, 241–242, 243
  aortic aneurysm surgery, 264
  cardiac surgery, 261, 323
  in children, 308
  local anaesthesia, 238
  patient controlled analgesia (PCA),
      241
  pulmonary collapse with heavy
      analgesia, 41
  transcutaneous electrical nerve
      stimulation (TENS), 162–163
Postoperative patient
  active cycle of breathing, 121
    chest compression/wound support,
        126

adult respiratory distress syndrome
    (ARDS), 41–42
analgesia *see* Postoperative pain relief
assessment, 243
bronchial secretions clearance, 203,
    222
cardiac surgery, 259–260, 323
chest auscultation, 18
collapse of lung tissue, 41, 140, 203,
    205
  with obesity, 11
cough, 6, 224
deep vein thrombosis/pulmonary
    embolus, 43, 242–243
drains, 11–12, 242
early ambulation, 203, 243
functional residual capacity
    reduction, 242
general surgery, 243–247
gynaecological surgery, 247–248
incentive spirometry, 141, 142
incisional site, 241
intermittent positive pressure
    breathing (IPPB), 243
lung function impairment, 57, 202
lung volume reduction, 201–203
  management, 202–203
  treatment outcome monitoring,
      203
mechanical ventilation, elective, 85
periodic continuous positive airway
    pressure (PCPAP), 140, 203,
    243
positioning, 201, 203, 243
renal function, 243
stress, 243
thoracic imaging, 39–43
  aspiration pneumonia, 41
  cardiac failure, 42–43
  extrapulmonary air, 42
  pneumonia, 42
  pulmonary collapse, 41
  pulmonary embolism, 43
  see also Intensive care unit (ICU)
Postoperative respiratory complications
  alcohol abuse, 241
  bullous emphysema, 256
  cardiac surgery, 260
  cardiovascular disease, 240
  cholecystectomy, 244
  with chronic airflow limitation, 246
  with chronic respiratory disease, 240
  elderly patients, 240
  malnutrition, 240–241
  myasthenia gravis, 270
  obesity, 240
  prevention in children, 308–309
  respiratory infection, 202, 205, 227,
      260
  smokers, 240
  upper abdominal surgery, 241
Postural drainage *see* Gravity-assisted
    positioning
Postural drainage frame, 400
Postural hypotension, 10

Posture exercises
  asthma, 303
  cardiac surgery, 262, 314
  children, 303, 309, 314
  cystic fibrosis, 413
  head and neck surgery, 264
  lobectomy patients, 255
  thoracoplasty patients, 257
Potassium levels, 78
Potassium supplements, 221
Pregnancy
  cystic fibrosis, 415
  reduction in lung volume, 206
Preoperative assessment, 243
Pressurized aerosol (metered dose)
    inhalers, 142–143
  asthma, 302
  breath-actuated, 143
  in childhood, 143, 302
  spacers, 142, 143, 302
Preterm infant
  causes of preterm birth, 293
  chest auscultation, 285
  chest percussion, 286
  chest vibration/shaking, 286
  infection, 295
  jaundice, 295
  manual hyperinflation, 288
  neonatal intensive care, 293
    problems, 293–294
  nutrition, 296
  periventricular
      haemorrhage/leucomalacia,
      294–295
  pneumothorax complicating
      ventilatory support, 300
  position for physiotherapy, 287
  positive pressure ventilation, 298
  pulmonary haemorrhage, 296
  pulmonary interstitial emphysema,
      300
  respiratory assessment, 284
  respiratory distress, 293–294
    pneumonia, 294
  respiratory rate, 285
  retinopathy of prematurity, 299,
      300
  suction, 289
  temperature control, 295
Preventive medicine, 182, 184
Primary ciliary dyskinesia, 307,
    402–404
  bronchial secretions clearance, 225
  clinical features, 403
  investigations, 403
  medical management, 403
  physiotherapy, 403–404
    evaluation, 404
Problem list, POMR, 3, 20–21
Problem orientated medical records
    (POMR), 3, 4
  database, 3–20
  discharge summary, 3, 22
  initial plan/goals, 3, 21
  problem list, 3, 20–21

progress notes, 3, 21
  subjective assessment, 5–9
Problem orientated medical system
    (POMS), 3, 199
Process audit, 22
Progress notes, POMR, 3, 21
Prone position
  oxygen transport effects, 103
    abdomen free/restricted, 103, 104
    three-quarters prone, 104
Proprioceptive neuromuscular
    facilitation
  immunodeficient states, 425
  shoulder joint movement in
    lobectomy patients, 254
Prothrombin time (PTT), 76
  international normalized ratio (INR),
    76, 79
Pseudomonas aeruginosa
  bronchiectasis, 224
  with cystic fibrosis, 225, 406
Pseudomonas cepacia, 406
Pseudomonas infection
  burns patients, 276
  inhaled antibiotics, 145, 146
Psychological aspects
  breathlessness, 221
  cardiac rehabilitation, 321
  cardiorespiratory dysfunction,
    173–175
    anxiety, 173–174
    defence mechanisms, 174
    family relationships disruption,
      174
    reactive depression, 174
    stigmatization, 174
    care/treatment, 174–175
  immunodeficient patients, 426
  mastectomy, 246
  spinal cord injury, 359
Psychosocial care, 175
Pulmonary agenesis, 43
Pulmonary angiography, 242
Pulmonary arteriovenous
    malformation, 26
Pulmonary artery catheterization, 71
  with positive end expiratory pressure
    (PEEP), 86
Pulmonary artery pressure
  intensive care patient monitoring, 11
  normal values, 431
Pulmonary artery wedge pressure, 64
  following cardiac surgery, 260
Pulmonary capillary wedge pressure
  monitoring, 71
    radiographic check of catheter
      position, 40
    normal values, 431
Pulmonary embolism, 323
  acid-base status, 77
  breathlessness, 219–220
  cardiac catheterization, 71
  clinical features, 220, 242
  electrocardiogram (ECG), 64
  embolectomy, 242

fibrinolysis, 242
gas exchange impairment, 54
immobilized patient, 93
inferior vena caval filter, 242
management, 220, 242
pleural effusion, 208
postoperative patient, 242–243
  imaging, 43
prophylaxis, 243
pulmonary arteriography, 26
Pulmonary haemorrhage, preterm/low
    birth weight infants, 296
Pulmonary hypertensive crises,
    postoperative, 314
Pulmonary hypoplasia, 298, 299
Pulmonary interstitial emphysema
  complicating asthma, 45
  high frequency jet ventilation/high
    frequency oscillation, 299
  imaging, postoperative, 42
  neonatal complicating ventilatory
    support, 300
Pulmonary mass
  imaging, 38
  percutaneous needle biopsy, 26, 38
Pulmonary nodule
  chest radiography, 24, 38
  computed tomography (CT), 26, 38
  histoplasmosis, 38
  imaging, 38–39
  metastatic deposits, 38, 39
  miliary, 38–39
  multiple, 38
  percutaneous needle biopy, 38
Pulmonary oedema, 209–211
  alveolar, 209, 211
  breathlessness, 211, 220, 221
  cardiac catheterization, 71
  cardiogenic, 220, 221
    continuous positive airway
      pressure (CPAP), 221
  causes, 209
  clinical features, 211
  fluid accumulation, 209
  stages, 209–210
  following cardiac surgery, 260
  impaired clearance/excess bronchial
    secretions, 227–228
  inspiratory crackles, 18
  interstitial, 209, 211
  lung function, 211
  management, 211
  mechanical ventilation, 85
  obstructive component, 211
  restrictive component, 211
  role of physiotherapist, 211
Pulmonary stenosis, 309, 313
  exercise tolerance following repair,
    337
  surgery, 313
Pulmonary vascular resistance (PVR)
    estimation, 71
Pulse deficit, 10
Pulse oximetry, 68–69
  chest clapping, 124

oxygen saturation (SaO$_2$)
  measurement, 54–55
  oxygen therapy monitoring, 155, 156
  ventilatory failure during sleep, 56
Pulse rate
  following cardiac surgery, 259
    exercise monitoring, 262
  objective assessment, 10
Pulsus paradoxus, 10, 390
Pursed-lip breathing, 14, 115

Quality of life
  cardiac rehabilitation, 333
    with cardiac failure, 335
  cardiopulmonary rehabilitation, 165
  palliative care, 368
Questionnaires, 192–193, 196
  functional activity with respiratory
    disease, 214
  lung disease assessment, 59

Radiant warmers, 291, 295
Radionuclide techniques, 242
  cardiac imaging, 62, 63
    ^{201}Tl scan, 63
    ^{99m}Tc red blood cell scan, 63
    ejection fraction measurement, 63
  pulmonary embolism, 43
Râles *see* Crackles
Rapid shallow breathing index, 86
Rating of perceived exertion (RPE),
    214, 326, 332
  cardiac rehabilitation exercise
    programme monitoring, 329,
    332
  cardiopulmonary transplantation
    rehabilitation, 354
Rebreathing therapy, 384–385
Recession, 285
Rectocele repair, 248
Recurrent laryngeal nerve, lung cancer
    involvement, 253
Relaxation techniques
  breathlessness with fear/anxiety, 221
  cardiac rehabilitation, 320
  cardiopulmonary transplantation
    postoperative care, 353
  hyperventilation syndrome, 379,
    386
Renal failure, acute
  following cardiac surgery, 260–261
  with inhalational burns, 275
  postoperative, 243
  renal support, 89, 91
Renal failure, chronic
  daily weight, 11
  metabolic acidosis, 77
  renal support, 89, 91
Renal function
  postoperative patients, 243
  tests, 78
Renal support, 89–91
  aims, 89
  continuous forms, 89–90
    continuous haemofiltration, 89–90

Renal support (contd)
    continuous haemofiltration with
        dialysis, 90
    dialysis, 89
    hazards for physiotherapists, 91
    indications, 91
    peritoneal dialysis, 90
Research, 187–197
    convergent/divergent thinking, 188
    data analysis, 197
    data collection, 196
    definition of question, 188–189
    design, 190–193
        censuses/surveys, 192
        clinical trials, 191
        descriptive studies, 190–191
        observational studies, 190
        questionnaires, 192–193
        single case study designs, 191–192
    ethical committees, 194
    fieldwork organization, 196
    literature review, 187–188
        reading articles, 187–188
        search, 187
        writing review, 188
    mind maps, 188, 189
    objectives/hypotheses, 189–190
    obtaining grants, 193
    patient consent, 194
    pilot work, 196–197
    proposal, 193–194
        background, 193–194
        plan of investigation, 194
        title, 193
    publication, 197
    questionnaires, 196
    reports, 197
    stages, 187
    statistical tests, 197
    subject availability, 196
    subject numbers, 196
    variables measurement, 194–196
        objectivity, 194
        reliability, 194–195
        scales, 195–196
        statistical tests, 195
        validity, 195
Residual volume (RV), 51
    in children, 58
Respiratory arrest
    recognition, 94
    risk situations, 93
Respiratory distress syndrome
    acquired lobar emphysema/lung
        cysts, 298
    extracorporeal membrane
        oxygenation, 87
    high frequency jet ventilation/high
        frequency oscillation, 299
    preterm/low birth weight infants,
        293–294
    surfactant therapy, 294
    ventilatory support
        complications, 300
        patient-triggered, 299

Respiratory failure
    definition, 56, 83
    lung function tests, 56
    respiratory support see Respiratory
        support
Respiratory function
    developmental aspects, 57, 283–284
    general anaesthesia effect, 200
    patient mobilization effect, 105
    patient positioning effect, 103
    postoperative, 57, 202, 242
    spinal cord injury, 358–359
    supine position effects, 103
    see also Airway function tests; Lung
        function tests
Respiratory infection
    bronchiectasis, acute exacerbation,
        402
    with chronic airflow limitation, 216,
        217
    with gas exchange impairment, 219
    immunodeficient patients, 420, 423,
        424
    mucus secretions viscosity, 150
    myasthenia gravis, 270
    postoperative, 202, 205, 227, 260
    primary ciliary dyskinesia, 403
    with sputum retention, 222
Respiratory movements, 14, 15, 357
    infants/children, 283, 285
Respiratory muscle weakness/paralysis
    breathlessness, 218–219
    with cardiac failure, 220
    cough reflex inhibition, 224
    hypercapnic respiratory failure, 213
    lung function abnormalities,
        212–213
    lung volume reduction, 200,
        212–213
    management, 213, 219
    mechanical ventilation, 85, 213
    myasthenia gravis, 270
    nasal intermittent positive pressure
        ventilation (NIPPV), 85
    neonatal negative extrathoracic
        pressure ventilation (NEPV),
        299
    nocturnal hypoventilation, 212–213
    poliomyelitis, 273
    quantification, 212
Respiratory muscles, 357
    function tests, 51–53
        endurance capacity tests, 53
    level of innervation, 357
    spasm in tetanus, 272
    spinal cord injury effects, 358
    training, 164–165
Respiratory rate
    infant/neonate, 283, 285
    monitoring, 67, 68
        cardiac rehabilitation exercise
            programme, 332
    normal values, 431
    objective assessment, 10
    physiotherapy effects, 68

Respiratory support, 83–88
    acid-base status, 77
    acute epiglottitis, 306
    adult respiratory distress syndrome
        (ARDS), 276
    aims, 85
    asthma, severe acute, 394–395
    barotrauma, 41, 42, 86
    bronchiolitis, 304
    cardiac surgery, 260, 261
    cardiopulmonary transplantation,
        354
    children, 290–291, 301
    complications, 86
    continuous positive airway pressure,
        83–84
    conventional mechanical ventilation,
        84–85
    extracorporeal carbon dioxide
        removal, 87
    extracorporeal membrane
        oxygenation, 87
    Guillain–Barré syndrome, 271
    high frequency jet ventilation,
        87–88
    indications, 85
    inspiratory pressure support (IPS),
        84–85
    intensive care patient, 9, 237
    intravascular oxygenation (IVOX),
        87
    neonate see Neonatal intensive care
    non-invasive, 85
    oxygen see Oxygen therapy
    poliomyelitis, 273
    principles, 84
    respiratory muscle weakness, 85,
        213, 299
    spinal cord injury, 358, 363–365
    tetanus, 272
    tracheal aspirate, 79
    weaning, 86–87, 159, 363–365
        criteria, 86
        difficult, 87
        predictors, 86
Respiratory syncytial virus (RSV)
    bronchiolitis, 303
    pneumonia, 305
Respiratory walking frame, 217
Retinopathy of prematurity, 300
    prevention, 299, 300
    treatment, 300
Retrosternal line, 30
Rhonchi see Wheezes
Rib fracture
    blunt chest injury, 265
    cough fracture, 6
    pain relief, 163, 229, 265
    paradoxical breathing, 15
    with pneumothorax, 208
    posteroanterior radiograph, 29
    with spinal cord injury, 359, 361
Rib springing, 126
Ribavirin, 304
Rickets, 286

Right atrial pressure
  following cardiac surgery, 259
  normal values, 431
Right ventricular pressure, normal
    values, 431
Road traffic accident, 267, 268

St George's Questionnaire, 59
Salbutamol, 144, 148
Saline instillation
  airway suction, 160, 162, 289
  inhalational burns, 276
  with manual hyperinflation, 158, 269
  mucociliary clearance stimulation,
    222, 423
Sarcoidosis, 39
Scalenes, respiratory function, 51, 357
Scapulae, lateral view, 29–30
Scoliosis, 14
  respiratory function effects, 51
Segmentectomy, 255
Self-treatment
  active cycle of breathing techniques,
    121
  bronchiectasis, 400
  bronchitis, chronic, 226
  chest clapping, 122, 123–124
  chest compression, 125
  chest vibrations, 125
  cystic fibrosis, 409
  post-laryngectomy, 224
Self-help groups, 184
Sepsis
  cardiac catheterization, 71
  microbiological investigations, 79, 80
  toxic psychosis, 241
Serum albumin, 79
Severity of illness scoring system, 237
Shock
  cardiogenic, 71, 88
  metabolic acidosis, 76–77
Shoulder girdle exercises
  aortic aneurysm surgery, 265
  cardiac surgery, 262
    in children, 314
  lobectomy, 254
  mastectomy, 246
  thoracoplasty, 257
Shuttle walk test, 20, 61
Side lying
  bronchial secretions clearance, 126
  bronchiectasis, acute exacerbation,
    402
  intermittent positive pressure
    breathing, 137, 138
  lobectomy patients, 253
  manual hyperinflation, 157
  postoperative patient, 203, 242
    children, 308–309
Side-to-side positioning, 103
Silhouette sign, 31
Single case study designs, 191–192
Sinus bradycardia, 73
Sinus tachycardia, 73
Sitting position

aortic aneurysm surgery, 264
inhalational burns, 276
intermittent positive pressure
    breathing, 137
postoperative patient, 203, 242, 243
  children, 309
Six minute walk test, 20, 60
  cardiac rehabilitation, 327
  chronic airflow limitation, 217
  oxygen therapy with portable oxygen,
    156
Skin-prick tests, 392
Sleeping positions, breathlessness, 221
Smoking, 12
  chronic airflow limitation, 217
  cough, 6, 222
  deep vein thrombosis risk, 242
  lung cancer risk, 252
  lung function impairment following
    anaesthesia, 57
  mucociliary clearance effect, 222
  postoperative lung function, 201
  postoperative respiratory
    complications, 202, 227, 240
  spontaneous pneumothorax, 258
SOAP, progress notes, 3, 21
Sodium bicarbonate
  advanced life support, 97
  metabolic acidosis, 77
Sodium cromoglycate, 145, 215, 302,
    392
Sodium levels, 78
Soft tissue stretching
  cardiopulmonary transplantation
    postoperative care, 353
  Guillain–Barré syndrome, 271
  poliomyelitis, 273
Spinal cord injury, 357–365
  abdominal binders, 361
  associated trauma, 268, 359
  battery-driven ventilator, 363
  cough, 358, 360
    assisted, 360, 361, 362, 363
  home ventilation, 364
  physiotherapy techniques, 360–365
    non-ventilated patients, 361, 363
    prophylactic treatment, 360–361
    ventilator dependent patient, 363
  posture effects, 359
  psychological aspects, 359
  respiratory assessment, 359–360
    vital capacity measurement, 360
  respiratory muscle effects, 358–359
  with rib fracture, 359, 361
  ventilator weaning, 363–365
  ventilator dependent patient, 358,
    363
    diaphragmatic pacing, 364–365
    ethical aspects, 364
    psychological support, 363, 364
Spirometry, 48–49, 51
  lung volume measurement, 51
  results evaluation, 20
Sputum retention, 224–228
  clinical features, 222–223

cough reflex failure, 223–224
inspiratory crackles, 18
physiotherapy evaluation, 228
wheezes, 18
Sputum specimen, 6, 7, 19, 222
  airway suction, 160
  asthma, 391
  bronchiectasis, 399
  microbiological investigations, 79–80
  nebulized hypertonic saline
    induction, 147
  Pneumocystis carinii pneumonia
    diagnosis, 423
  subjective assessment, 6–7
Stabbing injury, 267
Stair climbing exercise
  with breathing control, 116, 217,
    218, 256
  bronchiectasis, 402
  bullous emphysema, 256
  chronic airflow limitation, 217
  fibrotic lung conditions, 218
  postoperative
    cardiac surgery, 262
    cardiopulmonary rehabilitation,
      166
    cardiopulmonary transplantation,
      353
    lobectomy, 254
    pneumonectomy, 256
Staphylococcus
  bronchiectasis, 224
  cystic fibrosis, 225, 406
  lung abscess, 227
  pneumonia, 305
    burns patients, 276
    cavitating pulmonary lesions, 39
    complicating pertussis, 305
Steam inhalations, 152
Sternal thump, 97
Sternocleidomastoid
  respiratory function, 51, 357
  spinal cord injury effects, 358
Sternotomy, 252
  cardiac surgery, 259, 262, 310
  delayed healing, 261, 262
Stethoscope, 17
Strangulated hernia, 246
Streptococcus
  acute exacerbation of chronic
    bronchitis, 225
  pneumonia, 80, 305
    group B in preterm infants, 294
Stress ulcer, postoperative, 243
Stridor, 7
  children, 289
  infant/neonate, 285
Subglottic stenosis, 300
Subphrenic fluid collection, 25
Suction see Airway suction
Superior vena caval obstruction, 373
  stent insertion, 27
  superior vena cavography, 27
Superior vena cavography, 27
Supine chest radiograph, 30–31

Supine position
  haemodynamic effects, 103
  respiratory function effects, 103
  respiratory muscle
      weakness/paralysis, 219
Surfactant
  developmental aspects, 282, 283
  in respiratory distress syndrome, 293
  therapy, 294, 296
Surgical emphysema, 15–16
  blunt chest injury, 266
  following lung surgery, 256
Surgical patients, 238–277
  anaesthesia, 200, 238
  in children, 307–309
      postoperative care, 308–309
      preoperative preparation, 308
  general surgery, 243–247
  gynaecological surgery, 247–248
  high risk factors, 240–241
      alcohol abuse, 241
      cardiovascular disease, 240
      chronic respiratory disease, 240
      diabetes, 241
      elderly patients, 240
      haemophilia, 240
      mental changes, 241
      nutritional status, 240–241
      obesity, 240
      smoking, 240
  incisional sites, 238, 239
  lung function impairment, 57
  postoperative assessment, 243
  postoperative period see
      Postoperative patients
  preoperative assessment, 243
  reduction in lung volume, 199,
      200–203
      operation site, 200
  sutures, 238–240
  thoracic procedures, 200, 202, 224,
      248–258
Sutures, 238–240
  recommended times for removal, 239
Swabs, microbiological investigations,
      80
Swallowing reflex impairment, 269–270
Swan–Ganz catheter, 64
  radiographic check of position, 40
Synchronized intermittent mandatory
      ventilation (SIMV), 84
Systemic vascular resistance (SVR)
      estimation, 71

T-tube drainage, 244
Tachycardia, 10
Tachypnoea, 10
Teaching stethoscope, 17
Temperature control, preterm/low
      birth weight infants, 295
Tension pneumothorax, 35, 41, 208,
      265
  with closed intercostal drainage, 250
  with multiple trauma, 267
  neonate, 300

Terbutaline, 148
Tetanus, 93, 271–273
  muscle rigidity, 271
  physiotherapy, 272–273
  respiratory muscle effects, 272
Tetralogy of Fallot, 259, 309, 310–312
  Blalock-Taussig shunt, 259, 311
  exercise tolerance following repair,
      337
  surgery, 311
Tetraplegic patients
  abdominal binders, 361
  glossopharyngeal breathing,
      360–361
  respiratory function, 358
      posture effects, 359
      in spinal shock, 358
  respiratory training, 360
  ventilator dependent patient, 363,
      364
      diaphragmatic pacing, 364–365
      ethical aspects, 364
      psychological support, 364
Theophylline, 302, 303
Thoracic expansion exercises, 116,
      118–119
  bronchiectasis, 400
  with chest clapping, 123, 124
  with chest shaking/vibrations, 124
  pain relief, 162
  postoperative, 203
      cardiopulmonary transplantation,
          353
      pneumonectomy, 255
  preoperative instruction, 243
Thoracic imaging, 23–46
  bronchiectasis, 43–45
  chronic airflow limitation, 45–46
  computed tomography, 25–26
  cystic fibrosis, 43, 44
  fluoroscopy, 25
  interventional procedures, 26–27
  kyphoscoliosis, 43
  linear tomography, 23, 25
  magnetic resonance imaging, 26
  postoperative/critically ill patient,
      39–43
  radiography, 23–25
  ultrasonography, 25
Thoracic surgery, 248–258
  breathing patterns following, 202
  lung function effects, 200
Thoracoplasty, 256–257
  physiotherapy, 257
Thoracotomy
  anterolateral incision, 252
  cardiac surgery, 259
  congenital heart disease, 310, 313
  lung function impairment, 57
  oesophagectomy, 263
  penetrating chest injury, 266, 267
  posterolateral incision, 252
  postoperative pain relief, 229
  TENS, 163
Thrombocytopenia, 75

Thrombocytosis, 75
Ticarcillin, 146
Tidal volume (V_T)53
Tietze's syndrome see Costochondritis
Tilt table, 166
Total lung capacity (TLC), 51
Total red cell mass, 75
Toxic psychosis, 241
Trachea
  bifurcation, surface landmarks, 13
  deviation in elderly, 29
  lateral view, 29
  palpation, 15
  rupture, 266
Tracheal aspirate, microbiological
      investigations, 79–80
Tracheal suctioning
  hypoxaemia during, 68–69
  ineffective cough, 224
  risk of cardiac arrest, 93
  sinus bradycardia, 73
Tracheitis, 7
Tracheo-oesophageal fistula, 297
Tracheostomy
  acute epiglottitis, 306
  airway suction, 159
      self-treatment, 160
  complications, 41
  Guillain–Barré syndrome, 271
  head injured patients, 269–270
  humidification of inspired air, 150,
      153, 160
  ineffective cough, 223
  inhalational burns, 275
  with laryngectomy, 263
  neonatal following subglottic
      stenosis, 300
  radiographic check of tube position,
      41
  spinal cord injury, 363
  tetanus, 272
  weaning from ventilator/removal of
      tube, 159
Transcutaneous electrical nerve
      stimulation (TENS), 163–164,
      229, 230
  chest wall pain
      following cardiac surgery, 262
      lobectomy patients, 255
  contraindications, 164
  conventional application, 163
  nerve pain in lung cancer, 372
Transcutaneous PO_2/PCO_2
      monitoring, 67, 292
  paediatric patients, 69
Transplantation surgery see
      Cardiopulmonary
      transplantation
Transposition of great arteries, 309,
      311–312
  surgery, 312
Transtracheal catheter, 156
Trapezius
  in inspiration, 357
  spinal cord injury effects, 358

Treatment plan, 21
Tricuspid atresia, 309, 311
  surgery, 311
Trunk mobility exercises
  following cardiac surgery, 262
  lobectomy patients, 255
Tuberculosis, 7
  bronchiectasis, 45, 399
  cavitating pulmonary lesions, 39
  impaired clearance/excess bronchial
    secretions, 227
  miliary pulmonary nodules, 39
  pleuritic pain, 228
  thoracoplasty, 256

Ultrasonic nebulizer, 145, 148
  for humidification, 151, 153
  sputum induction for *Pneumocystis
    carinii* pneumonia diagnosis, 423
Ultrasonography, 25
  elevation of diaphragm, 37
  pleural disease, 37, 38
Umbilical hernia, 246
Upper abdominal surgery
  breathing patterns following, 202
  lung function following, 200, 202
  pleural effusion, 207
  postoperative respiratory
    complications, 241
Upper airway obstruction
  cardiac/respiratory arrest, 94
  Heimlich manoeuvre, 94
  infant/neonate, 282, 285
Upper gastrointestinal tract
  obstruction, 77
Upper limb weight programme, 353
Urea serum levels, 78
Urinary catheterization, 248
Urine specimens, microbiological
  investigations, 80
Uterine prolapse repair, 248
Uterovaginal prolapse, 248

Vagal nerve damage, 224
Vaginal prolapse, 248
Valvular heart disease, 259
  cardiac catheterization, 64

cardiac rehabilitation, 335–336
  heart sounds, 19
  surgery, 258, 259
Varicose veins, 242
Vascular surgery, 264–265
  aortic aneurysm, 264–265
  lower limb ischaemia, 265
Vasodilators, cardiovascular effects,
  221, 324
Venous lines, 11
  advanced life support, 96
  invasive monitoring, 69
Venous stasis, 242
Ventilation/perfusion ($\dot{V}/\dot{Q}$) imbalance,
  53, 54
  with abdominal distension, 205, 206
  asthma, 215, 391
  chronic airflow limitation, 216
  cystic fibrosis, 406
  fibrotic lung conditions, 218
  obese patients, 205
  pleural effusion, 207
  pneumothorax, 208
  postoperative period, 202
  pulmonary embolism, 220
  with sputum retention, 223
Ventilation/perfusion ($\dot{V}/\dot{Q}$) ratio
  mobilization effect, 105
  normal values, 431
  positioning effects, 102
Ventilatory failure
  definition, 56
  gas exchange impairment, 54
Ventilatory support *see* Respiratory
  support
Ventricular assist device (VAD),
  88–89
  complications, 89
  indications, 89
Ventricular fibrillation
  defibrillation, 97
  sternal thump, 97
Ventricular septal defect (VSD), 309,
  310
  exercise tolerance following repair,
    337
  surgery, 258, 310

Venturi mask, 152, 154
Vibratory jackets, 127
Visual analogue scales
  breathlessness, 214, 219
  pain, 196
Vital capacity (VC)
  diaphragm function testing, 52
  in supine position, 56
Vocal cord palsy
  cough reflex inhibition, 224
  lung cancer patients, 253
Vocal fremitus, 16
Vocal resonance, 19

Walking exercise programme
  bronchiectasis, 402
  bronchitis, chronic, 226
  cardiac rehabilitation, 166, 328
  chronic airflow limitation, 217
Walking tests, 59, 60, 61
  cardiac rehabilitation, 327
  exercise tolerance measurement,
    215
  oxygen therapy with portable oxygen,
    156
Warfarin
  deep vein thrombosis, 242
Weaning from ventilator, 86–87, 159
  criteria, 86
  predictors, 86
  spinal cord injury, 363–365
Weight-training, 328
Wheeze
  allergic bronchopulmonary
    aspergillosis, 396
  asthma, 393, 394
  chest auscultation, 18
  subjective assessment, 7
Whispering pectoriloquy, 19
White blood cell count (WCC), 75, 80
Wound support
  postoperative
    cardiac surgery, 261–262
    in children, 309
    preoperative instruction, 243

Xanthines, 392